Evidence-based Management of the Acute Coronary Syndrome

Evidence-based Management of the Acute Coronary Syndrome

Edited by

Roque Pifarré, MD
Professor and Chairman Emeritus
Department of Thoracic
    and Cardiovascular Surgery
Loyola University of Chicago
Stritch School of Medicine
Maywood, Illinois

Patrick J. Scanlon, MD
Professor of Medicine
Division of Cardiology
Loyola University of Chicago
Stritch School of Medicine
Maywood, Illinois

Hanley & Belfus, Inc. / Philadelphia

Publisher: HANLEY & BELFUS, INC.
                    Medical Publishers
                    210 South 13th Street
                    Philadelphia, PA 19107
                    (215) 546-7293; 800-962-1892
                    FAX (215) 790-9330
                    Web site: http://www.hanleyandbelfus.com

Note to the reader: Although the information in this book has been carefully reviewed for correctness of dosage and indications, neither the authors nor the editor nor the publisher can accept any legal responsibility for any errors or omissions that may be made. Neither the publisher nor the editor makes any warranty, expressed or implied, with respect to the material contained herein. Before prescribing any drug, the reader must review the manufacturer's current product information (package inserts) for accepted indications, absolute dosage recommendations, and other information pertinent to the safe and effective use of the product described.

Library of Congress Cataloging-in-Publication Data

Evidence-based management of the acute coronary syndrome / edited by Roque Pifarre, Patrick J. Scanlon.
        p. ; cm.
    Includes bibliographical references and index.
    ISBN 1-56053-458-3 (alk. paper)
        1. Coronary heart disease. 2. Evidence-based medicine. I. Pifarré, Roque.
    II. Scanlon, Patrick J., 1938–
        [DNLM: 1. Myocardial Infarction—drug therapy. 2. Angina, Unstable—drug therapy.
    3. Angina, Unstable—surgery. 4. Myocardial Infarction—surgery. 5. Myocardial
    Ischemia—drug therapy. 6. Myocardial Ischemia—surgery. WG 300 E89 2000]
    RC685.C6 E85 2000
    616.1'2306—dc21

                                                                        00-063240

**Evidence-based Management of the
Acute Coronary Syndrome**   ISBN 1-56053-458-3

Last digit is the print number: 9 8 7 6 5 4 3 2 1

Dedication

To our dear wives Marianne Scanlon and Teresa Pifarré

Contents

*INTERVENTIONAL MANAGEMENT OF
THE ACUTE CORONARY SYNDROME*

SURGICAL MANAGEMENT OF THE ACUTE CORONARY SYNDROME

Contributors

Fundador L. Adajar, MD
Cardiology Fellow (third year), Division of Cardiology, Department of Medicine, Loyola University Medical Center, Maywood, Illinois

Morton F. Arnsdorf, MD
Professor of Medicine, University of Chicago Pritzker School of Medicine, University of Chicago Hospitals, Chicago, Illinois

Peter Bacher, MD
Clinical Assistant Professor and Head of Antithrombotic Clinical Development, Knoll AG, Germany

Bradford P. Blakeman, MD
Professor, Department of Thoracic and Cardiovascular Surgery, Loyola University of Chicago Stritch School of Medicine, Maywood, Illinois

Martin C. Burke, DO
Assistant Professor of Medicine, University of Chicago Hospitals, Chicago, Illinois

Mark A. Chaney, MD
Associate Professor, Department of Anesthesia and Critical Care, University of Chicago Pritzker School of Medicine, Chicago, Illinois

Sudhakar B. Chennareddy, MD
Fellow, Interventional Cardiology, University of Alabama at Birmingham, Birmingham, Alabama

Kevin J. Cochran, MD
Fellow, Division of Cardiology, Loyola University Medical Center, Maywood, Illinois

Gregory J. Dehmer, MD, FACP, FACC, FSCA&I
Professor of Medicine, University of North Carolina at Chapel Hill School of Medicine; Director, Cardiac Catheterization Laboratory, University of North Carolina Hospitals, Chapel Hill, North Carolina

Ahmet Muzaffer Demir, MD
Visiting Hematologist and Assistant Professor of Medicine, Department of Pathology, Loyola University Medical Center, Maywood, Illinois

Henry DeMots, MD
Professor of Medicine, Division of Cardiology, Oregon Health Sciences University School of Medicine, Portland, Oregon

Elaine L. Enger, MS
Director, Midwest Heart Research Foundation, Lombard, Illinois

Mark H. Ereth, MD
Assistant Professor, Department of Anesthesiology, Mayo Clinic and Foundation, Rochester, Minnesota

Jawed Fareed, PhD, FACB
Professor of Pharmacology and Pathology, Loyola University Medical Center, Maywood, Illinois

James J. Ferguson, III, MD
Assistant Professor, Department of Internal Medicine, Baylor College of Medicine; Clinical Assistant Professor, Department of Internal Medicine, University of Texas Health Science Center at Houston, Houston, Texas

Bryan K. Foy, MD
Associate Professor, Surgical Director of Heart Transplantation, and Fellowship Training Program Director, Department of Thoracic and Cardiovascular Surgery, Loyola University Medical Center, Maywood, Illinois

Eric D. Grassman, MD, PhD
Associate Professor of Medicine, Department of Cardiology, Loyola University Medical Center, Maywood, Illinois

G. Steinar Gudmundsson, MD
Cardiology Fellow, Division of Cardiology, Loyola University Medical Center, Maywood, Illinois

Joseph R. Hartmann, MD
Clinical Associate Professor of Medicine, Loyola University Medical Center, Maywood, Illinois

David R. Holmes, Jr., MD
Professor of Medicine, Mayo Medical School; Consultant in Cardiovascular Diseases, and Director, Cardiac Catheterization Lab, Mayo Clinic Foundation, Rochester, Minnesota

Debra A. Hoppensteadt, PhD
Assistant Professor of Pathology, Loyola University Medical Center, Maywood, Illinois

Omer Iqbal, MD
Assistant Professor of Pathology and Clinical Trials Coordinator, Loyola University Medical Center, Maywood, Illinois

Richard J. Kaplon, MD
Assistant Professor of Clinical Surgery, Codirector of Artificial Heart Program, and Medical Director of Perfusion Services, University of Miami School of Medicine, Miami, Florida

Paul Kim, MD
Fellow and Clinical Instructor, Division of Cardiology, Baylor College of Medicine, Houston, Texas

Gary E. Lane, MD
Assistant Professor of Medicine, Cardiovascular Division, Mayo Clinic, Jacksonville, Florida

Donald F. Leon, MD
Distinguished Professor of Medicine, Division of Cardiology, Georgetown University School of Medicine, Washington, DC

Fred Leya, MD
Professor of Medicine, Division of Cardiology, Loyola University Medical Center, Maywood, Illinois

Patrick M. McCarthy, MD
Surgical Director, Kaufmann Center for Heart Failure; and Program Director, Heart Transplantation, Department of Thoracic and Cardiovascular Surgery, Cleveland Clinic, Cleveland, Ohio

Louis S. McKeever, MD
Midwest Heart Specialists, Ltd., Elmhurst, Illinois; Clinical Professor of Medicine, Division of Cardiology, Loyola University of Chicago Stritch School of Medicine, Maywood, Illinois

Thomas L. McKiernan, MD
Associate Professor of Medicine, Division of Cardiology, Loyola University Medical Center, Maywood, Illinois

Keith A. McLean, MD
Assistant Professor of Medicine, Division of Cardiology, Loyola University Medical Center, Maywood, Illinois

Harry L. Messmore, Jr., MD, FACP
Professor of Medicine, Loyola University of Chicago Stritch School of Medicine, Maywood, Illinois

Alvaro Montoya, MD
Chicago Cardiac Surgeons, Chicago, Illinois

John F. Moran, MD
Professor of Medicine, and Director, Division of Cardiology, Loyola University Medical Center, Maywood, Illinois

Gregory A. Nuttall, MD
Assistant Professor, Department of Anesthesiology, Mayo Clinic and Foundation, Rochester, Minnesota

John B. O'Connell, MD
Professor and Chairman, Department of Internal Medicine, Wayne State University School of Medicine, Detroit, Michigan

William C. Oliver, Jr., MD
Assistant Professor, Department of Anesthesiology, Mayo Clinic and Foundation, Rochester, Minnesota

Roque Pifarré, MD
Professor and Chairman Emeritus, Department of Thoracic and Cardiovascular Surgery, Loyola University of Chicago Stritch School of Medicine, Maywood, Illinois

Venkatesh K. Raman, MD
Fellow, Division of Cardiology, Georgetown University Medical Center, Washington, DC

Patrick J. Scanlon, MD
Professor of Medicine, Division of Cardiology, Loyola University of Chicago Stritch School of Medicine, Maywood, Illinois

David L. Smull, DO
Cardiology Fellow, Department of Medicine, Division of Cardiology, Loyola University Medical Center, Maywood, Illinois

J. Michael Tuchek, DO, FACS
Assistant Clinical Professor, Department of Cardiovascular and Thoracic Surgery, Loyola University Medical Center, Chicago, Illinois

Diane E. Wallis, MD
Midwest Heart Specialists, Downers Grove, Illinois; Clinical Associate Professor of Medicine, Loyola University Medical Center, Maywood, Illinois

William H. Wehrmacher, MD, FACP, FACC
Clinical Professor, Departments of Medicine and Physiology, Loyola University of Chicago Stritch School of Medicine, Maywood, Illinois

James M. Wilson, MD
Clinical Assistant Professor of Medicine, Department of Internal Medicine, Baylor College of Medicine, Houston, Texas

Preface

The unstable coronary syndrome, which includes unstable angina pectoris, non–Q-wave myocardial infarction, and ST elevation/Q wave infarction, is one of the two most common clinical entities requiring admission of a patient to an inpatient cardiology service, the other being congestive heart failure. In the past, evaluation and treatment options for patients with the unstable coronary syndrome were either empirical or based on observational reports of clinical outcomes. It is now generally agreed that in order to acquire meaningful and reproducible clinical data, a *randomized* clinical trial is the best method of clinical research.[1] Over the past few years, an ever-increasing number of randomized clinical trials have resulted in a much deeper *evidence-based* understanding of the pathophysiology, presentation, risk assessment, and management of the unstable coronary syndrome and its subsets.

This book organizes the data gleaned from these trials in a fashion that allows the reader to better understand the evidence-based best use of individual forms of evaluation and therapy, and how individual forms of treatment can be best combined to result in optimal patient outcomes. Unfortunately, data from randomized trials are still incomplete and many questions regarding the proper uses of drugs, interventions, and surgery are unanswered. In chapters where there is a relative lack of randomized trial data, the authors have relied on observational information and consensus recommendations.

We appreciate the willingness of the contributors to provide their expertise and authoritative critical insights on this exceedingly important subject, and hope that the reader will find it to be a useful resource.

Acknowledgments

We thank the authors for their efforts, expertise, and cooperation. We thank Ms. Bernice Krause for her invaluable assistance with the manuscript processing and correspondence. Ms. Linda Belfus is gratefully acknowledged for her editorial assistance.

Roque Pifarré, MD
Patrick J. Scanlon, MD

---

[1]Pocock SJ, Elbourne DR: Randomized trials or observational tribulations? N Engl J Med 342;1907–1909, 2000.

Pathophysiology of the Acute Coronary Syndrome

LOUIS S. MCKEEVER, MD

ELAINE L. ENGER, MS

Coronary atherosclerosis is ubiquitous in western society. Despite its frequency, most patients are asymptomatic. Although the earliest lesions may be present early in life, it usually takes decades for atherosclerosis to evolve into mature plaques responsible for the symptoms of ischemic heart disease. Slow plaque growth due to lipid accumulation, smooth muscle cell proliferation, and matrix synthesis gradually narrows the arterial lumen, ultimately limiting blood flow and altering coronary dynamics. This relatively innocuous, benign plaque that develops in the majority of patients is responsible for the chronic ischemic episodes that characterize stable angina pectoris.

A simplistic view of the nature of the ischemic syndrome pervaded cardiology literature for years, beginning with William Heberden's first description of angina pectoris in 1772 in a paper entitled, "Some Account of a Disorder of the Breast." Heberden pointed out that the condition was common and occurred while walking, especially uphill or after a meal. He added that this chest discomfort vanishes with standing still. We now recognize this syndrome as classic stable angina pectoris, resulting from an imbalance of oxygen supply and demand due to fixed coronary stenosis. The opposite end of the spectrum was first described by Herrick in the early part of the twentieth century.[1] He described survival of a patient with acute coronary thrombosis. It was reasoned that progressive stenosis of an atherosclerotic lesion led to decreased blood flow, stagnation, and subsequent thrombosis.

The advent of coronary arteriography in the latter half of the past century allowed the precise diagnosis of coronary stenosis due to atherosclerosis in living patients.[2] This, in turn, led to the development of strategies to revascularize the heart, first with surgery and then with coronary angioplasty.

As coronary angiography became more widely accepted with fewer associated risks, DeWood and colleagues studied patients during the early hours of an acute myocardial infarction and conclusively demonstrated that the vast majority had total coronary occlusion due to thrombosis.[3] According to the traditional view of the pathogenesis of an acute ischemic event, when the coronary arterial lumen narrows to the degree that only a few platelets can obstruct the vessel, the innocuous plaque can become obstructive, resulting in the clinical manifestations of unstable angina or acute myocardial infarction, depending on the nature of the resultant thrombus. Consequently, the severity of stenosis has been the focus of attention, with the assumption that the greater the stenosis, the higher the risk of a significant coronary event.

Emerging evidence, however, has redefined the transition process from the chronic to the unstable, acute atheroma. It now appears that plaque vulnerability and thrombogenic potential are much more critical factors than plaque size and stenosis in determining whether an acute ischemic event will occur. First, even in the presence of a significant atheromatous plaque, the size of the coronary lumen may remain substantial as a result of vascular remodeling, which occurs as a compensatory mechanism to allow the vessel to expand outward and accommodate the growth.[4] In addition, the results of four trials[5–8] reveal that less than 15% of patients with myocardial infarction have flow-limiting stenoses on a previous angiogram[9] (Fig. 1). Moreover, aggressive lipid lowering trials aimed at regression of atherosclerosis have produced greater clinical benefit than one would expect on the basis of angiographic improvement in the degree of stenosis.[10] These observations indicate that a high-grade luminal stenosis due to atheroma growth does not cause most acute ischemic coronary events. Instead, thrombosis, often on a noncritical stenosis, due to lesion disruption precipitates most events. Intracoronary thrombus has been found in 70% of cases of sudden death.[11,12] Coronary thrombosis occurs only in arteries containing atherosclerosis.[13] The initiating event for thrombosis is the rupture of the surface of an atherosclerotic plaque.[11,13–23] Davies and Thomas found ruptured atherosclerotic plaques underlying 103 (90%) of 115 episodes of coronary thrombosis that they observed in 74 patients dying of ischemic heart disease.[15] As a result, attention now has been focused on which intrinsic plaque characteristics contribute to its vulnerability to rupture, which extrinsic events may trigger this rupture, and which factors influence the extent of thrombus formation.

Ischemic heart disease includes a wide spectrum of conditions ranging from silent ischemia and chronic, stable, exertion-induced angina through unstable angina, non–Q-wave myocardial infarction, and acute Q-wave myocardial infarction. The term *acute coronary syndrome* describes the latter three conditions, which are differentiated primarily by clinical, electrocardiographic, and laboratory presentations correlating with the duration and extent of thrombotic occlusion as a

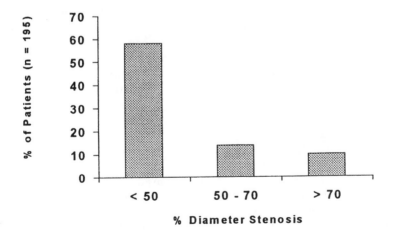

Figure 1.   Prevalence of flow-limiting coronary stenoses on angiograms obtained before acute myocardial infarction in four studies.[5–8]

consequence of plaque rupture. Q-wave myocardial infarction is the most frequent cause of mortality in the United States as well as in most western countries. Fortunately, Q-wave acute myocardial infarction is the most easily identified syndrome; persistent angina and ST-segment elevation are characteristic of sudden total or near-total thrombotic arterial occlusion. The distinction between unstable angina and non–Q-wave, non-ST segment elevation myocardial infarction is often not clear when patients first present. Diagnosis may take hours to days, depending on when the results of cardiac enzyme tests become available. Unstable angina accounts for more than 1 million hospital admissions annually,[24] and 6–8% of patients have nonfatal myocardial infarctions or die within 1 year of diagnosis.[25,26] For years the definition of unstable angina varied, making comparative studies difficult to analyze.

In 1989, Braunwald suggested a classification system to ensure uniformity[27] of diagnostic and prognostic information. The categories are defined as acute angina while at rest (within 48 hours before presentation), subacute angina while at rest (within the previous month but not within 48 hours before presentation), or new onset of accelerated (progressively more severe) angina. Furthermore, the clinical circumstances in which unstable angina develops is defined as either angina in the presence or absence of other conditions (i.e., anemia, fever, hypoxia, tachycardia, or thyrotoxicosis) or angina within 2 weeks after an acute myocardial infarction in the presence or absence of electrocardiographic abnormalities.[24] It is now thought that the chest pain syndromes associated with ischemic heart disease are a continuum, beginning with the most benign, chronic stable angina, and ending with the most deadly, acute myocardial infarction.[28]

Central to the initiation of acute coronary syndrome is disruption of a formed atheromatous plaque and consequent development of thrombus. This chapter explores the pathophysiology of the "unstable plaque" that leads to the clinical development of acute coronary syndrome. The risk of plaque disruption depends on the intrinsic properties of individual plaques and the extrinsic forces acting on these plaques. The intrinsic properties predispose plaques to rupture, whereas the extrinsic forces may precipitate disruption in the presence of "vulnerable" plaque. To understand more clearly the etiology and mechanism of plaque rupture, this chapter first begins with a discussion of atherogenesis and the intrinsic and extrinsic factors that may lead to rupture. This discussion is followed by examination of the effects of plaque rupture on the coagulation system. This chapter is not meant to be an exhaustive review of the subject, but to provide a framework for understanding acute coronary syndrome and, therefore, the strategies for treatment.

Atherogenesis: An Overview

Atherosclerosis is the result of a dynamic interaction between blood elements, disturbed flow, and the vessel wall characterized by a series of highly specific cellular and molecular responses that are best described in aggregate as an inflammatory process.[29] Early lesions tend to develop at specific arterial sites, such as branches, bifurcations, and curvatures, that cause characteristic alterations in blood flow and hemodynamics.[30,31] Numerous pathophysiologic observations by Ross and others[29] have led to the formation of the "response-to-injury" hypothesis, which proposes that endothelial dysfunction is the first step in atheroma development. Endothelial dysfunction results in the release of specific molecules that promote the adherence, migration, and accumulation of monocytes and T-cell lymphocytes. Once in the subendothelial space, recruited monocytes become macrophages, which imbibe lipid to become foam cells. Foam cells and, to a lesser extent, T lymphocytes compose the fatty streak, the first lesion of atherosclerosis. Endothelial dysfunction also results in a series of compensatory responses that alter the normal homeostatic properties of the endothelium. The adhesiveness of the endothelium to leukocytes and platelets as well as its permeability is enhanced. In addition, the dysfunction induces the endothelium to demonstrate procoagulant properties and to form a series of highly vasoreactive molecules, growth factors, and cytokines. If the injurious stimulation is not effectively neutralized or the offending agent removed, the inflammatory process continues indefinitely. Persistent inflammatory response stimulates migration and proliferation of smooth muscle cells that become intermixed with the inflammatory cells, forming an intermediate lesion. The immediate response to the thickened arterial wall is a compensatory mechanism called remodeling, during which the artery gradually dilates to maintain arterial lumen diameter. However, the unabated inflammatory response results in increased numbers of macrophages and lymphocytes, which multiply in the lesion. Activation of these cells leads to the release of cytokines, hydrolytic enzymes, chemokines, and growth factors, which intensify the arterial damage and eventually promote focal necrosis. Migration and proliferation of smooth muscle cells, accumulation of mononuclear cells, and formation of fibrous tissue result in further enlargement and restructuring of the lesion. It becomes covered by a fibrous cap that overlies a soft lipid-laden and necrotic tissue core. When the artery can no longer dilate in compensation, the lesion protrudes into the lumen, giving rise to the mature plaque.

Because atherosclerosis has been defined as a chronic inflammatory process, attention has focused on the measurement of inflammatory markers as a method of predicting the risk of development of significant cardiovascular disease in addition to some of the more traditional lipoprotein assays. Several plasma markers of inflammation have been proposed for use in screening. Among them are markers of systemic inflammation produced by the liver (C-reactive protein, serum amyloid A), cytokines (interleukin-6), and adhesion molecules (ICAM-1).[32–35] The rationale for the measurement of these markers should become more apparent after reviewing the following discussion. However, their clinical value is yet to be determined.

Endothelial Dysfunction

Early in the process of atheroma development, endothelial dysfunction occurs in lesion-prone areas. The predominant cause of this dysfunction appears to be elevated and modified, oxidized, low-density lipoproteins (LDLs).[36–38] Another potential cause is free radical formation secondary to cigarette smoking, hypertension, and diabetes mellitus.[38] High plasma concentrations of homocysteine also are toxic to the endothelium. Homocysteine decreases nitrous oxide availability, increases collagen production, and is prothrombotic.[39,40] Several recent reports have described a correlation between infectious organisms and development of atherosclerosis. *Chlamydia pneumoniae*, cytomegalovirus, and other herpesviruses have been identified in atheromatous lesions, and increased titers of their antibodies have been evaluated as a method of predicting outcome in patients suffering an acute myocardial infarction. The infectious process may be a distant infection that induces immune activation, cross-reactive antibodies, cytokine release, endothelial damage, and thrombogenesis or a local infection of endothelial cells, smooth muscle cells, or macrophages that results in endothelial dysfunction. Alternatively, the bacteria may be an innocent bystander.[41] Two pilot studies, however, have suggested that antibiotic therapy can improve prognosis after an acute coronary syndrome. In one trial, roxithromycin administered to 202 patients with unstable angina or non–Q-wave myocardial infarction for 30 days reduced the 6-month rate of death or myocardial infarction from 4% to 0%.[42] A second trial screened 220 men after myocardial infarction and randomized 80 patients with elevated antibody titers to either placebo or azithromycin for 3–6 days. The odds of an event in patients treated with placebo was 4 times higher than in nonrandomized patients with negative titers and azithromycin-treated patients with positive titers.[43]

Endothelial dysfunction is characterized by four distinct responses:

1. An increase in endothelial permeability to lipoproteins and other plasma constituents

2. Upregulation of endothelial adhesion molecule secretion, including E-selectin, P-selectin, intracellular adhesion molecule-1 (ICAM-1), and vascular-cell adhesion molecule-1 (VCAM-1)

3. Upregulation of leukocyte adhesion molecules, including L-selectin, integrins, and platelet-endothelial cell adhesion molecule 1 (PECAM-1)

4. Migration of leukocytes into the arterial wall, mediated by oxidized LDL, monocyte chemotactic protein 1, interleukin-8, platelet derived growth factor, and macrophage colony-stimulating factor.[29,44]

Development of Early Lesions

Endothelial dysfunction, characterized by the processes described above as well as other processes that are not completely understood, promotes the adherence, migration, and accumulation of monocytes and T-cell lymphocytes to the disturbed endothelium. Once in the subendothelial space, recruited monocytes engulf lipid and change morphologically to a macrophage structure. Fatty streaks, the first lesion of atherosclerosis, consist of these lipid-laden macrophages (foam cells) together with T-lymphocytes.[29] The intracellular cholesterol is derived primarily from modified LDLs that undergo progressive oxidation (modification) when they become trapped and accumulate in the extracellular subendothelial space of arteries. Oxidized LDL becomes internalized by macrophages by means of scavenger receptors on their surfaces. This internalization stimulates the formation of lipid peroxides and facilitates the accumulation of cholesterol esters to continue to form foam cells and to elicit their repetitive activation (Fig. 2).

In contrast to the uptake of native, nonoxidized LDL by macrophages, the uptake of the oxidized form by the scavenger pathway has no negative feedback regulation.[13,36,45–47] The upregulation of critical endothelial adhesion molecules (e.g., chemotactic protein-1) and ICAM-1 and VCAM-1 induced by lysophospalidycholin production in oxidized LDLs continue to promote enhanced attraction of monocytes to the site to undergo transformation. The results are massive uptake and activation of macrophages. As the formed foam cells accumulate and become activated, they release a series of hydrolytic enzymes that have a cytotoxic effect on vascular cells. These enzymes intensify the

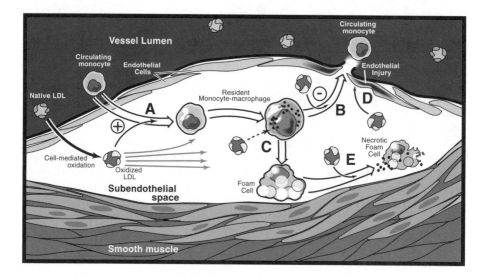

Figure 2. Early events in atherogenesis. Native low-density lipoprotein (LDL) becomes trapped in the subendothelial space, where it can be oxidized by resident vascular cells such as smooth muscle cells, endothelial cells, and macrophages. Oxidized LDL stimulates (plus sign) monocyte chemotaxis (A) and inhibits (minus sign) monocyte egress from vascular wall (B). Monocytes differentiated into macrophages then internalize oxidized LDL, leading to foam cell formation (C). Oxidized LDL also causes endothelial dysfunction and injury (D) as well as foam cell necrosis (E), resulting in the release of lysosomal enzymes and necrotic debris. Broken arrows indicate adverse effects of oxidized LDL. (Adapted from Diaz MN, Frei B, Vita JA, Keaney JF: Mechanisms of disease: Antioxidants and atherosclerotic heart disease. N Engl J Med 337:408–416, 1997.)

arterial damage and promote focal necrosis, giving rise to the lipid-rich necrotic core of the plaque.[48–53]

T-cell lymphocytes also are recruited to a lesser extent to the site of endothelial dysfunction. Immunohistochemical studies have revealed that T cells constitute up to 20% of the cells in regions of more advanced atherosclerotic plaques. Most of these cells accumulate at the vulnerable "shoulder" region of the plaque. T cells in atherosclerotic lesions bear markers of chronic activation, contributing to the sustained inflammatory environment in the plaque.[49] T-cell activation is believed to be mediated by tumor necrosis factor α, interleukin-2, macrophage colony-stimulating factor, and oxidized LDL in general.[29]

Development of Mature Lesions

Simultaneous with or subsequent to the massive recruitment and activation of macrophages and T cells at the site of endothelial dysfunction, platelets begin to adhere to the formed lesion. Activation of these platelets leads to the formation of free arachidonic acid, which can be transformed into prostaglandins such as thromboxane A_2 or leukotrienes. Thromboxane A_2 is one of the most potent vasoconstrictive and platelet-aggregating substances known. Leukotrienes, in contrast, are capable of amplifying the inflammatory response.[29] Activation of these platelets also causes them to release their granules, which contain cytokines and growth factors, including platelet-derived growth factor, epidermal growth factor, transforming growth factor, and somatomedin C.[54,55]

Stimulated by the platelet growth factors, smooth muscle cells migrate from the media to the intima and stimulate the production of collagen type I and type III, elastin, and glycoproteins. These proteins collectively provide the connective tissue matrix of the plaque and give it structural strength. Extracellular cholesterol crystals and esters derived from LDL or extruded by necrotic foam cells accumulate within this matrix and compose the core of the plaque.[56] A combination of smooth muscle cells, collagen, and a monolayer of endothelial cells forms a fibromuscular cap that walls off the lipid core and matrix from the arterial lumen.[57] This cap formation actually represents a type of healing response to the injury. The final lesion typically consists of a lipid-rich core in the central portion of an eccentrically thickened intima. This lipid core is bound on its luminal aspect by the fibrous cap, at its edges by the "shoulder" region, and on its abluminal aspect by the base or matrix. However, the composition of the intact developed atheroma is highly variable and contributes significantly to the vulnerability of plaque rupture[47] (Fig. 3).

Cholesterol is constantly transported in and out of the plaque. Cholesterol enters the plaque in the form of LDL and lipoprotein (a). Lipoprotein (a) is similar to LDL but contains an additional alipoprotein, apolipoprotein (a),[58–60] and has been shown to be an independent risk factor for coronary artery disease.[61] High-density lipoproteins (HDL) remove cholesterol from foam cells, then re-enter the circulation and transfer it to LDL and very low-density lipoproteins. Finally, the cholesterol is transported to the liver. The incidence of myocardial infarction is related directly to serum levels of LDL and inversely to the levels of HDL.[62]

Anatomy of a Vulnerable Plaque

Plaque composition and vulnerability have emerged as the most important determinants of plaque rupture. In fact, plaque disruption is common but often asymptomatic. Disrupted plaques are present in as many as 9% of healthy people

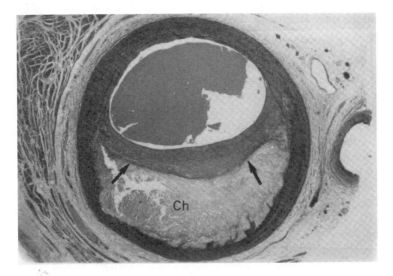

Figure 3. Transverse section of an eccentric lipid-rich plaque not causing significant stenosis in a coronary artery. The lumen is circular, and the crescent-shaped area contains cholesterol (ch). The lipid pool is separated by a fibrous tissue cap *(arrows)*. Opposite the plaque is a quadrant of normal vessel wall.

and in 22% of diabetic atherosclerotic patients coming to autopsy after noncoronary deaths.[12] In addition, this type of disruption probably accounts for the sudden, unpredictable, and nonlinear progression of coronary lesions commonly observed on coronary angiography. In general, however, the patient's odds of an event-free survival are excellent as long as the plaque rupture is not associated with major thrombotic complications. If, however, thrombosis is superimposed on the rupture of mature plaques, a relatively benign, stable chronic ischemic syndrome can quickly transform into a life-threatening acute coronary syndrome.[9] The three basic features of ruptured plaques are intimal rupture, intimal hemorrhage, and intraluminal thrombosis.[14–16] Nonocclusive thrombosis most likely precipitates unstable angina and non–Q-wave acute myocardial infarction, whereas a totally occlusive thrombosis results in Q-wave myocardial infarction (Fig. 4).

Rupture of the plaque surface typically occurs at points where the protective fibrous cap is thin, necrotic, and infiltrated by macrophages. These weakened areas are commonly at the margins or "shoulder" of the cap. Richardson et al.[65] demonstrated that plaques rupture at the junction of the fibrous cap and adjacent normal tissue in 64% of cases. Because this cap is all that stands between many patients and an acute coronary event, it is now regarded as the Achilles' heel of the plaque. Specifically, the fibrous cap ordinarily protects the blood from contact with the thrombogenic material in the lipid-rich core of the atheroma. Disruption of the cap allows proteins of the coagulation system in the blood to interact with the highly thrombogenic lipid core, thus unleashing the thrombotic cascade that promotes vessel occlusion. Clearly, the thrombogenicity of the plaque goes hand-in-hand with the lability of the fibrous cap as determinants of acute coronary syndrome.[66] It is believed that external stresses imposed on plaques play a pivotal role in plaque disruption by triggering rupture at the weak points. As such, plaque disruption is probably the result of a dynamic interaction between intrinsic plaque features (composition promoting vulnerability) and extrinsic stressors (rupture triggers). The former predispose a plaque to rupture, whereas the latter may precipitate rupture.

Intrinsic Determinants of Plaque Vulnerability

Atherosclerotic plaques prone to rupture have certain characteristic structural, cellular, and molecular features (Table 1, Fig. 5). The three major structural determinants are (1) core size, (2) fibrous cap thickness, and (3) matrix collagen content. The larger the lipid core, the higher the risk for plaque rupture.[67,68] Gertz and Roberts[69] examined the lipid composition of plaques from 17 infarct-related arteries on autopsy. They noted that the lipid cores were much larger in the segments with plaque rupture (39 segments) than in the segments with intact surfaces (229 segments). The nature of the lipid within the core also may be significant. Lipid in the form of cholesteryl ester softens the plaque. Crystalline cholesterol appears to have the opposite effect.[67] Although the thickness, cellularity, matrix strength, and stiffness of the fibrous cap vary significantly, cap thinning, decreased collagen content, and decreased smooth muscle cell proliferation increase plaque vulnerability[70] (Tables 2 and 3). The caps of eccentric lesions are typically thinnest at their shoulder regions. The shoulder regions are also the sites where macrophage foam cells and T lymphocytes most frequently infiltrate. An inflammatory cell infiltrate thus may

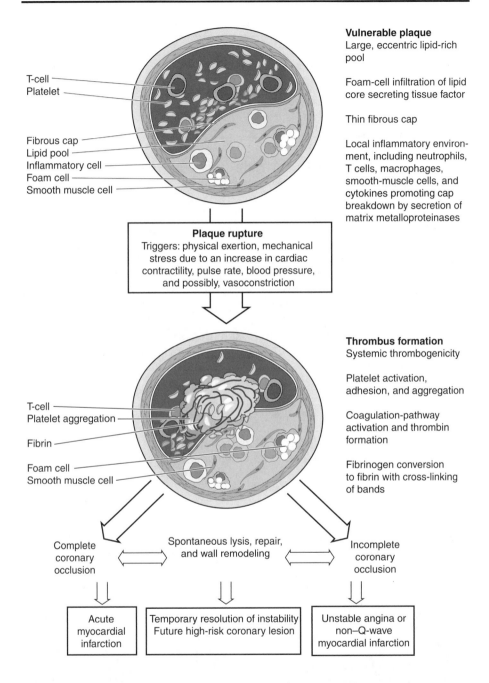

Vulnerable plaque
Large, eccentric lipid-rich pool

Foam-cell infiltration of lipid core secreting tissue factor

Thin fibrous cap

Local inflammatory environment, including neutrophils, T cells, macrophages, smooth-muscle cells, and cytokines promoting cap breakdown by secretion of matrix metalloproteinases

T-cell
Platelet

Fibrous cap
Lipid pool
Inflammatory cell
Foam cell
Smooth muscle cell

Plaque rupture
Triggers: physical exertion, mechanical stress due to an increase in cardiac contractility, pulse rate, blood pressure, and possibly, vasoconstriction

Thrombus formation
Systemic thrombogenicity

Platelet activation, adhesion, and aggregation

Coagulation-pathway activation and thrombin formation

Fibrinogen conversion to fibrin with cross-linking of bands

T-cell
Platelet aggregation

Fibrin

Foam cell
Smooth muscle cell

Complete coronary occlusion

Spontaneous lysis, repair, and wall remodeling

Incomplete coronary occlusion

Acute myocardial infarction

Temporary resolution of instability
Future high-risk coronary lesion

Unstable angina or non–Q-wave myocardial infarction

Figure 4. Pathophysiologic events culminating in acute coronary syndrome. Numerous triggers initiate the rupture of a vulnerable plaque. Rupture leads to adhesion, activation, and aggregation of platelets as well as to the activation of the clotting cascade, resulting in the formation of an occlusive thrombus. If this process leads to complete occlusion of the coronary artery, acute myocardial infarction with ST-segment elevation occurs. Alternatively, if the process leads to an incomplete occlusion, unstable angina or non–Q-wave myocardial infarction occurs. (Adapted from Yeghiazarians Y, Braunstein JB, Askari A, Stone PH: Unstable angina pectoris. N Engl J Med 342:101–114, 2000.)

Table 1. Characteristics of Ruptured Atherosclerotic Plaques

Structural	Cellular	Molecular
Thin fibrous caps	Abundant macrophage-derived foam	Expression of inflamma-
Large lipid pools	cells	tory markers/adhesion
High circumferential stress	T-lymphocyte accumulation at site of	molecules
at site of cap rupture	cap rupture	Cytokine release
Reduced collagen content	Paucity of vascular smooth muscle cells	Expression of matrix
Flow separation region	Evidence of chronic, local inflammation	degrading proteases

well be a marker of plaque vulnerability. One study revealed that the site of rupture in a thrombosed artery was characterized by an inflammatory infiltrate, regardless of plaque composition and structure.[71] Influx of activated cells as part of the chronic inflammatory reaction may incite the elaboration of matrix-degrading proteins, called metalloproteinases, as well as cytokines such as tumor necrosis factor and interferon-γ that inhibit collagen synthesis and proliferation of smooth muscle cells. This results in a weakening of the connective-tissue framework of the plaque.[47] Consequently, three mechanisms link inflammation with vulnerability: (1) decreased matrix synthesis, (2) increased matrix degeneration, and (3) cell death (apoptosis).

Extrinsic Stressors Contributing to Plaque Rupture

Coronary plaques are constantly stressed by various mechanical and hemodynamic forces that may precipitate or "trigger" disruption of vulnerable plaques.[72] Rupture occurs when these forces exceed the plaque's tensile strength.

The blood pressure inside an artery exerts a radial force across the arterial wall as well as a circumferential force. To prevent rupture of the vessel wall, these forces must be counteracted by tension within the wall, as described by the law of Laplace: $t = pr$, where t = wall tension (dynes/cm), r = vessel radius (cm), and p = intraluminal pressure (dyne/cm^2) (Fig. 6).

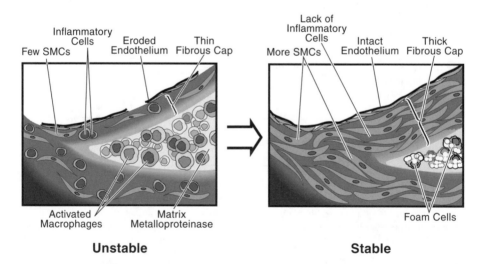

Unstable   **Stable**

Figure 5. Characteristics of stable vs. unstable plaques. (Adapted from Libby P: Molecular basis of the acute coronary syndromes. Circulation 91:2844–2850, 1995.)

Table 2. Biochemical Analysis of Protein and Extracellular Lipid Content of Ulcerated and Intact Human Aortic Plaque Caps

	Ulcerated Plaques (n = 24)	Nonulcerated plaques (n = 31)
Total protein	54.8 ± 1.2	57.2 ± 2.2
Collagen	35.4 ± 8.4	56.8 ± 1.4*
Elastin	0.87 ± 0.87	1.17 ± 0.31
Glycosoaminoglycan	0.9 ± 0.20	1.9 ± 0.2*
Extracellular lipid (% plaque volume)	54.9 ± 3.8	22.1 ± 2.4†

Valus are mean values ± SEM.
* $p = 0.05$.
† $p < 0.001$
Adapted from Davies MJ, Woolf N, Katz DR: The role of endothelial denudation injury, plaque fissuring, and thrombosis in the progression of human atherosclerosis. In Weber PC, Leaf A (eds): Atherosclerosis: Its Pathogenesis and the Role of Cholesterol. New York, Raven Press, 1991, pp 105–113.

The average circumferential wall stress (σ) can be calculated as follows:
$$\sigma = pr/h$$
where h = wall thickness of the artery. These equations provide evidence that larger-diameter blood vessels, higher intraarterial pressures, and thinner arterial walls lead to increased wall stress. This, in turn, may explain why less severe atherosclerotic lesions are more likely to rupture than more severe lesions. If intracoronary pressure is kept constant, the wall tension on a 50% stenosis is 5 times greater than that on a 90% stenosis.[73]

Richardson et al.[65] used a finite-element computer model to study the effects of plaque configuration on the distribution of wall stress. They found that circumferential stress is greatest at the arterial intima and falls across the vessel wall. Local variation and tissue components can lead to marked alterations in the distribution of stress. Areas with decreased load-bearing capabilities lead to increased stress elsewhere in the vessel wall. For example, because a lipid pool in a plaque has minimal tensile strength, all of the stress that normally would be borne by that area is displaced to the overlying fibrous cap. Therefore, plaque rupture tends to occur when the circumferential stress on the atherosclerotic cap exceeds its tensile strength.[73] Tensile strength depends on the various structural components of the cap itself and can be altered by factors that increase or decrease the fibrous matrix of the cap. Using finite-element modeling of the coronary artery with a lipid pool, Richardson[65] showed that the highest circumferential stress is on the cap at the edge of the lipid pool (Fig. 7). Thus, the greatest circumferential stress on the arterial wall tends to occur at the "shoulder" of the lesion, a site particularly prone to rupture.

Table 3. Cellular Content of Ulcerated and Intact Human Aortic Plaque Caps

	Ulcerated Plaques (n = 24)	Nonulcerated Plaques (n = 31)
Density of smooth muscle cells (SMC)	65.2 ± 13.2	174.0 ± 11.9*
Density of monocytes (MO)	122.1 ± 13.3	62.2 ± 8.8*
SMC/MO ratio (% plaque volume)	1.2	5.8*

Values are mean values ± SEM.
* $P < 0.001$.
Adapted from Davies MJ, Woolf N, Katz DR: The role of endothelial denudation injury, plaque fissuring, and thrombosis in the progression of human atherosclerosis. In Weber PC, Leaf A (eds): Atherosclerosis: Its Pathogenesis and the Role of Cholesterol. New York, Raven Press, 1991, pp 105–113.

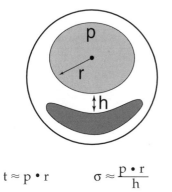

Figure 6. Circumferential tension of the fibrous cap of an atherosclerotic plaque containing a lipid pool (hatched area) is determined by the law of Laplace, which relates tension (t) to intralumen pressure (p) and intralumen radius (r). The mean circumferential stress (σ) on the fibrous cap is related to circumferential tension and cap thickness (h).

$$t \approx p \bullet r \qquad \sigma \approx \frac{p \bullet r}{h}$$

With an understanding of the biomechanics of stresses imposed on vulnerable plaques, clinical reports temporally relating myocardial infarction to strenuous physical activity and emotional stress seem more logical.[74–79] Although a causal link between such stresses and acute myocardial infarction has not been established, it is intuitive that common to such stresses are a rise in blood pressure and potential induction of coronary vasospasm as a result of a sudden surge of sympathetic activity. Vasospasm can produce endothelial damage and has been linked to plaque rupture and myocardial infarction.[80–82]

Hemodynamic forces also may play a significant role in the rupture of vulnerable plaque because the endothelium is constantly exposed to the influence of passing blood. The rate at which velocity of blood rises at the center of the vessel is termed shear rate. This velocity gradient creates shear stress on the endothelium that is parallel to blood flow and proportional to viscosity. Poiseuille's law dictates that shear stress in a vessel is directly proportional to blood velocity and inversely proportional to the cube of the vessel radius. Consequently, a small change in vessel diameter produces a large change in shear stress.[73] The normal response of a coronary artery to increased shear stress is vasodilation to counteract the effect of the stress and thereby reduce it. However, because atherosclerotic segments of an artery cannot dilate, the traditional hypothesis proposes that the narrowing of the artery radius imposed by a lesion produces a large change in shear stress. This increase in shear stress

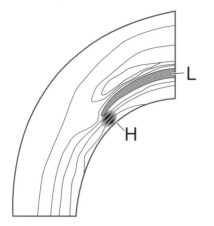

Figure 7. Map showing the contours of circumferential stress in a computer model of a 90% segment of a coronary artery with a lipid pool (L). The highest tensile circumferential stress (H) is on the cap at the edge of the lipid pool, where the contour lines lie close together. (Adapted from Richardson PA, Davies MJ, Born GV: Influence of plaque configuration and stress distribution on fissuring of coronary atherosclerotic plaques. Lancet 2:941–944, 1989.)

then serves as a physical abrasion that contributes to endothelial dysfunction and plaque rupture. However, if shear stress is a predominant factor causing plaque rupture, one would expect that lesions with the highest shear stress, such as those with high flow through a tight stenotic segment, would rupture most frequently. Current evidence contradicts this assumption because lesions of smaller magnitude appear more rupture-prone.[5,6,83,84]

Reevaluation of the role of hemodynamic factors in plaque rupture has led some to believe, in contrast, that a decrease in shear stress may contribute to plaque rupture by modulation of macrophage-borne proteases. More specifically, this alternative explanation holds that when flowing blood encounters a sudden increase in lumen diameter, streamlines of flow lose attachment to the wall, creating a jet.[73] A stagnant flow region can develop between the jet and the vessel wall where velocity is low and, consequently, shear stress is abnormally low. This type of flow separation can occur at abruptly branching vessels, bifurcations, and curvatures. Because early atherosclerotic lesions tend to form at these arterial sites, this flow separation phenomenon with decreased shear stress may be an important inciting factor to the endothelial dysfunction that represents the first step in atheroma development.[85] Of greater importance, because flow separation also can occur as blood exits from a stenosis, decreased shear stress in these stagnant flow regions may contribute to the adherence of inflammatory cells and platelets, which, when activated, may release powerful degradation proteases that trigger plaque rupture. In addition, stagnant flow would provide an appropriate environment for propagation of thrombi subsequent to rupture.[86]

Although the specific mechanisms by which hemodynamic factors influence plaque rupture may be incompletely understood, their influence is probably of a smaller magnitude than that of mechanical forces such as blood pressure. Nonetheless, a complex interplay of these extrinsic factors most likely results in a level of stress that exceeds the tensile strength of the fibrous cap, resulting in rupture and an environment that precipitates thrombus formation.[73]

Consequences of Plaque Rupture

Advances in understanding the etiology of acute coronary syndrome have forced cardiologists to study in greater depth the field of hematology. A cursory knowledge of the clotting cascade is no longer adequate. The final discussion of this chapter explores the nuances of coronary thrombosis. This information provides the building blocks to understand the use of modern antiplatelet and anticoagulant agents discussed in later chapters.

Plaque rupture may result in an acute ischemic event or may be asymptomatic. The extent of coronary thrombosis determines the degree of alteration in coronary blood flow. If coronary flow is reduced and collateral vessels are inadequate, an acute coronary syndrome is likely to result.[87] However, if coronary flow is maintained, the patient may remain asymptomatic. In fact, asymptomatic coronary plaque rupture was found in 9% of patients dying from noncardiac causes.[12] The extent of coronary thrombosis depends on the degree of the thrombogenic stimulators as well as the state of the coagulation system. The arterial media is more thrombogenic than the intima. A plaque rupture extending deep into the media, therefore, is more likely to produce an occlusive thrombus than a rupture that is more superficial and limited to the intima.[88]

The activity of the coagulation and thrombotic systems also influences the tendency to thrombosis.[89,90] Abnormalities leading to a prothrombotic state increase the risk of myocardial infarction when plaque rupture occurs. High concentrations of fibrinogen, factor VI, circulating von Willebrand factor, thrombocytosis, and increased platelet aggregation rates are associated with an increased risk of infarction and death.[91-95]

Impaired Fibrinolysis

Impaired fibrinolysis leads to a prothrombotic state. Plasmin, produced by plasminogen, mediates fibrinolysis.[96] Plasminogen is activated by tissue plasminogen activator (tPA) and rapidly inactivated by plasminogen activator inhibitor (PAI). High levels of PAI and low levels of tPA are associated with increased risk of recurrent myocardial infarction.[97,98] Although a crucial amino acid substitution of serum for arginine lipoprotein (a) has no enzymatic activity, it can compete with serum plasminogen for binding sites. Therefore, lipoprotein (a) may inhibit the activation of plasminogen by tPA and serve as a procoagulant by inhibiting fibrinolysis. Of interest, lipoprotein (a) is associated with both atherogenesis and thrombogenesis.[99]

Enhanced Thrombosis

Rupture of a vulnerable plaque allows exposure of circulating blood to the highly thrombogenic components of the subendothelial layers of the arterial walls as well as the extremely thrombogenic lipid core. Lipid-laden macrophages in the lesion's core express "tissue factor," which is a potent procoagulant. Tissue factor gains contact with circulating precursors of the activated clotting factors and triggers thrombin generation. Platelet glycoprotein 1a binds directly to subendothelial collagen, and glycoprotein 1b combines with subendothelial von Willebrand factor, leading to platelet adhesion to the wall of the artery.[100] This adhesion, as well as the presence of thrombin and other platelet agonists within the microenvironment, stimulate platelet activation with the release of adenosine diphosphate, serotonin, and thromboxane A_2. All of these factors trigger further recruitment and activation of surrounding platelets.

Multiple events occur during platelet activation, including a change in platelet shape, release of alpha and dense platelet granule contents, and induction of platelet coagulant activity. Platelet activation also initiates conformational changes in the inactivated, platelet glycoprotein (GP) IIb/IIIa receptor, transforming it into an activated, ligand-receptive state. GPIIb/IIIa is the most abundant receptor on the platelet surface; each platelet contains 50,000–100,000 GPIIb/IIIa receptors. As such, it mediates the final common step leading to platelet aggregation by binding the fibrinogen ligand, which then crosslinks receptors on adjacent platelets and forms a platelet aggregate, regardless of the platelet agonist responsible for the platelet activation. The GPIIb/IIIa receptor belongs to the integrin family of heterodimeric adhesion molecules, which are formed by the noncovalent interaction of a series of α and β subunits. Integrins are found on virtually all cell types and mediate a diversity of physiologic responses. The recognition specificity of the GPIIb/IIIa receptor is defined by two peptide sequences, the RGD and the KQAGDV sequences. The KQAGDV sequence is found only in fibrinogen. The RGD sequence is recognized by several other integrins and is present not only in fibrinogen but also in fibronectin, von Willebrand factor, and vitronectin ligands.[101] As such, although fibrinogen is the principal ligand binding to the receptor, it is not the exclusive adhesive ligand. These other adhesive proteins, however, appear to play only minor roles in the process of aggregation. Once aggregated at the site of plaque rupture, these platelets form the nidus of the thrombus, inciting the development of acute coronary syndrome[102] (Fig. 8).

Summary

The devastating clinical consequences of rupture of an atherosclerotic plaque usually result from thrombotic complications. Local thrombosis after plaque rupture results from complex interactions among the lipid core of the plaque, smooth muscle cells, macrophages, and collagen.[103–105] The lipid-rich core is extremely thrombogenic. Smooth muscle cells and foam cells within the lipid core express "tissue factor," a potent procoagulant. Once exposed to blood, tissue factor interacts with factor VIIa, which triggers thrombin generation and thus leads to platelet activation and thrombus formation. As platelets aggregate, they release granular contents that further propagate platelet aggregation, vasoconstriction, and thrombus formation.[106]

Conclusion

Although the traditional approach stressing the control of conventional risk factors for the development of atherosclerosis, including smoking cessation, control of hypertension, aggressive lowering of LDL cholesterol, and promotion of physical fitness, remains the cornerstone of current prevention of ischemic heart disease, atheroma development may occur early in life. The

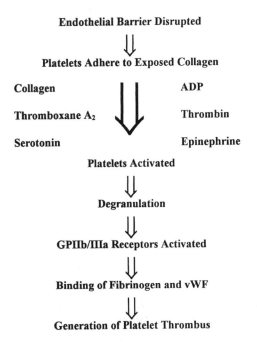

Figure 8. Physiology of platelet activation and aggregation. ADP = adenosine disphosphate, GP = glycoprotein, vWF = von Willebrand factor.

factors promoting the transition from a chronic to an acute state are highly unpredictable. Consequently, management of stable angina needs to be viewed separately from the prevention of thrombus-based events. Atherosclerosis represents a chronic inflammatory process, and plaque rupture and thrombogenicity are much more critical factors than plaque size or stenosis in determining whether a life-threatening acute coronary syndrome will occur. Aggressive medical management may lessen the need for invasive procedures focused simply on mechanically increasing the size of the vessel lumen. Systematic control of the inflammatory process may well be the key to preventing plaque activation and thrombus formation. Potentially useful interventions may include inhibitors of potent inflammatory products such as leukotrienes, thromboxane A_2, metalloproteinases, monocytes/macrophages, cytokines, and adhesion molecules. There is also a large potential for correcting the triggers to inflammation and the biologic offenders such as oxidized LDL, free radicals, and viruses and bacteria. In contrast, cardiovascular research focused on addressing the following critical questions may well offer the possibility of prevention of acute coronary syndrome in the future:

1. What early markers of inflammation may best facilitate the identification of patients at high risk for atherosclerotic development?

2. How can the vulnerability of a particular plaque best be identified and assessed?

3. What pharmacologic or molecular therapies may be used to modify the composition of a plaque and render it more stable?

4. What systemic or local therapies may be used to increase the tensile strength of the plaque or reduce the mechanical/hemodynamic forces exerted on the plaque, thus minimizing the triggers for disruption?

5. What strategies may be developed to modify the response of the fibrolytic and coagulation systems to plaque rupture and thus control the extent of thrombosis?

Many of these issues are already being addressed in research laboratories, and the transition from bench to bedside is under way. These efforts have led to the development of many exciting, new screening techniques and treatment strategies that may well continue to translate into reduced morbidity and mortality for patients with acute coronary syndrome.

References

1. Herrick J: Certain clinical features of sudden obstruction of the coronary arteries. Trans Am Assoc Physicians 27:100–116, 1912.
2. Sones FM Jr, Shirey EK, Prondfit WL, et al: Line coronary arteriography [abstract]. Circulation 20:773, 1959.
3. DeWood MA, Spores J, Notske R, et al: Prevalence of total coronary occlusion during the early hours of transmural myocardial infarction. N Engl J Med 303:897–902, 1980.
4. Glagov S, Weisenberg E, Zarins CK, et al: Compensatory enlargement of human atherosclerotic coronary arteries. N Engl J Med 316:1371–1375, 1987.
5. Ambrose J, Tannenbaum M, Alexopoulos D, et al: Angiographic progression of coronary artery disease and the development of myocardial infarction. J Am Coll Cardiol 12:56–62, 1988.
6. Little WC, Constantinescu M, Applegate RJ, et al: Can coronary angiography predict the site of a subsequent myocardial infarction in patients with mild to moderate coronary artery disease? Circulation 78:1157–1166, 1988.
7. Davies MJ, Richardson PD, Woolf N, et al: Risk of thrombosis in human atherosclerotic plaques: Role of extracellular lipid, macrophages, and smooth muscle cell content. Br Heart J 69:377–381, 1993.

8. Giroud A, Li JM, Urban P, et al: Relation of the site of myocardial infarction to the most severe coronary arterial stenosis at prior angiography. Am J Cardiol 68:729–732, 1992.
9. Falk E, Shah PK, Fuster V: Coronary plaque disruption. Circulation 82:657–671, 1995.
10. Brown BG, Albers JJ, Fisher LA, et al: Regression of coronary artery disease as a result of intensive lipid-lowering therapy in men with high levels of apolipoprotein B. N Engl J Med 323:1289–1298, 1990.
11. El Farual MA, Berg GA, Wheatley DJ, et al: Sudden coronary death in Glasgow: Nature and frequency of acute coronary lesions. Br Heart J 57:329–335, 1987.
12. Davies M, Blund J, Hangartner J, et al: Factors influencing the presence or absence of acute coronary thrombi in sudden ischaemic death. Eur Heart J 10:203–208, 1989.
13. Constantinides P: Causes of thrombosis in human atherosclerotic arteries. Am J Cardiol 66:37G–40G, 1990.
14. Constantinides P: Plaque fissures in human coronary thrombosis. J Atheroscler Res 61:1–17, 1966.
15. Davies MJ, Thomas A: Thrombosis and acute coronary artery lesions in sudden cardiac ischemic death. N Engl J Med 310:1137–1140, 1984.
16. Chapman I: Morphology of occluding coronary artery thrombosis. Arch Pathol 80:256–261, 1965.
17. Friedman M, Van Den Boilenkamp GJ: Role of thrombus in plaque formation in the human diseased coronary artery. Br J Exp Pathol 47:550–557, 1966.
18. Ridolfi RL, Hutchins GM: The relationship between coronary artery lesions and myocardial infarcts: Ulceration of atherosclerotic plaques precipitating coronary thrombus. Am Heart J 93:468–486, 1977.
19. Gertz SD, Kragel AH, Kalan JM, et al: Comparison of coronary and myocardial morphologic findings in patients with and without thrombolytic therapy during fatal first acute myocardial infarction. The TIMI Investigators. Am J Cardiol 66:904–909, 1990.
20. Gorlin R, Fuster V, Ambrose JA: Anatomic-physiologic links between acute coronary syndromes. Circulation 74:6–9, 1986.
21. Ambrose JA, Winters SL, Stern A, et al: Angiographic morphology and pathogenesis of unstable angina pectoris. J Am Coll Cardiol 5:609–616, 1985.
22. Wilson RF, Holida MD, White CE: Quantitative angiographic morphology of stenoses leading to myocardial infarction or unstable angina. Circulation 73:286–293, 1986.
23. Ambrose JA, Hjemdahl-Monsen CD: Arteriographic anatomy and mechanisms of myocardial ischemia in unstable angina. J Am Coll Cardiol 9:1397–1402, 1987.
24. Yeghiazarians Y, Braunstein JB, Askari A, Stone PH: Unstable angina pectoris. N Engl J Med 342:101–114, 2000.
25. Lincoff AM, Tcheng JE, Califf RM, et al: Sustained suppression of ischemic complications of coronary intervention by platelet GPIIb/IIIa blockade with abciximab: One year outcome in the EPILOG Trial. Circulation 99:1951–1958, 1999.
26. Gibson CM, Goel M, Cohen DJ, et al: Six month angiographic and clinical follow-up of patients prospectively randomized to receive either tirofiban or placebo during angioplasty in the RESTORE Trial. J Am Coll Cardiol 32:28–34, 1998.
27. Braunwald E: Unstable angina: A classification. Circulation 80:410–414, 1989.
28. Stary HC: Evolution and progression of atherosclerotic lesions in children and young adults. Atherosclerosis 99 (Suppl I):I19–I32, 1989.
29. Ross R: Atherosclerosis - an inflammatory disease. N Engl J Med 340:115–126, 1999.
30. McMillan DE: Blood flow in the localization of atherosclerotic plaques. Stroke 16:582–587, 1985.
31. Nakashima Y, Raines EW, Plump AS, et al: Upregulation of VCAM-1 and ICAM-1 at atherosclerosis-prone sites on the endothelium in the ApoE-deficient mouse. Arterioscler Thromb Vasc Biol 18:842–851, 1998.
32. Kuller LH, Tracy RP, Shaten J, Mellahn EN: Relationship of C-reactive protein in coronary artery disease in the MRFIT nested case-control study: Multiple Risk Factor Intervention Trial. Am J Epidemiol 144:537–547, 1996.
33. Tracy BP, Lemaltre RN, Pasty RM, et al: Relationship of C-reactive protein to risk of cardiovascular disease in the elderly: Results from the Cardiovascular Health Study and Rural Health Promotion Project. Arterioscler Thromb Vasc Biol 17:1121–1127, 1997.
34. Ridker PM, Cushman M, Stampfer MJ, et al: Inflammation, aspirin, and the risk of cardiovascular disease in apparently healthy men. N Engl J Med 336:973–979, 1997.
35. Ridker PM, Hennekens CH, Buring JE, Rifai N: C-reactive protein and other markers of inflammation in the prediction of cardiovascular disease in women. N Engl J Med 342:836–843, 2000.
36. Navab M, Berliner JA, Watson AD, et al: The ying and yang of oxidation in the development of the fatty streak: A review based on the 1994 George Lyman Duff memorial lecture. Arterioscler Thromb Vasc Biol 16:831–842, 1996.

37. Morel DW, Hessler JR, Chisholm GM: Low density lipoprotein cytotoxicity induced by free radical peroxidation of lipid. J Lipid Res 24:1070–1076, 1983.
38. Griendling KK, Alexander RW: Oxidative stress and cardiovascular disease. Circulation 96:3264–3265, 1997.
39. Majors A, Ehrhart LA, Pezacka EH: Homocysteine as a risk factor for vascular disease: Enhanced collagen production and accumulation by smooth muscle cells. Arterioscler Thromb Vasc Biol 17:3074–3081, 1997.
40. Upchurch GR Jr, Welch GN, Fabian AJ, et al: Homocysteine decreases bioavailable nitric oxide by a mechanism involving glutathione peroxidase. J Biol Chem 272:7012–7017, 1997.
41. Libby P, Egan D, Skarlatos S: Role of infectious agents in atherosclerosis and restenosis. Circulation 96:4095-4103, 1997.
42. Gurfinkel E, Bozovich G, Daroc AA, Beck E, Mautner B, for the ROXIS Study Group: Randomized trial of roxithromycin in non–Q-wave coronary syndromes. ROXIS Pilot Study. Lancet 350:404–407, 1997.
43. Guptka S, Leatham EW, Carrington D, et al: Elevation of Chlamydia pneumoniae antibodies, cardiovascular events, and zithromycin in male survivors of myocardial infarction. Circulation 96:404–407, 1997.
44. Springer TA, Sybulski MI: Traffic signals on the endothelium for leukocytes in health, inflammation, and atherosclerosis. In Fuster V, Ross R, Topol EJ (eds): Atherosclerosis and Coronary Artery Disease, vol 1. Philadelphia, Lippincott-Raven, 1996, pp 511–538.
45. Diaz MN, Frei B, Vita JA, Keaney JF: Mechanisms of disease: Antioxidants and atherosclerotic heart disease. N Engl J Med 337:408–416, 1997.
46. Goldstein JL, Ho YJ, Basu SK, et al: Binding sites on macrophages that mediate uptake and degradation of acetylated low density lipoproteins producing massive cholesterol deposition. Proc Natl Acad Sci USA 76:333–337, 1979.
47. Libby P: Molecular basis of the acute coronary syndromes. Circulation 91:2844–2850, 1995.
48. Steinberg A, Parthasarthy S, Carew TE, et al: Beyond cholesterol: Modifications of low-density lipoprotein that increase atherogenicity. N Engl J Med 320:915–924, 1989.
49. Wang JM, Sika A, Peri G, et al: Expression of monocyte chemotactic protein and interleukin-8 by cytokine-activated human vascular smooth muscle cells. Arterioscler Thromb 11:1166–1174, 1991.
50. Navab M, Imes SS, Hama SY, et al: Monocyte transmigration induced by modification of low-density lipoprotein in coculture of human aortic wall cells is due to the induction of monocyte chemotactic protein, synthesis, and abolished by high-density lipoprotein. J Clin Invest 88:2039–2046, 1991.
51. Cushing SA, Berliner JA, Valente AJ, et al: Minimally modified low-density lipoprotein induces monocyte chemotactic protein in human endothelial and smooth muscle cells. Proc Natl Acad Sci USA 87:5134–5138, 1990.
52. Geng Y-J, Libby P: Evidence for apoptosis in advanced human atheroma: Colocalization with interleukin-1-B-converting enzyme. Am J Pathol 147:251–266, 1995.
53. Collin P, Fox K: The pathogenesis of atheroma and the rationale for its treatment. Eur Heart J 13:560–565, 1992.
54. Ross R, Raines EW, Bowen-Pope DF: The biology of platelet derived growth factors. Cell 46:155–169, 1986.
55. Davies MJ, Woolf N, Katz DR: The role of endothelial denudation injury, plaque fissuring, and thrombosis in the progression of human atherosclerosis. In Weber PC, Leaf A (eds): Atherosclerosis: Its Pathogenesis and the Role of Cholesterol. New York, Raven Press, 1991, pp 105–113.
56. Davies MJ, Woolf N, Rowles PM, et al: Morphology of the endothelium over atherosclerotic plaques in human arteries. Br Heart J 60:459–464, 1988.
57. Hangartner JG, Charleston AJ, Davies MJ, et al: Morphological characteristics of chemically significant coronary artery stenosis in stable angina. Br Heart J 56:507–508, 1986.
58. Kragel AH, Reddy SG, Wiltes JT, et al: Morphometric analysis of the composition of coronary arterial plaques in isolated unstable angina pectoris with pain at rest. Am J Cardiol 66:562–567, 1990.
59. Kragel AH, Reddy SG, Wiltes JT, et al: Morphometric analysis of the composition of atherosclerotic plaques in four major epicardial coronary arteries in acute myocardial infarction and in sudden coronary death. Circulation 80:1747–1756, 1989.
60. Ress A: Lipoprotein(a): A possible link between lipoprotein metabolism and thrombosis. Br Heart J 65:2–3, 1991.
61. Danhlen G, Guyton JR, Attar M, et al: Association of levels of lipoprotein Lp(a), plasma lipids, and other lipoproteins with coronary artery disease documented by angiography. Circulation 74:758–765, 1986.

62. Stampfer MJ, Sacks FM, Salvini S, et al: A prospective study of cholesterol, apolipoproteins, and the risk of myocardial infarction. N Engl J Med 325:373–381, 1991.
63. Loree HM, Kamm RD, Stringfellow RG, Lee RT: Effects of fibrous cap thickness on peak circumferential stress in model atherosclerotic vessels. Circ Res 71:850–858, 1992.
64. Fuster V, Lewis A: Connor Memorial Lecture: Mechanisms leading to myocardial infarction: Insights from studies of vascular biology. Circulation 90:2126–2146, 1994.
65. Richardson PD, Davies MJ, Born GV: Influence of plaque configuration and stress distribution on fissuring of coronary atherosclerotic plaques. Lancet 2:941–944, 1989.
66. Libby P, Schoenbeck U, Mach F, et al: Current concepts in cardiovascular pathology: The role of LDL cholesterol in plaque rupture and stabilization. Am J Med 104:14S–18S, 1998.
67. Loree HM, Tobias BJ, Gibson LJ, et al: Mechanical properties of model atherosclerotic lesion lipid pools. Arterioscler Thromb 14:230–234, 1994.
68. Davies MJ, Richardson PD, Woolf N, et al: Risk of thrombosis in human atherosclerotic plaques: Role of extracellular lipid, macrophage, and smooth muscle cell content. Br Heart J 69:377–381, 1993.
69. Gertz SP, Roberts WC: Hemodynamic shear force in rupture of coronary arterial atherosclerotic plaques. Am J Cardiol 66:1368–1372, 1990.
70. Kullo IJ, Edwards WD, Schwartz RS: Vulnerable plaque: Pathobiology and clinical implications. Ann Intern Med 129:1050–1060, 1998.
71. van der Wal AC, Becker AE, van der Loss CM, Das PK: Site of intimal rupture or erosion of thrombosed coronary atherosclerotic plaques is characterized by an inflammatory process irrespective of the dominant plaque morphology. Circulation 89:36–44, 1994.
72. Muller JE, Abela GS, Nestro RW, Tofler GH: Triggers, acute risk factors, and vulnerable plaques. The lexicon of a new frontier. J Am Coll Cardiol 23:809–813, 1994.
73. MacIsaac A, Thomas JD, Topol EJ: Toward the quiescent coronary plaque. J Am Coll Cardiol 22:1228–1241, 1993.
74. Tofler GH, Stone PH, Maclurere M, et al: Analysis of possible triggers of acute myocardial infarction (The MILIS Study). Am J Cardiol 66:22–27, 1990.
75. Ciampricotti R, El Ganral M, Relic T, et al: Clinical characteristic and coronary angiographic findings of patients with unstable angina, acute myocardial infarction, and survivors of sudden ischemic death occurring during and after sport. Am Heart J 120:1207–1209, 1990.
76. Ciampricotti R, El Ganral M: Unstable angina, myocardial infarction, and sudden death after an exercise stress test. Int J Cardiol 24:211–218, 1989.
77. Gerlernt MD, Hochman JS: Acute myocardial infarction triggered by emotional stress. Am J Cardiol 69:1512–1513, 1992.
78. Meisel SR, Kutz I, Dayan K, et al: Effect of Iraqi Missiles War on incidence of acute myocardial infarction and sudden death in Israeli civilians. Lancet 338:660–661, 1992.
79. Muller JE, Tofler GH, Edelman E: Probable triggers of onset of acute myocardial infarction. Clin Cardiol 12:473–475, 1989.
80. Josis I, Majno G: Endothelial changes induced by arterial spasm. Am J Pathol 102:346–358, 1981.
81. Lin C-S, Penka PG, Zak FG, et al: Morphodynamic interpretation of acute coronary thrombosis with special reference to volcano-like eruption of atheromatous plaque caused by coronary artery spasm. Angiology 88:535–547, 1988.
82. Alpert JS: Coronary vasomotion, coronary thrombosis, myocardial infarction, and camel's back. J Am Coll Cardiol 5:617–618, 1985.
83. Singh RN: Progression of coronary atherosclerosis: Clues to pathogenesis from serial angiography. Br Heart J 12:56–62, 1988.
84. Hackett D, Davies G, Maseri A: Pre-existing coronary stenoses in patients with 1° MI are not necessarily severe. Eur Heart J 9:1317–1323, 1988.
85. Ku DN, Zairns CK, Glagov S: Pulsatile flow and atherosclerosis in the human carotid bifurcation: Positive correlation between plaque location and low and oscillating shear stress. Arteriosclerosis 5:293–302, 1995.
86. Tritton DJ: Physical Fluid Dynamics. Oxford, Clarendon Press, 1988, pp 7–19, 106.
87. Kolibasch AJ, Bush CA, Websic RA: Coronary collateral vessels: Spectrum of physiological capabilities with respect to providing rest and stress myocardial perfusion, maintenance of left ventricular function, and protection against infarction. Am J Cardiol 50:230–238, 1982.
88. Lam JTY, Chesebro JH, Steele PM, et al: Deep arterial injury during experimental angioplasty: Relation to a positive indium III, labeled platelet scintigram, quantitative platelet deposition, and mural thrombus. J Am Coll Cardiol 8:1380–1386, 1986.
89. Jansson JH, Nilsson TK, Olofsson BO: Tissue plasminogen activator and other risk factors as predictors of cardiovascular events in patients with severe angina pectoris. Eur Heart J 12:157–161, 1991.

90. Aznar J, Estelles A, Tormo G, et al: Plasminogen activator inhibitor activity and other fibrinolytic variables in patients with coronary artery disease. Br Heart J 59:535–541, 1988.

91. Meade TW, Brozovic M, Chakabarotic RR, et al: Hemostatic function and ischemic heart disease: Principal results of the Northwick Pork Heart Study. Lancet 2:533–537, 1986.

92. Cortellaro M, Boschett C, Lofzancesco E, et al: The PLAT Study: Hemostatic function in relation to atherothrombotic ischemic events in vascular disease patients. Arteriol Thromb 12:1063–1070, 1992.

93. Jansson JH, Nilsson TK, Johnson O: von Willebrand Factor in plasma: A novel risk factor of recurrent myocardial infarction and death. Br Heart J 66:351–355, 1991.

94. Thaulow E, Erikssen J, Sandvik L, et al: Blood platelet count and function are related to total and cardiovascular death in apparently healthy men. Circulation 84:613–617, 1991.

95. Wilhelmsen L: Thrombocytes and coronary heart disease. Circulation 84:936–938, 1991.

96. Prins MH, Hirsh J: A critical review of the relationship between impaired fibrinolysis and myocardial infarction. Am Heart J 122:545–551, 1991.

97. Hamsten A, de Faire U, Walldius G, et al: Plasminogen activator inhibitor in plasma: Risk factor for recurrent myocardial infarction. Lancet 2:3–9, 1987.

98. Gram J, Jespersen JA: A selective depression of tissue plasminogen activator (t-PA) activity in euglobin characterizes a risk group among survivors of acute myocardial infarction. Thromb Haemost 57:137–139, 1987.

99. Scott J: Thrombogenesis linked to atherogenesis at last? Nature 341:22–23, 1989.

100. Haviger J: Formation and regulation of platelets and fibrin hemostatic plug. Hum Pathol 18:111–122, 1987.

101. Lefkovitz J, Plow EF, Topol EJ: Platelet glycoprotein IIb/IIIa receptors in cardiovascular medicine. N Engl J Med 332:1553–1559, 1999.

102. Fuster V, Adams PC, Badimon JJ, et al: Platelet-inhibitor drugs role in coronary artery disease. Prog Cardiovasc Dis 29:325–346, 1987.

103. Fernandez-Ortiz A, Badimon JJ, Falk E, et al: Characterization of the relative thrombogenicity of atherosclerotic plaque components: Implications for consequences of plaque rupture. J Am Coll Cardiol 23:1562–1569, 1994.

104. Moreno PR, Bernardi VH, Lopez-Cullar J, et al: Macrophages, smooth muscle cells, and tissue factor in unstable angina: Implications for cell mediated thrombogenicity in acute coronary syndromes. Circulation 94:3090–3097, 1996.

105. Wilcox JN, Smith KM, Schwartz SM, Gordon D: Localization of tissue factor in the normal vessel wall and in the atherosclerotic plaque. Proc Natl Sci USA 86:2839–2843, 1989.

106. Patrons C, Renda G: Platelet activation and inhibition in unstable coronary syndromes. Am J Cardiol 80:17E–20E, 1997.

Clinical Presentation and Diagnosis (Including Triggering)

KEITH McLEAN, MD

JOHN F. MORAN, MD

Acute coronary syndrome (ACS) is now the most prevalent presentation of ischemic heart disease in Europe.[1] ST-segment elevation myocardial infarctions (MIs) are still more prevalent in the National Registry of Myocardial Infarctions than non–ST-segment elevation MIs (54.6% vs. 45.4%).[2] Successful treatment strategies that improve survival include anticoagulant, antiplatelet, thrombolytic, and interventional approaches. The initiation of these treatments requires accurate prompt diagnosis of ACS as the cause of chest pain.

Chest Pain

Chest pain is classically defined as the major physical symptom associated with ACS or acute MI. The differential diagnosis of chest pain is made by historical analysis, serial physical examinations, interpretation of electrocardiographic (EKG) findings, cardiac enzyme analysis, nuclear scans, and echocardiographic studies. The presentation of chest pain may vary and does not always reflect the spectrum of coronary artery disease (Fig. 1). Nonobstructive plaques in the coronary arteries may split and thrombose, turning mild obstruction into complete occlusion. The pathophysiology of this vulnerable plaque is a focus of current research (see Chapter 1).[3] Research in the area of chest pain has focused on computer algorithms, rapid assessment of cardiac enzymes, serum myoglobin analysis, diagnosis of the EKG, nuclear imaging, and the two-dimensional echocardiogram.

Ischemic chest pain can be retrosternal, squeezing, suffocating, or pressure-like with or without radiation to the arms in an ulnar distribution. William Heberden offered the best description of angina based on 100 patients[4]:

> But there is a disorder of the breast marked with strong and peculiar symptoms, considerable for the kind of danger belonging to it, and not extremely rare, which deserves to be mentioned more at length. The seat of it and sense of strangling and anxiety with which it is attended may make it not improperly called Angina Pectoris.
>
> They who are afflicted with it are seized while they are walking (more especially with the uphill and soon after eating) with a painful and most disagreeable sensation

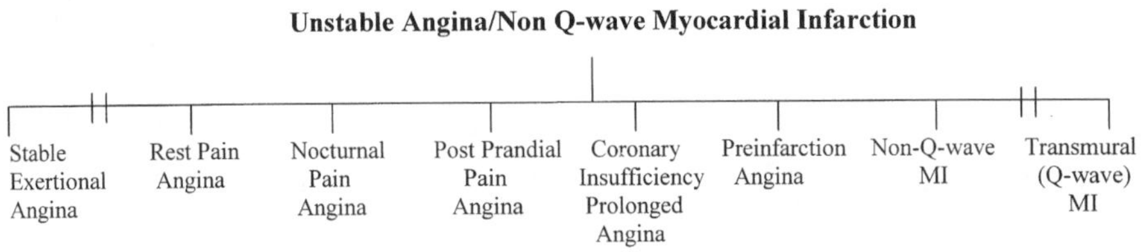

Unstable Angina/Non Q-wave Myocardial Infarction

Stable Exertional Angina	Rest Pain Angina	Nocturnal Pain Angina	Post Prandial Pain Angina	Coronary Insufficiency Prolonged Angina	Preinfarction Angina	Non-Q-wave MI	Transmural (Q-wave) MI

Figure 1.   Spectrum of coronary artery disease.

in the breast which seems as if it would extinguish life if it were to increase or continue. But the moment they stand still, all this uneasiness vanishes.

In all other aspects, patients are at the beginning of this disorder perfectly well and in particular have no symptoms of shortness of breath from which it is totally different. The pain is sometimes situated in the upper part, sometimes in the middle, sometimes at the bottom of the os sterni, and often more inclined to the left than to the right side. It likewise very frequently extends from the breast to the middle of the left arm. The pulse is at least sometimes not disturbed by this pain as I have had opportunities of observing by feeling the pulse during the paroxysm. Males are most liable to this disease especially if such as half past their 50th year.

Heberden had no idea that the disorder of the breast was related to the heart. However, he appreciated the fact that worsening angina eventually caused the death of the patient.

Brunwald's classification for unstable angina[5] takes into account severity of the pain, intensity of therapy, and clinical presentation. Class 1 is defined as angina of < 2 months' duration, severe or accelerated, with no rest pain in the preceding 2 months. Class 2 is defined as subacute angina at rest longer than 48 hours to 1 month previously. Class 3 is defined as acute angina at rest with at least one episode in the preceding 48 hours. The clinical classifications include class A, defined as secondary unstable angina triggered by anemia, infection, or thyrotoxicosis; class B, primary unstable angina; and class C, postinfarction unstable angina less than 2 weeks after documented MI. Therapy was divided into three parts: no or minimal therapy, angina in the presence of standard therapy, and angina despite maximal therapy. Later the guidelines for unstable angina were shown to support management for all aspects of the diagnosis and treatment of unstable angina in both inpatient and outpatient settings.[6]

Chest pain with radiation to the left arm increases the likelihood of ischemic pain by a factor of two. Radiation to the right arm increases the likelihood of ischemic pain by a factor of three. If radiation extends to both arms, the likelihood of ischemic disease is increased by a factor of seven.[7] The chest pain may last for 5-20 minutes and usually is relieved with sublingual nitroglycerin.

Diaphoresis, dyspnea, and vomiting also may occur with ACS. Patients sometimes clench their fist while describing the type of discomfort in their chest (Levine's sign). This sign may imply some heightened sense of acuity. Other characteristics that may portray a worse prognosis include rest pain or prolonged pain.

In a prospective study of 140 patients with unstable angina,[8] Gazes et al. found that the probability of survival at 1 year was significantly decreased from 96% in patients without persistent chest pain to 57% in 54 patients who had persistent angina within 48 hours of hospital admission. Rest pain has been shown to be associated with higher risk.[9]

Differential Diagnosis of Chest Pain

The differential diagnosis of chest pain in the emergency room can be a problem. The following disorders should be kept in mind:

- Costochondritis typically is associated with chest wall pain with a point tenderness. It often is exacerbated by movement, such as coughing or twisting. It seems to be more common in cigarette smokers and may even respond to smoking cessation. Pleuritic, positional, or stabbing chest pain is less likely to be ischemic.[10]
- The chest pain of pericarditis is typically precordial and located more commonly on the left side. It often is pleuritic, worsening with inspiration. The pain may be described as sharp and may radiate more toward the deltoid ridge. Classically, sitting up and leaning forward relieve the pain.
- Congenital absence of the pericardium may present with chest pain, described by Constant[11] as "a pain produced by lying on the left side that lasts only seconds or minutes."
- Aortic dissection pain is usually more severe at its onset than myocardial infarction or anginal pain, which gradually builds in a crescendo-type pattern. The pain with aortic dissection is often described as tearing and typically radiates toward the back.
- Patients with mitral valve prolapse may complain of an atypical type of chest pain, frequently with palpitations and some component of anxiety.
- Chest pain due to herpes zoster may be sharp and may occur before any of the typical dermatalogic manifestations, but it is often an easy diagnosis if a certain dermatome pattern is recognized on physical examination. Stress, emotional instability, exercise, or cold weather may exacerbate herpes zoster.

Other noncardiac causes of chest pain are possible, including gallbladder disease, peptic ulcer disease, anxiety, pulmonary embolism, pneumothorax, pulmonary hypertension, and esophageal reflux disease.

Silent Ischemia and Atypical Presentation of Acute Coronary Syndromes

Some patients with acute MI may not present with the classic symptom of crushing chest pain that radiates to the arm or jaw. In a national cohort study, Canto et al.[12] compared presenting characteristics, treatments, and outcomes of patients with MI. They found that one-third of all patients with the diagnosis of acute MI did not have chest pain on initial presentation to the hospital. Patients less likely to have chest pain were more often older, female, and non-white; they also had a higher prevalence of diabetes and congestive heart failure. Patients without chest pain were more likely to delay presentation at the hospital and thus were more likely to be diagnosed with acute MI at the time of admission. They also were less likely to receive thrombolysis (18.7% vs. 56.4%; p < 0.001), primary angioplasty (6.2% vs. 16.6%; p < 0.001),[12] aspirin, beta blockers, or heparin. Patients without chest pain had a twofold risk of hospital death compared with patients who presented with chest pain. The authors concluded that the one-third of patients who present with acute MI without chest pain often are treated less aggressively and thus are at increased risk for hospital death.[12]

The role of silent ischemia in patients who present with unstable angina cannot be overlooked. Gottlieb et al.[13] evaluated a series of 70 patients with unstable angina. Thirty-three had no evidence of silent ischemia, whereas 37 had evidence of silent ischemia on EKG monitoring. Patients with silent ischemia had a 5-fold increase in the relative risk of sustaining acute MI or needing bypass surgery for recurrent angina at 30 days. Patients with 60 minutes or more of silent ischemia in a 24-hour period had a significantly higher cumulative probability of unfavorable outcome than patients who had less than 60 minutes of ischemia. All patients were receiving three-drug treatment: propranolol, nitrates, and nifedipine.

Certain subpopulations are notorious for atypical presentations of ACS: women, elderly people, and patients with diabetes. Chiariello et al.[14] suggest that the symptoms of coronary artery disease are less likely to be present in patients with diabetes, probably because of sensory neuropathy. Dyspnea is the most common anginal equivalent in diabetic patients. Because of their atypical presentations, diabetics, elderly people, and women often present later in the course of the disease. Their symptoms may be attributed to some other disorder, such as bronchitis, emphysema, or asthma, often despite the lack of a prior history of such primary pulmonary processes. Other presenting symptoms for acute MI include confusion or abdominal or epigastric pain. Diagnosis may be delayed for tests such as ultrasounds of the liver or abdomen.

Methods of Diagnosing Acute Coronary Syndrome

Physical Examination

The physical examination has limited usefulness in the diagnosis of ACS. Findings may include increased autonomic nervous system activity, bradycardia (as part of the Bezold-Jarish reflex with acute inferior wall MI), and hypertension (due to acute anterior ischemia). Severe left ventricular dysfunction may be accompanied by a paradoxically split second heart sound, and transient or persistent apical murmur, often holosystolic, may accompany papillary muscle dysfunction or rupture associated with ischemia or infarction. Rales or a prominent S3 may be evident in patients with significant cardiac decompensation. An S4 is typically noted in the presence of ischemia.

Chest Radiograph

Chest radiographs also have limited usefulness. Unless the patient has had a previous infarction or presents with evidence of cardiac tamponade, the heart size remains normal in ACS. Widening of the mediastinum may be seen with aortic dissection, and various pulmonary changes may be seen with pulmonary sources of chest pain.

Laboratory Evaluation

Laboratory testing may show a slightly elevated white blood cell count as a stress response to the ischemic event. Anemia should be ruled out as a precipitating cause of unstable ischemia, as should hypoxemia and hyperthyroidism. Primary risk factors should be assessed in all patients suspected of having ACS, including evaluation for hyperlipidemia, diabetes, and increased levels of homocystine.

Electrocardiography

The first test usually done on a patient with chest pain suspicious of acute ischemic disease is the EKG. If the EKG interpretation is incorrect, high-risk patients may be misclassified. To improve diagnosis with EKG, Selker et al. used a computerized format incorporating age, sex, Q waves, and a more detailed analysis of ST-segment and T-wave changes.[15] They called this probability analysis of chest pain in the emergency room an acute cardiac ischemia–time-insensitive predictive instrument (ACI-TIPI). The ACI-TIPI was installed in the EKG machines of 10 participating hospitals. All patients with symptoms suggestive of ischemia were evaluated. The percentage probability for acute cardiac ischemia was then printed out on the EKG report. The trial was carried out over 7 alternating months of control and intervention. The 10,689 patients were divided into a control group (5951) and ACI-TIPI group (4738). For nonischemic patients, coronary care unit admission decreased from 15% to 12%, and discharges home increased from 49% to 52% (p < 0.09). For patients believed to be ischemic, coronary care unit admissions fell from 14% to 10% and telemetry admissions fell from 39% to 31%.[15] When fewer coronary care unit beds were available, more patients in the low-risk group were admitted to telemetry units. For patients with acute ischemia or acute MIs, admissions to the coronary care or telemetry unit were not reduced. Moreover in the months without ACI-TIPI, triage performance returned to baseline. No adverse influence on emergency room performance was observed.[15]

Cannon et al. examined the TIMI-III registry of patients with unstable angina or non–Q-wave MI to see whether prognostic information was available from the admission EKG.[16] Of 14,016 patients, 14.3 % had new ST-segment deviation (> 1 mm), 9% had complete left bundle-branch block (LBBB), 0.4% had new-onset complete LBBB, 21.9% had T-wave changes, and 54.9% had none of these changes. Of the patients with ST-segment deviation, 1.6% had ST elevation and 12.6% had ST depression. New ST-segment deviation and LBBB were associated with a 15.8% incidence of death or MI at 1 year.[16]

In a consecutive series of 265 patients who presented to the emergency department with chest pain, dyspnea, or both, Villaneuva et al. found that patients with a normal EKG were 6 times less likely to have a cardiac event during early and late follow-up than patients with an abnormal EKG.[17] ST elevation was associated with an 8-fold increased risk for a cardiac event. Serial EKGs are particularly important in evaluating such patients, especially if an EKG can be done during an episode of chest pain.

Langer et al.[18] noted ST-segment shifts on the admission EKG in 60 of 135 patients who had angina at rest or prolonged angina. In the group with ST-segment shifts, the incidence of death, MI, or need for urgent revascularization during hospital stay was 55% compared with 25% in the group without ST-segment changes (p < 0.005). They also showed that symptomatic or silent ST-segment changes on Holter monitoring indicated a poor prognosis, with a 48% rate of unfavorable events compared with a 20% rate in patients without ST-segment shifts (p < 0.005).

Cohen et al.[19] also showed that ST-segment changes during pain were reliable predictors of adverse events, such as recurrent ischemia, infarction, or need for revascularization. The positive predictive value for clinical events for ST-segment deviation > 1 mm in at least 2 or more leads was 89%.

Goldman et al.[20] predicted the need for intensive care in patients who come to the emergency department with acute chest pain by examining the rate of adverse events in relation to presenting EKG. They found that ST-segment elevation was associated with a 21% incidence of adverse events compared with a 9.4% incidence in patients with ST-segment depression or T-wave inversion.

Biochemical Markers in the Acute Coronary Syndromes

In addition to EKG changes, serum markers for myocardial necrosis also have prognostic importance in patients with ACS. These markers may be particularly important if the patient presents with no ST-segment deviation. Serial measurements of the serum cardiac enzymes creatinine kinase (CK), creatinine kinase MB (CK-MB), myoglobin, and cardiac troponin T or I are used to diagnose myocardial necrosis as well as to estimate prognosis (Table 1).

Cardiac Troponins

Troponin has become the standard of care in terms of myocardial markers. A certain number of patients have elevated troponins in the absence of significant CK elevation. Several studies have shown that despite nondiagnostic CK levels, an elevated troponin often indicates a poor prognosis. Antman et al.[21] showed that troponin-positive patients were at increased risk for adverse outcome even when CK-MB was below threshold values. At 42 days the CK-MB–negative group with a positive troponin test had a 2.5% chance of death, whereas the troponin-negative group had an 0.8% chance of death. Troponin may be so sensitive that it creates a new class of patients with ACS.

Troponin T and I are more sensitive than CK-MB and may begin to rise as early as 3 hours after the onset of ischemia. Antman et al.[21] found that the mortality rate was significantly higher in the 573 patients with elevation of cardiac troponin I levels of at least 0.4 ng/ml compared with the 831 patients with cardiac troponin I levels < 0.4 ng/ml. The risk ratio for death increased with each increase of 1 ng/ml in the cardiac troponin I level.

Ohman et al.[22] found troponin T to be a powerful independent risk marker in patients with acute myocardial ischemia. In GUSTO-IIa, 289 of 801 patients with baseline serum samples showed elevated troponin T levels. The mortality rate in the first 30 days was higher in these patients than in patients with troponin T levels < 0.1 ng/ml.

Olatidoye et al.[23] compared the prognostic roles of troponin T and troponin I in patients with unstable angina pectoris. They showed that the two markers were essentially equal in sensitivity, and both had high specificities (91% for troponin T vs. 92% for troponin I). They also performed a meta-analysis of 12 clinical trials in 2,847 patients with unstable angina and found essentially no significant differences between the sensitivities and specificities of the two enzymes.

Table 1.   Biochemical Markers for Acute Coronary Syndromes

Creatinine kinase MB	Matrix metalloprotease (MMP-9)
Troponins	Urinary fibrinopeptide-A
C-reactive protein	Protein C resistance
Chlamydia pneumoniae titers	Von Willebrand factor
Lymphocyte count	

Inflammatory Markers

Because inflammation is suspected to play a key role in the development of ACS, C-reactive protein also has been studied. Ting-Hsing Chao et al.[24] hypothesized that C-reactive protein can be used as a potential marker for ACS in patients with chest pain. In 214 patients with acute chest pain, C-reactive protein and troponin I were measured at 4, 8, 12, and 12–24 hours after onset. Patients were divided clinically into two groups: an ACS group and a non-ACS group. In the ACS group they found higher levels of C-reactive protein (1.2 ± 1.4 vs. 0.7 ± 1.7 mg/dl; $p < 0.01$) and cardiac troponin I (21.8 ± 32.1 vs. 0.8 ± 1.0 µg/L; ($p < 0.001$). C-reactive protein showed a 92% sensitivity and cardiac troponin I a 78% sensitivity. C-reactive protein had a 71% specificity and cardiac troponin I a 93% specificity. In the earlier stages of ACS (i.e., < 4 hours), serum levels of C-reactive protein were more sensitive than serum levels of cardiac troponin I (81% vs. 15%, respectively). The authors concluded that C-reactive protein is a sensitive marker in detecting ACS and may be used as an adjunct to EKG criteria for its early diagnosis.

Conversely, Baird et al.[25] found that in patients with unstable angina cardiac troponin I improves risk stratification, whereas the addition of a positive C-reactive protein yielded no further diagnostic benefit.

Berk[27] and his group tried to measure the presence of inflammation in active atherosclerotic lesions. They measured C-reactive protein in 37 patients with unstable angina, 30 patients with nonischemic illnesses, and 32 patients with stable coronary artery disease. They found that C-reactive protein levels were significantly elevated in 90% of the unstable angina group compared with 20% of the nonischemic group and 13% of the stable angina group. The average levels of C-reactive protein were significantly different for the unstable angina group (2.2 ± 2.9 mg/dl) compared with the nonischemic group (0.9 ± 0.7 mg/dl) and the stable angina group (0.7 ± 0.2; $p < 0.001$). The patients with unstable angina who had ST/T-wave abnormalities had higher C-reactive protein levels than patients without these changes.

Serum amyloid A protein also may be a marker of inflammation and a potential prognosticator in ACS. Liuzzo et al.[26] measured C-reactive protein, serum amyloid A protein, CK, and cardiac troponin T in 32 patients with chronic stable angina, 31 with severe unstable angina, and 29 with acute MI. At the time of hospital admission, CK and troponin were normal in all patients, but C-reactive protein and serum amyloid A protein were > 0.3mg/dl in 13% of the stable angina group, 65% of the unstable angina group, and 76% of the acute MI group. Patients with unstable angina and levels > 0.3 mg/dl. had more subsequent ischemic episodes than patients with levels < 0.3 mg/dl (4.8 ± 2.5 vs. 1.8 ± 2.4, p= 0.004). No deaths or MIs occurred in 11 patients with levels of the acute phase reactants < 0.3mg/dl, and only two of the 11 required coronary revascularization. Based on this study, it seems reasonable to conclude that elevation of C-reactive protein and serum amyloid A protein at the time of admission to the hospital may predict poor outcome in patients with unstable coronary syndrome. This finding underscores the inflammatory component of the disease and emphasizes that patients with higher levels of acute-phase reactants may convert from unstable angina to acute MI.

Although not generally used at this time, the inflammatory markers C-reactive protein and serum amyloid A may add diagnostic and prognostic power to troponin abnormalities and EKG changes in patients with ACS.

Chlamydia pneumoniae

Infection with *Chlamydia pneumoniae* and subsequent inflammation of the coronary arteries have been a controversial topic. Chandra et al.[28] examined *C. pneumoniae* and inflammatory markers in ACS. This prospective study included 814 patients admitted to a chest pain center. Clinical information and blood tests were obtained at the time of admission, and outcome data were collected. Multivariate analysis showed that a *C. pneumoniae* IgG level > 1:1024 was associated with a 1.47 relative risk of ACS. The authors concluded that ACS was strongly associated with a high level of seropositivity to *C. pneumoniae* in patients admitted with chest pain. A possible hypothesis is that recent reinfection with *C. pneumoniae* or an exaggerated immune response may be an etiologic factor for ACS.

Lymphocyte Count

Other novel markers of ACS may include the lymphocyte count in the peripheral blood. Zouridakis et al.[29] analyzed the lymphocyte count in peripheral blood and how it improved risk stratification in 71 patients with unstable angina. Cardiac troponin I levels and lymphocyte counts were measured within 24 hours of admission. During 12 ± 2 months of follow-up, 20 patients developed an adverse cardiac event—readmission for unstable angina and revascularization, MI, or cardiac death. Patients with a cardiac troponin I level > 0.4 mg/l had a relative risk 3.9 times higher than patients with normal levels of cardiac troponin I. Combined with a low lymphocyte count, this finding predicted a 6.5-fold increase in risk of adverse cardiac events during follow-up ($p = 0.003$). The authors concluded that a low lymphocyte count provides initial prognostic information beyond that of an abnormal troponin I alone and suggested that it may help in risk stratification.

Soluble Matrix Metalloprotease

Son et al.[30] noted that in atherosclerotic plaques prone to rupture, matrix metalloprotease (MMP-9) is induced in vascular smooth muscle cells and infiltrating macrophages. The authors evaluated MMP-9 in patients with variant angina, patients with atrial pacing and stable exertional angina, and patients with acute MI. Blood was sampled from the coronary sinus and aortic root before and after inducible ischemia and from venous blood in patients with acute MI. MMP-9 levels were significantly increased in patients with acute MI compared with other groups ($p = 0.005$). The authors concluded that higher levels of MMP-9 in acute MI may indicate that MMP-9 plays an important role in plaque rupture at the onset of acute MI.

Urinary Fibrinopeptide A

Another novel biochemical marker for ACS or intracoronary artery thrombus formation is urinary fibrinopeptide A, a polypeptide cleaved from fibrinogen by thrombin. It is a sensitive marker for thrombin activity and fibrin generation. Wilensky et al.[31] examined the level of urinary fibrinopeptide A and presence or absence of angiographic intracoronary thrombus in patients with unstable angina. The angiographic incidence of thrombus was significantly higher in patients with new onset of rest angina (67%, $p < 0.001$) and crescendo angina (50%, $p < 0.001$) than in patients with stable angina or chest pain without coronary artery disease. The angiographic incidence of thrombus was also significantly higher in patients with elevated levels of fibrinopeptide A (p = 0.002). Fibrinopeptide-A levels correlated significantly with the presence of a filling defect or contrast staining. However, a significant number of patients with unstable angina had no angiographic or biochemical evidence of thrombus. The authors concluded that elevated fibrinopeptide-A levels in unstable angina reflected active intracoronary thrombosis. Patients who did not have angiographic or biochemical evidence of thrombosis were believed to have had transient platelet aggregation without fibrin thrombus formation.

Activated Protein C Resistance and von Willebrand Factor

Activated protein C-resistance and von Willebrand factor also can be used for prognostication in patients with ACS. Ledon et al.[32] hypothesized that activation of the coagulation system may persist beyond the initial period of ACS. They analyzed the 1-year prognostic value of activated protein C resistance and von Willebrand factor in 214 patients treated with aspirin. Twelve patients died of cardiac cause. Activated protein C-resistance values were lower in nonsurvivors than in survivors (0.83 ± 0.1 vs 1.0 ± 0.1; $p < 0.001$) by the time of hospital discharge and at 3 months. The values also remained lower in the 6 patients who died at a later time. The authors also noted a trend toward higher levels of von Willebrand factor at discharge in nonsurvivors than in survivors (299 ± 94 vs $249 \pm 87\%$; p = nonsignificant). Higher levels at 3 months correlated significantly with a poorer outcome (p = 0.04). The authors concluded that in nonsurvivors, activated protein C-resistance values are persistently reduced during at least the first 3 months after discharge, whereas levels of von Willebrand factor remain increased. These findings suggest that coagulation derangements may continue beyond the initial period of ACS and may contribute to long-term mortality.

Triggers of Acute Coronary Syndromes

Much discussion and research have focused on the triggers of acute MI (Table 2). Triggering includes any activity of the patient that produces acute physiologic or pathophysiologic changes culminating in acute cardiac events.[33] Do acute MIs happen spontaneously, or are they triggered by an emotional or physical event?

Circadian Variation

Patients suffer acute MI at all times of the day, but the incidence is highest during the morning.[34] Much evidence suggests that the onset of acute MI can be attributed to both endogenous and exogenous daily rhythms.[34] An increase in adrenergic activity, coagulability, and hormone levels may create a transient risk state and thus precipitate acute MI.[34] Morning increases in ischemia are related, at least in part, to the increase in myocardial oxygen consumption (MVO_2) secondary to adrenergic increases in heart rate, blood pressure, and

Table 2. Triggers of Acute Coronary Syndrome

Circadian rhythm	Exertion
• Adrenergic surge	Job stress
• Increased platelet aggregability	Sexual activity
• Day of the week	Cocaine
Gender	Plaque rupture

myocardial contractility upon awakening, accompanied by a reduction in available myocardial oxygen secondary to increases in coronary vascular resistance.[35] An exception to this pattern has been observed in diabetic patients with autonomic nervous system dysfunction, who do not show an increase in morning ischemic episodes.[36] This exception suggests that alterations in the sympathovagal balance, which characterizes diabetic autonomic dysfunction, may influence the circadian pattern of ischemia.[36]

Behar et al.[37] studied 1818 consecutive patients hospitalized with acute MI in Israel and found that 32% experienced MI between 6 AM and noon (p < 0.01) compared with the other three 6-hour intervals. He concluded that endogenous changes in the morning hours are probably responsible for the higher rate of AMI after awakening.[37] Other acute coronary syndromes also have demonstrated significant circadian variation. In both TIMI-III and TIMI-IIIB, an increased number of patients experienced the onset of unstable angina or non–Q-wave MI between the hours of 6 AM and noon (p < 0.001).[38]

It has been proposed that platelet aggregability differs during specific times of the day. Tofler et al.[39] measured platelet activity at 3-hour intervals for 24 hours in 15 healthy men. This study showed that in vitro platelet responsiveness to either adenosine diphosphate or epinephrine was lower at 6 AM, before the men arose, than at 9 AM, 60 minutes arising. The period from 6 AM to 9 AM was the only 3-hour period during which the platelet aggregability was shown to be increased significantly. The authors also showed that the morning increase in platelet aggregation was not observed if the men remained inactive and supine. Based on this information, the authors concluded that platelet aggregability was increased in the morning hours but could not conclude that the increase in platelet aggregability was a causal factor in the increased frequency of morning MIs.

Although sleep protects an individual from ordinary day-to-day stressors such as job, exertion, anger, or sexual activity, Muller et al.[40] found that 12–15% of all cardiac events and almost 36,000 deaths occur annually during sleep. These events may tend to occur during rapid-eye-movement (REM) sleep, when sympathetic stimulation is closer to the levels perceived during daytime hours. Increases in sympathetic nervous system activity may trigger ischemic episodes and/or ventricular dysrhythmias. Further studies are needed to evaluate the possible causes or potential triggers of cardiac events during sleep.

In addition to circadian effects, other factors can be triggers in determining the timing of acute MI. A German study conducted by Spielberg et al.[41] looked at 2906 consecutive men and women with a confirmed diagnosis of acute MI over an 8-year period. The time of onset of MI (based on symptom onset) was known in 1901 cases. The authors also noted whether the patient was employed or retired. The study revealed that MI occurred more frequently between 7:00 AM and 10:00 AM, on Mondays, and during the winter months from January to March. Employed patients had a second peak in the afternoon at 4:00 PM (p < 0.05) and a trend toward an additional seasonal peak in September (p = not significant). The authors concluded that circadian rhythm, day of week, and seasonal variations markedly affect the occurrence of MI, with minor differences in employed and retired populations.[41]

Gender

Culic et al.[42] evaluated the role of gender in the onset of acute MI. Women had a higher rate of infarctions between 6 AM and noon than men (p = 0.0002).

The independent predictors of morning infarction included female sex (odds ratio [OR] = 1.3; 95% confidence interval [CI] = 1–1.7), previous angina (OR = 1.24, 95% CI = 1–1.9), presence of diabetes mellitus (OR = 1.4, 95% CI = 1.1–2.1), and no use of an anti-ischemic drug in the previous 24 hours (OR = 1.52, 95% CI = 1.1–2.5). The same circadian pattern also was seen more often in patients with no triggers than in patients with triggers (p = 0.01). Men were more likely to have triggered infarctions than women (45.2 vs. 37.3%, p = 0.009). By multivariate analysis, the independent predictors of triggered MIs included the absence of diabetes (OR = 1.4, 95% CI = 1.2–1.8), no previous angina (OR = 1.2, 95% CI = 1–1.6), normal serum cholesterol in women (OR = 1.5, 95% CI = 1.1–2.1), and no use of anti-ischemic drug in the previous 24 hours (OR = 1.6, 95% CI = 1.4–2.1).[39] This study further revealed a lower mortality rate in patients with triggered acute MI. Physical exertion as a trigger of AMI was roughly equal in both women and men. Women were more likely to recall mental stress as a possible trigger of acute MI.

Exertion

In the Myocardial Infarction Onset Study (MIOS),[43] 4.4% of patients reported heavy exertion within an hour before the onset of infarction. Heavy exertion was defined as 6 or more METS of work and was regarded as at least vigorous with panting or sweating. This study found that the relative risk of infarction onset in the hour after strenuous exercise was 5.9%. If the patient was sedentary and exercised less than once per week, the relative risk was 107%. If the patient participated in regular physical exertion once or twice per week, the relative risk fell to 19.4%. If the patient exercised 3–4 times per week, it fell to 8.6%, and if the patient exercised 5 times or more per week, it fell to 2.4%.

Several theories have been proposed to determine why physical exertion may precipitate MI, including hemodynamic shear stress, endothelial dysfunction (in which exercise induces vasoconstriction instead of vasodilatation), and increased coagulability.

Exertion has been reported to increase the risk of sudden coronary death, but the underlying mechanisms are unclear.[43] In an autopsy study, Burke et al. examined the frequency of plaque rupture in sudden deaths related to exertion compared with sudden deaths not related to exertion. In 141 men with severe coronary artery disease, 116 deaths occurred at rest and 25 deaths during strenuous physical activity or emotional stress. The mean number of vulnerable plaques was 1.6 in the men in the exertional group and 0.9 in the at-rest group (p = 0.03). The culprit plaque in the exertional MI group had ruptured in 17 of 25 (68%) men vs. 27 of 116 (23%) men in the at-rest MI group.[44] The authors concluded was that in men with severe CAD, sudden cardiac death related to exertion was associated with acute plaque rupture.

Job Stress

A Swedish study conducted by Theorell et al. examined the role of decision latitude and job stress in the etiology of a first MI in blue-collar men aged 45–64 years.[45] Low decision latitude was associated with increased risk of first MI, as was a decrease in decision latitude during the 10 years preceding MI. The combination of job stress and low decision latitude was found to be an important risk factor for MI in blue-collar men less than 55 years of age.

Johnson et al. investigated the relationship between work environment and prevalence of cardiovascular disease in a sample of Swedish male and female workers. An age-adjusted prevalence ratio of 2.17 was observed among a group of workers who had high demands, low control, and low social support compared with a group of workers with low demand, high control, and high social support.[46]

Sexual Activity

Patients often inquire about sexual activity after recovering from acute MI. Most patients are embarrassed to ask this personal question, and their fears feed into their imagination about repeat heart attacks or death during or after sexual activity. This topic also has been overrated in the media, movies, and television. In reality, Muller et al. reported that the frequency of acute MI related to sexual activity is very low.[47] Of a total of 1663 patients recovering from acute MI, only 858 were sexually active 1 year before MI, and only 27 of the 858 had engaged in sexual activity within 2 hours before MI. Sexual activity was the trigger event in only 0.9% of cases. The incidence of sexually induced MI was higher in sedentary people than in people who engaged in regular physical exercise (relative risk = 3.0 and 1.2, respectively). Of the 27 reported cases of MIs induced by sexual activity, 23 occurred in the sedentary group.

Preliminary data from the MIOS study indicated that sexual activity can trigger MI. Three percent of patients reported sexual activity within 2 hours preceding MI. The relative risk for infarction within 2 hours after sexual activity was 2.1.

Cocaine

Cocaine may trigger ACS through several possible mechanisms. Cocaine causes a dose-related increase in heart rate and blood pressure. Fischman et al.[48] showed that intravenous cocaine can increase heart rate up to 34% and blood pressure up to 15%. Both effects peak at 10 minutes. Lange et al.[49] showed that on coronary angiography small doses of cocaine intranasally (2mg/kg) induced an acute but mild diffuse reduction in coronary caliber (8–12 % compared with baseline), a significant reduction of 17% in coronary sinus blood flow, and a significant increase of 33% in coronary vascular resistance. Heart rate and blood pressure also increased modestly. The alpha blocker phentolamine prevented increased coronary vascular resistance and reduction in coronary caliber. The authors also reported that intracoronary beta blockade with propanolol may exacerbate the effects of cocaine on coronary vasculature and further reduce coronary flow.[50] Flores et al.[51] observed that the magnitude of vasoconstriction due to intranasal cocaine was greater in coronary artery segments narrowed by atherosclerosis (29%) than in nondiseased segments (13%). All of these factors may explain how cocaine can trigger ACS. Patients with cocaine-induced MI may have normal coronary arteries, which suggests spasm as the precipitating cause. However, two-thirds of patients have some form of atherosclerotic coronary artery disease.

Mental Stress

Atherosclerosis causes endothelial dysfunction in the coronary arteries and alters their reactivity to such stimuli as acetylcholine and exercise. Yeung et al.[52] studied the effect of mental stress on the vasomotor response of coronary arteries in 26 patients who performed mental arithmetic under stressful conditions during cardiac catheterization. Four patients who did not perform the arithmetic served as controls. Mental stress caused constriction of 24 ± 4% in narrowed coronary segments and constriction of 9± 3% in irregular segments without narrowing. Smooth segments were substantially unchanged or had mild dilatation. The authors concluded that the vasomotor response of normal epicardial coronary arteries to mental stress is either no change or limited dilatation. Atherosclerosis, however, causes a disruption in this normal response and results in paradoxic vasoconstriction, providing a potential trigger for ACS.

Plaque Rupture

Other potential triggers include a vulnerable plaque, which is characterized by a lipid-rich pool covered by a thin fibrous cap that is often infiltrated by macrophages and inflammatory cells. Lipid- and macrophage-rich plaques may be more prone to rupture and subsequent thromboses, but this hypothesis has not been proved in trials. Although it seems reasonable to consider "vulnerable plaque" as a potential trigger for ACS, at present there is no specific way to diagnose a vulnerable or nonvulnerable plaque.

A potential trigger for plaque rupture may be elevated systemic arterial pressure. This conclusion seems logical based on the pathophysiology of ACS, but it has no direct support. Inferential data may include the observation that the circadian cycle of blood pressure seems to correlate with the timing of ACS. Despite the lack of evidence for acute sheer forces or hemodynamic forces in plaque rupture, these elements are important in the development of chronic arterial occlusion and plaque formation.

Cost-effective Ways of Diagnosing Acute Coronary Syndromes

Over 5 million patients per year present to the emergency department for acute chest pain. Early diagnosis and treatment are of utmost importance. Early reperfusion is essential in ST-segment MI. Because not all patients have ST-segment elevation, the physician must determine which patients have chest pain of cardiac origin and which patients have chest pain due to a noncardiac cause. Some clinical algorithms and diagnostic strategies have been studied. Currently this issue is particularly important because of the need for cost-effective medical care.

Classically the 4Ds have emphasized the importance of early reperfusion. The first D represents the time when the patient reaches the **d**oor of the hospital; the second D, the amount of time required for **d**ata collection; the third D, the time when the **d**ecision is made for institution of primary treatment; and the fourth D, the time of **d**rug administrastion (thrombolytic therapy). The fourth D also can be used to represent the time of primary angioplasty.

Correct identification of patients with non–ST-segment elevation ACS is important and often results in admission to the hospital to rule out coronary artery disease. A strategy to evaluate patients with chest pain was developed by the Multicenter Chest Pain Study.[54] Factors associated with major cardiac events include older age, male sex, and chest pain similar to a previous MI or worse than usual angina. In addition, blood pressure < 110 mmHg, bibasilar crepitant rales extending more than halfway up the chest, and EKG findings of ischemia or infarction defined the high-risk patients.[54] Recently Shah et al.[53]

reviewed the GUSTO-IIb database and found that patients who develop heart failure with ACS are more likely to have a history of MI, hypertension, and diabetes and are more likely to be female.

In a later study, Nichol et al. developed a critical pathway for patients with acute chest pain and low risk for complications of ischemic heart disease.[54] Forty-eight percent of patients were admitted to the hospital and considered at low risk. Ninety-three percent of these had a benign clinical course and a mean length of stay of 2.8 days compared with 5.5 days for high-risk patients. Four of 1068 low-risk patients had an acute MI after 12 hours of observation, and 163 had unstable angina (15%). Overall, life-threatening complications occurred in 5 patients (0.5%) after 12 hours of observation. If patients who were stable after 6 or 12 hours of observation were discharged, significant resources could be saved. Recently, Reilly et al.[55] confirmed the value of this approach in a smaller patient cohort (n = 207). Faroghi et al. further characterized the low-risk patient with chest pain.[56]

A cost-effective standardized approach for patients with ACS may lower the cost of initial hospital evaluations and the frequency and cost of admissions, prevent unnecessary discharges from the emergency department, and improve the overall quality of care. Many hospitals have developed their own protocols for patients with ACS. Most protocols assess short-term risk of death based on clinical characteristics, such as duration of pain, presence or absence of pulmonary edema, EKG findings, age, and other cardiac risk factors (e.g., vascular disease, diabetes). Such information puts patients in perspective and may lead the physician to make an assumption about the likelihood of coronary artery disease. Relevant parameters can be placed on pocket cards or flowcharts, and algorithms placed in the emergency department to standardize patient evaluation in a specific institution may become the standard of care. Such protocols may reduce unnecessary inpatient admissions for nonischemic chest pain syndromes and lead to a substantial decrease in the cost of the rule-out evaluation.

Noninvasive Testing in the Evaluation of the Acute Coronary Syndromes

Understanding the ischemic cascade (Fig. 2) is important in determining which diagnostic modalities should be used in protocols to rule out MI. The ischemic cascade indicates that perfusion abnormalities are the first detectable objective evidence of ischemia. Hauser et al.[57] showed that echo wall motion changes may occur before pain or significant ST-segment changes in the process of an acute coronary event. EKG changes are the next step in the ischemic cascade, followed by chest pain. Understanding this cascade can lead to appropriate use of nuclear imaging, echocardiography, and serial EKGs and improve diagnostic accuracy.

Nuclear imaging may be used in the emergency department to improve diagnostic accuracy for ACS. Perfusion abnormalities should be the first objective evidence of ischemia. A normal perfusion scan in a symptomatic patient can prevent hospital admission and decrease the cost of care. Hilton et al. examined 102 patients who presented to the emergency department with chest pain and had a normal and/or nondiagnostic EKG.[59] Patients with a positive perfusion scan had a 71% incidence of a recurrent event, which was defined as cardiac death, nonfatal MI, percutaneous transluminal coronary angioplasty, surgery, or thrombolysis compared with 1.4% of patients with a negative scan (p < 0.001).

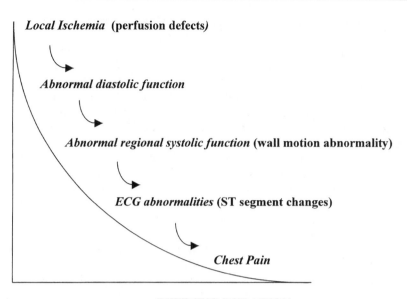

EXERCISE DURATION

Figure 2.   Indices of ischemia. (From Topol EJ (ed): Cardiovascular Medicine Version 2. Enhanced Multimedia CD-ROM. Philadelphia, Lippincott Williams & Wilkins, 2000, with permission.)

Peels et al.[58] examined the role of echocardiography in detecting coronary ischemia in the emergency department and found that it had 92% sensitivity and 53% specificity for acute MI as well as 88% sensitivity and 78% specificity for myocardial ischemia excluding MI. Patients should be imaged when they are having pain because the sensitivity is lower when patients are pain-free. The major pitfall is that body habitus may not allow an adequate echocardiographic window to make certain diagnostic conclusions. The endocardium must be imaged to determine accurately the presence or absence of normal systolic thickening.

In some cases, a stress test to evaluate myocardial ischemia may be ordered without an accompanying imaging modality. Certain subgroups of patients, however, may have false-positive EKG responses and require some sort of imaging modality along with the stress test. Possible causes for a false-positive EKG portion of the stress test may include left ventricular hypertrophy, preexisting ST-segment depression, Wolff-Parkinson White syndrome, concomitant use of digoxin, and mitral valve prolapse.

Chest Pain Evaluation Units

Chest pain evaluation units have been developed with defined protocols in an attempt to admit to the hospital only patients who truly need admission and to stratify risk in patients who may be at lower risk for cardiac complications. The shift in this paradigm has been toward ruling out MI in the emergency department instead of admitting every patient. Certainly MIs should not be missed if all patients with symptoms that could be construed as ACS were admitted, but this approach entails a high financial burden on the health care system. Patients who do not show clear-cut signs of ACS on initial admission are often kept in a unit for 8–12 hours while follow-up EKGs and cardiac enzyme tests are done. If the results prove negative, the patient often is set up for a predischarge functional exercise test, whether it is pharmacologic or exercise with or without some sort of imaging modality.

The basic idea behind the chest pain evaluation unit or chest pain center is to combine three key elements: initial rapid assessment, new biologic markers, and imaging modalities. These elements may improve diagnostic accuracy and quality of care. Integral to this system is the rapidity with which the information can be obtained. The other important factor is the sensitivity of the information on which decisions are based. With the newer cardiac markers, which are more sensitive for myocardial injury, a streamlined approach often can be used for patients visiting the emergency department. Troponin plays a key role because it is a highly sensitive and specific marker of myocardial injury. Myoglobin may be more useful for ruling out (but not for ruling in) MI. The previous standard of care, which has rapidly been replaced by troponin, was the measurement of CK with isoenzymes. The timing of ACS in relation to the release of enzymes into the serum is important to understand. Enzymes that can be interpreted at relatively short intervals may allow stress testing on the same day. Myoglobin may rule out MI at 4 hours after presentation. CK and MB isoenzymes require at least 8 hours. One strategy is to use an early marker, such as myoglobin, in combination with a late marker, such as troponin or CK. Myoglobin is used early to expedite the rule out of MI. If the myoglobin is abnormal, the clinician must rely on subsequent enzymes, such as CK and troponin, to ensure that the elevated myoglobin was specific for myocardial release. Serial EKGs should not be overlooked during this period.

Although chest pain evaluation units have been shown to provide cost-effective medical care, it is not certain whether they actually improve care and outcome in patients with MI. Canto et al.[60] compared 25,645 patients in the NRMI-III study who presented to hospitals with chest pain evaluation units and 102,377 patients who presented to hospitals without chest pain evaluation units. Several variables were studied, including time to first EKG, door to thrombolytic time, door to balloon inflation time, percent of patients receiving aspirin, percent of patients receiving beta blockers, percent of patients receiving any reperfusion, and crude hospital mortality rate. The data showed no significant differences in outcomes between the two groups. Chest pain evaluation units did not seem to be directly associated with improved process of care or lower hospital mortality rates.

References

1. Fox KAA, on behalf of the ENACT investigators. The ENACT Study. J Am Coll Cardiol 35(Suppl A):352A, 2000.
2. Barron HV: NRMI 3 and acute coronary syndromes. NRMI 3 News, Dec. 1999.
3. Fuster V: The Ventricle Atheroscleratic Plaque: Understanding, Identification and Modification. Armonk, NY, Futura, 1999.
4. Willus FA, Keyes TE: Classics of Cardiology, vol. 1. New York, Dover, 1941.
5. Braunwald E: Unstable angina: A classification. Circulation 80:410–414, 1989.
6. Braunwald E, et al: Diagnosing and managing unstable angina. Circulation 90:613–622, 1994.
7. Paujes A, et al: A critical appraisal of the cardiovascular listing and physical exam. In Yusuf S, Cairns JA, Camm AJ, et al (eds): Evidence Based Cardiology. London, BMJ Books, 1998.
8. Gazes PC, et al: Preinfarctional unstable angina: A prospective study 10 year follow up. Circulation 48:331–337, 1973.
9. Betriu A, et al: Unstable angina outcomes according to clinical presentation. J Am Coll Cardiol 19:1659–1663, 1992.
10. Pozen MW, et al: A predictive instrument to improve coronary care unit admission practices in acute ischemic heart disease. N Engl J Med 310:1273–1278, 1984.

11. Constant J: Bedside Cardiology, 4th ed. Boston, Little, Brown, 1993.
12. Canto JG, Shilpak MG, Rogers WJ, et al: Chest pain and myocardial infarction: Is it time to re-define the classical clinical presentation? Observations from the NRMI 2. J Am Coll Cardiol 35(Suppl A):380, 2000.
13. Gottlieb SO, et al: Silent ischemia: A marker for early unfavorable outcomes in patients with unstable angina. N Engl J Med 314:1214–1219, 1986.
14. Chiariello M, Indolfi C: Silent myocardial ischemia in patients with diabetes mellitus. Circulation 93:2089–2091, 1996.
15. Selker H, et al: Use of the acute cardiac ischemia–time-insensitive predictive instrument (ACI-TIPI) to assist with triage of patients with chest pain or other symptoms suggestive of acute cardiac ischemia. Ann Intern Med 129:845–855, 1998.
16. Cannon CP, et al, for the TIMI III Registry ECG Ancillary Study investigators: The electrocardiogram predicts one year outcome of patients with unstable angina and non-Q wave myocardial infarction. J Am Coll Cardiol 30:133–140, 1997.
17. Villaneuva FS, et al: Value and limitations of current methods of evaluating patients presenting to the emergency room with cardiac related symptoms for determining long term prognosis. Am J Cardiol 69:746–750, 1992.
18. Langer A, Freeman MR, Armstrong PW: ST-segment shift in unstable angina: Pathophysiology and association with coronary anatomy and hospital outcome. J Am Coll Cardiol 13:1495–1502, 1989.
19. Cohen M, et al: Usefulness of ST-segment changes in greater than two leads on the emergency room electrocardiogram in either unstable angina pectoris or non–Q-wave myocardial infarction in predicting outcome. Am J Cardiol 67:1368–1373, 1991.
20. Goldman L, Cook EF, Johnson P: Predicting the need for ICU in patients who come to the emergency department with acute chest pain. N Engl J Med 334:1498–1504, 1996.
21. Antman EM, Tanasijevic MJ, Thompson B, et al: Cardiac-specific troponin I levels to predict the risk of mortality in patients with acute coronary syndromes. N Engl J Med 335:1342–1349, 1996.
22. Ohman EM, Armstrong PW, Christenson RH, et al: Cardiac troponin I levels for risk stratification in acute myocardial ischemia. N Engl J Med 335:1333–1341, 1996.
23. Olatidoye AG, Wu AH, Feng YJ, Waters D: Prognostic role of troponin T versus troponin I in unstable angina pectoris for cardiac events with meta-analysis comparing published studies. Am J Cardiol 81:1405–1410, 1998.
24. Chao TH, Li YH, Tsai WC, et al: C-reactive protein as a useful marker for acute coronary syndrome manifested with acute chest pain. J Am Coll Cardiol 35(Suppl A):388–389, 2000.
25. Baird SH, Trouten TG, Ryan M, et al: Evaluation of cardiac troponin I kinetics profile in patients with acute coronary syndrome. J Am Coll Cardiol 35:(Suppl A):389, 2000.
26. Liuzzo G, Biasucci LM, Gallimore JR, et al: The prognostic value of C-reactive protein and serum amyloid A in severe unstable angina. N Engl J Med 331:417–424, 1994.
27. Berk BC, Weintraub W, Alexander RW: Elevation of C-reactive protein in "active" coronary artery disease. Am J Cardiol 65:168–172, 1990.
28. Chandra HR, Choudhary N, O'Neill C, et al: Chlamydia pneumoniae and inflammatory markers in acute coronary syndrome. J Am Coll Cardiol 35(Suppl A):359, 2000.
29. Zouridakis EG, Garcia-Moll X, Kaski JC: Lymphocyte count in peripheral blood improves risk stratification in unstable angina patients. J Am Coll Cardiol 35(Suppl A):360, 2000.
30. Son JW, Koh KK, Kim W, et al: Soluble matrix matalloprotease (MMP)-9 levels in systemic and coronary circulation in patients with variant angina and acute coronary artery syndrome (ACS). J Am Coll Cardiol 35(Suppl A):388, 2000.
31. Wilensky RL, Bourdillon PD, Vix VA, Zeller JA: Intra-coronary artery thrombus formation in unstable angina: A clinical, biochemical and angiographic correlation. J Am Coll Cardiol 21:692–699, 1993.
32. Lidon R, Figueras J, Angles A, et al: Activated protein C resistance and von Willebrand factor are useful markers for 1 year mortality after acute coronary syndromes. J Am Coll Cardiol 35(Suppl A):411,, 2000.
33. Muller JE, Abela GS, Nesto RW, Tofler GH: Triggers, acute risk factors and vulnerable plaques: The lexicon of a new frontier. J Am Coll Cardiol 23:809–813, 1994.
34. Culic V, Eterovic D, Miric D, et al: Gender differences in triggering of acute myocardial infarction. Am J Cardiol 85:753–756, 2000.
35. Fugita M, Fronklin D: Diurnal changes in coronary blood flow in conscious dogs. Circulation 76:488–491, 1987.
36. Zarich S, Waxman S, Freeman RT, et al: Effect of autonomic nervous system dysfunction on the circadian pattern of myocardial ischemia in diabetes mellitus. J Am Coll Cardiol 24:956–962, 1994.
37. Behar S, Halabi M, Reicher-Reiss H, et al: Circadian variation and possible external triggers of onset of myocardial infarction. Am J Med 94:395–400, 1993.

38. Cannon CP, McCabe CH, Stone PH, et al: Circadian variation in the onset of unstable angina and non–Q-wave acute myocardial infarction (the TIMI III registry and TIMI IIIB). Am J Cardiol 79:253–258, 1997.

39. Tofler GH, Brezinski D, Schafer AI, et al: Concurrent morning increase in platelet aggregability in the risk of myocardial infarction and sudden cardiac death. N Engl J Med 316:1514–1518, 1987.

40. Muller JE, Kaufmann PG, Luepker RV, et al: Mechanisms precipitating acute cardiac events: Review and recommendations of an NHLBI workshop. Circulation 96(9):3233–3239, 1997.

41. Speilberg C, Falkenhahn D, Willich S, et al: Circadian, day-of-week, and seasonal variability in myocardial infarction: Comparison between working and retired patients. Am Heart J 132:579–585, 1996.

42. Culic V, Eterovic D, Miric D, et al: Gender differences in triggering of acute myocardial infarction. Am J Cardiol 85:753–756, 2000.

43. Mittleman MA, Maclure M, Tofler GH, et al, for the Determinants of Myocardial Infarction Onset Study Investigators: Triggering of acute myocardial infarction by heavy physical exertion: Protection against triggering by regular exertion. N Engl J Med 329:1677–1683, 1993.

44. Burke AP, Farb A, Malcom GT, et al: Plaque rupture and sudden death related to exertion in men with coronary artery disease. JAMA 281:921–926, 1999.

45. Theorell T, Tsutsumi A, Hallquist J, et al: Decision latitude, job strain and myocardial infarction: A study of working men in Stockholm. Am J Public Health 88:382–388, 1998.

46. Johnson JV, Hall EM: Job strain, workplace, social support and cardiovascular disease: A cross-sectional study of a random sample of the Swedish working population. Am J Public Health 78:1336–1342, 1988.

47. Muller JE, Mittleman MA, Maclure M, et al, for the Determinants of Myocardial Infarction Onset Study Investigators: Triggering myocardial infarction by sexual activity: Low absolute risk and prevention by regular physical exertion. JAMA 275:1405–1409, 1996.

48. Fischman MW, Schuster CR, Resnekov L, et al: Cardiovascular and subjective effects of intravenous cocaine administration in humans. Arch Gen Psychiatry 33:983–989, 1976.

49. Lange RA, et al: Cocaine-induced coronary artery vasoconstriction. N Engl J Med 321: 1557–1562, 1989.

50. Lange RA, et al: Potentiation of cocaine-induced coronary vasoconstriction by beta adrenergic blockade. Ann Intern Med 1990; 112:897–903, 1990.

51. Flores ED, et al. The effect of cocaine on coronary artery dimensions in atherosclerotic coronary artery disease: Enhanced vasoconstriction at sites of significant stenosis. J Am Coll Cardiol 16:74–79, 1990.

52. Yeung AC, Verkshtein VL, Krantz DS, et al: The effect of atherosclerosis on the vasomotor response of coronary arteries to mental stress. N Engl J Med 325:1551–1556, 1991.

53. Shah SS, Tokarski GF, McCord JK, et al: Impact of an emergency department cardiac clinical decision unit on population of patients with episodic chest discomfort. J Am Coll Cardiol 35:212, 2000 [abstract].

54. Nichol G, et al: A critical pathway for management of patients with acute chest pain who are at low risk for myocardial ischemia: Recommendation and potential impact. Ann Intern Med 127:996–1005, 1997.

55. Reilley B, et al: Performance and potential of a chest pain prediction rule in a large public hospital. Am J Med 106:285–291, 1999.

56. Faroghi A, Kontos MC, Jesse RL, et al: Are cardiac risk factors predictive in low risk emergency department chest pain patients who have chest pain? J Am Coll Cardiol 35(Suppl A):379, 2000.

57. Hauser AM, et al: Sequence of mechanical, EKG, and clinical effects of repeated coronary occlusions in human beings. J Am Coll Cardiol 5:193–197, 1985.

58. Peels CH, Visser CA, Kupper AJ, et al: Usefulness of two-dimensional echocardiography for immediate detection of myocardial ischemia in the emergency room. Am J Cardiol 65:687–691, 1990.

59. Hilton TC, Thompson RC, Williams HS, et al: Technetium 99 M sestamibi myocardial perfusion imaging in the emergency room: Evaluation of chest pain. J Am Coll Cardiol 23:1016–1022, 1994.

60. Canto JG, Ornato JP, Zalenski R, et al: Chest pain emergency units and their impact on processes of care and outcome: Observations room the National Registry of Myocardial Infarction. J Am Coll Cardiol 35(Suppl A):337, 2000.

Risk Factor Stratification and Acute Coronary Syndromes

DAVID L. SMULL, DO
THOMAS L. McKIERNAN, MD

In the early 1970s Fowler, Scanlon, and others coined the term unstable angina to describe the clinical syndrome of chest pain and electrocardiographic changes that precedes myocardial infarction (MI).[1,2] Acute MI was defined clinically, based on history and presence or absence of ST-segment changes and Q-waves on the electrocardiogram, and serum markers. These definitions were used commonly in the practice of cardiology until a recent paradigm shift to the concept of the acute coronary syndromes (ACSs) as a spectrum of disease including unstable angina, non–Q-wave MI, and Q-wave MI. The concept of plaque fissure and thrombosis put forth by Davies, Ambrose, and others and the results of the Thrombolysis in Myocardial Infarction (TIMI)-IIIB Trial have given us a new clinical classification.[3–5]

The ACSs are now described based on the electrocardiogram as non–ST-segment elevation or ST-segment elevation. These new groupings include unstable angina and non–Q-wave MI in the non–ST-segment elevation group and Q-wave MI in the ST-segment elevation group. In the TIMI-IIIB Trial, no benefit from thrombolytic therapy was seen in the non–ST-segment elevation group,[3] but many trials have shown that thrombolysis clearly benefits the ST-segment elevation group. Similar treatment plans, including aspirin, glycoprotein (GP) IIb–IIIa agents, antithrombins, calcium channel blockers, beta blockers, and interventional devices have made the distinction between unstable angina and non–Q-wave MI less important. It now appears that the two classifications identified by electrocardiographic ST-segment change should be used in determining prognosis and directing therapy. Excellent complete reviews of ACS risk stratification can be found in *Acute Coronary Syndromes* edited by Topol and in *Contemporary Cardiology: Management of Acute Coronary Syndromes*, edited by Cannon.[6,7] This chapter reviews the current factors that determine the risk stratification for both non–ST-segment elevation and ST-segment elevation ACSs and discusses how stratification affects prognosis and helps to place patients in the proper treatment categories.

Non–ST-Segment Elevation Acute Coronary Syndrome

Clinical Factors

Early indicators of risk for non–ST-segment elevation ACS include clinical history and physical examination, electrocardiogram, biochemical markers, echocardiography, and nuclear scanning. All of these tools provide important risk assessment data. The baseline characteristics of patients as they present with non–ST-segment elevation should be considered in predicting outcome. Recently, the PURSUIT investigators found that in a multivariate logistic regression analysis of 9461 patients with ACS without ST-segment elevation the most important determinants of death at 30 days were age, heart rate, systolic blood pressure, ST-segment depression, signs of heart failure, and cardiac enzymes. These determinants of mortality were also predictive of a broader endpoint of death or myocardial (re)infarction.[8]

Other important risk factors in the PURSUIT analysis were diabetes mellitus, prior MI, previous anginal symptoms and creatine kinase (CK)-MB level at enrollment (MI vs. unstable angina). Patients taking cardiac medications had a worse prognosis than patients not taking such medications before enrollment.[8]

The same investigators developed a simple score tool to estimate 30-day risk for complications. Points are given for age, gender, prior angina, heart rate and systolic blood pressure, signs of heart failure, and ST depression on EKG. The points provide a risk score that can be converted to a probability of adverse events with the help of the graph in Figure 1.[8]

The most obvious presentation of ACS is angina pectoris. It is difficult to distinguish unstable angina from non–Q-wave MI by patient history. Although several classifications of angina are available, the most commonly used are the Canadian classification system, Braunwald's classification, and Rizik's classification.[9,10,12] In Braunwald's classification,[9] patients are grouped according to severity as follows:

Type I   New onset or accelerated angina without pain at rest
Type II   Angina at rest but not within the preceding 48 hours
Type III   Angina at rest within 48 hours

And according to clinical circumstances:

Type A   Secondary to an extracardiac condition (fever, tachycardia, anemia)
Type B   No extracardiac condition (primary unstable angina)
Type C   Postinfarction angina

The patient is also classified according to the presence or absence of changes on the resting EKG and according to intensity of medical treatment:

Type 1   Minimal therapy
Type 2   Extreme oral therapy
Type 3   Maximal therapy (intravenous nitroglycerin)

In validations of this system, progression to infarction, death, angiography, or percutaneous transluminal coronary angioplasty (PTCA)/coronary artery bypass grafting (CABG) during the in-hospital period was most frequently observed in type III-C patients (postinfarction angina at rest).[10] In a multivariate analysis, elderly age, male gender, hypertension, and type C were independent predictors of death.[10] Unstable angina scores also have been developed from the Braunwald classification and used to predict outcome in patients. Dangas et al. correlated clinical presentation of unstable angina with angiographic morphology and found angina type III was associated with complex lesions

		Score	
		Mortality only	Mortality or infarction
Age (year)	50	0	8 (11)
	60	2 (3)	9 (12)
	70	4 (6)	11 (13)
	80	6 (9)	12 (14)
Gender	Female	0	0
	Male	1	1
Worst CCS-class in previous 6 weeks	No angina; I or II	0	0
	III or IV	2	2
Heart rate (bpm)	80	0	0
	100	1 (2)	0
	120	2 (5)	0
Systolic blood pressure (mmHg)	120	0	0
	100	1	0
	80	2	0
Signs of heart failure (rales)	No	0	0
	Yes	3	2
ST-depression on presenting ECG	No	0	0
	Yes	3	1

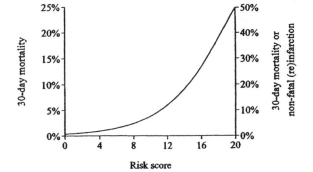

Figure 1. Simple scheme to estimate risk of 30-day complications. Points are given for each predictive factor. With respect to age and heart rate, there are separate points for enrollment diagnosis of unstable angina and MI (between parentheses). Summed points provide a risk score, which can be converted into a probability with the help of the graph. CSS = Canadian Cardiovascular Society. (From Boersma E, Pieper K, Steyerberg E, et al: Predictors of outcome in patients with acute coronary syndromes without persistent ST-segment elevation. The PURSUIT Investigators. Circulation 101:2557–2567, 2000, with permission.)

and decreased TIMI flow, whereas type C correlated with complex lesions and intracoronary thrombus.[11]

In a prospective validation of the Braunwald system, Calvin et al. found four clinical factors that were predictive of in-hospital major cardiac complications:

(1) MI within less than 14 days, (2) need for IV nitroglycerin, (3) absence of beta blockers or calcium blockers before admission, and (4) baseline ST-segment depression.[13] In addition, increasing age and diabetes were also predictive of in-hospital complications, although these characteristics are not part of the Braunwald classification system.[13] Emre et al. also showed type III-C-3 to be associated with a greater size and intensity of perfusion defect and wall motion abnormality on scintigraphic evaluation.[14] Hemodynamic deterioration during angina (manifested by pulmonary edema, new mitral regurgitation, or a third heart sound) or hypotension also predicts a more serious prognosis.

The classification system of Rizik et al.[12] is divided into the following groups:

Group IA Accelerated angina without EKG changes
Group IB Accelerated angina with EKG changes
Group II   New onset of exertional angina
Group III New onset of resting angina
Group IV Protracted rest angina with EKG changes

Risk of MI, death, or intractable angina was evaluated in 1387 consecutive patients using this system. The trend in cardiac events increased significantly with higher group classification (p < 0.001).[12] Group IV patients showed a high rate of in-hospital adverse events (42.8%).[12]

Electrocardiographic Findings

The EKG is the cornerstone and most objective tool for the classification of the non–ST-segment elevation ACS. Transient EKG changes, specifically ST-segment elevation or depression, predicts a higher short-term risk of death or MI.[15–17] In a TIMI III substutdy, ST-segment deviation on the initial EKG was one of four predictors of non–Q-wave MI.[18] In GUSTO-IIa, Ohman et al. correlated 30-day mortality rate and incidence of MI with EKG changes. They found that a normal EKG or an EKG with only T-wave inversions had a 1.2% mortality rate and a 50.9% incidence of MI; ST-segment depression on EKG was associated with an 8% mortality rate and a 56.8% incidence of MI. ST-segment elevation was associated with a 7.4% mortality rate and an 84% incidence of MI, and EKG abnormalities such as left ventricular hypertrophy, permanent pacemaker, and left bundle-branch block demonstrated the highest risk with an 11.6% mortality rate and 66.7% incidence of MI.[19]

Savonitto showed that in GUSTO-IIb the baseline EKG correlated with mortality at 6 months. Patients with T-wave inversion had the lowest mortality rate (3.4%), followed by ST-segment elevation (6.8%), ST-segment depression (8.9%), and combined ST-segment elevation and depression (9.1%).[20] In TIMI-IIIB dynamic ST-segment depression was associated with an increase in the likelihood of death, MI, ischemia at rest, or provokable ischemia during a test to stratify risk.[21] Krone et al. demonstrated that at 4 years patients with acute MI and ST depression had a 10.3% mortality rate compared with 5.6% in patients without ST depression.[22] Hamm et al. correlated EKG changes with troponin T and I (rapid test) in patients presenting to the emergency department with chest pain. Among 158 patients with ST-segment depression, 32% had at least one positive troponin T test and 56% at least one positive troponin I test. Among the 197 patients with T-wave inversion, 6% had a positive troponin T tests, and 5% had at least one positive troponin I test. Among 331 patients with normal EKGs, 10% had a positive troponin T test and 10% a positive troponin I test. Of patients with a nondiagnostic EKG (paced rhythm or bundle-branch block), 32% had at least one elevated troponin T and 47% at least one elevated troponin I test.[23] Despite such important data, the initial 12-lead EKG is limited because it provides only a brief picture of what is occurring. It does, however, have the advantages of availability and low cost. Thus, patients with ST-segment depression or elevation have a worse prognosis in ACS.

Serum Cardiac Markers

Acute coronary syndromes pathologically consist of varying degrees of myocardial injury. It is thought that larger infarcts convey poorer prognosis. In addition, territory at risk also may define subsets of populations that have worse outcomes. Although EKG evidence may provide information about territory, a large proportion of EKGs are equivocal, thus making the identification of patients at increased risk of death and recurrent cardiac morbidity an important challenge. Patients presenting to the emergency department with chest pain present a clinical and financial problem. Of the estimated 5 million presentations to emergency departments annually, only about 10% are diagnosed with MI. With the goal of cost reduction and reduced hospitalizations, determining which patients are at highest risk is a major objective. Accordingly, serum markers of myocardial necrosis have become integral to the diagnosis and risk stratification of patients with ACS.

Recent series have demonstrated that serum cardiac markers have prognostic value in unstable angina. The most commonly used markers of myocardial necrosis include creatine kinase (CK), cardiac-specific CK-MB, CK-MB subforms, myoglobin, and cardiac troponins T and I. Ideally, these markers should be highly sensitive and specific. They should be absent in noncardiac tissue and serum but elevated in the serum soon after the onset of injury. They should remain elevated for a prolonged period. The degree of elevation should correlate with the degree of myocardial injury. In addition, they should be inexpensive and have rapid laboratory turn-around times. Although none of the currently available serum markers are ideal, combinations of assays may be sufficient. Currently, potentially more sensitive markers of myocardial necrosis are under development.

Myoglobin

Myoglobin is a heme protein found in all striated muscle. Its small size (17.5 kDa) allows early detection in serum, but it is rapidly cleared in the kidneys within 12–15 hours. It is a nonspecific marker of muscle necrosis and injury. It is often elevated after trauma or exercise and in patients with renal failure. In 305 patients evaluated for suspicion of MI, an elevated myoglobin was found to be highly sensitive (72% on admission, 98% after 4 hours, and 100% at 15 hours); thus, a negative myoglobin test had excellent negative predictive value for diagnosis of infarction.[24] Patients with postinfarction complications, including arrhythmia, circulatory problems, and death, also had significantly higher serum myoglobin levels. Data from the BIOMACS study[25] compared myoglobin with CK-MB and troponin T in 142 patients presenting within 12 hours of pain and a nondiagnostic EKG. The sensitivity of serum myoglobin drawn on admission for the diagnosis of MI was 83% compared with 41% and 24% for CK-MB and troponin T, respectively. The combination of myoglobin and CK-MB afforded the best combination of sensitivity and specificity for the early diagnosis of MI. Myoglobin, although an early sensitive marker of myocardial necrosis, has limited use for risk stratification because of its poor specificity.

Creatine Kinase

CK is an 85-kDa enzyme that catalyzes phosphorylation of creatine to creatine phosphate. It is found in all striated muscle and separated into three isoenzymes. CK-MM is the predominant form in all striated muscle, CK-MB is found in highest concentrations within the myocardium, and CK-BB is found predominantly in the brain, gut, and kidney. CK and its isoforms have been the gold standard for diagnosis of MI for over 30 years. Although CK may be a sensitive marker for myocardial necrosis, approaching > 95%[24] at 15 hours, it may be falsely elevated in many pathologic conditions; thus its specificity is limited.

CK-MB is relatively specific to cardiac tissue. Although it may be increased after skeletal trauma or during inflammatory conditions, it is a much more specific marker for myocardial necrosis than CK. An increase in CK-MB correlates well with infarct size and thus has prognostic value.[26] Because CK-MB appears to represent necrosis rather than ischemia, patients with elevated levels are at risk for clinical events, including death.[27] CK-MB becomes elevated within 3–4 hours after the onset of ischemic injury and returns to baseline within 24–36 hours—ideal timing for a cardiac-specific marker. However, CK-MB may miss low levels of myocardial necrosis, thus decreasing its sensitivity. Sensitivities of only 50–75% within the first 6 hours have been documented.[28,29]

The role of appropriately diagnosing acute MI in its early stages has diagnostic, therapeutic, and financial implications. In TIMI-IIIB,[3] patients with unstable angina who received thrombolytic therapy had an increased rate of death and MI, whereas patients diagnosed with non–Q-wave MI had similar outcomes whether or not they received thrombolytics. However, the mean time from symptoms to treatment was 9 hours, which may have decreased the efficacy of therapy. An early marker for myocardial injury may benefit such patients.

CK-MB exists as two forms in equilibrium, tissue form (MB2) and seroconverted form (MB1). When the myocyte becomes injured and its membrane loses integrity, the MB2 subform is released and converted to MB1 in the serum. This process increases the MB2:MB1 ratio as well as the absolute amount of circulating MB2. CK-MB subforms are highly sensitive and can detect myocardial injury as early as 3 hours after the onset of symptoms. In the Diagnostic Marker Cooperative Study,[28] CK-MB subforms, CK-MB (activity and mass), myoglobin, troponin T, and troponin I were evaluated in 955 patients presenting to an emergency department for chest pain. At 6 hours from admission, MB subforms (MB2 > 2.5 IU/L or MB2:MB1 > 1.6 IU/I) were the most sensitive diagnostic markers (91.5%), followed by myoglobin (positive predictive value = 97%). Cardiac troponin T and troponin I were highly cardiac-specific and accurate for late diagnosis of MI. However, CK-MB subforms carry the same limitations in specificity as CK-MB. Puleo and colleagues[29] showed that CK-MB subforms were elevated in patients with MI within 4 hours of onset of symptoms. Patients with positive CK-MB subforms had a significantly higher incidence of diagnosis of MI within 6 hours of onset of symptoms. CK-MB subforms, alone or in combination with cardiac troponins, can reliably identify patients with ACS.

Cardiac Troponins

The troponins consist of a group of three proteins (C, T, and I) that make up the calcium-sensitive contractile apparatus of all striated muscle. Troponin T binds the troponin complex to tropomyosin, troponin I binds to actin and regulates the actin-myosin interaction, and troponin C responds to changes in intracellular calcium. Cardiac-specific monoclonal antibody-based immunoassays have been developed to detect cardiac troponin T and I. Because troponin C is identical in both cardiac and skeletal muscle, no specific immunoassay is currently available for clinical use.

Early risk assessment is essential for the appropriate application of therapy in patients with ACS. Cardiac troponins are now regularly used because conventional markers, serum CK, and CK-MB lack sufficient sensitivity and specificity. Because cardiac troponins are not normally detected in the blood of healthy people, the cut-off value for elevated troponin is set slightly above the noise level of the assay, permitting the test to be more sensitive to lesser degrees of myocardial injury. In addition, recent data suggest that cardiac troponins identify patients at risk for further events with greater accuracy, even in the face of normal CK values.

Troponin T is thought to be a highly specific marker of myocardial necrosis. A substudy of GUSTO-IIa[19] examined the usefulness of troponin T vs. CK-MB and EKG abnormalities in risk stratification of patients with acute myocardial ischemia. Troponin T elevation on admission was associated with an independent increase in risk of death at 30 days. Even in patients with ST-segment elevation, an elevated troponin T increased the 30-day mortality rate to 13% compared with 4.7% in patients with normal troponin T values. Of interest, this increased risk held true whether the EKG indicated infarction or ischemia or was nondiagnostic. For patients without ST-segment elevation, an elevated troponin T level was associated with a 30-day mortality rate of 7.6% compared with 1.2% in patients with normal troponin values. These data are supported by a TRIM substudy.[30] Elevated troponin T also predicted higher mortality rates in patients with and without CK-MB elevations. However, because troponin T may remain elevated for 10–14 days after an infarct, the authors could not rule out delayed diagnosis of a recent infarct, which places the patient at high risk for adverse outcomes. In addition, all patients were selected on the basis of high risk for acute ischemic syndromes; thus, one may question the ability of troponin T to predict adverse outcomes in a more heterogeneous population.

Hamm and colleagues evaluated 773 consecutive patients presenting to the emergency department with chest pain of less than 12 hours' duration and without ST-segment elevation.[23] A bedside immunoassay was used to determine qualitative positive or negative status of troponin T and I at admission and at 6 hours from onset of symptoms. Troponin T identified 94% of patients diagnosed with acute MI, whereas troponin I was 100% sensitive within 4 hours. The negative event rates at 30 days for patients with negative troponin T and I tests were 1.1% and 0.03%, respectively. Thus, in this population troponin T and troponin I identified patients at risk for further cardiac events. The prognostic value of troponin T at 5 months was evaluated in a substudy of FRISC.[27] FRISC examined the use of dalteparin sodium, a low-molecular-weight heparin, in 1506 patients with unstable angina or non–Q-wave MI. The 5-month risk of cardiac death or MI significantly increased from lower to higher quintiles of troponin T levels (4.3%, 10.5%, and 16.1%, respectively). Similarly, Stubbs and colleagues[31] showed that patients with ST-segment elevation and positive troponin T tests had increased mortality rates after 3 years (32% vs. 13%).

Troponin T is an inexpensive, independent method for early and late risk assessment in patients with ACS. Patients with low levels of troponin T have favorable outcomes, whereas elevated levels identify patients at increased risk of adverse outcomes.

Troponin I also has been shown to predict adverse events in patients suffering from ACS.[30–33] In a substudy of TRIM,[30] troponin T and troponin I identified patients without ST elevation at risk for cardiac death at 30 days. The composite endpoint of acute MI and cardiac death was 11.5% and 12.5% in the groups with elevated troponin T and troponin I compared with 3.2% and 4.0% in patients with negative troponin tests. The close correlation between troponin T and troponin I for both mortality and cardiac events supports the theory that these markers represent the same pathologic process. Data from TIMI-IIIB[3] revealed that 41% of 1404 patients had elevated troponin I levels. Troponin I elevation was a predictor of mortality at 42 days whether the patient was enrolled early or late in relation to onset of symptoms, although the prognostic value was greater for patients after 6 hours. Furthermore, elevated levels of troponin I conveyed increased mortality even when CK-MB measurements were normal. Progressively higher levels of troponin also appeared to predict increased risk of mortality, presumably due to larger amounts of myocardial necrosis.

These results indicate that the cardiac troponins appear to provide early identification of a subgroup of patients with ACS who are at increased risk. Thus, they may be useful in identifying patients who would benefit from a more aggressive treatment strategy.

The FRISC study indicated that troponin-positive patients received greater benefit from treatment with dalteparin than their troponin-negative counterparts.[34] Troponin T-positive patients had a significant (14.2% vs. 7.4%) reduction in 40-day mortality rate with long-term use (5 weeks) of low-molecular-weight heparin compared with placebo. Troponin T-negative patients had no difference in outcomes with treatment. In the CAPTURE Study,[35] analysis of the 518 Troponin T-positive patients showed that patients with troponin T > 0.1ng/ml had a significantly greater number of cardiac events before and up to 6 months after PTCA compared with patients with low troponin levels (< 0.1ng/ml). The rate of events in the troponin T-positive group, however, was significantly reduced with abciximab before and after PTCA (23.9% vs. 9.5% at 6 months). In patients with low levels of troponins, there was no difference between placebo and treatment arms at any of the time points. Mortality was not affected in any of the groups.

Although cardiac troponins may help to identify patients at risk for negative outcomes, the mechanism by which it does so is unclear. In the TIMI-IIIB trial,[3] 1150 patients underwent coronary angiography. In this group there was no significant difference in angiographic findings, either in the number of vessels occluded or thrombus grade, between patients with elevated and patients with normal troponin I levels. This finding suggests that elevated troponins do not necessarily represent epicardial thrombosis. Whether cardiac troponin elevations represent necrosis, possibly at a microvascular level, or ischemia without infarction has yet to be delineated. In addition, prognostic information demonstrated in the individual studies needs to be interpreted with caution. Differences in assays and measurement precision between studies may corrupt their ability to stratify risk. However, the ability of troponins to identify high-risk patients during ACS provides an opportunity to enact aggressive therapeutics and cost-effective care.

Inflammation and Novel Cardiac Markers

The genesis of atherosclerosis is linked strongly to inflammation. Studies of the development of the so-called fatty streak (lesions that are common to small infants and children) demonstrate significant inflammatory responses involving macrophages and T lymphocytes.[36] If left unabated over time, this milieu of recurrent inflammation and injury, endothelial dysfunction, low-density lipoprotein modification, and free radical formation results in the formation of atherosclerotic plaques. Additional risk factors for endothelial dysfunction, including diabetes, hypertension, smoking, plasma homocysteine, and infectious microorganisms, contribute to the development of the advanced atherosclerotic lesion. Such lesions are most prominent at the branches and bifurcations of the vascular tree, where alterations in blood flow, sheer stress, and turbulence promote the accumulation of inflammatory monocytes and T cells. In addition, increasing data support the role of inflammation in the development of ACS. Plaque inflammation (causing cytokine secretion), endothelial activation, a procoagulant nidus, and thinning of the fibrous atherosclerotic cap (leading to rupture) are among the many mechanisms thought to be responsible.[37] Much research is directed at recognition of the inflammatory response and its role in the pathogenesis of ACS.

C-reactive protein (CRP), a nonspecific marker of low-grade systemic inflammation, is the prototypical acute-phase reactant. It is synthesized in the liver after stimulation by monocyte-derived interleukin 6. CRP has received much attention, and several studies support a strong link between CRP elevation and future cardiac events in reportedly healthy men and women.[38-40] These data hold true even for patients with known coronary disease. In a substudy of CARE[41] that involved 391 patients who developed recurrent cardiac events after a recent MI and a matched cohort, CRP was higher in the 391 patients with recurrent cardiac events. Patients with levels in the highest quintile had a 75% increase in relative risk for cardiac events. Tommasi and colleagues[42] reported similar data in 64 patients followed for 1 year after an uncomplicated MI. The levels of CRP in patients who suffered cardiac mortality or a combined endpoint were significantly increased (relative risk [RR] = 3.55) compared with patients who did not.

In addition to its value as a long-term predictor of cardiac events in healthy people and patients with prior infarction, highly sensitive tests for CRP appear to be valid as means of stratifying risk in patients with ACS. In the ECAT study, 2121 patients with stable and unstable angina were followed for 2 years.[43] Using an ultrasensitive immunoassay for CRP, the researchers found that patients with elevated levels of CRP at entry into the study had a greater relative risk of coronary events (RR = 1.45, confidence interval [CI] = 1.15–1.83) than patients with normal levels of CRP. Patients with the highest concentrations (> 3.6mg/L) had the highest rate of coronary events. Contrasting data about the ability of CRP to predict short-term outcomes in patients with ACS have led to speculation that the specificity of CRP is not adequate to identify the inflammation associated with acute plaque rupture in the presence of the systemic inflammation surrounding an ischemic event.[44,45] Whether elevations in CRP are related to coronary plaque inflammation or represent a systemic inflammatory response to ischemia and injury is not yet known.

Currently, other markers of inflammation are under investigation for their value as predictors of coronary risk. Cytokines such as interleukin (IL) 6, tumor necrosis factor-α, and IL-1 are under examination as representatives of the proinflammatory state. However, the source of these cytokines remains unclear. Regardless of whether they represent inflammation at the plaque itself or an extravascular source (e.g, chronic infection), emerging evidence supports the theory of an inflammatory pathway associated with acute coronary events. Recently, several studies focusing on IL-6 suggest that it correlates well with adverse outcomes. In a substudy of the Physicians Health Study,[46] 202 healthy men who later experienced cardiac events had significantly higher IL-6 levels at baseline than age-matched controls. This finding, which suggests an enhanced inflammatory response in people with susceptibility to unstable plaques, may allow screening years in advance of the first infarction. Data also suggest that IL-6 is useful in defining patients with unstable angina at risk for negative outcomes.[47,48] Although studies confirm an increase in the cytokine response during ACS, one must interpret them with caution. The small number of samples collected cannot account for diurnal variations in IL-6. In addition, of all the current markers of inflammation, only CRP has an established World Health Organization standard that allows consistently reliable results.

Inflammatory markers provide essential insight into the pathology of coronary atherosclerosis and atherothrombosis. Although initial results seem promising, their utility needs to be better established. Reliable, reproducible assays are mandatory. In addition, the use of inflammatory markers must add to our current ability to predict risk. Finally, whether inflammation is a modifiable risk factor needs to be determined.

As our understanding of the pathophysiology of ACS increases, our ability to predict reliably which patients are at risk for future morbidity will allow us to institute effective preventive strategies.

Echocardiography

In the setting of ACS without ST-segment elevation, echocardiography may be helpful in risk assessment. Small studies in highly selective populations of patients without known coronary artery disease or prior infarction have shown sensitivities of 86–92%, and specificities of 53–90% depending on the endpoint.[49] Two-dimensional echocardiography consistently localized impaired wall motion associated with anterior and inferior infarcts in more than 90% of patients.[50] Wall motion abnormalities can be detected by technically adequate studies, but they are not specific for ACS. Jaarsma et al. showed that a normal wall motion index can identify a low-risk subgroup of acute MIs that remain free of complication with a negative predictive accuracy of 95%.[51] Echocardiography is highly operator- and interpreter-dependent, however, and it is not clear that it adds to the diagnostic and prognostic accuracy of simpler tests such as enzyme markers and EKG. It may be of particular importance when electrographic findings are nondiagnostic.

Predischarge Noninvasive Testing

The prognostic value of an exercise test after an episode of ACS is well established. The diagnostic and prognostic value is greater for symptom-limited stress tests than for rate-limited tests, without an increase in adverse events.[52] The recently published VANQUISH Trial established that predischarge stress testing can play an important role in risk stratification of patients with non–ST-segment elevation ACS.[53] Symptom-limited stress testing in patients with non–Q-wave MI has a > 75% positive predictive value for critical stenosis of one vessel or more in the presence of 2-mm ST-segment depression.[54] The conservative strategy in the VANQUISH Trial recommended coronary angiography only if one or more of the following criteria were met: (1) postinfarction angina with EKG changes, (2) > 2 mm of ST depression on an EKG at peak exercise, (3) redistribution defects in two or more different vascular regions on thallium scintigraphy, (4) or one redistribution defect with increased uptake of thallium by the lung.[53] Criteria for earlier exclusion from randomization in this trial included persistent ischemia or significant congestive heart failure despite maximal medical therapy. During 23 months of follow-up, the number of patients with one of the components of the primary endpoint (death or nonfatal MI) and the number who died were significantly higher in the group undergoing the invasive strategy. Overall mortality rates, however, did not differ between the two groups.[53] Patients with anterior infarction, ST-segment depression on EKG at entry, reduced ejection fraction, or prior infarction did not fare better with routine invasive management. The TIMI-IIIb investigators performed a subgroup analysis of 476 patients with non–Q-wave MI randomly assigned to invasive vs. conservative treatment after thrombolytic therapy. They found no significant differences in the rates of death or recurrent infarction at 6 weeks.[3]

In contrast, the FRISC II Trial showed that an invasive approach should be preferred in patients with unstable angina and non–Q-wave MI. At 1-year follow-up, the mortality rate in the invasive group was 2.2% vs. 3.9% in the noninvasive group (p = 0.016). MI occurred in 8.6% vs. 11.6% (p = 0.015), and the composite rates of death or MI were 10.4% vs. 14.1% (p < 0.001). Invasive treatment also was associated with a lower risk of readmission and revascularization after initial admission.[55]

This controversy over risk stratification will continue in the near future. Proponents of interventional cardiology and the "open artery theory" favor catheterization in all patients with non–ST-segment elevation ACS, whereas more conservative physicians follow the VANQWISH protocol of noninvasive testing. In our opinion, a low threshold for cardiac catheterization is indicated in this group because of the evidence of the FRISC trial, the lack of use of stents and GPIIb/IIIa inhibitors in the invasive arm of VANQWISH, and the fact that 29% of the conservative arm underwent angiography for objective ischemia within 30 days. Larger studies and newer modalities of treatment may answer this question more clearly.

Summary

In the non–ST-segment elevation form of ACS we can obtain important risk factor information from stratification and categorization of the patients into three groups; low, moderate, and high risk. Clinically, patients with new exertional angina are at low risk and generally have a low unstable angina score and no significant physical signs of clinical compromise. The EKG is generally normal or shows minimal ST-segment change. Serum markers are also normal, and echocardiography or nuclear testing demonstrates good or normal left ventricular function. Such patients generally can be evaluated on an outpatient basis within 72 hours and have an extremely low risk for advancing to MI. The intermediate-risk group has a greater likelihood for developing a cardiac event. Pain at rest usually has been briefly present, but there are no signs of physical or hemodynamic instability. The EKG may show borderline ST depression and

T-wave changes, and cardiac enzymes are slightly elevated or often in a "high-risk" range. Analysis of left ventricular function may show fixed dysfunction. Such patients are best admitted to a coronary care unit or to telemetry and often need an invasive study. However, a conservative approach, as recommended by the VANQWISH investigators, may be appropriate in clinically stable cases. The high-risk group consists of patients with protracted rest angina, often intermittent, and patients with postinfarction angina. They usually have transient ST-segment changes, either elevation or depression, and echocardiography may show transient wall motion abnormalities, particularly with pain. Elevated cardiac enzymes are to be expected, usually in the MI range. Such patients are candidates for aggressive medical treatment along with invasive study (Table 1).

ST-Segment Elevation Acute Coronary Syndrome

Risk stratification in ST-segment elevation ACS is different from that in non–ST-segment elevation ACS. Most importantly, patients are now treated early in the event process with either thrombolysis or primary angioplasty. Much of the risk stratification data published before the thrombolytic era is no longer applicable. The in-hospital mortality rate in the prethrombolytic era was 10–15% with an additional 10% of patients dying within 1 year after hospital discharge.[56,57] In the postthrombolytic era, outcome has improved significantly. In the GISSI Trial the mortality rate was 8–10%[58]; in the GUSTO trial it was 6.3–7.3% at 35 days[59]; and in TIMI-II it was 2.0–3.3% at 1 year.[60] The late mortality rates also have decreased markedly. In the SWIFT Trial, the mortality rate at 1 year was 2.5–3.3%; at 2 years, 1.3%; and at 3 years, 1.7%.[61] If risk stratification

Table 1. General Guidelines for Risk Evaluation and Tailored Therapy

	Risk		
Risk Evaluation	*High*	*Intermediate*	*Low*
Likelihood of disease	Documented	Suspect	Low
Severity of ischemia	Prolonged pain, recurrent angina Hemodynamic deterioration	Rest pain	New-onset, effort angina
Unstable angina score (background and severity)	6, 5	4, 3	2, 1
Electrocardiogram	New, transient ST-segment shift	Borderline change	Normal
Blood tests	Elevated CK-MB, troponin I, troponin T	(Admission and 8–12 hr after onset of pain)	Normal
LV function/perfusion	Transient dysfunction or perfusion defect	Fixed dysfunction or perfusion defect	No regional dysfunction No perfusion defect
Other	Gradient in risk with age, LV dysfunction, previous bypass surgery, and associated other medical conditions		
Patient orientation	Coronary care unit	Coronary care unit, wards	Emergency department, home, wards

CK-MB = creatine kinase, myocardial bound; LV = left ventricular.
From Theroux P, Fuster V: Acute coronary syndromes: Unstable angina and non–Q-wave myocardial infarction. Circulation 97:1195–1206, 1998, with permission.

is defined as the ability to identify patients at increased risk of adverse outcome, in whom intervention will lower the risk, the problem is how to detect high-risk patients in a group in which the overall mortality rate after thrombolysis is very low.

Clinical Factors

In the prethrombolytic era, the key risks were anterior myocardial necrosis, recurrent ischemia, electrical instability, and extensive coronary artery disease.[62] Other risks after MI were prolonged symptoms, ejection fraction < 40%, pulmonary rales, pulmonary congestion on chest radiograph, prior MI, abnormal exercise testing, abnormal signal-averaged EKG, > 10 ventricular ectopic beats/hour, and abnormal heart rate variability.[63] In the TIMI-II Trial, Hillis et al. demonstrated that after thrombolysis the 6-week mortality rate was 1.5% in patients with no risk factors and 17.5% in patients with ≥ 4 risk factors. Eight variables in this study were associated with an increased mortality risk:[64] age > 70 years, previous infarction, anterior infarction, atrial fibrillation, rales in more than one-third of the lung fields, hypotension and sinus tachycardia, female gender, and diabetes mellitus.[64] Essentially, these clinical markers support the concept that mortality rates increase with the severity of left ventricular dysfunction. This concept has not changed from the pre- to postthrombolytic era and remains the key factor in patient outcome after ST-segment elevation ACS or acute MI.

Electrocardiographic Factors

Acute MI presents with and is diagnosed by ST-segment elevation in the appropriate and contiguous leads. This finding, in a typical clinical setting of chest pain and serum cardiac markers, necessitates thrombolysis or primary angioplasty on an urgent basis. ST-segment elevation generally correlates well with coronary anatomy and thrombosis as opposed to ST-segment depression. Early resolution of ST-segment elevation is associated with a more favorable outcome.[65] A decrease > 50% in the sum of the ST-segment elevation in all EKG leads is considered a cut-off for predicting coronary patency.[65] EKG findings associated with increased mortality include (1) anterior ST-segment elevation, (2) left bundle-branch block, (3) advanced atrioventricular block, and (4) atrial fibrillation.[66] Evidence of right ventricular infarction complicating inferior MI, as manifest by elevated ST segments in V4R, also carries a higher mortality rate than inferior MIs without right ventricular infarction.[67] In GUSTO-I, the 30-day mortality rate was 9.9% in patients with anterior ST-segment elevation vs. 5.0% in patients with inferior ST-segment elevation.[68] Persistent ST-segment depression in the 12-lead EKG is a high-risk variable predictive of a worse outcome.[22] Not all ST-segment elevation is predictive of Q-wave MI.

Left Ventricular Assessment

In most MIs, an ejection fraction below 40% is associated with an increased risk of mortality and morbidity. In a comparison of pre-thrombolytic and post-thrombolytic ejection fractions in postinfarction patients, Volpe et al. showed that thrombolytic treatment shifted the curvilinear relation between ejection fraction and mortality to the left. A 30% ejection fraction in the prethrombolytic period was associated with a 14% mortality rate at 1 year, whereas the same 30% ejection fraction after thrombolytic therapy was associated with an 8%

mortality at 6 months.[69] Although these studies compared radionucleide ejection fraction with echocardiographically determined ejection fraction, they demonstrate the correlation between low ejection fraction and an increased mortality in both the pre- and postthrombolytic periods. Multiple studies involving echocardiography and associated wall motion abnormalities and severely depressed left ventricular dysfunction in the prethrombolytic period showed a sensitivity of 79–100% and specificity of 19–90% for cardiovascular end-points that included cardiogenic shock, death, severe heart failure, serious arrhythmias, and angina.[51,70–73] Increased left ventricular volume also has been identified as a high risk for increased mortality in postinfarction patients. Zaret and colleagues showed that a left ventricular ejection fraction < 30%, as demonstrated by radionuclide angiography, was still predictive of mortality in patients treated with thrombolytic therapy.[74] White and colleagues performed contrast left ventriculography and found that end-systolic volume > 130 ml was a better predictor of mortality after MI than an ejection fraction < 40% or increased end-diastolic volume.[75]

Exercise Testing after Myocardial Infarction

A real question in the risk stratification of patients after ST-segment elevation MI involves the value of exercise testing. Patients now are less likely to have three-vessel coronary disease, and many have smaller infarcts 1 year after thrombolysis.[76,77] Because patients with recurrent angina and heart failure after MI are selected for aggressive management, the population eligible for predischarge exercise testing is far different from that in the prethrombolytic era. Predictive accuracy, therefore, of early exercise testing is reduced. ST-segment depression, inability to perform more than 5 METS of exercise, or inability to exercise at all have a negative predictive value after MI.[78,79] The American College of Cardiology/American Heart Association (ACC/AHA) guidelines state that exercise testing to 5 METS or greater and to 70% of maximal predicted heart rate or to a clinical indicator is preferable to symptom-limited stress testing.[80] Testing is safe at 3–5 days after MI in patients without complications. High-risk subsets of patients should be referred directly to angiography before discharge. Data suggest that nuclear imaging is less valuable now than it was in the prethrombolytic era for risk assessment because of the low number of cardiac event rates after thrombolytic therapy.[81–83] Myocardial perfusion imaging with either thallium 201 or technetium 99 can assess infarct size,[84,85] which is significantly associated with mortality risk. Figure 2 summarizes the ACC/AHA guidelines for risk stratification after ST-segment elevation ACS. This strategy is based on clinical risk presentation and utilizes cardiac catheterization, symptom-limited exercise testing at 14–21 days, or submaximal exercise testing at 5–7 days to stratify risk. High-risk patients include those with cardiogenic shock, mechanical complications, or failed reperfusion, in addition to those with congestive heart failure, postinfarction angina, ischemia, or malignant arrhythmias. Such patients require cardiac catheterization before discharge (strategy I).

For patients at low risk at time of discharge after MI, two strategies for performing exercise testing can be used. Strategy II is symptom-limited testing at 14–21 days. Patients taking digoxin or with a baseline EKG change that prevents ST interpretation require an imaging study. Markedly positive exercise testing results can then be used to predict the need for invasive studies.

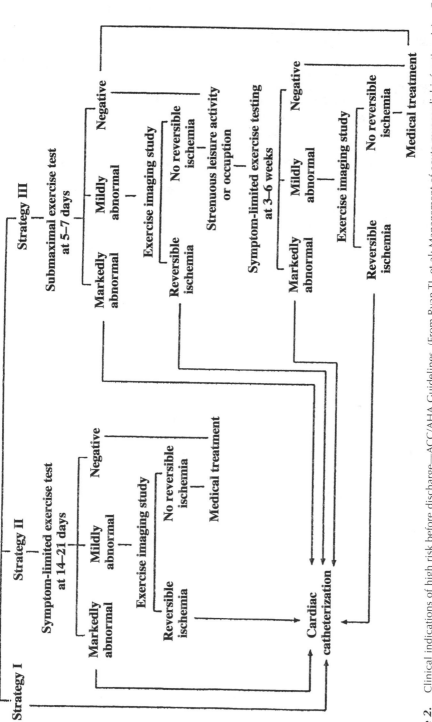

Figure 2. Clinical indications of high risk before discharge—ACC/AHA Guidelines. (From Ryan TJ, et al: Management of acute myocardial infarction. J Am Coll Cardiol 28:1328–1428, 1996, with permission.)

Strategy III is a submaximal exercise test at 5–7 days after MI. If the test is negative, it should be followed by a second symptom-limited test in 3–6 weeks if the patient undertakes strenuous leisure activity or work.

Despite the ACC/AHA guidelines, several studies from the postthrombolytic era contradict the prognostic value of post-MI stress testing with or without imaging. Stevenson et al. studied 254 patients with submaximal exercise testing and found no prognostic value for the outcomes of death, MI, or ischemia.[86] The best predictive value in this study was exercise test rate-pressure product. Bowling et al. performed exercise thallium imaging before discharge in 84 patients, looking at the same outcome indicators, and found no prognostic value.[87] Hendel et al. studied 71 patients with the endpoints of death and MI at 2 years. Postdischarge dipyramidole thallium imaging had no prognostic value.[88] Zhu et al. examined death and MI for 3.5 years; multiple gated acquisition (MUGA) blood pool scan during exercise had no prognostic value except for the peak left ventricular ejection fraction.[89] These data demonstrate no ability to predict death or reinfarction by noninvasive testing.

In view of the above data, Reeder and Gibbons[90] offer a similar approach to the ACC/AHA guidelines for risk stratification after MI in the thrombolytic era. In patients who have received a thrombolytic agent or primary PTCA, the authors recommend angiography and revascularization for spontaneous ischemia or severe exercise-induced ischemia (similar to TIMI-II guidelines). Angiography should be considered in patients with high-risk clinical variables. In patients who received no thrombolytic or primary angioplasty, the classic postinfarction risk stratification with left ventricular testing and stress testing with or without imaging should be undertaken (Table 2).

Electrical Instability

Episodes of sustained or nonsustained ventricular tachycardia detected by Holter monitor or telemetry > 24 hours after MI are an independent predictor of poor prognosis.[91–99] Patients with sustained ventricular tachycardia (> 30 seconds or 3 beats or more with hemodynamic compromise) require coronary angiography and invasive electrophysiologic testing. Routine testing of patients with lower-grade arrhythmia, such as ventricular couplets, bigeminy, and nonsustained ventricular tachycardia, is more controversial.[100]

The Multicenter Automatic Defibrillation Implantation Trial evaluated patients within 3 weeks of MI who were thought to be at high risk for sudden cardiac death. Patients with ejection fractions < 35% with asymptomatic nonsustained

Table 2. Practical Approach to Postinfarct Management in the Thrombolytic Era

Patients who receive thrombolysis (or immediate reperfusion by PTCA)
    Treatment with aspirin, beta blocker, and ACE inhibitor if ejection fraction ≤ 40%
    Angiography and revascularization for spontaneous ischemia or severe exercise-induced ischemia
        (similar to TIMI-II guidelines)
    Angiography should be considered in patients with multiple high-risk clinical variables
Patients who receive no thrombolysis
    Immediate angioplasty
    If no thrombolysis or immediate angioplasty, nuclear stress testing should be done

PTCA = percutaneous transluminal coronary angioplasty, ACE = angiotensin-converting enzyme, TIMI-II = Thrombolysis in Myocardial Infarction Phase II trial.
From Reeder GS, Gibbons RJ: Acute myocardial infarction: Risk stratification in the thrombolytic era. Mayo Clin Proc 70:87–94, 1995, with permission.

ventricular tachycardia (3–30 beats) and inducible and nonsuppressible ventricular tachycardia had improved survival rates with a prophylactic automatic implantable cardioverter defibrillator (AICD).[101] The Multicenter Unsustained Tachycardia Trial also showed that in 704 patients with asymptomatic coronary artery disease, left ventricular ejection fraction < 40%, and inducible sustained ventricular arrhythmias, the risk of cardiac arrest or death from arrhythmia was significantly lower in those who received defibrillators than in those without defibrillators. The mortality benefit was seen with defibrillator treatment but not with EP-guided antiarrhythmic therapy.[102] Although these results are interesting, the potential costs of such a strategy are staggering; further studies and developments are needed.

The signal-averaged EKG is also an independent predictor of risk for developing arrhythmias after MI. Heart rate variability also can be measured and reflects the sympathovagal interaction regulating heart rate. Low heart rate variability, indicative of decreased vagal tone, is a predictor of sudden cardiac death in postinfarction patients.[103,104] All of these parameters are clearly worsened in the presence of left ventricular dysfunction. The overall positive predictive value of these tests is low and the therapeutic indications unclear. The ACC/AHA guidelines do not routinely recommend these tests with a class I indication, but further investigation in this area continues to be of interest.[80]

Summary

The value of early clinical risk factor identification from the history and physical examination and from assessment of left ventricular function remains constant in assessing prognosis for both non ST-segment elevation and ST-segment elevation ACSs in the postthrombolytic era. Dynamic changes in the EKG ST-segments consistently predict higher risk in ACS. Troponins probably will replace CK-MB to detect myocardial injury. Sensitive markers for early detection of myocardial necrosis and thus early identification of patients at high risk of MI who may need aggressive invasive testing and therapy still need to be developed. The exciting work with C-reactive protein and IL-6 as inflammatory markers will help us to understand and treat ACS in the future.

Finally, the use of noninvasive testing to stratify risk in patients with ACS remains unclear. One must consider costs and safety issues. Patients with non–ST-segment ACS are most dependent on selection and prognosis, but data remain unclear as to choice of an invasive or noninvasive strategy for patients at intermediate-to-low risk. In the ST-segment elevation group, aggressive postinfarction treatment with thrombolysis and primary angioplasty makes noninvasive testing in low-risk groups less predictive. The ACC/AHA guidelines with strategies I, II, and III are the best choices while we await further clinical data. The management and risk stratification of ACS will remain a difficult and continuing problem for cardiologists as the population ages.

References

1. Fowler N: Pre-infarction angina. Circulation 44:755–758, 1971.
2. Scanlon P, Nemickas R, Moran JF, et al: Accelerated angina pectoris: Clinical, hemodynamic, arteriographic and therapeutic experience in 85 patients. Circulation 47:19–26, 1973.
3. TIMI-IIIB Investigators: Effects of tissue plasminogen activator and a comparison of early invasive and conservative strategies in unstable angina and non Q-wave myocardial infarction: Results of the TIMI IIIB Trial. Circulation 89:1545–1556, 1994.

4. Davies MJ, Thomas AC: Plaque fissuring: The cause for acute myocardial infarction, sudden ischemic death, crescendo angina. Br Heart J 53:363–373, 1985.
5. Ambrose JA, Winters SL, Stern A: Angiographic morphology and the pathogenesis of unstable angina pectoris. J Am Coll Cardiol 5:609–616, 1985.
6. Topol EJ: Acute Coronary Syndrome. New York Marcel Dekker, 1998.
7. Cannon CP: Contemporary Cardiology: Management of Acute Coronary Syndrome. Totowa, NJ, Humana Press, 1999.
8. Boersma E, Pieper K, Steyerberg E, et al: Predictors of outcome in patients with acute coronary syndromes without persistent ST-segment elevation. The PURSUIT Investigators. Circulation 101:2557–2567, 2000.
9. Braunwald E: Unstable angina: A Classification. Circulation 80:410–414, 1989.
10. Van-Mittenburg-VanZijl A, Simoons M, Veerhoek R, Bossuyt P: Incidence and follow up of Braunwald subgroups in unstable angina pectoris. J Am Coll Cardiol 25:1286–1292, 1995.
11. Dangas G, Mettran R, Wallenstein S, et al: Correlation of angiographic morphology and clinical presentation in unstable angina. J Am Coll Cardiol 29:519–525, 1997.
12. Rizik DG, Healy S, Margulis A, et al: A new clinical classification for hospital prognosis of unstable angina pectoris. Am J Cardiol 75:993–997, 1995.
13. Calvin JE, Klein LW, VandenBerg BJ, et al: Risk stratification in unstable angina: Prospective validation of the Braunwald classification. JAMA 273:136–141, 1995.
14. Emre A, Ersek B, Gursurer M, et al: Angiographic and scintigraphic (perfusion and electrocardiogram–gated-SPECT) correlates of clinical presentation in unstable angina. Clin Cardiol 23:495–500, 2000.
15. Langer A, Freeman WR, Armstrong PW: ST-Segment shift in unstable angina: Pathophysiology and association with coronary anatomy and hospital outcome. J Am Coll Cardiol 13:1495–1502, 1989.
16. Schectman KB, Capone RJ, Kleiger RE, et al: Risk stratification of patients with non–Q-wave myocardial infarction: The critical role of ST-segment depression. Circulation 80:1148–1158, 1989.
17. Willich SN, Stone PH, Muller JE et al: High risk subgroups of patients with non–Q-wave myocardial infarction based on direction and severity of ST-segment deviation. Am Heart J 114:1110–1119, 1987.
18. Cannon CP, Thompson B, McCabe CH, et al, for the TIMI-III Investigators: Predictors of non–Q-wave myocardial infarction in patients with acute ischemic syndromes: An analysis from the Thrombolysis in Myocardial Infarction III Trial. Am J Cardiol 75:977–981, 1995.
19. Ohman EM, Armstrong PW, Christenson RH, et al, for the GUSTO IIa Investigators: Cardiac troponin T for risk stratification in acute myocardial ischemia. N Engl J Med 335:1333–1341, 1996.
20. Savonitto S, Ardissino D, Ottain F, el al: Prognostic value of the admission electrocardiogram in acute coronary syndrome: Results from the GUSTO IIb trial. Eur Heart J 18(Suppl):124, 1997 [abstract].
21. Stone PH, Thompson B, Zaret BL, et al: Factors associated with failure of medical therapy in patients with unstable angina and non–Q-wave myocardial infarction: A TIMI-IIIB data base study. Eur Heart J 20:1084–1093, 1999.
22. Krone RJ, Greenberg H, Dwyer EM, et al: Long-term prognostic signficance of ST-segment depression during acute myocardial infarction. The Multicenter Diltiazem Postinfarction Trial Research Group. J Am Coll Cardiol 22:361–367, 1993.
23. Hamm C, Goldman B, Heeschen C, et al: Emergency room triage of patients with acute chest pain by means of rapid testing for cardiac troponin T or troponin I. N Engl J Med 337:1648–1653, 1998.
24. Roxin LE, Cullhed I, Groth T, et al: The value of serum myoglobin determinations in the early diagnosis of acute myocardial infarction. Acta Med Scand 215:417–425, 1984.
25. Lindahl B, Venge P, Wallentin L: Early diagnosis and exclusion of acute myocardial infarction using biochemical monitoring. The BIOMACS Study Group. Biochemicals Markers of Acute Coronary Syndromes. Coron Artery Dis 6:321–328, 1995.
26. Grande P, Hansen BF, Christiansen C, Naestoft J: Estimation of acute myocardial infarct size in man by serum CK-MB measurements. Circulation 65:756–764, 1982.
27. Lindahl B, Venge P, Wallentin L: Relation between troponin T and the risk of subsequent cardiac events in unstable coronary artery disease. The FRISC study group. Circulation 93:1651–1657, 1996.
28. Zimmerman J, Fromm R, Meyer D, et al: Diagnostic marker cooperative study for the diagnosis of myocardial infarction. Circulation 99:1671–1667, 1999.
29. Puleo PR, Meyer D, Wathen C, et al: Use of a rapid assay of subforms of creatine kinase-MB to diagnose or rule out acute myocardial infarction. N Engl J Med 331:561–566, 1994.

30. Luscher MS, Thygesen K, Ravkilde J, Heickendorff L: Applicability of cardiac troponin T and I for early risk stratification in unstable coronary artery disease. TRIM Study Group. Thrombin Inhibition in Myocardial Ischemia. Circulation 96:2578–2585, 1997.
31. Stubbs P, Collinson P, Moseley D, et al: Prognostic significance of admission troponin T concentrations in patients with myocardial infarction. Circulation 94:1291–1297, 1996.
32. Antman EM, Tanasijevic MJ, Thompson B, et al: Cardiac-specific troponin I levels to predict the risk of mortality in patients with acute coronary syndromes. N Engl J Med 335:1342–1349, 1996.
33. Galvani M, Ottani F, Ferrini D, et al: Prognostic influence of elevated values of cardiac troponin I in patients with unstable angina. Circulation 95:2053–2059, 1997.
34. Lindahl B, Venge P, Wallentin L: Troponin T identifies patients with unstable coronary artery disease who benefit from long-term antithrombotic protection. Fragmin in Unstable Coronary Artery Disease (FRISC) Study Group. J Am Coll Cardiol 29:43–48, 1997.
35. Hamm CW, Heeschen C, Goldmann B, et al: Benefit of abciximab in patients with refractory unstable angina in relation to serum troponin T levels. c7E3 Fab Antiplatelet Therapy in Unstable Refractory Angina (CAPTURE) Study Investigators. N Engl J Med 340:1623–1629, 1999 [published erratum appears in N Engl J Med 341:548, 1999].
36. Stary HC, Chandler AB, Glagov S, et al: A definition of initial, fatty streak, and intermediate lesions of atherosclerosis: A report from the Committee on Vascular Lesions of the Council on Arteriosclerosis, American Heart Association. Circulation 89:2462–2478, 1994.
37. Crea F, Biasucci LM, Buffon A, et al: Role of inflammation in the pathogenesis of unstable coronary artery disease. Am J Cardiol 80:10E–16E, 1997.
38. Ridker PM, Buring JE, Shih J, et al: Prospective study of C-reactive protein and the risk of future cardiovascular events among apparently healthy women [see comments]. Circulation 98:731–733, 1998.
39. Ridker PM, Cushman M, Stampfer MJ, et al: Inflammation, aspirin, and the risk of cardiovascular disease in apparently healthy men. N Engl J Med 336:973–979, 1997 [published erratum appears in N Engl J Med 337:356, 1997].
40. Koenig W, Sund M, Frohlich M, et al: C-reactive protein, a sensitive marker of inflammation, predicts future risk of coronary heart disease in initially healthy middle-aged men: Results from the MONICA (Monitoring Trends and Determinants in Cardiovascular Disease) Augsburg Cohort Study, 1984 to 1992. Circulation 99:237–242, 1999.
41. Ridker PM, Rifai N, Pfeffer MA, et al: Inflammation, pravastatin, and the risk of coronary events after myocardial infarction in patients with average cholesterol levels. Cholesterol and Recurrent Events (CARE) Investigators. Circulation 98:839–844, 1998.
42. Tommasi S, Carluccio E, Bentivoglio M, et al: C-reactive protein as a marker for cardiac ischemic events in the year after a first, uncomplicated myocardial infarction. Am J Cardiol 83:1595–1599, 1999.
43. Haverkate F, Thompson SG, Pyke SD, et al: Production of C-reactive protein and risk of coronary events in stable and unstable angina. European Concerted Action on Thrombosis and Disabilities Angina Pectoris Study Group. Lancet 349:462–466, 1997.
44. Benamer H, Steg PG, Benessiano J, et al: Comparison of the prognostic value of C-reactive protein and troponin I in patients with unstable angina pectoris. Am J Cardiol 82:845–850, 1998.
45. Rebuzzi AG, Quaranta G, Liuzzo G, et al: Incremental prognostic value of serum levels of troponin T and C-reactive protein on admission in patients with unstable angina pectoris. Am J Cardiol 82:715–719, 1998.
46. Ridker PM, Rifai N, Stampfer MJ, Hennekens CH: Plasma concentration of interleukin-6 and the risk of future myocardial infarction among apparently healthy men. Circulation 101:1767–1772, 2000.
47. Biasucci LM, Vitelli A, Liuzzo G, et al: Elevated levels of interleukin-6 in unstable angina. Circulation. 1996;94:874–877, 1996.
48. Biasucci LM, Liuzzo G, Fantuzzi G, et al: Increasing levels of interleukin (IL)-1Ra and IL-6 during the first 2 days of hospitalization in unstable angina are associated with increased risk of in-hospital coronary events. Circulation 99:2079–2084, 1999.
49. Selker HP, Zalenski RJ, Antman EM, et al: An evaluation of technologies for identifying acute cardiac ischemia in the emergency department: Executive summary of a National Heart Attack Alert Program Working Group Report. Ann Emerg Med 29:1–87, 1997.
50. Reeder GS, Seward JB, Tajik AJ: The role of two-dimensional echocardiography in coronary artery disease. Mayo Clin Proc 57:247–258, 1982.
51. Jaarsma W, Visser CA, Eenige van MJ, et al: Predictive value of two dimensional echocardiographic and hemodynamic measurements on admission with acute myocardial infarction. J Am Soc Echocardiogr 1:187–193, 1988.

52. Jain A, Myer GH, Sapin PM, O'Rourke RA: Comparison of symptom limited and low-level exercise tolerance tests early after myocardial infarction. J Am Coll Cardiol 22:1816–1820, 1993.

53. Boden WE, O'Rourke R, Crawford M, et al, For the Veteran Affairs Non–Q–wave Infarction Strategies in Hospital (VANQWISH) Trial Investigators: Outcomes in patients with acute non–Q–wave myocardial infarctions randomly assigned to an invasive or compared with a conservative management strategy. N Engl J Med 338:1785–1792, 1998.

54. Zaacher S, Liebson P, Calvin J, et al: Unstable angina and non–Q-wave myocardial infarction: Does the clinical diagnosis have therapeutic implications? J Am Coll Card 33:107–118, 1999.

55. Walleub L, Lagerquist B, Husted, Steen, et al: Outcome at one year after an invasive compared with noninvasive strategy in unstable coronary artery disease: The FRISC II invasive randomized trial. Lancet 356:9–16, 2000.

56. Cooperative Study: Death rate among 795 patients in first year after myocardial infarction. JAMA 197:906–908, 1966.

57. Moss AJ, DeCaiolla J, Davis H: Cardiac death in the first 6 months after myocardial infarction: Potential for mortality reduction in the early post-hospital period. Am J Cardiol 39:816–820, 1977.

58. Gruppo Italiano per lo Studio della Sopravvivenza nell'Infarto Miocardico (GISSI-2): Effectiveness of intravenous thrombolytic treatment in acute myocardial infarction. Lancet 1:397–401, 1986.

59. GUSTO Investigators: An international randomized trial comparing four thrombolytic strategies for acute myocardial infarction. N Engl J Med 329:673–682, 1993.

60. William DO, Braunwald E, Knatteund G, et al: One year results of the Thrombolysis in Myocardial Infarction (TIMI) phase II trial. Circulation 85:533–542, 1992.

61. SWIFT (Should We Intervene Following Thrombolysis) Trial Study Group: SWIFT trial of delayed elective intervention v. conservative treatment after thrombolysis with anistreplase in acute myocardial infarction. BMJ 302:555–560, 1991.

62. Sauz G, Castaier A, Betrice A: Determinants of prognosis in survivors of myocardial infarction with a prospective clinical angiographic study. N Engl J Med 306:1065–1070, 1982.

63. Krone RJ: The role of risk stratification in the early management of a myocardial infarction. Ann Intern Med 116:223–237, 1992.

64. Hillis LD, Forman S, Braunwald E: Thrombolysis in Myocardial Infarction (TIMI) Phase II Coinvestigation. Risk stratification before thrombolytic therapy in patients with acute myocardial infarction. J Am Coll Cardiol 16:313–315, 1990.

65. Mauri F, Maggioni AP, et al, for the GISSI-2 investigators: A simple electrocardiographic predictor of the outcome of patients with acute myocardial infarction treated with a thrombolytic agent: A Gruppo Italiano per lo Studio della Sopravvivenza nell'Infarto Miocardico (GISSI-2)-derived analysis. J Am Coll Cardiol 29:600–607, 1994.

66. Lee KL, Woodlief LM, Topol EJ, et al: Predictors of 30-day mortality in the era of reperfusion for acute myocardial infarction: Results from an international trial of 41,021 patients. Circulation 91:1659–1668, 1995.

67. Berger PB, Ryan TJ: Inferior myocardial infarction: High-risk subgroups. Circulation 81:401–411, 1990.

68. GUSTO I Investigators: An international randomized trial comparing four thrombolytic strategies for acute myocardial infarction. N Engl J Med 329:673–682, 1993.

69. Volpe A, DeVita C, Franzosi MG, et al: The Ad-hoc Working Group of the Gruppo Italiano per lo Studio della Sopravvivenza nell'Infarto Miocardico (GISSI)-2 database: Determinants of the six month mortality in survivors of myocardial infarction after thrombolysis: Result of the GISSI-2 database. Circulation 88:416–429, 1993.

70. Gibson RS, Bishop HL, Stanon RB, et al: Value of early two dimensional echocardiography in patients with acute myocardial infarction. Am J Cardiol 49:1110–1119, 1982.

71. Horowitz RS, Morganroth J: Immediate diagnosis of acute myocardial infarction by two dimensional echocardiography. Circulation 65:323–329, 1982.

72. Nishimara RA, Tajik AJ, Shub C, et al: Role of two dimensional echocardiography in the prediction of in-hospital complications after acute myocardial infarction. J Am Coll Cardiol 4:1080–1087, 1984.

73. Saabia P, Abbott RD, Afrokteh A, et al: Importance of two dimensional echocardiographic assessment of left ventricular function in patients presenting to emergency room with cardiac related symptoms. Circulation 84:1615–1624, 1991.

74. Zaret BL, Wackers FJ, Terrin M, et al: Does left ventricular ejection fraction following thrombolytic therapy have the same prognostic impact described in the prethrombolytic era? Results of the TIMI II Trial. J Am Coll Cardio 17:214A, 1991 [abstract].

75. White HD, Norris RM, Brown MA, et al: Left ventricular end-systolic volume as the major determinant of survival after recovery from myocardial infarction. Circulation 76:44–51, 1987.

76. Rogers WJ, Babb JD, Baim DS, et al: Selective versus routine predischarge coronary arteriography after therapy with recombinant tissue-type plasminogen activator, heparin and aspirin for acute myocardial infarction: TIMI-II Investigators. J Am Coll Cardiol 17:1007–1016, 1991.

77. Ritchie JL, Cerqueira M, Maynard C, et al: Ventricular function and infarct size: The Western Infarction Trial. J Am Coll Cardiol 11:689–697, 1988.

78. Mark DB, Shaw L, Harrell FE, et al: Prognostic value of a treadmill exercise score in outpatients with suspected coronary artery disease. N Engl J Med 325:849–853, 1991.

79. Piccalo G, Pirelli S, Massa D, et al: Value of negative predischarge exercise testing in identifying patients at low risk after acute myocardial infarction treated by systemic thrombolysis. Am J Cardiol 70:31–33, 1992.

80. Ryan TJ, Anderson JL, Antman EM, et al: ACC/AHA Guidelines for the Management of Patients with Acute Myocardial Infarction (A report of the ACC/AHA Task Force in Practice Guidelines). J Am Coll Cardiol 28:1328–1428, 1996.

81. Tilkemeier PL, Guiney TE, LaRaia PJ, Boucher CA: Prognostic value of predischarge low-level exercise thallium testing after thrombolytic treatment of acute myocardial infarction. Am J Cardiol 66:1203–1207, 1990.

82. Hendel RC, Gore JM, Alpert JS, Leppo JA: Prognosis following interventional therapy for acute myocardial infarction: Utility of dipyridamole thallium scintigraphy. Cardiology 79:73–80, 1991.

83. Miller TD, Gersh BJ, Christian TF, et al: Limited prognostic value of thallium-201 exercise treadmill testing early after myocardial infarction in patients treated with thrombolysis. Am Heart J 130:259–266, 1995.

84. Cerqueira MD, Maynard C, Ritchie JL, et al: Long-term survival in 618 patients from the Western Washington Streptokinase in Myocardial Infarction trials. J Am Coll Cardiol 20:1452–1459, 1992.

85. Miller TD, Christian TF, Hopfenspirger MR, et al: Infarct size after acute myocardial infarction measured by quantitative tomographic ^{99m}Tc sestamibi imaging predicts subsequent mortality. Circulation 92:334–341, 1995.

86. Stevenson RN, Unach Andion V, Ranjadayalan K, et al: Post infarction exercise testing is of limited value for risk stratification in the thrombolytic era. Circulation 86(Suppl I):I-13C, 1992 [abstract].

87. Bowling BA, Ajluni SC, Puchrowicz S, et al: Assessing the utility of exercise nuclear scintigraphy after reperfusion following myocardial infarction. Circulation 86(Suppl I):I-136, 1992 [abstract].

88. Hendel RC, Gore JM, Alpert JS, Leppo JA: Prognosis following interventional therapy for acute myocardial infarction: Utility of dipyridamole thallium scintigraphy. Cardiology 79:73–80, 1991.

89. Zhu W, Barley KR, Gibbons RJ: Prognostic value of predischarge radionuclide angiography in post infarct patients treated with thrombolytic therapy. Circulation 82(Suppl III):III-160, 1990 [abstract].

90. Reeder GS, Gibbons RJ: Acute myocardial infarction: Risk stratification in the thrombolytic era. Mayo Clin Proc 70:87–94, 1995.

91. Ruberman W, Weinblatt E, Goldberg JD, et al: Ventricular premature beats and mortality after myocardial infarction. N Engl J Med 297:750–757, 1977.

92. Moss AJ, Davis HT, DeCamilla J, Bayer LW: Ventricular ectopic beats and their relation to sudden and nonsudden cardiac death after myocardial infarction. Circulation 60:998–1003, 1979.

93. Bigger JT Jr, Fleiss JL, Kleiger R, et al: The relationships among ventricular arrhythmias, left ventricular dysfunction, and mortality in the 2 years after myocardial infarction. Circulation 69:250–258, 1984.

94. Mukharji J, Rude RE, Poole WK, et al: Risk factors for sudden death after acute myocardial infarction: Two-year follow-up. Am J Cardiol 54:31–36, 1984.

95. Kostis JB, Byington R, Friedman LM, et al: Prognostic significance of ventricular ectopic activity in survivors of acute myocardial infarction. J Am Coll Cardiol 10:231–242, 1987.

96. McClements BM, Adgey AA: Value of signal-averaged electrocardiography, radionuclide ventriculography, Holter monitoring and clinical variables for prediction of arrhythmic events in survivors of acute myocardial infarction in the thrombolytic era. J Am Coll Cardiol 21:1419–1427, 1993.

97. Hohnloser SH, Franck P, Klingenheben T, et al: Open infarct artery, late potentials and other prognostic factors in patients after acute myocardial infarction in the thrombolytic era: A prospective trial. Circulation 90:1747–1756, 1994.

98. Farrell TG, Bashir Y, Cripps T, et al: Risk stratification for arrhythmic events in postinfarction patients based on heart rate variability, ambulatory electrocardiographic variable and the signal-averaged electrocardiogram. J Am Coll Cardiol 18:687–697, 1991.

99. Califf RM, Topol EJ, Van de Werf F, et al, for the GUSTO Investigators: One year follow-up from the GUSTO I Trial. Circulation 90(Suppl I):I-325, 1994 [abstarct].
100. Stevenson WG, Ridker PM: Should survivors of myocardial infarction with low ejection fraction be routinely referred to arrhythmia specialists? JAMA 276:481–485, 1996.
101. Moss AJ, Hall WJ, Cannon DS, et al: Improved survival with an implanted defibrillator in patients with coronary artery disease at high risk for ventricular arrhythmia. N Engl J Med 335:1933–1940, 1996.
102. Buxton AE, Lee KL, Kisher JD, et al: A randomized study of the prevention of sudden death in patients with coronary artery disease. N Engl J Med 341:1882–1890, 1999.
103. Bigger JT, Fleiss JL, Rolnitzky LM, Steinman RC: The ability of several short-term measures of RR variability to predict mortality after myocardial infarction. Circulation 88:927–934, 1993.
104. Kleiger RE, Miller JP, Bigger JT Jr, Moss AJ: Decreased heart rate variability and its association with increased mortality after acute myocardial infarction. Am J Cardiol 59:256–262, 1987.
105. Ohman EM, Granger CB, Harrington RA, Lee KL: Risk stratification and therapeutic decision making in acute coronary syndromes. JAMA 284:876–878, 2000.

Antiplatelet Agents in Acute Coronary Syndromes

JAMES M. WILSON, MD

PAUL KIM, MD

JAMES J. FERGUSON III, MD

Thrombotic complication of coronary artery lesions is the most common cause of morbidity and mortality in patients with atherosclerotic cardiovascular disease. As a result, treatment and prevention of coronary thrombosis is among the most rewarding and intensely studied aspects of modern cardiology. Driven by clinical experience and improved understanding of the physiology of arterial thrombosis, antiplatelet therapy has taken center stage. A number of drugs have been developed that are capable of influencing each of the major steps in platelet-mediated thrombus formation, adhesion, activation, and aggregation. However, theoretical capabilities of individual drugs are not uniformly accompanied by clinical benefit. Therefore, the increased availability of new options for pharmacologic intervention has created a growing need for clinical trials to guide the rational use of antiplatelet agents.

The contents of an advanced atherosclerotic lesion are an intense stimulus for platelet accumulation and thrombosis. Exposure of these contents by endothelial cell loss or spontaneous intimal rupture initiates thrombus formation whose presence may critically limit coronary blood flow, producing the clinical syndromes of unstable angina or acute myocardial infarction.[1-6] Thrombus volume is determined by a dynamic equilibrium between stimulus intensity, blood flow characteristics, and platelet and coagulation enzyme function on one hand and intrinsic thrombolytic capacity and thrombosis regulatory function on the other.[2,3,7] The goal of antiplatelet therapy is to influence this equilibrium by limiting thrombus growth or favoring its dissolution.

Platelet Function

Arterial thrombosis has four component processes: platelet adhesion to connective tissue surfaces, activation and granule release, platelet-platelet aggregation, and thrombin generation, resulting in interstitial fibrin deposition. Complex glycoprotein molecules found on the surface of the platelet membrane act as receptors that mediate attachment to collagen and other platelets through intermediary molecules. An exposed connective tissue surface containing collagen or adherent von Willebrand factor or an adherent platelet with exposed glycoprotein (GP) IIb/IIIa receptors binding fibrinogen or vWF offers a site of attachment for the passing platelet. Upon attaching to such a site, the platelet undergoes a metamorphosis, becoming spiculated in appearance and altering its membrane to act as a catalyst for coagulation enzymes. Release of storage granules is initiated, and the surface density of GP IIb/IIIa is increased, allowing the attachment of additional platelets.[7,8] Platelet shape change, membrane alteration, granule release, and receptor exposure are termed the activation process.

Antiplatelet drugs are loosely classified according to their main target of inhibition. The only inhibitor of adherence, aurintricarboxylic acid, has not been commercially developed. Inhibitors of the activation process include aspirin, ticlopidine, and clopidogrel. Drugs specifically affecting platelet aggregation inhibit the GP IIb/IIIa–fibrinogen interaction and are referred to collectively as GP IIb/IIIa inhibitors. Examples include abciximab, eptifibatide, and tirofiban (Fig. 1).

Inhibitors of Activation

Increased cytosolic calcium concentrations promote alterations in the platelet cytoskeleton, storage granule release, and activation of phospholipase A_2. Platelet calcium concentrations are determined by the influence of second messengers, cyclic adenosine monophosphate (cAMP), and cyclic guanosine monophosphate (cGMP). Occupation of receptors for thromboxane A_2 (TXA$_2$), adenosine diphosphate (ADP), epinephrine, thrombin, platelet-activating factor, serotonin, and collagen inhibits the production of cAMP, thus reducing calcium sequestration and increasing free calcium concentrations. Cyclic GMP, whose production is stimulated by adenosine and prostacyclin, prevents calcium release from storage sites as well as entry through the platelet membrane. Activation pathways are redundant. Therefore, inhibition of only one pathway does not completely inhibit platelet function and may be overcome in the presence of potent stimuli.[9–11] Meanwhile, the clinical effectiveness of even partial inhibition of platelet function has been clearly established.

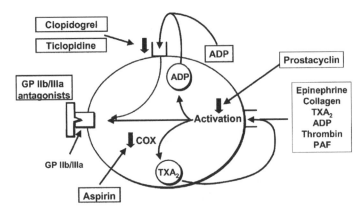

Figure 1.   Antiplatelet agents: molecular sites of action. TXA$_2$ = thromboxane A_2, ADP = adenosine diphosphate, PAF = platelet-activating factor, GP IIb/IIIa = glycoprotein IIb/IIIa.

Aspirin

Arachidonic acid that is liberated from membrane storage pools by phospholipase A_2 is modified by cyclooxygenase (COX) to produce prostaglandin (PG) G_2 and PGH_2. PGH_2 may be further modified to produce prostacyclin or TXA_2. COX exists in two forms, the first of which, COX-1, is found on the endoplasmic reticulum of virtually every cell and is important in the regulation of normal physiologic functions. COX-2, on the other hand, is typically induced by exposure to cytokines and is more important in orchestrating defense functions and inflammation.

Aspirin acetylates a serine moiety of COX-1 at very low doses and COX-2 at doses greater than 300 mg/day. This modification obstructs entry of arachidonic acid to the active site of the enzyme. Covalently altered, both platelet and endothelial COX are forever prevented from producing PGH_2 or PGI_2. The anucleate platelet cannot produce additional COX, rendering it incapable of producing TXA_2 for the remainder of its lifespan after exposure to a single dose of aspirin. Meanwhile, endothelial cells are able to produce additional enzyme and may recover some capability to produce PGH_2 and thereby PGI_2. This differential effect of aspirin, hinging on the absence of a platelet nucleus, is believed to be the primary mechanism by which "upstream" inhibition of the prostanoid pathway may result in an antiplatelet effect.[12-14]

The onset of antiplatelet effect is apparent within 15–20 minutes after ingestion of a single aspirin dose.[15] Effects may be hastened by chewing the aspirin tablet before ingestion.[16] As little as 10–20 mg/day is sufficient to reduce serum thromboxane production in healthy volunteers.[17] Significant prolongation of the bleeding time requires doses of 30 mg/day or more. Theoretically, COX-2, whose presence is induced by inflammation near advanced atherosclerotic lesions, may act as a donor of PGH_2 for adherent platelets. Aspirin therapy produces little or no inhibition of COX-2 at doses below 300 mg/day. However, no clinical evidence indicates that inhibition of COX-2 is required for the clinical benefit of aspirin therapy to be realized.

Unstable Angina

The use of aspirin as a routine part of the treatment of unstable angina is supported by the results of four randomized clinical trials and one meta-analysis (Table 1). One of the first large-scale clinical trials supporting the use of aspirin in unstable angina was the Veterans' Administration Cooperative Study.[18] Between 1974 and 1981, 1266 men, hospitalized for unstable angina, were randomized to treatment with either 324 mg buffered aspirin or placebo. Medication was administered within 48 hours of admission to the hospital and continued daily for 3 months. Patients with evolving ST-segment elevation myocardial infarction were excluded. At the conclusion of the study, the incidence of death or myocardial infarction was reduced from 10.1% in the placebo arm to 5.0, in patients randomized to aspirin therapy. This finding translates to an overall 50% relative risk reduction (p = 0.0005). At 1-year follow-up, a 43% relative survival benefit persisted (9.6% placebo vs. 5.5% aspirin, p = 0.008) despite cessation of therapy at 3 months. No adverse gastrointestinal complications were observed in the aspirin arm.

The Canadian Multicenter Trial was a placebo-controlled study that examined the efficacy of aspirin, sulfinpyrazone, or both in the setting of unstable angina.[19]

Table 1.   Aspirin in Unstable Angina

	VA Cooperative Study[18] at 3-mo Follow-up		Canadian Multicenter Trial[19] at 18-mo Follow-up				Antiplatelet Trialists' Collaboration[114] at 6-mo Follow-up		Theroux I[22] at Follow-up of 6 ± 3 d		RISC[25] at 3-mo Follow-up	
	ASA	*Placebo*	*ASA*	*ASA + Sulf.*	*Sulf.*	*Placebo*	*ASA*	*Placebo*	*ASA*	*Placebo*	*ASA*	*Placebo*
Daily dose	325 mg		1300 mg	1300 mg + 800 mg	800 mg		75–325 mg		650 mg		75 mg	
No. of patients	625	641	139	137	140	139	1991	2027	121	118	399	397
Death/MI	31 (5.0%)	65 (10.1%)	8 (5.7%)	9 (6.6%)	18 (12.9%)	18 (12.9%)	182 (9.1%)	285 (14.0%)	4 (3.3%)	16 (13.5%)	26 (6.5%)	68 (17.1%)
All MI	22 (3.5%)	50 (7.8%)							4 (3.3%)	14 (11.0%)		
Death	10 (1.6%)	21 (3.3%)	3 (2.2%)	3 (2.2%)	10 (7.1%)	12 (8.6%)			0 (0.0%)	2 (1.7%)	6 (1.5%)	10 (2.5%)
NNT (death, MI)	20		8*				20		10		9	

ASA = aspirin, MI = myocardial infarction, Sulf. = sulfinpyrazone, NNT = number needed to treat.
* All aspirin-treated patients ± sulfinpyrazone vs. all patients not receiving aspirin ± sulfinpyrazone.

Patients admitted to coronary care units for unstable angina were randomized to aspirin, 325 mg 4 times daily; sulfinpyrazone, 200 mg 4 times daily; both; or neither for up to 2 years. Patients could be entered into the study up to 8 days after admission to the hospital. After a mean follow-up period of 18 months, 6% of aspirin-treated patients and 12.9% of patients receiving placebo or sulfinpyrazone alone suffered death or myocardial infarction. In analyzing cardiac death alone, the relative risk reduction was a striking 70.6% with aspirin therapy (p = 0.004).

The Antiplatelet Trialists' Collaboration meta-analysis analyzed the results of 145 randomized clinical trials of prolonged antiplatelet therapy in 70,000 high-risk patients (defined as having vascular disease or other conditions implying an increased risk of occlusive vascular disease) and 30,000 low-risk patients from the general population.[20] Among high-risk patients, antiplatelet therapy provided an overall risk reduction of 27% in vascular events (nonfatal myocardial infarction, stroke, or vascular death). An analysis of all aspirin trials demonstrated a 25% odds reduction in vascular events. The collaboration examined seven trials involving 4018 patients with the diagnosis of unstable angina. At 6 months the vascular event rate was 9% (182 of 1991 patients) in the treatment arm and 14% (285 of 2027 patients) in the placebo arm (relative risk reduction = 35%, 95% CI = 21–49%). Doses of aspirin ranged from 75–325 mg/day. Larger doses did not confer additional benefit but led to a greater number of untoward side effects.

Aspirin and Heparin

A separate body of literature details the usefulness of anticoagulant therapy with either heparin or warfarin in unstable angina[21] (Table 2). Theroux and coworkers performed a double-blind, placebo-controlled study involving 479 patients with unstable angina randomized to either aspirin, 325 mg twice/day; heparin, 5000 IU bolus plus an infusion of 1000 IU/hour; or both.[22] After 6 days, myocardial infarction was observed in 12% of patients treated with placebo, 3% of patients randomized to aspirin, 0.8% of patients randomized to heparin, and 1.6% of patients randomized to both agents.

Again the value of aspirin therapy was confirmed. In addition, anticoagulation with heparin was shown to reduce the likelihood of myocardial infarction with a suggestion of superiority over aspirin. Combination therapy, although effective compared with placebo, did not appear to be superior to monotherapy with either agent and was associated with a greater number of bleeding complications. Although heparin appeared to be more effective in reducing events early after its application, this benefit was lost after treatment was discontinued. In 13% of patients treated with heparin alone, clinical evidence of reactivation was observed. This finding was not observed in the remaining treatment groups, suggesting that concurrent therapy with aspirin prevented the heparin withdrawal effect.[23]

Pursuing a more definitive comparison between aspirin and heparin, the same group performed a randomized, double-blind comparison of aspirin, 325 mg twice/day, with heparin, 5000 IU intravenous bolus followed by an infusion adjusted to the activated partial thromboplastin time (aPTT), in 484 patients with unstable angina.[24] The same endpoints were analyzed at 5.7 ± 3.3 days after randomization. Myocardial infarction occurred in 2 (0.8%) of the 240 patients randomized to heparin and in 9 (3.7%) of the 244 randomized to aspirin (p = 0.035), translating to a 2.9% absolute and 78% relative risk reduction with heparin.

Table 2.   Aspirin With or Without Heparin in Unstable Angina and Non–Q-wave Myocardial Infarction

	Theroux I[22] at Follow-up of 6 ± 3 d		Theroux II[24] at Follow-up of 5.7 ± 3.3 d		RISC[25] at 90-day Follow-up			ATACS[26] at 14-day Follow-up (Intention-to-Treat)	
	ASA	*ASA + Heparin*	*ASA*	*Heparin*	*ASA*	*Heparin*	*ASA + Heparin*	*ASA*	*ASA + Heparin + Warfarin*
No. of patients	121	122	244	240	189	198	210	109	105
Daily doses	650 mg	650 mg + 5000 U + 1000 U/hr	650 mg	5000 U + adjunctive infusion to aPPT	75 mg	5000 U IV q 6 hr for 24 hr + 3750 U IV q 6 hr for 4 d	75 mg + 5000 U IV q 6 hr for 24 hr + 3750 U IV q 6 hr for 4 d	162.5 mg	162.5 mg + 100 U/kg and infusion + INR 2.0–3.0
MI/death	4 (3.3%)	2 (1.6%)	9 (3.7%)	2 (0.8%)	14 (7.4%)	33 (16.6%)	12 (5.7%)	29 (27%)	11 (10%)*
NNT MI/death vs. ASA alone		59		23			59		NA

ASA = aspirin, MI = myocardial infarction, NNT = number needed to treat, aPTT = activated partial thromboplastin time, INR = international normalized ratio.
* Includes recurrent angina.

The Research Group on Instability in Coronary Artery Disease in Southeast Sweden (RISC) examined the effects of aspirin (75 mg/day), intermittent bolus heparin, neither, or both in 796 men with unstable angina or non–Q-wave myocardial infarction.[25] The study was a two-by-two design with approximately 200 patients in each randomization arm. At 30 days the incidence of death and myocardial infarction was 14% in the placebo group, 12.6% in the heparin group, 4.8% in the aspirin group, and 3.8% in the group that received both. At 90-day follow-up, the incidence of death and myocardial infarction was 17.6% in the placebo group, 16.7% in the heparin group, 7.4% in the aspirin group, and 5.7% in the group that received both. There was no statistically significant difference between the groups that received aspirin and combination therapy either at 30- or 90-day follow-up. Of interest, at 5 days there was little difference between the groups that received monotherapy, in contrast to the data presented by Theroux, et al.[24] The unusual dosing regimen for heparin, lack of standardized anticoagulant monitoring, and entry of many patients beyond the first 24 hours of admission weaken conclusions about heparin monotherapy or combination therapy. However, the results provide further confirmation of the benefit of aspirin.

The Antithrombotic Therapy in Acute Coronary Syndromes Research Group (ATACS) sought to compare the effect of aspirin vs. the combination of aspirin and heparin followed by warfarin anticoagulation in patients with unstable angina and non–Q-wave myocardial infarction. Primary endpoints were recurrent angina with electrocardiographic changes, myocardial infarction, and total deaths during a 12-week treatment period.[26] Both groups (n = 214) took aspirin, 162.5 mg daily, and the group randomized to receive anticoagulation also received a 100-U/kg bolus of heparin followed by an infusion set to keep the aPTT at twice the control value for 3–4 days. Warfarin also was given for the remainder of the trial period at doses titrated to keep international normalized ratios between 2.0 and 3.0.

There was a significant withdrawal rate in the combination therapy group (45%) compared with the aspirin-only group (31%). Intention-to-treat analysis of the data at 14 days (before most of the withdrawals) revealed that 27% of the patients assigned to aspirin vs. 10% of patients assigned to combination therapy experienced a primary endpoint. No major bleeding complications were reported in the aspirin-only group. In patients assigned to combination therapy, 2.6% experienced major hemorrhage. Minor bleeding was observed in 2.8% of patients treated with aspirin and 6.7% of patients treated with combination therapy.

To explore further the value of combined aspirin and anticoagulant therapy, Yusuf and coworkers performed a meta-analysis of trials that used aspirin or a combination of aspirin and unfractionated heparin (UFH), administered as a bolus with continuous infusion guided by the aPTT, or low-molecular-weight heparin (LMWH) for treatment of unstable coronary syndromes.[27] Their findings are in agreement with the results reported by Theroux and ATACS. The combination of aspirin and anticoagulation with heparins reduces the incidence of death and myocardial infarction when used early after the diagnosis of unstable coronary syndrome. Beyond the first week of therapy, the addition of anticoagulant therapy provides no additional benefit and increases the risk of bleeding side effects.[28]

Acute Myocardial Infarction

Aspirin is a relatively weak antiplatelet drug and does not accentuate thrombolysis.[29] However, its benefit in the setting of acute myocardial infarction is profound. A pilot study of the value of heparin, aspirin, and streptokinase for the treatment of acute myocardial infarction in 619 patients reported a 42% reduction in in-hospital mortality with aspirin therapy.[30] In the full-scale trial, ISIS-2, 17,187 patients presenting within 24 hours of the onset of a suspected acute myocardial infarction were randomized to intravenous streptokinase (1.5 MU), 162.5 mg of enteric-coated aspirin daily for 30 days, both, or neither (Table 3).[30] After 5 weeks, vascular death occurred in 11.8% of patients assigned to placebo and 9.4% of those assigned to aspirin therapy. This absolute 2.4% reduction in vascular death represented a 23% relative risk reduction and was accompanied by a 50% reduction in the risk of nonfatal reinfarction. The groups receiving either aspirin or streptokinase had a similar incidence of vascular mortality (10.7% vs. 10.4%). The combination of streptokinase and aspirin resulted in an 8.0% incidence of vascular death, representing a 40% relative risk reduction compared with placebo. Aspirin therapy was not associated with an increase in major bleeding complications. The survival benefit of aspirin therapy was maintained through 10 years of follow-up.[31]

The survival benefit accompanying aspirin therapy in ISIS-2 is the result of preventing infarct-related artery reocclusion rather than promoting thrombolysis. Heparin is far more effective in enhancing the lytic effect of newer-generation thrombolytic agents. In the Heparin-Aspirin Reperfusion Trial, the combination of recombinant tissue-type plasminogen activator (tPA) and heparin was associated with a 24-hour infarct-related artery patency of 82% compared with 52% in patients treated with aspirin and recombinant tPA (p < 0.0001).[32] Treatment with aspirin is associated with a reocclusion rate of 11% compared with 29% in patients who are not treated with aspirin (p < 0.001). This finding holds true regardless of the thrombolytic agent used. Recurrent ischemia is reduced from 45% in patients treated with thrombolytic therapy only to 28% in patients who receive adjunctive aspirin therapy (p < 0.001).

Clinical Use

Gastrointestinal side effects may limit the use of aspirin in some patient populations. Aspirin therapy can induce bleeding ulcers and/or erosions even at low doses, although the clinical importance of this effect appears to be dose-dependent. Buffered aspirin does not lessen gastric toxicity, and enteric-coated preparations seem to be protective only in short-term use.[33] An analysis of clinical trials using higher doses of aspirin (900–1300mg/day) found that the incidence of stomach pain, heartburn, and nausea was 40–60% higher than in

Table 3.   Aspirin in Acute Myocardial Infarction at 35-Day Follow-up

	Placebo	SK	Aspirin	SK + Aspirin
Dose		1.5 MU	162.5mg	1.5 MU + 162.5 mg
No. of patients	4300	4300	4295	4292
Vascular death	568 (13.2%)	448 (10.4%)	461 (10.7%)	343 (8.0%)
NNT compared with placebo		40	40	19

Sk = streptokinase, NNT = number needed to treat.
From Baigent C, Collins R, Appleby P, et al: ISIS-2: 10 year survival among patients with suspected acute myocardial infarction in randomised comparison of intravenous streptokinase, oral aspirin, both, or neither. The ISIS-2 (Second International Study of Infarct Survival) Collaborative Group. BMJ 316:1337–1343, 1998, with permission.

patients receiving placebo (24–44% vs. 15–32%).[12,34] At a dose of 75 mg/day for 1–4 years, the frequency of gastrointestinal symptoms is 11–13% compared with 3–4% in placebo-treated patients.[35–37]

Clinical benefit in avoidance of drug-related morbidity and improved compliance with therapy may be expected by using the lowest effective dose of aspirin. In normal volunteers, aspirin doses as low as 40 mg/day are sufficient to produce a measurable antiplatelet effect.[38] However, limited evidence suggests that such low doses have clinical efficacy in patients with vascular disease.[39] Randomized, controlled clinical trials have established clearly the efficacy of aspirin therapy at doses of 162 and 325 mg/day for myocardial infarction and 75, 324, 650, and 1300 mg/day for unstable angina.

Only one adequately sized trial has compared the efficacy of two aspirin dosing regimens. The Dutch TIA trial compared aspirin doses of 30 mg/day with 283 mg/day and found no significant difference in event rates.[40] However, this trial was relatively small and did not address specifically the group of patients with active intracoronary thrombus. It cannot be used for guidance in the treatment of myocardial infarction and unstable angina. In their review of available clinical trials of aspirin therapy, the Antiplatelet Trialists' Collaboration concluded that clinical evidence suggests that medium-dose aspirin (75–325 mg/day) is a reasonable first choice for antiplatelet therapy except in the rare patient with a genuine aspirin allergy or in patients with severe gastric side effects.[20]

Angiotensin-converting enzyme (ACE) inhibitors have proved an effective means of impeding disease progression and reducing mortality in patients with impaired left ventricular systolic function. It has been proposed that one mechanism of this benefit is enhanced production of vasodilator prostaglandins, which may be inhibited by concomitant aspirin therapy. Indeed, aspirin therapy may mitigate some of the hemodynamic effects of ACE inhibitor therapy.[41] However, clinical evidence suggests that the addition of aspirin to ACE inhibitor therapy provides additional clinical benefit. In a cohort study from the Bezafibrate Infarction Prevention Trial, 1247 patients were treated with ACE inhibitors, and 618 also received aspirin.[42] Although clinical characteristics and other therapies were similar, patients taking aspirin experienced a lower mortality rate than patients who did not (19% vs. 27%, p = 0.001). In an overview of trials involving 98,496 patients with acute myocardial infarction in whom the effect of ACE-inhibitor therapy was tested, concomitant aspirin therapy did not reduce the benefits of ACE inhibition.[43] Taken together, these observations argue against any clinical correlate to the theoretical drug interaction.

There is an absolute 0.2–0.3% increase in the risk of hemorrhagic stroke in aspirin-treated patients.[20] This risk is not appreciably altered by aspirin dose or the clinical setting in which it is used. There is currently no contraindication to use of low-dose aspirin in patients with mild renal impairment or essential hypertension. In patients with aspirin allergy, as little as 30 mg can provoke bronchospasm. For such patients, a thienopyridine should be used for the treatment of unstable angina or acute myocardial infarction.

Thienopyridines

Ticlopidine and clopidogrel are thienopyridine derivatives that inhibit ADP-induced platelet activation. The importance of this pathway in platelet function is reflected in the ability of thienopyridines to inhibit platelet aggregation in response to a variety of stimuli.[44,45] Inhibition of fibrinogen binding to GP IIb/IIIa receptors is observed after treatment with these agents and is believed to be a secondary effect of ADP receptor blockade.[46] In contrast to aspirin, the antiaggregatory effects of the thienopyridines are not reduced by epinephrine or shear stress.[47,48] Antiaggregatory effects cannot be reproduced by direct application of the parent drug in vitro, suggesting that a metabolite is responsible for observed clinical effects. Maximal effect on bleeding time is seen after 5 days of ticlopidine or 3–5 days of clopidogrel and can be hastened by application of a loading dose. The effects on bleeding time persist for about 1 week after discontinuation of the drug.[45,49]

Ticlopidine

Although efficacy is clearly established for reducing intracoronary thrombotic events after stent implantation, few clinical trials have examined the use of ticlopidine as medical therapy in the setting of an acute coronary syndrome. Only one small trial has examined its efficacy after acute myocardial infarction. Inadequate power and a low event rate render results unenlightening.[50] In an open-label trial, 652 patients with unstable angina were randomized within 48 hours of admission to receive 250 mg ticlopidine twice daily or conventional therapy without aspirin. At 6 months the rate of fatal and nonfatal myocardial infarction was reduced from 13.6% in the placebo arm to 7.3% in the group taking ticlopidine, a 46% absolute reduction (CI = 0.12–0.81).[51,52] The number needed to treat (NNT) was 16, which echoes the NNT for aspirin (see Table 1). This effect, however, took 2 weeks to become evident, presumably reflecting the time required to achieve steady-state levels and maximal inhibition of platelet function. No study to date has compared ticlopidine with aspirin in the treatment of either unstable angina or acute myocardial infarction.

The use of ticlopidine has been limited by its side effects, particularly rare but severe neutropenia, which occurs in about 0.8% of patients. Neutropenia tends to occur within 3 months of the initiation of treatment and is usually reversible after discontinuation. Thrombotic thrombocytopenic purpura (TTP) may occur within the first month of therapy in 0.02% of patients. The mortality rate is 50% unless the patient is treated with plasmapheresis, which reduces the mortality rate to 24%.[53] The specter of hematologic aberrations with ticlopidine requires regular screening with a complete blood count. Current recommendations are for monitoring every 2 weeks for the duration of therapy. Other common side effects include nausea, vomiting, diarrhea, increased serum cholesterol, and abnormal liver function tests.[45]

Clopidogrel

The molar potency of clopidogrel in the inhibition of ADP-induced platelet aggregation is greater than that of ticlopidine.[49] Clopidogrel appears to have a faster onset of action than ticlopidine. A 75-mg, once-daily dose inhibits ADP-induced platelet aggregation within 2 hours of the first dose and reaches steady state within 3–7 days. A 375-mg loading dose of clopidogrel, followed by 75 mg/day for 10 days, inhibits ADP-induced platelet aggregation by 55% (± 8.2%) at 1 hour and 80% (± 3.6%) at 5 hours.[54]

The Clopidogrel vs. Aspirin in Patients at Risk of Ischemic Events (CAPRIE) Trial was designed to assess the relative safety and efficacy of clopidogrel in reducing the risk of vascular events in patients with a recent ischemic stroke or myocardial infarction or symptomatic peripheral artery disease. Over 19,000 patients were randomized to clopidogrel, 75 mg/day, or aspirin, 325 mg/day, and followed for 1–3 years (mean = 1.9 years).[55] Clopidogrel was associated with a slight (5.32% vs. 5.83%, p = 0.043) reduction in the annual risk of fatal or nonfatal ischemic stroke, myocardial infarction, or other vascular death. Specifically, clopidogrel therapy provided a 19.2% relative risk reduction for myocardial infarction.[56] Therefore, in a population of atherosclerotic patients similar to CAPRIE, clopidogrel would be expected to prevent an additional 5 major clinical events (ischemic stroke, myocardial infarction, vascular death) per 1000 patients per year compared with aspirin.

The only available data for the use of clopidogrel in myocardial infarction come from a small safety trial in which clopidogrel was substituted for aspirin in 116 patients treated with thrombolytic therapy. The mortality rate (3.6%) and severe bleeding rate (1.7%) compare favorably with historical data.[57]

The side effects of clopidogrel are generally mild, and tolerability is similar to that of aspirin. In the CAPRIE trial, the most commonly reported adverse effects in clopidogrel-treated patients were gastrointestinal upset, bleeding disorders, rash, and diarrhea. Gastrointestinal hemorrhage occurred in 2.0% of patients treated with clopidogrel compared with 2.7% of those treated with aspirin (p < 0.05), whereas intracranial hemorrhage occurred in 0.35% of patients in the clopidogrel group compared with 0.49% for those taking aspirin (p = NS). The incidence of neutropenia (< $1200/mm^3$) in the clopidogrel group (0.10%) was similar to that in the group taking medium-dose aspirin (0.17%). Thrombocytopenia occurred in 0.26% of patients in both treatment groups. There was no effect on liver function tests, and no clinically significant pharmacodynamic drug interactions have been reported to date.[55] Like ticlopidine, clopidogrel has been associated with TTP, albeit with a lower incidence.[58] Whereas most cases of TTP in ticlopidine-treated patients occurred in the first 2–12 weeks of therapy, most cases of clopidogrel-associated TTP occurred within the first 2 weeks. In addition, TTP in the setting of clopidogrel usage was associated with greater need for plasma exchange as well as with a higher recurrence rate. There is no current recommendation for formal hematologic monitoring as there is in ticlopidine.

Two trials testing the value of combination therapy with clopidogrel and aspirin in unstable coronary syndromes are under way. One trial will randomize 9000 patients with unstable angina and non–ST-elevation myocardial infarction to combined therapy with clopidogrel and aspirin or aspirin alone. A second trial under way at 1100 sites in China will examine the outcome of 30,000 patients with acute myocardial infarction randomized to combination therapy or aspirin alone. Until the results of these trials have been reported, clopidogrel should be reserved for use only in patients who are aspirin-intolerant or who have undergone coronary stent implantation.

Glycoprotein IIb/IIIa Antagonists

Exposure of additional GP IIb/IIIa receptors to facilitate platelet aggregation is the final common denominator of platelet activation and a principal determinant of arterial thrombus volume and strength. Inhibition of GP IIb/IIIa function cripples platelet hemostatic function, prevents thrombus growth, and favors its dissolution.[59] Currently four intravenous GP IIb/IIIa antagonists are undergoing clinical trials worldwide. Three are commercially available in the United States. The first to be developed was abciximab, a chimeric monoclonal antibody derived from murine antibody against the GP IIb/IIIa receptor. Eptifibatide is a cyclic heptapeptide; tirofiban and lamifiban are small molecule peptidomimetic agents that occupy the fibrinogen-binding site of GP IIb/IIIa. In addition, a number of orally administered GP IIb/IIIa agents are under investigation. Unfortunately, dosing uncertainty and poor results in early clinical trials have prevented the commercial introduction of oral agents.

The use of GP IIb/IIIa antagonists as an addition to medical therapy for unstable angina was tested in the PURSUIT, PRISM, PRISM (PLUS), and PARAGON trials. In the setting of percutaneous revascularization, data for patients with unstable coronary syndromes are available from the EPIC, EPILOG, EPISTENT, CAPTURE, IMPACT II, and RESTORE trials. The use of GP IIb/IIIa antagonists as an adjunct to thrombolytic therapy has been examined in IMPACT-AMI, TAMI-8, SPEED, and TIMI-14.

Abciximab

The pharmacokinetics of abciximab (ReoPro) have been described in some detail.[60] After intravenous administration, abciximab binds avidly to the platelet GP IIb/IIIa receptor. Free drug is cleared rapidly from plasma with an initial-phase half-life of less than 10 minutes and a second-phase half-life of approximately 30 minutes.[61] In patients receiving only a bolus of abciximab (0.25 mg/kg), receptor blockade decreases to 50% at 24 hours after infusion.[62] Continuous intravenous infusion of abciximab produces a maximal GP IIb/IIIa receptor blockade of 93% that falls to 68% at 12 hours after cessation of the infusion. Platelet function recovers gradually over 48 hours after completion of abciximab therapy. Flow cytometry at 8 and 15 days, a time beyond the normal circulating platelet life span, reveals 29% and 13% GP IIb/IIIa receptor blockade, suggesting that abciximab is transferred to newly released platelets.[63] Abciximab is not specific for the GP IIb/IIIa receptor. It also may associate with the vitronectin receptors that participate in cell migration and proliferation responses.

Unstable Angina

A number of trials have explored the use of abciximab in the setting of an unstable coronary syndrome managed with percutaneous coronary revascularization (Table 4).

The EPIC (Evaluation of 7E3 in Preventing Ischemic Complications) trial was a randomized, controlled study of abciximab in patients undergoing high-risk angioplasty or atherectomy.[64] A total of 2099 patients were randomized to one of three treatment arms: (1) bolus of abciximab plus 12-hour abciximab infusion; (2) bolus of abciximab and placebo infusion; or (3) placebo bolus and placebo infusion. The primary endpoint was the composite incidence of death, nonfatal myocardial infarction, and urgent intervention at 30 days. Of this group of patients, 23% had unstable angina, 3% had myocardial infarction, and 74% had high-risk lesion morphology.

In patients with unstable angina (n = 489) treated with bolus plus infusion of abciximab, the 30-day composite endpoint of death, myocardial infarction, or urgent intervention was reduced from 12.8% to 4.8%.[65] At 6-month follow-up, abciximab bolus plus infusion showed an even more dramatic effect on

Table 4. Abciximab in Patients with Unstable Angina

	Pilot Study[69] in Refractory USA during Hospital Stay		EPIC Substudy[65] in USA with PCI at 6-mo Follow-up			CAPTURE Trial[70] in USA with PCI at 6-mo Follow-up	
	Placebo	*Abciximab*	*Placebo*	*Preprocedural Abciximab Bolus*	*Preprocedural Abciximab Bolus + Infusion for 12 hr*	*Placebo*	*18–24 hr Preprocedural Abciximab to 1 hr after PCI*
No. of patients (treated)	30	30	153	161	156	635	630
Dose	ASA + heparin	0.25 µg/kg bolus + 10 µg/kg/min + ASA + heparin	ASA + heparin	0.25 µg/kg bolus + ASA + heparin	0.25 µg/kg bolus 10 µg/kg/min + ASA + heparin	ASA + heparin	0.25 µg/kg bolus + 10 µg/kg/min + ASA + heparin
Primary endpoint	Death, MI, urgent revascularization		Death, MI, urgent intervention			Death, MI, intervention	
Incidence of primary endpoint	12 (23%)	1 (3%) p = 0.03	(35.0%)	(26.8%)	(24.3%)	193 (30.8%)	193 (31.0%)
Death only			(6.7%)	(1.2%)	(0.7%)	14 (2.2%)	17 (2.8%)
MI only			(11.3%)	(6.9%)	(1.3%)	59 (9.3%)	41 (6.6%)
NNT (death/MI)		NS			6*		NS

USA = unstable angina, PCI = percutaneous coronary intervention, MI = myocardial infarction, ASA = aspirin, NNT = number needed to treat, NS = not significant.
* Compared with placebo group.

the incidence of death (1.8% vs. 6.6%) and myocardial infarction (2.4% vs. 11.1%). In contrast to the overall EPIC cohort, abciximab had no effect on the incidence of revascularization in this subgroup.

Within the cohort of patients with myocardial infarction (n = 64) who underwent angioplasty within 12 hours, 42 underwent direct PTCA and 22 had rescue PTCA after failed thrombolysis (Table 5).[66] Treatment with abciximab bolus plus infusion was associated with a 91% decrease in 6-month composite endpoints (4.5% vs. 47.8% in the placebo group; p = 0.002) and a trend toward lower 30-day endpoints (4.5% vs. 26.1%; p = .058).

The EPILOG Trial (Evaluation in PTCA to Improve Long-term Outcome with abciximab GP IIb/IIIa blockade) followed the EPIC Trial, using a lower dose of heparin in an attempt to reduce bleeding side effects.[67] Similar to the results of EPIC, abciximab therapy was associated with a reduction in the 30-day risk of death or myocardial infarction from 9.1% in the placebo arm to 4% in the treatment arm. In the EPISTENT (Evaluation of Platelet IIb/IIIa Inhibitor for Stenting) Study, patients scheduled to undergo coronary stent implantation were randomized to standard therapy or standard therapy with the addition of abciximab and reduced-dose heparin (similar to that in the EPILOG study). Troponin-T (TnT) values were determined preoperatively and appeared to be a powerful predictor of treatment benefit. TnT-positive patients who underwent stent alone suffered a 20.6% incidence of death or myocardial infarction at 30 days compared with 4.3% in stent patients who received abciximab.[68]

In a pilot study, 60 patients with refractory unstable angina underwent diagnostic angiography and, after a culprit lesion suitable for angioplasty was found, were randomized to standard care or standard care plus abciximab for 18–24 hours until 1 hour after completion of second angiography and intervention.[69] During drug infusion, recurrent ischemia occurred in 9 abciximab-treated and 16 placebo-treated patients (p = 0.06).

The multicenter, randomized trial, CAPTURE (C7E3 AntiPlatelet Therapy in Unstable REfractory Angina), studied the effect of abciximab on 1266 patients with refractory unstable angina undergoing coronary intervention.[70] The primary endpoint was the 30-day combined incidence of death, myocardial infarction, and urgent intervention. During the 24 hours that pharmacologic therapy only was employed, the rate of death or nonfatal myocardial infarction was reduced in the treatment arm compared with placebo (1.3% vs. 2.8%, p = 0.032). At 30 days the primary combined endpoint was reduced from 15.9% in the placebo group to 11.3% in the treatment arm; death and myocardial infarction alone were similarly reduced from 9.0% to 4.8%. All of the individual events included in the primary endpoint also were reduced (death, from 1.3% to 1.0%; myocardial infarction, from 8.2% to 4.1%; and urgent intervention, from 10.9% to 7.8%). The benefits of the CAPTURE dosing regimen of abciximab were lost at 6 months. There was a 31.0% incidence of the combined clinical endpoint in the abciximab arm compared with 30.8% in the placebo group.

As shown in the EPISTENT Study, elevated TnT concentrations identify a subgroup of patients who are at a high risk for adverse events and derive clear benefit from abciximab treatment.[70] In a substudy of CAPTURE, TnT concentrations were determined in randomly selected patients.[71] TnT concentrations were > 0.1ng/ml in 275 patients (30.9%). The 6-month cumulative event rate was 23.9% in this group and only 7.5% in patients with normal troponin values. Treatment with abciximab completely abolished the increased risk associated

Table 5. Abciximab with Primary Angioplasty

	EPIC Substudy[66] AMI with PTCA within 12 hr, 6-mo Follow-up		RAPPORT[72] Primary PTCA in AMI, 6-mo Follow-up		ADMIRAL[73] Primary PTCA with Stent in AMI, 30-day Follow-up	
	Heparin + ASA	*Abciximab + Heparin + ASA*	*Heparin + ASA*	*Abciximab for 12 hr + Heparin + ASA*	*Heparin + ASA + Ticlopidine*	*Heparin + ASA + Ticlopidine*
No. of patients	64		242	241	150	150
Dose	Heparin at operator discretion	0.25 µg/kg bolus ± 10 µg/kg/min + heparin + ASA	100 U/kg bolus + infusion (ACT > 300) + ASA	0.25 µg/kg bolus + 10 µg/kg/min + 100 U/kg bolus + infusion (ACT > 300) + ASA	NA	NA
Primary endpoint	Death, reinfarction, revascularization		Death, reinfarction, target-vessel revascularization (urgent, elective)		Death, reinfarction, urgent target-vessel revascularization	
Incidence of primary endpoint	(47.8%)	(4.5%)	(28.1%)	(28.2%)	(20.0%)	(10.7%)
Death only					(4.7%)	(3.3%)
MI only					(4.7%)	(2.0%)

PTCA = percutaneous transluminal coronary angioplasty, AMI = acute myocardial infarction, ASA = aspirin.

with elevated TnT values (9.5% in TnT-positive patients vs. 9.45% in patients with normal TnT, p = NS).

Primary Percutaneous Coronary Intervention

Several trials have supported the use of abciximab in acute myocardial infarction either as an adjunct to percutaneous intervention or as an adjunct to thrombolytic therapy (see Table 5). The RAPPORT (ReoPro and Primary PTCA Organization and Randomized Trial) and ADMIRAL (Abciximab before Direct angioplasty and stenting in Myocardial Infarction Regarding Acute and Long-term follow-up) Trials explore the use of abciximab with angioplasty with or without stent deployment. The TAMI-8 (Thrombolysis and Angioplasty in Myocardial Infarction), SPEED (Strategies for Patency Enhancement in the Emergency Department) and TIMI-14 (Thrombolysis in Myocardial Infarction) Trials investigate the use of abciximab with thrombolytic drugs.

The RAPPORT trial examined the efficacy of abciximab in the setting of primary percutaneous transluminal coronary angioplasty (PTCA) for acute myocardial infarction.[72] In this study 483 patients presenting within 12 hours of an acute myocardial infarction and deemed to be candidates for primary PTCA were randomized to receive an abciximab bolus plus a 12-hour infusion (n = 241) or placebo (n = 242). All patients received aspirin. Heparin was administered in all patients as a 100-U/kg bolus, with activated clotting time (ACT) titrated to > 300 seconds, and could be continued for up to 48 hours after the procedure.

The primary endpoint was the composite incidence of death, reinfarction, or target-vessel revascularization (urgent or elective) at 6 months. Although there was no significant difference in the primary endpoint at 6 months (28.1% placebo, 28.2% abciximab by intention-to-treat analysis), abciximab significantly reduced the combined incidence of death, reinfarction, and *urgent* target-vessel revascularization at all time points: 9.9% vs. 3.3% at 7 days; 11.2% vs. 5.8% at 30 days, and 17.8% vs. 11.6% at 6 months. The need for unplanned ("bailout") stenting also was reduced significantly from 20.4% with placebo to 11.9% with abciximab. There was a significant increase in major bleeding (predominantly at the arterial access site) with abciximab (from 9.5% to 16.6%), probably reflecting the impact of "high-dose" heparin therapy. As shown in the EPILOG trial, lowering the target for anticoagulation to an ACT of 200–300 seconds markedly reduces this risk.

The ADMIRAL study examined the use of abciximab with primary angioplasty and stenting in the presence of myocardial infarction with ST-segment elevation.[73] Patients were randomized to abciximab or placebo as soon as an infarction was diagnosed. All patients received aspirin, ticlopidine, and heparin. The composite endpoint of death, recurrent myocardial infarction, and urgent revascularization at 30 days was reduced from 20% to 10.7% with abciximab (p < 0.03). Urgent revascularization was reduced from 14.0% to 6.0% (p = 0.03), but the reductions in death and recurrent myocardial infarction (4.7% to 3.3%, p = 0.35, and 4.7% to 2.0%, p = 0.09, respectively) were not statistically significant. Angiographic results obtained 24 hours after the intervention revealed that abciximab-treated TIMI-3 flow rates were higher before (21% vs. 10%, p < 0.01) and 24 hours after stent implantation (86% vs. 78%, p < 0.05).

Thrombolysis

The thrombolytic literature demonstrates that timely restoration of infarct-related artery patency is required to realize treatment benefit and that brisk

(TIMI grade 3) flow is associated with the best prognosis (Table 6). Contemporary thrombolytic regimens restore patency in 60%–85% of patients with acute myocardial infarction,[74–76] but only slightly more than one-half of patients achieve TIMI grade 3 flow in the infarct-related artery. In addition, reocclusion, reinfarction, or both occur in roughly one-third of patients by 3 months.[77,78] Part of the inability of thrombolytics to achieve greater rates of vessel patency may be due to the fact that arterial thrombi are platelet-rich and their aggregation is not solely fibrin-dependent.[79,80]

In the TAMI-8 pilot study, patients with acute myocardial infarction, treated with recombinant tPA, aspirin, and heparin, were randomized to adjunctive therapy with abciximab or placebo.[81] Bolus injections of abciximab were given to 60 patients in ascending doses at 3, 6, and 15 hours after initiation of the thrombolytic infusion. Ten patients treated with recombinant tPA alone were studied as control subjects. Recurrent ischemia occurred in 13% of abciximab-treated patients and 20% of controls. Infarct-related coronary artery patency was 92% in patients receiving abciximab and 56% in control patients. Fifteen (25%) abciximab-treated patients and five (50%) control patients had major bleeding; eight of these events (seven in abciximab-treated patients and one in a control patient) occurred after coronary bypass surgery. Although this study was not designed to evaluate clinical benefit, it suggests that combination treatment with thrombolytic therapy and a GP IIb/IIIa antagonist may improve early patency rates without excessive bleeding risk.

The SPEED trial (see Table 6) evaluated the combination of recombinant plasminogen activator (Retavase) and abciximab in patients with acute myocardial infarction.[82] A total of 305 patients were randomized to treatment with abciximab alone or one of a number of different doses of Retavase plus abciximab. All patients received aspirin (150–325 mg) and heparin (60-U/kg bolus, maximum of 4000 U, followed by an 800-U/hr infusion). Catheterization and angiography were performed 60–90 minutes after initiation of therapy (median = 62–64 min.). The incidence of TIMI grade 3 flow at 60–90 minutes was 27% in the abciximab-only group, 55% in the 5-U Retavase bolus plus abciximab group, 44% in the 7.5-U Retavase bolus plus abciximab group, 46% in the 10-U bolus Retavase plus abciximab group, and 62% in the 5 + 5-U Retavase group. Analysis of cohorts receiving 5 + 5U Retavase with standard abciximab dosing but different heparin regimens showed that TIMI grade 3 flow was higher (61.1%) with 60 U/kg than with the lower 40-U/kg dose (51.4%). Although not the primary clinical endpoint, 30-day intention-to-treat outcomes were low in every category because the study was not powered to show such effect. The group receiving both abciximab and 5 + 5 U Retavase had a 6.1% incidence of the composite endpoint of death, reinfarction, and urgent revascularization compared with 11.0% in the Retavase-only group (p = 0.19). The rate of death or reinfarction alone was 3.5% in the combination arm compared with 8.3% in the Retavase-only group (p = 0.13). Hemorrhagic complications were not significantly increased with combination therapy.

The TIMI-14 study (see Table 6) was a prospective, multicenter, randomized, controlled trial of combined therapy with thrombolytic agents and abciximab in patients with acute myocardial infarction.[83] A total of 681 patients were randomized to standard front-loaded tPA (100 mg), streptokinase (500,000, 750,000, 1,250,000, or 1,500,000 U), and abciximab; low-dose tPA (20, 35, 50, or 65 mg) and abciximab; or abciximab alone. In the streptokinase groups, lytic

Table 6.   Abciximab with Thrombolysis

	SPEED[82] AMI with r-PA, 30-day Follow-up			TIMI-14[115] AMI with SK or tPA, 30-day Follow-up			
	Heparin + ASA + Abciximab	Heparin + ASA + r-PA	Heparin + ASA + Abciximab + r-PA (One-half Dose)	Heparin + ASA + tPA	Abciximab + Heparin + ASA	Abciximab + ASA + Heparin + SK	Abciximab + ASA + Heparin + tPA (One-half Dose)
No. of patients	48	98	100	163	32	51	34
Dose	40–60 U/kg bolus + infusion (ACT > 200 sec + aPTT 50–70 sec)	70 U/kg bolus + infusion (ACT > 200 sec + aPTT 50–70 sec) + 150–325 mg + 10 + 10 U	40–60 U/kg bolus + infusion (ACT > 200 sec + aPTT 50–70 sec) + 0.25 µg/kg +0.125 µg/min + 5 + 5 U	70 U/kg + 15 U/kg + 150–325 mg + 100 mg	0.25 µg/kg + 0.125 µg/kg/min for 12 hr + 60 U/kg + 7 U/kg/hr + 150–325 mg	0.25 µg/kg + 0.125 µg/kg/min for 12 hr + 60 U/kg + 7 U/kg/hr + 150–325 mg + 1250 U × 10³ for 50 min	0.25 µg/kg + 0.125 µg/kg/min for 12 hr + 60 U/kg + 7 U/kg + 150–325 mg + 50 mg
Primary endpoint	TIMI grade 3 flow at 60–90 minutes			TIMI grade 3 flow at 90 minutes			
Incidence of primary endpoint	(27%)	(47%)	(54%)	87 (57%)	10 (32%)	20 (46%)	22 (76%)
Death only	NA	NA	NA	5 (3%)	0	2 (4%)	1 (3%)
MI only	NA	NA	NA	5 (3%)	0	2 (4%)	0

AMI = acute myocardial infarction, r-PA = recombinant plasminogen activator, ASA = aspirin, ACT = activated clotting time, aPTT = activated partial thromboplastin time, NA = not available.   SK = streptokinase, tPA = tissue plasminogen activator.

therapy was administered as a 30- to 50-minute infusion. In the tPA groups, lytic therapy was administered as a bolus, a bolus plus a 30-minute infusion, or a bolus plus a 60-minute infusion.

The incidence of TIMI 3 flow at 90 minutes was 58% in the tPA-only group, 32% in the abciximab-only group, and 42%, 39%, 47%, and 80% (discontinued because of excessive bleeding and mortality) in the respective streptokinase-plus-abciximab groups. In the tPA-plus-abciximab groups, the incidence of TIMI 3 flow at 90 minutes was 53% (20-mg bolus), 38% (35-mg bolus), 62% (15-mg bolus, 20-mg infusion over 30 minutes), 54% (50-mg bolus), 61% (15-mg bolus, 35-mg infusion over 30 minutes), 79% (15-mg bolus, 35-mg infusion over 60 minutes), and 71% (15-mg bolus, 50-mg infusion over 60 minutes). A group that combined tPA (15-mg bolus, 35-mg infusion over 60 minutes) with higher-dose abciximab and reduced heparin had a 90-minute TIMI 3 flow rate of 69% (n = 36).

The incidence of major bleeding was 6% with tPA alone; 6% with abciximab alone; 5%, 8%, 14%, and 67% (discontinued arm) in the respective streptokinase groups; and 5%, 4%, 0%, 8%, 8%, 5%, and 0% in the respective tPA groups. Thus a combination of reduced-dose thrombolytic therapy and abciximab appears to augment appreciably the rate and extent of thrombolysis.

Eptifibatide

Eptifibatide (Integrilin) is a cyclic heptapeptide GP IIb/IIIa inhibitor derived from the venom of the Southeastern pygmy rattlesnake. It has less affinity for the GP IIb/IIIa receptor than abciximab.[84] Studies in normal subjects found that bolus doses of 180 and 135 µg/kg inhibit more than 80% of ADP-induced platelet aggregation in more than 75% of subjects, falling to 50% within 4 hours after discontinuation of the drug.[85] The short half-life of platelet inhibition with eptifibatide presumably reduces bleeding side effects and facilitates easier conversion to bypass surgery.

Unstable Angina

The first prospective, double-blind clinical trial involving eptifibatide in unstable angina sought the most effective dose for inhibiting ADP-dependent platelet aggregation.[86] Patients were treated with either of two doses of eptifibatide plus placebo or aspirin or with aspirin alone. No heparin was given. Infusions were continued for 24–72 hours (mean = 37.7 ± 1.4 hours) or until revascularization was performed. Eptifibatide therapy reduced the number and duration of ischemic episodes detected on ST-segment monitoring without increasing the risk of bleeding.

The PURSUIT Trial (Platelet Glycoprotein IIb/IIIa in Unstable Angina: Receptor Suppression Using Integrilin Therapy) examined the effect of higher doses of eptifibatide on clinical outcomes in patients with unstable coronary syndromes (Table 7).[87] Patients with ischemic chest pain and electrocardiographic abnormalities suggestive of ischemia were randomized to receive low-dose eptifibatide (180-µg/kg bolus followed by 1.3 µg/kg/min), high-dose eptifibatide (180-µg/kg bolus followed by 2 µg/kg/min) or placebo within 11 hours of presentation. Because of apparent lack of benefit, the lower-dose arm was discontinued prematurely. At 30 days, treatment with high-dose eptifibatide reduced the risk of death and myocardial infarction from 15.7% to 14.2% (p = 0.04). Treatment benefit was apparent only in patients who underwent percutaneous coronary intervention. Those who had

Table 7. Eptifibatide in Acute Coronary Syndromes

	PURSUIT[87] at 30-day Follow-up		IMPACT-AMI[89]: 90-min Angiography and In-hospital Outcomes	
	ASA + Heparin	Eptifibatide + ASA + Heparin	tPA + ASA + Heparin	Eptifibatide + tPA + ASA + Heparin
Daily dose	80–325 mg + 5000 U bolus + infusion (aPTT 50–70 sec)	180 µg/kg bolus + infusion 2 µg/kg/min + 80–325 mg + 5000 U BOLUS + infusion (aPTT 50–70 sec)	Accelerated tPA 100 mg once only + 325 mg + 40 U/kg bolus + 15 U/kg/hr (2–2.5 × control aPTT)	180 µg/kg + 0.75 µg/kg/min + accelerated tPA 100 mg once only + 325 mg +40 U/kg + 15 U/kg/hr (2–2.5 × control aPTT)
No. of patients	4739	4722	52 angiographic/13 clinical	49 angiographic/51 clinical
Primary endpoint	Death, recurrent MI		TIMI grade 3 flow at 90 min (secondary endpoint included in-hospital outcomes)	
Incidence of primary endpoint	See Death/MI		66%	39%
Death/MI	(15.7%)	(14.2%)	7.3%	7.8%
All MI	(13.5%)	(12.6%)	3.6%	0%
Death	(3.7%)	(3.5%)	3.6%	7.8%
NNT (death/MI)		67		NA (p = NS)

ASA = aspirin, tPA = tissue plasminogen activator (Alteplase), aPTT = activated partial thromboplastin time, MI = myocardial infarction, NNT = number needed to treat.

a revascularization procedure enjoyed a 31% relative risk reduction for death or myocardial infarction with treatment (11.6% vs. 16.7%, p = 0.010), whereas no treatment benefit was observed in patients who did not (14.6% eptifibatide vs. 15.6% placebo, p = NS).[88] Bleeding complications requiring transfusion were increased with treatment (11.6% vs. 9.2%); the incidence of stroke (0.7% vs. 0.8%) and thrombocytopenia (6.8% vs. 6.7%) was not affected.

Thrombolysis

In IMPACT-AMI (Integrilin to Minimize Platelet Aggregation and Prevent Coronary Thrombosis and Acute Myocardial Infarction)[89] (see Table 7), eptifibatide (180-µg/kg bolus with continuous infusion of 0.75 µg/kg/min) added to aspirin, low-dose heparin, and tPA improved the rate of TIMI grade 3 flow at 90 minutes from 39% in the placebo group to 66% in the treatment group (p = 0.006). However, treatment did not reduce the incidence of death or reinfarction (8.0% eptifibatide vs. 7.3% placebo). Bleeding complications were mild and occurred mostly at vascular access sites. The incidence of thrombocytopenia was not increased. This study was not sufficiently robust to assess clinical efficacy.[90]

Tirofiban

Tirofiban (Aggrastat) is a small-molecule GP IIb/IIIa inhibitor derived from the amino acid tyrosine.[91] It has a plasma half-life of 2 hours and is cleared predominantly through the kidney. Dosage adjustments are required in patients with impaired renal function. Ninety percent of platelet ADP-dependent aggregation is inhibited within 5 minutes after a bolus of 10 µg/kg followed by an infusion of 0.10–0.15 µg/kg/min. At 16–24 hours the inhibition remains at 80% with the 0.10-µg/kg/min infusion and 90% with the 0.15-µg/kg/min infusion. Inhibition falls to 50% 4 hours after therapy is discontinued.[92]

Unstable Angina

In the randomized, double-blind PRISM Trial (Platelet Receptor Inhibition in Ischemic Syndrome Management), patients with unstable angina were randomized to receive tirofiban or heparin in addition to aspirin[93] (Table 8). The primary endpoint was death, myocardial infarction, and refractory ischemia at 48 hours. Intervention before the end of 48 hours was discouraged. Treatment provided a 32% relative risk reduction for the primary endpoint. At 1-month follow-up, relative risk reduction for the primary endpoint had fallen to 7% (p = 0.34), primarily because of increased frequency of recurrent ischemia in the treatment group that, surprisingly, did not alter the survival benefit (2.3% vs. 3.6%, p = 0.02).

Treatment with tirofiban plus heparin was evaluated in 1915 patients with acute coronary syndromes in the PRISM-PLUS trial (Platelet Receptor Inhibition in Ischemic Syndrome Management—Patients Limited by Unstable Signs and Symptoms).[94] Patients were randomized to receive heparin, tirofiban, or both. Aspirin therapy was given to all patients as tolerated. The study was stopped prematurely for the group receiving tirofiban without heparin because of excessive mortality. Tirofiban-plus-heparin therapy reduced the combined risk of myocardial infarction and refractory ischemia by 23% at 30 days and the combined risk of myocardial infarction and death by 31% compared with the combination of heparin and aspirin. Major bleeding occurred in 6% of patients receiving tirofiban, and 3.9% required transfusions. There was no increase in the incidence of thrombocytopenia.

Table 8. Tirofiban in Acute Coronary Syndromes

| | PRISM[93] USA without Heparin or Urgent PTCA | | | | PRISM-PLUS[94] USA/Non-Q-wave MI | | | | RESTORE[95] USA + AMI with PTCA or DCA within 72 hr | |
| | 48-hr Follow-up | | 30-day Follow-up | | 30-day Follow-up | | 60-day Follow-up | | 30-day Follow-up | |
	Heparin + ASA	Tirofiban + ASA	Heparin + ASA	Tirofiban + ASA	Placebo + Heparin + ASA	Tirofiban + Heparin + ASA	Placebo + Heparin + ASA	Tirofiban + Heparin + ASA	Placebo + ASA + Heparin	ASA + Heparin + Tirofiban
Dose	2 × control aPTT	0.6 μg/kg bolus + 0.15 μg/kg/min	2 × control aPTT	0.6 μg/kg bolus + 0.15 μg/kg/min	2 × control aPTT	0.4 μg/kg bolus + 0.1 μg/kg/min + 2 × control aPTT	2 × control aPTT	0.4 μg/kg bolus + 0.1 μg/kg/min + 2 × control aPTT	Up to 10,000 U bolus + infusion (ACT 300–400 sec)	Up to 10,000 U bolus + infusion (ACT 300–400 sec) + 10 μg/kg followed by an infusion of 0.15 μg/kg/min
No. of patients	1616	1616	1616	1616	797	773	797	773	1070	1071
Death/MI/recurrent ischemia/readmission for USA	(5.6%)	(3.8%)	(17.1%)	(15.9%)	178 (22.3%)	143 (18.5%)	256 (32.1%)	214 (27.7%)	130 (12.2%)	110 (10.3%)
MI			(4.3%)	(4.1%)	73 (9.2%)	51 (6.6%)	84 (10.5%)	64 (8.3%)	61 (5.7%)	45 (4.2%)
Death			(3.6%)	(2.3%)	36 (4.5%)	28 (3.6%)	56 (7.0%)	53 (6.9%)	8 (0.7%)	9 (0.8%)
NNT (death, MI only)	NA		NA		29		41		71	

USA = unstable angina, PTCA = percutaneous transluminal coronary angioplasty, DCA = directed coronary atherectomy, MI = myocardial infarction, ASA = apsirin, NNT = number needed to treat, aPTT = activated partial thromboplastin time, ACT = activated clotting time.

Percutaneous Coronary Intervention in Acute Myocardial Infarction and Unstable Angina

In the RESTORE Trial (Randomized Efficacy Study of Tirofiban for Outcomes and Restenosis), tirofiban was tested in patients undergoing either PTCA or directional coronary atherectomy (see Table 8).[95] Of 2141 patients, two-thirds had unstable angina, and one-third had an acute myocardial infarction. Patients were randomized to receive either placebo or tirofiban (10 μg/kg followed by an infusion of 0.15 μg/kg/min) for 36 hours. All patients received aspirin and heparin given as a bolus followed by an infusion. The primary endpoint was the composite of death, myocardial infarction, stent placement for threatened or abrupt closure, coronary artery bypass surgery for failure of percutaneous intervention, or recurrent ischemia requiring repeat intervention within 30 days. An early 3.3% absolute reduction in the primary endpoint (8.7% vs. 5.4%, p = 0.005) did not persist at 30 days (10.3% tirofiban vs. 12.2% placebo, p = 0.160). Major bleeding complications were similar in both treatment groups (5.3% in the tirofiban group vs. 3.7% in the placebo group, p = 0.096). Thrombocytopenia was rare.

Lamifiban

Lamifiban is a synthetic, nonpeptide inhibitor of the GP IIb/IIIa receptor. Like other small-molecule antagonists, it has a relatively short pharmacologic half-life of approximately 4 hours and depends on renal excretion.

The Canadian Lamifiban Study was a phase-II dose-finding trial in which placebo or lamifiban was administered in varying doses to patients with unstable angina (86%) or myocardial infarction without ST segment elevation (14%).[96] The two highest dosing regimens provided 100% inhibition of ADP-dependent platelet aggregation and a reduction in the composite endpoint of death and myocardial infarction at 30 days (8.1% placebo vs. 2.5% lamifiban, p = 0.03).

The PARAGON-A Trial (Platelet IIb/IIIa Antagonism for the Reduction of Acute coronary syndrome events in a Global Organization Network) compared two doses of lamifiban with and without heparin to placebo with heparin in patients with acute coronary syndrome without persistent ST-segment elevation.[97] There was no difference between any lamifiban dose and placebo at 30 days. A slight divergence in event rates was observed during 6-month follow-up so that the composite endpoint was reached in 13.7% of the low-dose lamifiban group, 16.4% of the high-dose group, and 18.1% of the placebo group. The absence of dose-related benefits and the small effect of drug therapy render the results of PARAGON-A uncertain with respect to the value of lamifiban for patients with unstable coronary syndromes.

Thrombolysis

The PARADIGM Trial (Platelet Aggregation Receptor Antagonist Dose Investigation and Reperfusion Gain in Myocardial Infarction) was a dose-ranging trial of lamifiban in conjunction with thrombolytic drugs in patients presenting within 12 hours of an acute myocardial infarction.[98] Primary endpoints included safety, evidence supporting reperfusion, and clinical outcomes. Although the time to steady-state ST-segment resolution was faster than with placebo (88 min compared with 122 min, p = 0.003), there was no difference in clinical outcomes. There was however, a treatment-related increase in the incidence of intermediate-to-major bleeding complications (16.2% vs. 7.2%). Unlike other studies in which complications at vascular access sites predominated, the rate of gastrointestinal and intracranial hemorrhage was higher in the lamifiban-treated groups compared with placebo.

Oral Glycoprotein IIb/IIIa Receptor Antagonists

Because parenteral GP IIb/IIIa antagonists have demonstrated efficacy in the treatment of acute coronary syndromes, it is logical to assume that oral agents would have similar results, not only acutely, but also in secondary prevention of ischemic events. Three such agents—xemilofiban, sibrafiban, and orbofiban—have undergone clinical investigations with disappointing results. Other oral GP IIb/IIIa agents under evaluation are lotrifiban, lefradifiban, and roxifiban.

In the EXCITE trial, xemilofiban was compared with placebo before and after percutaneous coronary intervention in 4818 patients.[99] Despite the continuation of xemilofiban for up to 182 days after the procedure, there was no difference in the incidence of the composite endpoint or death, myocardial infarction, or urgent revascularization. Twice as many patients taking xemilofiban reported major bleeding episodes compared with placebo.

TIMI-12 (Thrombolysis in Myocardial Infarction) was a phase-II trial examining the use of sibrafiban for unstable angina or after myocardial infarction.[100] There were no deaths among the 323 patients, and the incidence of death, myocardial infarction, or recurrent ischemia was not significantly different across treatment groups. The incidence of major hemorrhage, defined as a drop in the hematocrit by 15%, was approximately the same with sibrafiban and aspirin (1.5% vs. 1.9%). Minor bleeding events were increased 20- to 30-fold with high-dose sibrafiban.

The SYMPHONY trial (Sibrafiban vs. aspirin to Yield Maximum Protection from ischemic Heart events post-acute cOroNary syndromes) randomized 9233 patients within 7 days after an acute coronary syndrome to either placebo (aspirin, 80 mg twice daily) or sibrafiban (3, 4.5, or 6 mg/day).[101,102] Doses were titrated according to renal function and body mass to achieve at least 25% platelet inhibition in the low-dose arm (3 or 4.5 mg/day) and at least 50% inhibition in the high-dose arm (6 mg/day). Patients taking sibrafiban were not allowed to take concomitant aspirin therapy. However, the use of ticlopidine was allowed after coronary stenting. The primary endpoints—death, nonfatal infarction, and severe recurrent ischemia—did not differ significantly among the three treatment groups (9.8% for aspirin, 10.1% for both low- and high-dose sibrafiban). Major bleeding was more common with high-dose sibrafiban (5.7%) than with aspirin (3.9%) or low-dose sibrafiban (5.2%).

The SYMPHONY-2 trial was designed to test a different dosing scheme and its efficacy in patients with angina or myocardial infarction. The trial was stopped because of disappointing results after 6400 patients had been randomized.[103] The primary endpoint of death, second heart attack, or recurrent ischemia occurred at 30 days in 9.3% of aspirin-treated patients, 9.2% of patients receiving low-dose sibrafiban, and 10.5% of patients receiving high-dose sibrafiban. Death was significantly increased in patients receiving high-dose sibrafiban (2.4%) compared with aspirin-treated patients (1.3%). In short, sibrafiban has not proved to be as effective as aspirin in preventing recurrent ischemia and death in the setting of unstable coronary syndromes.

The first clinical trial testing orbofiban for efficacy was the OPUS-TIMI-16 trial, in which 10,302 patients with either unstable angina or non–Q-wave myocardial infarction were randomized to one of three treatment arms.[104] One group received orbofiban, 50 mg twice daily; another received 50 mg twice daily for 30 days, followed by a reduction in the dose to 30 mg twice daily; and the third group received placebo. A 12-month follow-up was planned. The study was terminated early because of excessive mortality in the 50- and 30-mg dose group (2.3% for the group receiving 50/30 mg of orbofiban vs. 1.6% for patients receiving only 50 mg of orbofiban and 1.4% for placebo.

Clinical Use of Glycoprotein IIb/IIIa Agents

Available GP IIb/IIIa antagonists require intravenous administration, beginning with a loading dose. Side effects are uncommon and anaphylaxis extraordinarily rare. Because of its method of manufacture, abciximab requires filtration during administration. The primary risk accompanying the use of GP IIb/IIIa antagonists is bleeding. Transfusion is required for bleeding side effects in excess of the standard aspirin/heparin risk by roughly 0.6–1.5%. Bleeding events frequently are associated with an invasive procedure. After diagnostic angiography, the major bleeding risk is about 1%. This risk rises to about 10% when a revascularization procedure is performed. Experience with GP IIb/IIIa antagonists during percutaneous coronary intervention has taught that safety improves with meticulous attention during instrumentation and use of low-dose heparin targeting a procedural ACT of 200–300 seconds.

Intracranial hemorrhage is a rare occurrence across all GP IIb/IIIa trials. In the event of life-threatening hemorrhage or the need for emergency surgical referral, small-molecule agents afford some relief because of their short half-life. However, small-molecule, nonpeptide agents such as tirofiban are cleared by renal mechanisms, and in patients with hemodynamic instability and impaired renal perfusion, their half-life may be substantially prolonged. No antidote is available for any of the small-molecule GP IIb/IIIa antagonists. Conversely, abciximab has a long duration of effect, but it may be reversed almost completely by platelet transfusion. Therefore, when hemodynamic instability is probable or renal function is suspect, abciximab may be the GP IIb/IIIa antagonist of choice.

Thrombocytopenia occurs in 0.3–0.5% of patients treated with abciximab.[105] The mechanism is believed to be immune-related, resulting in antibody attachment and sequestration of treated platelets. The onset of thrombocytopenia is typically seen within 24 hours. Resolution is spontaneous and may take more than 1 week. Fortunately, life-threatening hemorrhage due to thrombocytopenia is rare. Treatment is conservative, including cessation of the GP IIb/IIIa agent, aspirin, and heparin. Aspirin may be resumed when platelet counts have normalized. Platelet transfusions may be given in the event of complicating hemorrhage or prophylactically for a platelet count less than 20,000/ml.

Readministration of abciximab is generally believed to be safe. No cases of allergic, hypersensitivity, or anaphylactic reactions were reported in 329 patients re-exposed to abciximab.[106] The incidence of thrombocytopenia is increased and onset more rapid after readministration of abciximab. Screening platelet count is recommended 6 hours after readministration. Treatment is the same as for thrombocytopenia after primary administration. To date, no antibodies have been detected with the use of tirofiban or eptifibatide.

Only unfractionated heparins have been used in conjunction with GP IIb/IIIa inhibitors in the trials reported to date. Unfractionated heparins given intravenously have a short half-life of elimination, and their effect may be reversed with the administration of protamine. Low-molecular-weight heparins (LMWHs) given subcutaneously have a long duration of effect, and reversal with protamine is incomplete. As yet there is little clinical experience with the combination of LMWH and GP IIb/IIIa antagonists. Therefore, when a GP IIb/IIIa antagonist is chosen for therapy, unfractionated heparins are the anticoagulant of choice.

Dipyridamole

Dipyridamole (Persantine) is a pyramidopyridine agent that exerts both antithrombotic and vasodilatory effects. It is thought that dipyridamole affects the platelet by increasing plasma concentrations of adenosine and nitric oxide. Adenosine, in turn, binds to platelet-membrane adenosine A_2 receptors, increasing cyclic AMP concentrations.[107] This effect, however, has been difficult to demonstrate in vivo.[108] Dipyridamole also inhibits degradation of cGMP. This effect has also been difficult to reproduce in vivo.[109]

No clinical trials examine the use of dipyridamole alone in acute coronary syndromes. Dipyridamole apparently does not add to the beneficial effects of aspirin.[110] In the Persantine-Aspirin Reinfarction Study (PARIS), the combination of dipyridamole and aspirin did not reduce total mortality, nonfatal myocardial infarction, or coronary mortality more than aspirin alone. In addition, dipyridamole has no additive beneficial effect in maintenance of patency in coronary bypass surgery.[20,111] Adverse events associated with dipyridamole such as gastrointestinal symptoms, nausea, headache, and a rare coronary steal that may induce myocardial ischemia, limit its usefulness as an antiplatelet agent.[112] No evidence supports the use of dipyridamole as an antiplatelet agent for patients with coronary artery disease.

Conclusion

Antiplatelet therapy reduces the risk of recurrent ischemia, first infarction, reinfarction, and death for patients with unstable coronary syndromes. Available antiplatelet therapies generally fall into two categories: (1) those that inhibit specific pathways to the activation process, limiting the platelet's ability to propagate the original thrombotic stimulus, and (2) those that impair platelet–platelet attachment, namely the GP IIb/IIIa inhibitors. The current place of individual drugs in the treatment of unstable coronary syndromes is summarized in Table 9 and Figure 2.

Aspirin is the prototypical activation inhibitor, preventing platelet TXA_2 production at doses as low as 30 mg/day. An abundance of clinical evidence using medium- and high-dose aspirin (75–1500 mg/day) attests to its efficacy in limiting the growth of coronary thrombi and preventing new occlusion in the setting of unstable angina and reocclusion in patients with acute myocardial infarction. Short-term use is associated with a 23% reduction in mortality rate in patients treated for myocardial infarction and a 50% reduction in the risk of death or myocardial infarction in patients with unstable angina. By virtue of its relatively weak antiplatelet effect, the risk of bleeding side effects is not substantially increased with medium-dose, short-term therapy. Common use of the prostanoid pathway in several biologic systems, particularly in the gastric mucosa, results in an increased incidence of gastrointestinal side effects and associated hemorrhage,

Table 9. Intravenous Glycoprotein IIb/IIIa Inhibitors

Generic (Brand)	Approved Uses	Dose in PCI	Dose in ACS
Abciximab (ReoPro)	Before and during PCI	0.25 µg/kg bolus + 0.125 µg/kg/min for 12 hr*	Not approved
Eptifibatide (Integrilin)	PCI and ACS	135 µg/kg bolus + 0.5 µg/kg/min for 24 hr[†]	180 µg/kg bolus + 2 µg/kg/min for up to 72 hr[‡]
Tirofiban (Aggrastat)	ACS	Not approved	0.4 µg/kg/min for 30 min 0.1 µg/kg/min for up to 72 hr[§]
Lamifiban (None)	Not approved	Not approved	Not approved

PCI = percutaneous coronary intervention, ACS = acute coronary syndrome.
* The infusion can be started up to 24 hr before the procedure and continued at the same rate through the procedure.
[†] This is the approved dosage for PCI but may change given the recent EPSRIT 30-day data, which support a double-bolus dose.
[‡] No specific recommendations have been made in patients with renal insufficiency.
[§] If the creatinine clearance is < 30 min/L, the infusion should be reduced by 50%.

especially with high-dose therapy. Therefore, medium-dose aspirin (75–325 mg/day) is recommended for the treatment of unstable coronary syndromes in all nonallergic patients.

Inhibition of the ADP pathway to platelet activation results in more intense inhibition of platelet function than inhibition of the TXA_2 pathway. Limited clinical experience attests to the safety and efficacy of the available inhibitors of the ADP activation pathway, ticlopidine and clopidogrel, for the treatment of unstable coronary syndromes. Available evidence suggests that their efficacy will prove to be similar to that of aspirin. Ticlopidine is associated with rash, gastrointestinal intolerance, and hematologic side effects that may limit its use. Clopidogrel is well tolerated with a slightly increased risk of hematologic side effects; it is a reasonable alternative to aspirin in patients with severe aspirin intolerance or allergy. The safety, efficacy, and role of combination therapy with aspirin and clopidogrel are currently under study.

GP IIb/IIIa inhibitors are unique in their ability to impair platelet–platelet aggregation, regardless of the type of stimulus or its intensity. Two types of GP

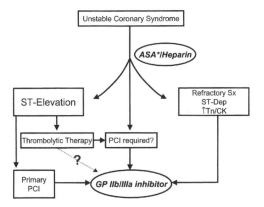

Figure 2. Algorithm for the use of antiplatelet agents in unstable coronary syndromes.

IIb/IIIa inhibitor are available: (1) an antibody derivative with high receptor affinity and long duration of effect that acts as a noncompetitive inhibitor and (2) small-molecule, competitive antagonists with a short duration of effect. The ability of these drugs to induce a temporary thrombasthenic state has reduced significantly the risk of percutaneous revascularization in the setting of unstable angina or acute myocardial infarction. Short-term use as an addition to medical therapy for unstable angina appears beneficial in patients with non–ST-elevation myocardial infarction or high-risk (refractory symptoms or ST-segment depression) unstable angina.[113]

By interfering with platelet–platelet attachment, GP IIb/IIIa inhibitors appear to augment the efficacy of thrombolytic drugs. Several small clinical trials have established that concurrent administration of eptifibatide or abciximab with fibrin-specific thrombolytic agents increases the 90-minute patency rate and improves the proportion of patients achieving TIMI-3 flow without substantially altering the risk of hemorrhage. Routine administration of the combination requires more robust clinical experience to confirm improved survival without excessive bleeding complications.

Oral GP IIb/IIIa inhibitors have met with disappointing results in clinical trials. Reasons for their relative failure are uncertain. Possibilities include difficulties in arriving at a dose that will provide adequate, consistent inhibition of platelet function and perhaps an increased risk of bleeding with long-term, high-intensity platelet inhibition.

In any patient in whom the diagnosis of unstable coronary syndrome is considered, aspirin therapy (75–325 mg/day) should be instituted immediately. Patients with aspirin allergy or intolerance may be treated with clopidogrel (75 mg/day). For the subset of patients with refractory symptoms, ST-segment depression, or abnormal cardiac marker determinations and patients in whom percutaneous therapy is planned, a GP IIb/IIIa inhibitor should be added to the medical regimen. GP IIb/IIIa inhibitor therapy may be continued until a treatment strategy has been defined or through the period of revascularization if percutaneous therapy is chosen.

References

1. Falk E: Coronary thrombosis: Pathogenesis and clinical manifestations. Am J Cardiol 68:28B–35B, 1991.
2. Folts JD, Crowell EB Jr, Rowe GG: Platelet aggregation in partially obstructed vessels and its elimination with aspirin. Circulation 54:365–370, 1976.
3. Fuster V, Badimon L, Badimon JJ, Chesebro JH: The pathogenesis of coronary artery disease and the acute coronary syndromes (2). N Engl J Med 326:310–318, 1992.
4. Fuster V: Coronary thrombolysis—a perspective for the practicing physician [editorial]. N Engl J Med 329:723–725, 1993.
5. DeWood MA, Spores J, Notske R, et al: Prevalence of total coronary occlusion during the early hours of transmural myocardial infarction. N Engl J Med 303:897–902, 1980.
6. Willerson JT, Golino P, Eidt J, et al: Specific platelet mediators and unstable coronary artery lesions: Experimental evidence and potential clinical implications. Circulation 80:198–205, 1989.
7. Fuster V, Verstraete M: Hemostasis, thrombosis, fibrinolysis, and cardiovascular disease. In Braunwald E (ed): Heart Disease: A Textbook of Cardiovascular Medicine, 5th ed. Philadelphia, W.B. Saunders, 1997, pp 1809–1842.
8. Schafer AI: Antiplatelet therapy with glycoprotein IIb/IIIa receptor inhibitors and other novel agents. Tex Heart Inst J 24:90–96, 1997.
9. Becker RC, Bovill EG, Corrao JM, et al: Platelet activation determined by flow cytometry persists despite antithrombotic therapy in patients with unstable angina and non–Q-wave myocardial infarction. J Thromb Thrombol 1:95–100, 1994.

10. Herbert JM, Tissinier A, Defreyn G, Maffrand JP: Inhibitory effect of clopidogrel on platelet adhesion and intimal proliferation after arterial injury in rabbits. Arterioscler Thromb 13:1171–1179, 1993.
11. Folts JD, Schafer AI, Loscalzo J, et al: A perspective on the potential problems with aspirin as an antithrombotic agent: A comparison of studies in an animal model with clinical trials. J Am Coll Cardiol 33:295–303, 1999.
12. Patrono C: Aspirin as an antiplatelet drug. N Engl J Med 330:1287–1294, 1994.
13. FitzGerald GA, Brash AR, Oates JA, Pedersen AK: Endogenous prostacyclin biosynthesis and platelet function during selective inhibition of thromboxane synthase in man. J Clin Invest 72:1336–1343, 1983.
14. FitzGerald GA, Maas RL, Lawson JA, et al: Aspirin inhibits endogenous prostacyclin and thromboxane biosynthesis in man. Adv Prostaglandin Thromboxane Leukot Res 11:265–266, 1983.
15. Dabaghi SF, Kamat SG, Payne J, et al: Effects of low-dose aspirin on in vitro platelet aggregation in the early minutes after ingestion in normal subjects. Am J Cardiol 74:720–723, 1994.
16. Feldman M, Cryer B: Aspirin absorption rates and platelet inhibition times with 325-mg buffered aspirin tablets (chewed or swallowed intact) and with buffered aspirin solution. Am J Cardiol 84:404–409, 1999.
17. Patrignani P, Filabozzi P, Patrono C: Selective cumulative inhibition of platelet thromboxane production by low-dose aspirin in healthy subjects. J Clin Invest 69:1366–1372, 1982.
18. Lewis HD Jr, Davis JW, Archibald DG, et al: Protective effects of aspirin against acute myocardial infarction and death in men with unstable angina: Results of a Veterans Administration Cooperative Study. N Engl J Med 309:396–403, 1983.
19. Cairns JA, Gent M, Singer J, et al: Aspirin, sulfinpyrazone, or both in unstable angina: Results of a Canadian multicenter trial. N Engl J Med 313:1369–1375, 1985.
20. Antiplatelet Trialists' Collaboration: Collaborative overview of randomised trials of antiplatelet therapy. I: Prevention of death, myocardial infarction, and stroke by prolonged antiplatelet therapy in various categories of patients. BMJ 308:81–106, 1994 [published erratum appears in BMJ 308:1540, 1994].
21. Williams DO, Kirby MG, McPherson K, Phear DN: Anticoagulant treatment of unstable angina. Br J Clin Pract 1986;40:114–116.
22. Theroux P, Ouimet H, McCans J, et al: Aspirin, heparin, or both to treat acute unstable angina [see comments]. N Engl J Med 319:1105–1111, 1998.
23. Theroux P, Waters D, Lam J, et al: Reactivation of unstable angina after the discontinuation of heparin. N Engl J Med 327:141–145, 1992.
24. Theroux P, Waters D, Qiu S, et al: Aspirin versus heparin to prevent myocardial infarction during the acute phase of unstable angina. Circulation 88:2045–2048, 1993.
25. RISC Group: Risk of myocardial infarction and death during treatment with low dose aspirin and intravenous heparin in men with unstable coronary artery disease. Lancet 336:827–830, 1990.
26. Cohen M, Adams PC, Parry G, et al: Combination antithrombotic therapy in unstable rest angina and non–Q- wave infarction in nonprior aspirin users. Primary end points analysis from the ATACS trial. Antithrombotic Therapy in Acute Coronary Syndromes Research Group. Circulation 89:81–88, 1994.
27. Eikelboom JW, Anand SS, Malmberg K, et al: Unfractionated heparin and low-molecular-weight heparin in acute coronary syndrome without ST elevation: A meta-analysis. Lancet 355:1936–1942, 2000.
28. Kaul S, Shah PK: Low molecular weight heparin in acute coronary syndrome: Evidence for superior or equivalent efficacy compared with unfractionated heparin? J Am Coll Cardiol 35:1699–1712, 2000.
29. Mruk JS, Zoldhelyi P, Webster MW, et al: Does antithrombotic therapy influence residual thrombus after thrombolysis of platelet-rich thrombus? Effects of recombinant hirudin, heparin, or aspirin. Circulation 93:792–799, 1996.
30. Randomized trial of intravenous streptokinase, oral aspirin, both, or neither among 17,187 cases of suspected acute myocardial infarction: ISIS-2. ISIS-2 (Second International Study of Infarct Survival) Collaborative Group. J Am Coll Cardiol 12:3A–13A, 1998.
31. Baigent C, Collins R, Appleby P, et al: ISIS-2: 10 year survival among patients with suspected acute myocardial infarction in randomised comparison of intravenous streptokinase, oral aspirin, both, or neither. The ISIS-2 (Second International Study of Infarct Survival) Collaborative Group. BMJ 316:1337–1343, 1998.
32. Hsia J, Hamilton WP, Kleiman N, et al: A comparison between heparin and low-dose aspirin as adjunctive therapy with tissue plasminogen activator for acute myocardial infarction. Heparin-Aspirin Reperfusion Trial (HART) Investigators. N Engl J Med 323:1433–1437, 1990.

33. Guslandi M: Gastric toxicity of antiplatelet therapy with low-dose aspirin. Drugs 53:1–5, 1997.
34. Hirsh J, Dalen JE, Fuster V, et al: Aspirin and other platelet-active drugs. The relationship between dose, effectiveness, and side effects. Chest 102:327S–336S, 1992.
35. Wallentin LC: Aspirin (75 mg/day) after an episode of unstable coronary artery disease: Long-term effects on the risk for myocardial infarction, occurrence of severe angina and the need for revascularization. Research Group on Instability in Coronary Artery Disease in Southeast Sweden. J Am Coll Cardiol 18:1587–1593, 1991.
36. Swedish Aspirin Low-Dose Trial (SALT) of 75 mg aspirin as secondary prophylaxis after cerebrovascular ischaemic events. The SALT Collaborative Group. Lancet 338:1345–1349, 1991.
37. Juul-Moller S, Edvardsson N, Jahnmatz B, et al: Double-blind trial of aspirin in primary prevention of myocardial infarction in patients with stable chronic angina pectoris. The Swedish Angina Pectoris Aspirin Trial (SAPAT) Group. Lancet 340:1421–1425, 1992.
38. Patrono C, Ciabattoni G, Pinca E, et al: Low dose aspirin and inhibition of thromboxane B_2 production in healthy subjects. Thromb Res17:317–327, 1980.
39. Hoffman W, Forster W: Two year Cottbus reinfarction study with 30 mg aspirin per day. Prostaglandins Leukot Essent Fatty Acids 44:159–169, 1991.
40. Koudstaal PJ, Algra A, Pop GA, et al: Risk of cardiac events in atypical transient ischaemic attack or minor stroke. The Dutch TIA Study Group. Lancet 340:630–633, 1992.
41. Spaulding C, Charbonnier B, Cohen-Solal A, et al: Acute hemodynamic interaction of aspirin and ticlopidine with enalapril: Results of a double-blind, randomized comparative trial. Circulation 98:757–765, 1998.
42. Leor J, Reicher-Reiss H, Goldbourt U, et al: Aspirin and mortality in patients treated with angiotensin-converting enzyme inhibitors: A cohort study of 11,575 patients with coronary artery disease. J Am Coll Cardiol 33:1920–1925, 1999.
43. Latini R, Tognoni G, Maggioni AP, et al: Clinical effects of early angiotensin-converting enzyme inhibitor treatment for acute myocardial infarction are similar in the presence and absence of aspirin: Systematic overview of individual data from 96,712 randomized patients. J Am Coll Cardiol 35:1801–1807, 2000.
44. Hass WK, Easton JD: Changing concepts of the pathophysiology of cerebral myocardial infarction. In Hass WK, Easton JD (eds): Ticlopidine, Platelets and Vascular Disease. New York, Springer-Verlag, 1993, pp 1–12.
45. Saltiel E, Ward A: Ticlopidine: A review of its pharmacodynamic and pharmacokinetic properties, and therapeutic efficacy in platelet-dependent disease states. Drugs 34:222–262, 1987.
46. Di Minno G, Cerbone AM, Mattioli PL, et al: Functionally thrombasthenic state in normal platelets following the administration of ticlopidine. J Clin Invest 75:328–338, 1985.
47. Cattaneo M, Lombardi R, Bettega D, et al: Shear-induced platelet aggregation is potentiated by desmopressin and inhibited by ticlopidine. Arterioscler Thromb 13:393–397, 1993.
48. Roald HE, Barstad RM, Kierulf P, et al: Clopidogrel—a platelet inhibitor which inhibits thrombogenesis in non-anticoagulated human blood independently of the blood flow conditions. Thromb Haemost 71:655–662, 1994.
49. Coukell AJ, Markham A: Clopidogrel. Drugs 54:745–750, 1997; discussion, 751.
50. Knudsen JB, Kjoller E, Skagen K, Gormsen J: The effect of ticlopidine on platelet functions in acute myocardial infarction. A double-blind, controlled trial. Thromb Haemost 53:332–336, 1985.
51. Balsano F, Rizzon P, Violi F, et al: Antiplatelet treatment with ticlopidine in unstable angina: A controlled multicenter clinical trial. Studio della Ticlopidina nell'Angina Instabile Group. Circulation 82:17–26, 1990.
52. Scrutinio D, Lagioia R, Rizzon P: Ticlopidine treatment for patients with unstable angina at rest. A further analysis of the study of ticlopidine in unstable angina. Studio della Ticlopidina nell'Angina Instabile Group. Eur Heart J 12(Suppl G):27–29, 1991.
53. Bennett CL, Weinberg PD, Rozenberg-Ben-Dror K, et al: Thrombotic thrombocytopenic purpura associated with ticlopidine: A review of 60 cases. Ann Intern Med 128:541–544, 1998.
54. Savcic M, Hauert J, Bachmann F, et al: Clopidogrel loading dose regimens: Kinetic profile of pharmacodynamic response in healthy subjects. Semin Thromb Hemost 25:15–19, 1999.
55. CAPRIE Steering Committee: A randomised, blinded, trial of clopidogrel versus aspirin in patients at risk of ischaemic events (CAPRIE). Lancet 348:1329–1339, 1996.
56. Gent M: Benefit of clopidogrel in patients with coronary disease [abstract]. Circulation 96:I–467, 1997.
57. Bassand JP, Cariou R, Grollier G, et al: Clopidogrel-rt-PA-heparin combination in the treatment of acute myocardial infarction. Semin Thromb Hemost 25:69–75, 1999.
58. Bennett CL, Connors JM, Carwile JM, et al: Thrombotic thrombocytopenic purpura associated with clopidogrel. N Engl J Med 342:1773–1777, 2000.
59. Du XP, Plow EF, Frelinger ALD, et al: Ligands "activate" integrin alpha IIb beta 3 (platelet GPIIb-IIIa). Cell 65:409–416, 1991.

60. Faulds D, Sorkin EM: Abciximab (c7E3 Fab). A review of its pharmacology and therapeutic potential in ischaemic heart disease. Drugs 48:583–598, 1994.

61. Bhattacharya S, Weisman H, Morris K, et al: Chimerization of monoclonal antibody 7E3 preserves the GP IIb/IIIa receptor-blockade and platelet functional inhibition of murine 7E3 [abstract]. Clin Res 39:196A, 1991.

62. Kleiman NS, Raizner AE, Jordan R, et al: Differential inhibition of platelet aggregation induced by adenosine diphosphate or a thrombin receptor-activating peptide in patients treated with bolus chimeric 7E3 Fab: Implications for inhibition of the internal pool of GPIIb/IIIa receptors. J Am Coll Cardiol 26:1665–1671, 1995.

63. Mascelli MA, Lance ET, Damaraju L, et al: Pharmacodynamic profile of short-term abciximab treatment demonstrates prolonged platelet inhibition with gradual recovery from GP IIb/IIIa receptor blockade. Circulation 97:1680–1688, 1998.

64. EPIC Investigation: Use of a monoclonal antibody directed against the platelet glycoprotein IIb/IIIa receptor in high-risk coronary angioplasty. N Engl J Med 330:956–961, 1994.

65. Lincoff AM, Califf RM, Anderson KM, et al: Evidence for prevention of death and myocardial infarction with platelet membrane glycoprotein IIb/IIIa receptor blockade by abciximab (c7E3 Fab) among patients with unstable angina undergoing percutaneous coronary revascularization. EPIC Investigators. Evaluation of 7E3 in Preventing Ischemic Complications. J Am Coll Cardiol 30:149–156, 1997.

66. Lefkovits J, Ivanhoe RJ, Califf RM, et al: Effects of platelet glycoprotein IIb/IIIa receptor blockade by a chimeric monoclonal antibody (abciximab) on acute and six-month outcomes after percutaneous transluminal coronary angioplasty for acute myocardial infarction. EPIC investigators. Am J Cardiol 77:1045–1051, 1996.

67. EPILOG Investigators: Platelet glycoprotein IIb/IIIa receptor blockade and low-dose heparin during percutaneous coronary revascularization. N Engl J Med 336:1689–1696, 1997.

68. EPISTENT Investigators: Randomised placebo-controlled and balloon-angioplasty-controlled trial to assess safety of coronary stenting with use of platelet glycoprotein-IIb/IIIa blockade. Evaluation of Platelet IIb/IIIa Inhibitor for Stenting [see comments]. Lancet 352:87–92, 1998.

69. Simoons ML, de Boer MJ, van den Brand MJ, et al: Randomized trial of a GPIIb/IIIa platelet receptor blocker in refractory unstable angina. European Cooperative Study Group. Circulation 89:596–603, 1994.

70. Randomised placebo-controlled trial of abciximab before and during coronary intervention in refractory unstable angina: the CAPTURE Study [published erratum appears in Lancet 1997 Sep 6;350(9079):744]. Lancet. 1997;349:1429–1435.

71. Hamm CW, Heeschen C, Goldmann B, et al: Benefit of abciximab in patients with refractory unstable angina in relation to serum troponin T levels. c7E3 Fab Antiplatelet Therapy in Unstable Refractory Angina (CAPTURE) Study Investigators. N Engl J Med 340:1623–1629, 1999.

72. Brener SJ, Barr LA, Burchenal JE, et al: Randomized, placebo-controlled trial of platelet glycoprotein IIb/IIIa blockade with primary angioplasty for acute myocardial infarction. ReoPro and Primary PTCA Organization and Randomized Trial (RAPPORT) Investigators. Circulation 98:734–741, 1998.

73. Montalescot G: ADMIRAL: Abciximab with PTCA and stent in acute myocardial infarction. Presented at the 48th Annual Scientific Session of the American College of Cardiology, New Orleans, 1999.

74. Thrombolysis in Myocardial Infarction (TIMI) Trial: Phase I findings. TIMI Study Group. N Engl J Med 312:932–936, 1985.

75. GUSTO Investigators: An international randomized trial comparing four thrombolytic strategies for acute myocardial infarction. N Engl J Med 329:673–682, 1993.

76. Bode C, Smalling RW, Berg G, et al: Randomized comparison of coronary thrombolysis achieved with double-bolus reteplase (recombinant plasminogen activator) and front-loaded, accelerated alteplase (recombinant tissue plasminogen activator) in patients with acute myocardial infarction. RAPID II Investigators. Circulation 94:891–898, 1996.

77. Verheugt FW, Meijer A, Lagrand WK, Van Eenige MJ: Reocclusion: The flip side of coronary thrombolysis. J Am Coll Cardiol 27:766–773, 1996.

78. Meijer A, Verheugt FW, Werter CJ, ete al: Aspirin versus coumadin in the prevention of reocclusion and recurrent ischemia after successful thrombolysis: A prospective placebo-controlled angiographic study. Results of the APRICOT Study. Circulation 87:1524–1530, 1993.

79. Moliterno DJ, Topol EJ: Conjunctive use of platelet glycoprotein IIb/IIIa antagonists and thrombolytic therapy for acute myocardial infarction. Thromb Haemost 78:214–219, 1997.

80. Coller BS: Platelets and thrombolytic therapy. N Engl J Med 322:33–42, 1990.

81. Kleiman NS, Ohman EM, Califf RM, et al: Profound inhibition of platelet aggregation with monoclonal antibody 7E3 Fab after thrombolytic therapy: Results of the Thrombolysis and Angioplasty in Myocardial Infarction (TAMI) 8 Pilot Study. J Am Coll Cardiol 22:381–389, 1993.

82. Trial of abciximab with and without low-dose reteplase for acute myocardial infarction. Circulation 101:2788–2794, 2000.

83. de Lemos JA, Antman EM, Gibson CM, et al: Abciximab improves both epicardial flow and myocardial reperfusion in ST-elevation myocardial infarction. Observations from the TIMI 14 trial. Circulation 101:239–243, 2000.

84. Scarborough RM, Kleiman NS, Phillips DR: Platelet glycoprotein IIb/IIIa antagonists: What are the relevant issues concerning their pharmacology and clinical use? Circulation 100:437–444, 1999.

85. Harrington RA, Kleiman NS, Kottke-Marchant K, et al: Immediate and reversible platelet inhibition after intravenous administration of a peptide glycoprotein IIb/IIIa inhibitor during percutaneous coronary intervention. Am J Cardiol 76:1222–1227, 1995.

86. Schulman SP, Goldschmidt-Clermont PJ, Topol EJ, et al: Effects of integrelin, a platelet glycoprotein IIb/IIIa receptor antagonist, in unstable angina: A randomized multicenter trial. Circulation 94:2083–2089, 1996.

87. PURSUIT Trial Investigators: Inhibition of platelet glycoprotein IIb/IIIa with eptifibatide in patients with acute coronary syndromes. Platelet Glycoprotein IIb/IIIa in Unstable Angina: Receptor Suppression Using Integrilin Therapy. N Engl J Med 339:436–443, 1998.

88. Kleiman NS, Lincoff AM, Flaker GC, et al: Early percutaneous coronary intervention, platelet inhibition with eptifibatide, and clinical outcomes in patients with acute coronary syndromes. PURSUIT Investigators. Circulation 101:751–757, 2000.

89. Ohman EM, Kleiman NS, Gacioch G, et al: Combined accelerated tissue-plasminogen activator and platelet glycoprotein IIb/IIIa integrin receptor blockade with Integrilin in acute myocardial infarction: Results of a randomized, placebo-controlled, dose-ranging trial. IMPACT-AMI Investigators. Circulation 95:846–854, 1997.

90. Simes RJ, Topol EJ, Holmes DR Jr, et al: Link between the angiographic substudy and mortality outcomes in a large randomized trial of myocardial reperfusion. Importance of early and complete infarct artery reperfusion. GUSTO-I Investigators. Circulation 91:1923–1928, 1995.

91. Peerlinck K, De Lepeleire I, Goldberg M, et al: MK-383 (L-700,462), a selective nonpeptide platelet glycoprotein IIb/IIIa antagonist, is active in man. Circulation 88:1512–1517, 1993.

92. Kereiakes DJ, Kleiman NS, Ambrose J, et al: Randomized, double-blind, placebo-controlled dose-ranging study of tirofiban (MK-383) platelet IIb/IIIa blockade in high risk patients undergoing coronary angioplasty. J Am Coll Cardiol 27:536–542, 1996.

93. PRISM Investigators: A comparison of aspirin plus tirofiban with aspirin plus heparin for unstable angina. Platelet Receptor Inhibition in Ischemic Syndrome Management Study. N Engl J Med 338:1498–1505, 1998.

94. PRISM-PLUS Investigators: Inhibition of the platelet glycoprotein IIb/IIIa receptor with tirofiban in unstable angina and non–Q-wave myocardial infarction. Platelet Receptor Inhibition in Ischemic Syndrome Management in Patients Limited by Unstable Signs and Symptoms Study. N Engl J Med 338:1488–1497, 1998 [published erratum appears in N Engl J Med 339:415, 1998].

95. RESTORE Investigators: Effects of platelet glycoprotein IIb/IIIa blockade with tirofiban on adverse cardiac events in patients with unstable angina or acute myocardial infarction undergoing coronary angioplasty. Randomized Efficacy Study of Tirofiban for Outcomes and REstenosis. Circulation. 96:1445–1453, 1997.

96. Theroux P, Kouz S, Roy L, et al: Platelet membrane receptor glycoprotein IIb/IIIa antagonism in unstable angina. The Canadian Lamifiban Study. Circulation 94:899–905, 1996.

97. PARAGON Investigators: International, randomized, controlled trial of lamifiban (a platelet glycoprotein IIb/IIIa inhibitor), heparin, or both in unstable angina. Platelet IIb/IIIa Antagonism for the Reduction of Acute coronary syndrome events in a Global Organization Network. Circulation 97:2386–2395, 1998.

98. PARADIGM Investigators: Combining thrombolysis with the platelet glycoprotein IIb/IIIa inhibitor lamifiban: Results of the Platelet Aggregation Receptor Antagonist Dose Investigation and Reperfusion Gain in Myocardial Infarction (PARADIGM) trial. J Am Coll Cardiol 32:2003–2010, 1998.

99. O'Neill WW, Serruys P, Knudtson M, et al: Long-term treatment with a platelet glycoprotein-receptor antagonist after percutaneous coronary revascularization. EXCITE Trial Investigators. Evaluation of Oral Xemilofiban in Controlling Thrombotic Events. N Engl J Med 342:1316–1324, 2000.

100. Cannon CP, McCabe CH, Borzak S, et al: Randomized trial of an oral platelet glycoprotein IIb/IIIa antagonist, sibrafiban, in patients after an acute coronary syndrome: Results of the TIMI 12 trial. Thrombolysis in Myocardial Infarction. Circulation 97:340–349, 1998.

101. Newby LK: Long-term oral platelet glycoprotein IIb/IIIa receptor antagonism with sibrafiban after acute coronary syndromes: Study design of the sibrafiban versus aspirin to yield maximum protection from ischemic heart events post-acute coronary syndromes (SYMPHONY) trial. Symphony Steering Committee. Am Heart J 138:210–218, 1999.

102. SYMPHONY Investigators: Comparison of sibrafiban with aspirin for prevention of cardio-vascular events after acute coronary syndromes: A randomised trial. Sibrafiban versus Aspirin to Yield Maximum Protection from Ischemic Heart Events Post-acute Coronary Syndromes. Lancet 355:337–345, 2000.

103. Newby K: A randomized comparison of sibrafiban, an oral glycoprotein IIb/IIIa antagonist, with and without aspirin versus aspirin after acute coronary syndromes: Results of the 2nd SYMPHONY trial. Anaheim, CA, American College of Cardiology, 2000.

104. Cannon CP, McCabe CH, Wilcox RG, et al: Oral glycoprotein IIb/IIIa inhibition with or-bofiban in patients with unstable coronary syndromes (OPUS-TIMI 16) trial. Circulation 102:149–156, 2000.

105. Ferguson JJ, Kereiakes DJ, Adgey AA, et al: Safe use of platelet GP IIb/IIIa inhibitors. Eur Heart J 19 Suppl D:D40–D51, 1998.

106. Tcheng JE, Kereiakes DJ, Braden GA, et al: Readministration of abciximab: Interim report of the ReoPro readministration registry. Am Heart J 138:S33–S38, 1999.

107. Dawicki DD, Agarwal KC, Parks RE Jr: Potentiation of the antiplatelet action of adenosine in whole blood by dipyridamole or dilazep and the cAMP phosphodiesterase inhibitor, RA 233. Thromb Res 43:161–175, 1986.

108. Edlund A, Siden A, Sollevi A: Evidence for an anti-aggregatory effect of adenosine at physio-logical concentrations and for its role in the action of dipyridamole. Thromb Res 45:183–190, 1987.

109. Bult H, Fret HR, Jordaens FH, Herman AG: Dipyridamole potentiates platelet inhibition by nitric oxide. Thromb Haemost 66:343–349, 1991.

110. Persantine-Aspirin Reinfarction Study Research Group: Persantine and aspirin in coronary heart disease. Circulation 62:449–461, 1980.

111. Schafer AI: Antiplatelet therapy. Am J Med 101:199–209, 1996.

112. FitzGerald GA: Dipyridamole. N Engl J Med 316:1247–1257, 1987.

113. Boersma E, Akkerhuis KM, Theroux P, et al: Platelet glycoprotein IIb/IIIa receptor inhibition in non-ST-elevation acute coronary syndromes: Early benefit during medical treatment only, with additional protection during percutaneous coronary intervention. Circulation 100: 2045–2048, 1999.

114. Collaborative overview of randomised trials of antiplatelet therapy. II: Maintenance of vascu-lar graft or arterial patency by antiplatelet therapy. Antiplatelet Trialists' Collaboration. BMJ 308:159–168, 1994

115. Antman EM, Giugliano RP, Gibson CM, et al: Abciximab facilitates the rate and extent of thrombolysis: Results of the thrombolysis in myocardial infarction (TIMI) 14 trial. The TIMI 14 Investigators. Circulation 99:2720–2732, 1999.

116. Roe MT, Sapp SK, Lincoff AM: Glycoprotein IIb/IIIa inhibitors in acute coronary syndromes. Cleve Clin J Med 67:131–140, 2000.

Heparin in Acute Coronary Syndromes

DIANE E. WALLIS, MD

JOSEPH HARTMANN, MD

Heparin has been a mainstay of therapy for acute coronary syndromes in clinical practice for the past few decades. The widespread use of heparin for myocardial ischemia and infarction is increasingly challenged by the development of newer anticoagulants. To understand better why there is so much interest in replacing heparin, it is important to review the historical context of heparin, which paralleled the understanding of the pathophysiology of acute coronary syndromes. This chapter examines the mechanisms of action of heparin, including the growing understanding of the importance of the relationship between drug efficacy, tissue factor pathway inhibitor, and von Willebrand factor. Clinical studies investigating heparin and low-molecular-weight heparin in unstable angina, non–Q-wave myocardial infarction, and transmural myocardial infarction are discussed. Understanding the disadvantages of heparin, including heparin rebound and heparin-induced thrombocytopenia, hopefully paves the way to understanding the search for a "better" anticoagulant, particularly in acute coronary syndromes.

The History of Heparin

Jay McLean, a second-year medical student at Johns Hopkins University, uncovered an endogenous anticoagulant while trying to isolate procoagulants in the laboratory of W. H. Howell in 1916.[1] This singular discovery changed the direction of cardiovascular medicine and offset the turmoil and disappointments that the discoverer of heparin faced throughout his life. McLean lost his physician father when he was four years of age. The family home and all accumulated assets were lost in the San Francisco earthquake in 1906, when he was fifteen. Denied financial support for college and medical school from his stepfather, he was forced to leave college for 15 months while he worked in a Mojave Desert gold mine. Any spare time at school was spent working in various part-time jobs, including analyzing blood and urine samples in a college infirmary, working in a museum of invertebrate zoology, scrubbing ferry boat decks, clerking in railroad mail cars, and working in oil fields. After completing the first year of medical school at the University of California at Berkeley in 1914, McLean left for Baltimore, despite being rejected for admission to Johns Hopkins Medical School. Later McLean remarked ruefully that the dean's letter stated that he was "not the kind of man Hopkins sought." By happenstance, he was informed on the day after his arrival in Baltimore of an unexpected vacancy in the second-year medical school class, and he was admitted.[2]

Wishing to devote a year to physiologic research, he approached Howell, a well-known physiologist at Hopkins, who assigned him a research project to determine what element of a crude brain extract had coagulant or "thromboplastic" activity. Testing the purity of this thromboplastic substance, known as "cephalin," involved the malodorous process of macerating brain tissue, spreading it on glass panes, and drying it in a gas-flame oven. The material was extracted with ether and precipitated with alcohol. McLean found that hearts and livers contained larger amounts of cephalin than brain and also noted that the extract degraded over time from contact with air. While determining whether these degraded substances still had thromboplastic activity, McLean observed that two phosphatides, "heparphosphatide" and "cuorin" (named by their origin from the ox heart and lung), retarded coagulation. Presenting the data to his initially skeptical preceptor, he was admonished not to include this observation in his paper until more careful studies were done.[2] Thus, there was no discussion of the discovery and how it related to theories of coagulation that were in vogue at that time. McLean managed to squeeze in three sentences as an aside, including the statements, "The heparphosphatide ... when purified by many precipitations in alcohol at 60 degrees has no thromboplastic action and in fact shows a marked power to inhibit the coagulation. The anticoagulating action of this phosphatide is being studied and will be reported on later."[1]

Unfortunately, there was no "later" for McLean. After a rather undistinguished clinical career in which he moved through surgery, pathology, radiology and oncology-based practices, the final years of his life were spent trying to obtain recognition for his role in the discovery of heparin. He died before this was achieved.[3-7] Howell continued to work on the purification of this substance, coining the name "heparin" in 1918 from the phosphatides, *hepar*phosphatide and cuor*in*, in which it was first isolated.[8]

The first clinical use of heparin was short-lived, marred by severe systemic reactions related to the primitive purification process when it was used in transfusing human blood in 1924. In addition, the clinical use of heparin was limited by expense and low potency. The original bottles of crystalline sodium salt heparin, prepared from dog livers by the laboratory supplier Hynson, Wescott, and Dunning, used Howell's original method and had a potency of only 5 units/mg. One unit of heparin was defined as the amount needed to prevent the coagulation of 5 ml of cat's blood. Charles H. Best in Toronto, the discoverer of insulin, needed purified heparin for experiments involving histamine that were hampered by the clotting of arterial cannulas needed to measure continuous arterial pressure.[3,9,10] Best, who was also assistant director of Connaught Laboratories in Toronto, was intimately involved with the preparation of insulin and liver extract for administration to humans. Seeing a similar advance in the use of heparin, he was able to interest a young organic chemist, Arthur F. Charles, and his colleague, David Scott, to devise a commercially practical method using more readily procurable sources from ox lung or porcine intestine. The difficulties in the purification of heparin are underscored by a researcher who reported that it took 80 kg of pig intestinal slime to be distilled into 112 mg of heparin, which had the anticoagulant activity of 56 units/mg.[11]

Refinements in the processing of heparin led to increasing potency, and when 1 mg of a new crystalline barium salt preparation was found to anticoagulate 110 ml of blood, the batch was labeled as 100 units/mg of heparin for simplicity in calculation, a standard that is still used today. The United States Pharmacopoeia now defines one USP unit of heparin as that which will prevent 1 ml of citrated sheep's plasma from clotting for 1 hour after the addition of a calcium chloride solution.[10]

Clinical trials involving heparin began concurrently in 1935 in Stockholm and Toronto. Surgeon Clarence Craaford was the first to report on the efficacy of heparin in the prevention of postoperative thrombosis and embolism in 1937. Toronto surgeon Gordon Murray reported the efficacy of heparin in preventing thrombosis one year later in 1938.[12-14] Charles A. Lindbergh, the pilot of the Spirit of St. Louis, had been working for several years on a mechanical heart pump in the laboratory of the Nobel Laureate Alexis Carrel at the Rockefeller Institute. His experiments became successful only after heparin from the Connaught Laboratories was made available.[11,15] Protamine was discovered inadvertently in 1937 during experiments designed to prolong the effects of insulin. The ability to reverse its anticoagulant action also paved the way to the clinical use of heparin.[6]

The History of Heparin for Acute Coronary Syndromes

Russian physicians W. P. Obrastzow and N.D. Straschesko published the first paper describing the typical clinical features of acute myocardial infarction in an obscure German journal of clinical medicine in 1910. Chicago physician James Herrick, however, is given the credit for convincing the English-speaking medical community that coronary thrombosis was not invariably fatal and could be recognized during life. His 1912 paper, "Certain Clinical Features of Sudden Obstruction of the Coronary Arteries," provided a detailed explanation for the spectrum of symptoms in acute coronary syndromes. By the 1920s it was generally accepted that sudden thrombotic occlusion of a diseased coronary artery was the triggering event.[16]

Almost immediately after heparin and dicoumarol became available to the medical community, the possibility of their use in the treatment of coronary thrombosis was considered. The initial use in acute coronary syndromes was with coumarin anticoagulation for the prophylaxis of thromboembolism following myocardial infarction. This was not an insignificant problem, given the common practice of prolonged bed rest at that time.[10] In 1938, Charles Best and another Canadian physiologist, Donald Solandt, described an experimental method of preventing canine coronary artery thrombosis with highly purified heparin and proposed the need for clinical studies to begin investigating the efficacy of heparin in myocardial infarction.[17]

In 1945, McLean made a prophetic statement on a nationwide radio program, *The Doctors Talk It Over*. The transcript of the broadcast was entitled "The Evidence for the Use of Heparin in Acute Coronary Thrombosis," by Jay McLean, M.D., Associate Professor of Research Surgery, Ohio State University and "Discoverer of Heparin." When asked to summarize the use of heparin, McLean stated, "The true evaluation of heparin in acute coronary occlusion must, of course, wait upon the results of clinical findings ... we know that it has the power to prevent the formation of clots ... we know that it can prevent a clot, once formed, from growing larger ... and it is reasonable to suppose that it has the effect of dissolving a fresh clot ... we can say that here heparin may prove of great value."[7,14]

Paul Wood was the first to report on the use of anticoagulation in 10 cases of "angina at rest" at the December, 1948, meeting of the Medical Society of London. Nichols, however, has been credited with the first paper (written in 1950) about the use of anticoagulants in the prevention of myocardial infarction in patients with unstable angina. Nichols and associates began treating their private patients with unstable angina with heparin for 1 week before beginning oral anticoagulation, stating that "relief of pain was often striking, coincident with full heparinization."[18] In a follow-up study, they reported their experience in 313 patients with unstable angina, describing a 6.3% rate of myocardial infarction vs. 60% in patients who abandoned anticoagulation before 60 days of therapy.[19] These observations were followed by multiple observational reports, leading to the belief of some that heparin's benefit was so evident that placebo-controlled randomized trials were unethical (P.J. Scanlon, personal communication). In 1981, Mitchell made a plea for "strict verification" by properly designed prospective trials.[20] Almost an entire generation had passed from the first use of heparin for acute coronary syndromes to the first randomized trial of heparin in patients with unstable angina in 1988.[21]

Heparin: Mechanism of Action

Pathophysiology of Acute Ischemic Syndromes

Disrupted atherosclerotic plaques are found beneath 75% of the thrombi responsible for acute coronary syndromes.[22,23] Following plaque rupture, thrombogenic components, such as collagen, lipids, macrophages, tissue factor, and surface-bound von Willebrand factor, are exposed to blood, leading to activation of the extrinsic pathway of the coagulation system.[24] Abundant stores of tissue factor are found in the lipid-rich core, as evidenced by high concentrations of tissue factor antigen and activity within atherectomy specimens in patients with acute coronary syndromes.[25,26] Tissue factor activates factor VII, forming a complex that leads to the formation of factor Xa.[27] Tissue factor pathway inhibitor, a potent protease inhibitor produced by healthy endothelial cells, scavenges this complex of factor Xa, factor VIIa, and tissue factor, leaving a reduced amount of activated factors to continue the coagulation process.[28,29] Ultimately, thrombin, or factor IIa, is produced to convert soluble fibrinogen into fibrin monomers and activates factor XIII to produce cross-linked fibrin. Thrombin promotes clot formation by activating factors V and VIII; promotes platelet adhesion, activation, and aggregation; and causes the release of the vasoconstrictor endothelin 1. Thrombin also potentiates the proliferative effects of multiple growth factors, including smooth muscle cells, that contribute to the formation of a platelet-rich thrombus.[30–32] Patients with clinically stable and unstable coronary artery disease and patients with acute myocardial infarction have evidence of increased thrombin activity and generation.[33–36] Depending on the extent of activation of coagulation and the degree of stasis in the affected artery, a fibrin and erythrocyte-rich thrombus may develop and propagate, leading to the clinical syndromes of angina, unstable angina, and non–Q-wave and Q-wave myocardial infarction.

Anticoagulant Action of Heparin

Heparin is a heterogeneous mucopolysaccharide made of alternating units of D-glucosamine and uronic acid, with an average molecular weight of 15,000 Daltons (range = 5,000–30,000 Daltons).[37] Heparin derives the majority of its anticoagulant activity from its interaction with antithrombin III (AT III), an endogenous thrombin inhibitor made in the liver.[38] A chain length of at least 18 saccharides is necessary to form a ternary complex of heparin, antithrombin III, and thrombin. A critical pentasaccharide sequence is required for the heparin fragment to attach to AT III, and an additional 13-saccharide sequence is required to allow the heparin fragment to attach itself simultaneously to the heparin-binding domain of thrombin. Approximately one-half of heparin molecules are ineffective as an anticoagulant, because no more than 30–50% have a saccharide chain of this length.[40]

By inducing a conformational change in AT III, heparin accelerates its ability to inactivate thrombin a thousand-fold, bringing thombin in close proximity to AT III.[41] The heparin-AT III complex binds avidly and reversibly to the active site of activated factors Xa, XIIa, XIa, and IXa and protein C (Fig. 1). Factor Xa inhibition is one-tenth that of thrombin inhibition, because it is protected by binding with a phospholipid complex.[37,41–43] Heparin effects independent of its anticoagulant activity include vessel wall permeability changes and the suppression of the proliferation of vascular smooth muscle cells, which also may contribute to antiischemic activity.[44,45]

The contribution of tissue factor to intravascular thrombotic events suggests that natural thromboresistance pathways, such as tissue factor pathway inhibitor, are extremely important.[46] Heparin-mediated tissue factor pathway inhibitor mobilization may be another important means to limit thrombosis.[47,48] Large quantities of tissue factor are exposed with vessel wall injury. Sandset et al. and others have demonstrated that tissue factor pathway inhibitor is released from vascular endothelial cells into the circulation after an intravenous or subcutaneous injection of either unfractionated or low-molecular-weight heparin.[47,49–51] Tissue factor pathway inhibitor released by heparin is not bound to lipoproteins and therefore is able to exert a strong anticoagulant effect.[52,53]

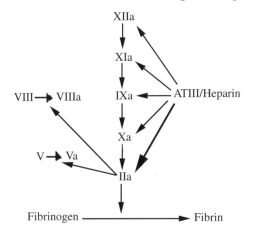

Figure 1. The heparin/antithrombin III (AT III) complex inactivates the coagulation enzymes factor XIIa, factor XIa, factor IXa, factor Xa, and thrombin (IIa). Thrombin and factor Xa are most sensitive to the effects of heparin/AT III.

Supplies of tissue factor pathway inhibitor appear to be limited, however. When tissue factor pathway inhibitor is depleted, unchecked coagulation may lead to propagation and the perpetuation of a coronary thrombosis.[54] In a study by Hanson et al., repeated injections of heparin at 4-hour intervals caused a progressive decrease in heparin-releasable tissue factor pathway inhibitor and a progressive shortening of the dilute prothrombin clotting time. During a 24-hour continuous infusion of heparin, tissue factor pathway inhibitor decreased by nearly 80% with a concomitant decrease in the contribution of tissue factor pathway inhibitor to the inhibition of tissue factor-mediated coagulation by heparin. These findings of a depletion of intravascular tissue factor pathway inhibitor by continuous unfractionated heparin administration may explain why heparin effectiveness decreases with the duration of administration.[55]

Pharmacokinetics of Heparin

Heparin can be administered both intravenously and subcutaneously. After subcutaneous injection, the anticoagulant effect is delayed for 1–2 hours, with peak levels at approximately 3 hours. High doses must be administered to compensate for reduced bioavailability.[56,57] The bioavailability of heparin is markedly enhanced by intravenous infusion, and an intravenous bolus is required for an immediate anticoagulant effect.[56] Heparin is cleared through a rapid saturable mechanism by the binding of heparin to receptors on endothelial cells and macrophages.[58] There is also a slower first-order mechanism of clearance due to renal elimination, and the biologic half-life of the drug can vary considerably. Thus, the anticoagulant action of heparin is not linear; both intensity and duration of anticoagulant effect increase with increasing doses.[58,59]

The anticoagulant effect of heparin is titrated by dividing the patient's activated partial thromboplastin time (aPTT) by the mean of the laboratory control aPTT to obtain a ratio of 1.5 to 2.5. Commercial activated partial thromboplastin time reagents vary considerably in responsiveness to heparin, according to their sensitivity. The reagents can be standardized by calibration against the heparin levels based on an anti-factor Xa chromogenic assay in a plasma system (therapeutic range = 0.3 –0.7 U/ml) or by protamine titration (therapeutic range = 0.2–0.4 U/ml). The chain length of the molecules influences the clearance of heparin; accumulation of the lower-molecular-weight species is due to slower clearance.[61]

Low-molecular-weight Heparin vs. Heparin

Preparations of low-molecular-weight heparin contain fewer than 18 saccharides but retain the critical pentasaccharide sequence to form a factor Xa–antithrombin III:heparin complex. The inactivation of factor Xa by heparin/AT III does not require ternary complex formation but is achieved solely through binding of heparin to AT III. Low-molecular-weight heparin has a reduced ratio of antithrombin to anti-factor Xa activity. The lower-weight species, measured in the anti-factor Xa assay, have a minimal effect on aPTT, which accounts for the differences observed between aPTT and heparin levels.[61] Advantages over heparin include enhanced anti-Xa activity, relative resistance to the neutralizing effect of platelet factor 4, ability to inhibit factor Xa located on platelet surfaces, inhibition of von Willebrand factor, and facilitation of tissue factor inhibitor release. Each low-molecular-weight heparin has a unique tissue factor pathway inhibitor release profile that is also distinct from its anti-Xa activity.[48]

Another important difference between low-molecular-weight heparin and unfractionated heparin may be their relative effects on von Willebrand factor, a heterogeneous plasma glycoprotein with two major functions:

1. It promotes platelet interaction with the damaged vessel wall under conditions of high shear stress by binding to the platelet glycoprotein Ib and IIb/IIIa receptors.

2. It is the carrier of factor VIII, an essential cofactor in the generation of factor Xa.

Binding of factor VIII to von Willebrand factor protects factor VIII from inactivation by activated protein C.[62] Von Willebrand factor also promotes platelet aggregation by cross-linking multiple activated platelets. Feedback loops promote the release of von Willebrand factor from the alpha granules of platelets and endothelial cells.[62] Also present in von Willebrand factor are heparin-binding sites, capable of inhibiting platelet interactions.[63,64] Thus, given its combined effects on platelet adhesion/aggregation and its procoagulant effect, von Willebrand factor plays an important role in thrombus formation and propagation,[30] as demonstrated by the findings that von Willebrand factor is an independent predictor of adverse clinical outcome at 14 and 30 days of follow-up in patients with unstable angina.[65]

The greater effect of low-molecular-weight heparins on von Willebrand factor may be important to their clinical benefits in acute coronary syndrome (see below). Enoxaparin has been shown to blunt the increase in von Willebrand factor compared with unfractionated heparin and may be more efficient than unfractionated heparin in binding to the heparin-binding domain of von Willebrand factor.[30] The results may be reduction in von Willebrand factor-dependent platelet adhesion and aggregation and release of less von Willebrand factor from platelet alpha granules. Alternatively, or in addition, the greater anti-Xa activity of enoxaparin compared with unfractionated heparin may result in less thrombin generation, which also may lead to less platelet activation and a reduction in release of von Willebrand factor from storage depots.[30]

Heparin in Unstable Angina

The natural history of unstable angina is quite bleak, with a reported 3-month myocardial infarction rate of 22–49% and a mortality rate of 16–24%.[66,67] Uncontrolled studies suggested that anticoagulation may improve the prognosis of unstable angina.[19,67] In 1980, Spokane cardiologist Marcus DeWood and his colleagues confirmed postmortem findings that thrombus was an important component of the ruptured plaque in 126 patients with acute coronary syndromes undergoing coronary angiography within 4 hours of the onset of symptoms. They reported an 87% angiographic prevalence of total coronary occlusion.[68,69] In 1981, one year after DeWood's landmark study, the first randomized, double-blind study investigating heparin in unstable angina was reported by Telford and Wilson.[70] Fifty-one patients with unstable angina received 7 days of 5,000 units of heparin every 8 hours and were compared with 54 patients on placebo and 60 patients on atenolol. An additional 49 patients received both heparin and atenolol. Heparin reduced death and myocardial infarction by 80% over 7 days—from 17% on placebo and 13% on atenolol to 2% on heparin and 4% on heparin and atenolol (p < 0.03). All five reported deaths occured in the non-heparin groups. Aspirin was not used. These results were not generally accepted because of concerns about study design and analysis.[71]

Heparin vs. Aspirin

The first study to conclusively demonstrate the benefit of heparin was done in 1988, when Theroux et al. randomized 479 patients with unstable angina to either intravenous heparin (5000-unit bolus followed by 1000 units/hour), aspirin (650-mg initial dose followed by 324 mg twice daily), or both.[72] Refractory angina was defined as the presence of recurrent anginal chest pain with ischemic ST-T changes on the electrocardiogram despite full medical therapy, including intravenous nitroglycerin plus beta or calcium channel blockade, or the need for urgent intervention (intraaortic balloon counterpulsaton, coronary angiography, angioplasty, or bypass surgery). This endpoint was reduced significantly with heparin (relative risk = 0.31; 95% confidence limits = 0.14–0.68; p = 0.002). Myocardial infarction was significantly reduced from 12% in the placebo group to 3% in the group receiving aspirin (p = 0.01), 0.8% in the group receiving heparin (p < 0.001), and 1.6% in the group receiving both aspirin and heparin (p = 0.003). Although death occurred in 1.7% of the placebo group, no deaths occurred in the active treatment groups. However, the study was underpowered to permit evaluation of the effect of treatment on this endpoint. The combination of aspirin and heparin had no greater protective effect than heparin alone but was associated with slightly more serious bleeding (3.3% vs. 1.7%). Overall, the addition of heparin to aspirin reduced the risk of myocardial infarction by 89% and refractory angina by 63%.[72]

In 1990, the RISC group reported a double-blind placebo-controlled trial in 945 men with unstable angina or non–Q-wave myocardial infarction. Patients were enrolled 1–3 days after admission and received aspirin, 75 mg/day for 3 or more months, and heparin, 5,000 units intravenously every 4 hours for the first 5 days. Aspirin reduced the risk of myocardial infarction and death at 5 days, 1 month, and 3 months (risk ratios = 0.43, 0.31, and 0.36, respectively). Heparin had no significant influence on event rate at 30- and 90- day follow-up, although the combined aspirin and heparin arm had the lowest number of events during the initial 5 days.[73]

The Montreal group reported a follow-up double-blind, randomized trial comparing aspirin (325 mg twice daily) and heparin (5,000 units intravenously followed by a constant infusion titrated to a partial thromboplastin time of 1.5–2.5 times control) in 484 patients with unstable angina. Fatal and nonfatal myocardial infarction occurred in 0.8% of heparin patients and 3.7% of aspirin patients (p = 0.0035), thus demonstrating the superiority of intravenous heparin over aspirin in the acute phase of unstable angina.[74] One of the arms of this trial also included the combination of heparin and aspirin. The two drugs together were not superior to heparin alone, although the study was underpowered to detect small significant differences.[74]

Neri Serneri et al. reported on the efficacy of a heparin infusion or bolus in 399 patients with unstable angina found to be refractory to conventional antianginal treatment after a 48-hour observation period. Heparin infusion significantly decreased the frequency of angina by 84–94%, episodes of silent ischemia by 71–77%, and duration of ischemia by 81–86%.[75] The Antithrombotic Therapy for Acute Coronary Syndromes (ATACS) Study Group randomized

214 non-aspirin users with unstable angina to 162.5 mg of aspirin alone, a combination of aspirin plus heparin, (adjusted to an aPTT of two times control) followed by aspirin and warfarin titrated to an international normalized ratio of 2–3. By 2 weeks, there was a significant reduction in total ischemic events (death, myocardial infarction, recurrent ischemia with electrocardiographic changes) in the combination group vs. the group treated with aspirin alone (10.5% vs. 27%, p = 0.004). At 12 weeks there was also a large reduction in total ischemic events (13% vs. 25%, p = 0.06).[76]

In a meta-analysis of 6 small trials, the overall relative risk of myocardial infarction or death during treatment with heparin and aspirin vs. aspirin alone in patients with unstable angina was 0.67 (95% confidence interval = 0.44–1.02, p = 0.06). For recurrent ischemic pain, the relative risk reduction was 0.68 (95% confidence interval = 0.40–1.17). For death or myocardial infarction occurring 2–12 weeks after randomization, the relative risk reduction was 0.82 (95% confidence interval = 0.56-1.20) (Fig. 2).[77]

Compared with the later mega trials of thrombolytics and glycoprotein IIb/IIIa inhibitors, these randomized studies, which constitute the basis of the current recommendations for heparin in unstable angina, were relatively small. Thus, while the overall 33% reduction in risk of myocardial infarction or death in patients with unstable angina treated with the combination compared with those treated with aspirin alone was not statistically significant, a strong trend supported the use of unfractionated heparin in high-risk patients.[77] The appreciation of the role of platelets in the pathogenesis of acute ischemic syndromes makes the earlier arguments of a relative superiority of heparin over aspirin of historical interest only.[78] Current clinical practice guidelines advocate the combination of both agents for initial therapy in unstable angina, particularly given the benefits of aspirin for the secondary prevention of cardiovascular events after acute ischemic syndromes.[79,80]

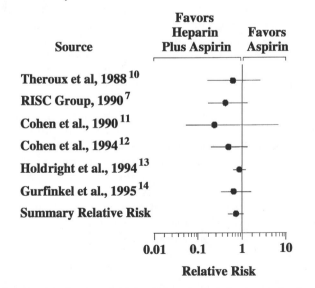

Figure 2. Relative risk of myocardial infarction or death during hospitalization: aspirin alone vs. aspirin plus heparin. (From Oler A, Whooley MA, Oler J, Grady D: Adding heparin to aspirin reduces the incidence of myocardial infarction and death in patients with unstable angina. A meta-analysis. JAMA 276:811–815, 1996, with permission.)

Low-molecular-weight Heparin vs. Heparin

Three low-molecular-weight heparins have been studied in patients with unstable angina: nadroparin, dalteparin, and enoxaparin. Each agent is pharmacodynamically unique, differing in the ability to inhibit thrombin and affect tissue factor pathway inhibitor and in anti-Xa and anti-IIa potency.[81,82] Nadroparin was the first low-molecular-weight heparin to be studied in unstable angina and non–Q-wave myocardial infarction. In a small open trial, nadroparin reduced the risk of ischemic outcomes compared with aspirin alone or a combination of aspirin and standard heparin.[83]

The efficacy of dalteparin in patients with unstable angina, in which only one-third received aspirin, was investigated in the placebo-controlled FRISC study (Fragmin During Instability in Coronary Artery Disease). The study reported a 3% absolute and a 63% relative risk reduction in death or new myocardial infarction at a dose of 120 IU/kg twice daily for 6 days. The benefit was attenuated when dalteparin was continued at a lower dose of 7,500 IU for the next 35–45 days.[84] Two other trials studied dalteparin (Fraxiparine in Ischaemic Syndromes; FRAXIS) and nadroparin (Fragmin in Unstable Coronary Artery Disease; FRIC) in acute coronary syndromes. Although they found no superiority of low-molecular-weight heparin over unfractionated heparin, they did show equivalency.[85,86] The FRAXIS trial randomized 3468 patients to twice-daily nadroparin or heparin and showed similar endpoints of death, myocardial infarction, or refractory angina at 6 days of treatment.[85] The FRIC trial, using a dalteparin regimen similar to that of the FRISC trial, randomized 1482 patients with unstable angina or non–Q-wave myocardial infarction in an open-label, 6-day comparison of dalteparin with dose-adjusted unfractionated heparin. The trial also included a prolonged treatment phase comparing dalteparin with placebo from day 6 to day 45. Short-term dalteparin showed possibly less favorable effects and no advantage over heparin; prolonged treatment showed no additional benefit compared with aspirin.[86]

Enoxaparin was compared to intravenous heparin in 3171 patients with unstable coronary disease for a mean of 2.6 days in the ESSENCE Trial (Efficacy and Safety of Subcutaneous Enoxaparin in Non–Q-Wave Coronary Events).[87] A weight-based heparin protocol was not used. The risk of a composite primary endpoint of death, myocardial infarction, or recurrent angina at 14 days was reduced by 16% (19.8% vs. 16.6%, odds ratio = 0.80, 95% confidence intervals = 0.67–0.96). No benefit was evident at 48 hours. The primary reduction in events was due largely to a reduction in recurrent angina, which became significant at 14 days and persisted at 30-day and 1-year follow-up.[88]

Enoxaparin was also studied in the TIMI 11B trial (Thrombolysis in Myocardial Infarction) in 3910 patients with unstable angina and non–Q-wave myocardial infarction.[89] A weight-based heparin nomogram was used for comparison. One-third of patients received intravenous unfractionated heparin for up to 24 hours before enrollment. Patients received 3 days of heparin vs. 4.6 days of enoxaparin. Concern about a lower-than-expected aggregate event rate prompted modification of the protocol so that all patients were required to have either ST-segment shift or positive cardiac markers in addition to a clinical diagnosis. Early evidence of benefit 48 hours after randomization was based on a triple composite endpoint of death, myocardial infarction, and urgent revascularization. The study reported a marginally significant risk reduction of 14.4% (p = 0.048), which equates to the avoidance of 21 events per 1000 patients treated, 13 of which would be either death or myocardial infarction. Subgroup analysis indicates a clear advantage for patients with definite electrocardiographic changes and no benefit for patients without. Of importance, continued therapy through 43 days with twice-daily, weight-adjusted enoxaparin did not produce additional benefit for patients with unstable coronary syndromes.

Neither enoxaparin trial was powered to test the effects on death and myocardial infarction alone. When both enoxaparin trials were combined in a meta-analysis of 7081 patients, the 20% reduction in death and myocardial infarction achieved statistical significance after day 8 and persisted through days 14–43. There was no significant difference in major hemorrhage between low-molecular-weight and unfractionated heparin (1.3% vs. 1.1%, p = 0.35), although the rate of minor hemorrhage was significantly higher with enoxaparin (10% vs. 4.3%, p < 0.0001).[90]

Thus, based on data from ESSENCE, TIMI-11B, and FRIC trials in patients with unstable angina and non–ST-segment elevation myocardial infarction, the short-term use of enoxaparin and dalteparin is as effective and safe as unfractionated heparin in reducing the hard endpoints of death and recurrent myocardial infarction (Fig. 3). Enoxaparin appears to have modest superiority over unfractionated heparin, primarily due to a reduction in recurrent angina (the softest endpoint, accounting for more than 70% of the composite endpoint) in high-risk patients.[91] When the added benefits of ease of use, reduced cost, elimination of anticoagulant monitoring, and reduction of thrombocytopenia are considered, low-molecular-weight heparin is a reasonable alternative to unfractionated heparin. Timing of dose needs to be coordinated with invasive and interventional procedures to prevent bleeding complications.[92]

Prior Aspirin Use vs. No Aspirin Use

Many patients with acute coronary syndromes have been on chronic aspirin therapy. Aspirin "resistance" can be seen in vitro in as many as 8% of aspirin users.[93] Patients who experience an event on aspirin may have a clinical course and outcomes that differ from those who had not previously used aspirin.[93,94] Lancaster et al. examined the efficacy of drug therapy in patients with unstable coronary syndromes based on aspirin use, comparing outcomes from the ESSENCE trial and PRISM-PLUS study, which compared heparin with tirofiban,

| Trial name | N | Follow-up | Death or MI | | |
			Asp + LMW Heparin	Asp + Std Heparin	
ESSENCE	3171	30 days	6.2%	7.7%	
Gurfinkel	138	in hosp	0.0%	5.7%	
FRIC	1482	6 days	3.9%	3.6%	
Crude Total	4791		5.3%	6.4%	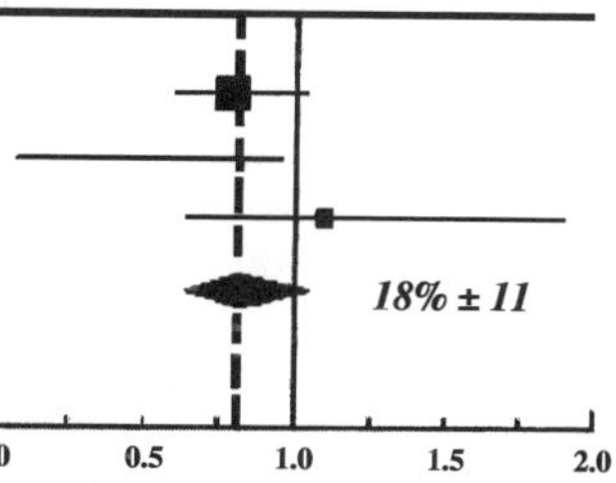 *18% ± 11*

Figure 3. Results of trials comparing the combination of aspirin and standard heparin with aspirin and low-molecular-weight (LMW) heparin in patients with unstable angina. The relative risk of death or nonfatal myocardial infarction (MI) and 95% confidence intervals are shown. X^2 heterogeneity = 4.4, 2df, p = 0.1. Treatment effect: 2p = 0.06. STD = standard (unfractionated) heparin.

a glycoprotein IIb/IIIa inhibitor. Patients who previously took aspirin were less likely to have a non–Q-wave myocardial infarction (16.0% vs. 29.2%, p < 0.001 in ESSENCE trial; 34.2% vs. 57.5%, p < 0.001 in PRISM-PLUS). However, they were more likely to fail standard medical therapy with heparin than patients without prior use of aspirin (21.5% vs. 16.5%, p = 0.017 in ESSENCE trial; 23.5% vs. 12.1, p < 0.001 in PRISM-PLUS). In addition, patients with prior use of aspirin were more likely to benefit from enoxaparin (21.5% vs. 16.8%; p = 0.009) and tirofiban with heparin (23.5% vs. 16.0%, p = 0.007) than from heparin alone. Although prior aspirin users with unstable coronary syndromes at first may appear to have a more benign presentation, they may be more likely to fail medical therapy with unfractionated heparin and should be considered a high-risk group. In patients who were not prior users of aspirin, there was no advantage to either enoxaparin or tirofiban over heparin.[95]

Heparin in Myocardial Infarction

There are three general approaches to the treatment of myocardial infarction: conservative, thrombolytic, and interventional. Heparin has played a role in all three approaches. Conservative therapy is indicated for patients who are not candidates for intervention or thrombolysis, such as those with completed infarctions who present more than 12 hours after the onset of chest pain or those with comorbid disease that precludes aggressive treatment. Most of the trials involving anticoagulation in the prethrombolytic era focused on the prevention of thromboembolic complications. In an overview of 26 randomized trials investigating anticoagulation in acute myocardial infarction in the absence of aspirin and fibrinolytic therapy, Collins et al. reported that heparin saves 35 lives per thousand patients, with mortality benefits provided by a reduction in reinfarction (15 per 1000 patient lives), stroke (10 per 1000 patient lives), and pulmonary embolism (19 per 1000 patient lives). Excessive morbidity due to major bleeding (13 per 1000 patient lives) was found in the highest-dose heparin regimens.[96,97] The ISIS-2 study, which compared the efficacy of streptokinase, aspirin, or both with placebo, included some information about the use of heparin in the placebo arm.[98] Heparin administration, while planned at entry, was not randomized, and details about the dosages or frequency of administration were not provided. With these limitations in mind, intravenous heparin was associated with a mortality rate of 8.3% vs. 9.0% for subcutaneous heparin and 10.1% for patients not receiving heparin.

Heparin and Thrombolytics

At least five randomized studies have evaluated the timing of heparin administration (delayed or at the same time as thrombolysis) with an endpoint of vessel patency. The largest studies, GUSTO-1, GISSI 2, and ISIS-3, used heparin in both subcutaneous and intravenous dosages and found no improvement in endpoints when streptokinase was the thrombolytic agent.[99–102] Overall, there were more bleeding complications and little evidence for a reduction in mortality. These findings contrast with the findings of studies using heparin in combination with tissue plasminogen activator. In ISIS-3 (Third International Study of Infarct Survival) 20,891 patients were randomized to either streptokinase or tissue plasminogen activator, followed by heparin, 12,500 units subcutaneously every 12 hours until hospital discharge.

The vascular mortality rate was 10.3% in the heparin group and 10.0% in the group without heparin at 35 days. During the early treatment phase, the trend for mortality reduction was 7.4% with heparin and 7.9% without heparin (p = 0.06). There was also a trend to reduce in-hospital reinfarction (3.2% with heparin vs. 3.5% without heparin, p = 0.09).[102]

The GUSTO trial randomized 41,021 patients into one of four groups: (1) accelerated tissue plasminogen activator plus aggressive intravenous heparin (5000-unit bolus followed by an infusion to maintain aPTT at 60–85 seconds); (2) streptokinase plus subcutaneous heparin according to the ISIS-3 protocol; (3) streptokinase plus intravenous heparin; and (4) intravenous heparin with nonaccelerated tissue plasminogen activator and a lower dose of streptokinase.[100] All patients received 160 mg of aspirin daily. Heparin in any form added to streptokinase showed no clinical benefits, but accelerated recombinant tissue plasminogen activator plus intravenous heparin resulted in an absolute reduction of 1.0%, from 7.3% to 6.3% compared with the other strategies. The mechanism appeared to be related to a rapid, complete, and maintained restoration of coronary blood flow in the infarct-related artery. In an analysis of studies primarily investigating streptokinase, Collins et al. found a modest benefit with heparin: 5 fewer deaths, 3 fewer reinfarctions, and 1 less pulmonary embolism per 1000 patient lives vs. 3 major bleeding episodes.[96]

Significant reocclusion rates have plagued the use of tissue plasminogen activator but not streptokinase or anisoylated plasminogen-streptokinase activator complex.[103,104] The combined use of heparin plus aspirin resulted in the lowest angiographic reocclusion rates reported to date.[105,120] The intensity of aPTT between 50 and 70 seconds was associated with the lowest 30-day rates of mortality, stroke, and bleeding complication. Taken together, these studies show that the main benefit of heparin in conventional doses appears to be in reducing early reocclusion rather than enhancing acute lytic effect of thrombolysis.

Heparin is an important agent to maintain late infarct-related patency 18 hours or more after thrombolysis with tissue plasminogen activator.[106–108] In the Heparin-Aspirin Reperfusion Trial (HART), tissue plasminogen activator was given to 205 patients presenting with acute myocardial infarction and randomized to receive either intravenous heparin (5,000 unit bolus followed by 1000 units/hr to maintain aPTT at 1.5–2 times normal) or aspirin (80 mg daily). Angiography 24 hours later showed that the heparin group had an 82% patency rate in the infarct-related artery vs. 52% in the aspirin group (p < 0.0001).[109] The mean aPTT was higher in the patients with a patent infarct-related artery (81 seconds vs. 54 seconds, p < 0.01).[109] Heparin given for 48 hours had no advantage over aspirin alone.[110]

Heparin in Infarct Angioplasty

Many hospitals are equipped with the technologic support required for acute intervention in patients with acute myocardial infarction. Although thrombolysis can be used successfully in centers without access to cardiac catheterization facilities, the preponderance of evidence supports emergency angioplasty and/or stenting for improved patient outcome.[111] The role of heparin in interventional procedures in general is in flux as experience with glycoprotein IIb/IIIa inhibitors and low-molecular-weight heparin increases.[92] Heparin is necessary for primary angioplasty of the culprit vessel causing acute myocardial infarction. When it is given and how it is dosed depend on several factors. If the angiographic team is not readily available, heparin should be given when the diagnosis of acute myocardial infarction is made. Most cardiologists give glycoprotein IIb/IIIa antagonists when performing primary angioplasty for myocardial infarction. Of note, heparin does not appear to be advantageous in unstable angina caused by restenosis after coronary angioplasty. Doucet et al. randomized 200 patients with unstable angina due to non-stent coronary restenosis to intravenous nitroglycerin, intravenous heparin, both, or placebo for 63 hours.[112] Angina recurred in 75% of the placebo group and heparin-only groups, 42.6% of the intravenous nitroglycerin group, and 41.7% of the intravenous nitroglycerin plus heparin group. A significantly greater number of patients in the heparin and placebo groups required urgent angiography compared with the two intravenous nitroglycerin groups. This finding underscores the difference in pathophysiology between de novo unstable angina and the cellular proliferation of restenosis.[112]

Disadvantages of Heparin

The anticoagulant response to heparin varies widely for many reasons. Heparin-binding proteins and receptor sites on endothelium must be saturated before therapeutic plasma levels of heparin can be achieved. The concentration of heparin-binding proteins varies greatly among different patients.[113,114] Natural inhibitors of heparin, such as platelet factor 4 from activated platelets and fibrin monomer II formed during the conversion of fibrinogen to fibrin, may be released from thrombus. The amounts vary with clot burden.[115] Heparin is relatively inaccessible to clot-bound thrombin and unable to neutralize effectively factor Xa-mediated procoagulant activity.[116] Fibrin-bound thrombin remains enzymatically active and causes thrombus growth by locally activating platelets and amplifying coagulation.[117–119] Heparin has only weak activity against platelet activation and deposition.[120] Using the Clot Signature Analyzer to measure platelet activity and soluble-phase coagulation, Dehmer et al. reported marked variation in platelet hemostasis time while the activated clotting time and aPTT were in the therapeutic range. In other words, the flow device identified a lack of effect in 43% of patients, suggesting a variable effect of unfractionated heparin on platelet function.[121] Low plasma levels of AT III are also associated with heparin-resistance.[122] Despite treatment with heparin, patients continue to exhibit increased thrombin generation.[33,46,123–125]

Heparin Rebound

Clinicians also remain concerned about a resurgence of symptoms and the development of thrombotic events after the cessation of heparin.[126–128] The precipitation of thrombotic coronary arterial events after unfractionated heparin cessation has been termed "heparin rebound" and may represent the removal of suppression of an underlying prothrombotic environment that has remained quiescent during treatment.[129] Granger et al. described 35 patients with unstable angina or acute myocardial infarction receiving at least 48 hours of heparin.[130] Thrombin generation measured in plasma increased transiently but significantly within 3–6 hours of heparin cessation, supporting the hypothesis that a rebound prothrombotic state develops rapidly when heparin is stopped.

Becker et al. demonstrated that thrombin generation was evident within 1 hour of heparin cessation in 30 patients with either unstable angina or non–ST-segment elevation myocardial infarction who had received a continuous intravenous infusion of heparin for 48 hours. Patients were assigned randomly to abrupt cessation, intravenous weaning, or subcutaneous weaning.[125] Thrombin generation nearly doubled at 24 hours (p = 0.002) and correlated inversely with the concentration of tissue factor pathway inhibitor (r = –0.61). Tissue factor pathway inhibitor fell by 30–40% after the heparin dose was modified, with an associated rise in generation of both factor VIIa and thrombin, suggesting either downregulation or depletion of endothelial cell tissue factor pathway inhibitor. Thrombin generation was greatest among patients randomized to abrupt cessation (1.6-fold increase at 24 hours) and least in those with intravenous weaning. Neither weaning strategy, however, prevented thrombin generation. The investigators concluded that abrupt cessation of heparin provokes a rapid decrease in the concentration of tissue factor pathway inhibitor, impairing natural thromboresistance and leading, in the presence of heightened factor Xa activity, to a sudden burst of thrombin generation. As long as even low doses of heparin are present, tissue factor pathway inhibitor is not cleared rapidly. Once heparin is no longer present, a transient prothrombotic state ensues in the absence of stores of tissue factor pathway inhibitor.

An additional explanation of heparin rebound is that a persistently unstable atheromatous plaque may consume tissue factor pathway inhibitor in the process of neutralizing factors VIIIa and Xa.[131,132] The provocation of impaired thromboresistance by heparin also may involve thrombin–thrombomodulin interactions and protein C activation.[133] If such were the case, suboptimal inhibition of factors Va, VIIa, VIIIa, and Xa and tissue factor would adversely affect the balance of coagulation and anticoagulation—not only after but also during treatment.

The clinical manifestation of heparin rebound is reflected in the findings of Granger et al., who reported that 33% of the myocardial infarctions in the GUSTO-1 study occurred within 10 hours of heparin discontinuation and nearly one-half within 20 hours, despite the universal use of aspirin.[134] The finding that the most likely time for reinfarction is 2–4 hours after stopping intravenous heparin suggests that patients should be observed carefully during this high-risk period and that methods are needed to protect patients from reinfarction. Both the American College of Cardiology/American Heart Association (ACC/AHA) Guidelines for the Management of Patients with Acute MI and the clinical practice guidelines for unstable angina sponsored by the American College of Chest Physicians and the National Heart-Lung-Blood Institute include concerns about heparin rebound and state that a gradual reduction in heparin dose may be preventive.[135,136]

Heparin-induced Thrombocytopenia

Heparin-induced thrombocytopenia (HIT) is an immunologic process in which complexes of heparin and platelet factor 4 form on the platelet surface, providing a site for antibody binding, platelet activation, and release of prothrombotic microparticles.[137–139] This process leads to platelet destruction and thrombosis. Heparin-induced platelet antibodies can be detected in 8–13% of patients receiving unfractionated heparin. A mortality rate of 25–37% and an equal morbidity rate are seen in the 2–3% of patients who develop thrombocytopenia.[140–142] HIT is seen predominantly in surgical or trauma patients and is relatively infrequent in medical patients with acute coronary syndromes.[143–145] Nonetheless, many patients who are exposed to heparin for interventional procedures or acute ischemic syndromes and later require cardiac surgery may be at risk for future antibody formation. Low-molecular-weight heparin may reduce this risk.[140]

The diagnosis of HIT is made on a clinical basis, given the problems with the sensitivity and specificity of currently available laboratory tests. Platelet aggregometry, the test most commonly used to diagnose HIT, is readily available but has the lowest sensitivity of the functional assays and is highly dependent on donor selectivity. Sensitivity has been reported as low as 30% and as high as 88%.[139,146] The more sensitive serotonin release assay requires radioisotope handling, a technically challenging and time-consuming technique, and has a false-negative rate of approximately 15%.[147,148] In addition, test specificity may be reduced in certain populations. Bauer et al. reported that 13% of patients who had a positive serotonin release assay after cardiopulmonary bypass failed to develop HIT.[149] Warkentin et al. detected HIT antibodies in 8% of patients who received subcutaneous unfractionated heparin after orthopedic surgery, but less than 3% developed HIT.[140] The enzyme-linked immunosorbent assay (ELISA) for heparin–platelet factor 4 complexes is the most sensitive (10% false-negative rate in patients with proven HIT) but least specific (with positive results in as many as 60% of patients undergoing open heart surgery).[148]

Immediate heparin cessation has been advocated as the mainstay of treatment for HIT, because platelet recovery generally does not occur until the antigenic stimulus is removed.[137,150,151] Data about the efficacy of heparin cessation as sole therapy for the prevention of morbid events are limited. Warkentin et al. reported that one-half of thrombotic events occurred in the 30 days after heparin cessation in a 14-year review of patients with heparin antibodies.[143] Laster et al. studied the complication rate of patients with HIT before and after an active surveillance program using daily platelet counts.[151] They reported a reduction in morbidity rate from 61% to 23% and in mortality rate from 23% to 12%. Almeida et al. reported that morbidity and mortality can be reduced as low as 7.4% and 1.1% , respectively, with aggressive screening and prompt heparin cessation in patients with any platelet decline from baseline.[151] Wallis et al. reported that heparin cessation at less than 48 hours of the onset of thrombocytopenia compared with more than 48 hours after the onset of thrombocytopenia did not decrease morbid or fatal events. More than one-third of patients developed thrombosis, and more than one-quarter died, regardless of the time to heparin cessation.

Once thrombosis ensues, therapy in addition to heparin cessation is indicated. Treatment of HIT with iloprost (a stable prostaglandin analog), low-molecular-weight heparin, thrombolytics, mechanical removal of thrombosis, gammaglobulin, plasmapheresis, ancrod (a defibrogenating agent), and danaparoid (a mixture of anticoagulant glycosaminoglycans) has been either limited by adverse reactions or examined only anecdotally.[141,152] More promising agents are the direct thrombin inhibitors such as argatroban, a synthetic antithrombin, and recombinant hirudin, an antithrombin produced by the leech, *Hirudo medicinalis*.[153–155] Direct thrombin inhibitors do not require AT III for activity and inactivate clot-bound thrombin that otherwise is inaccessible to heparin. In one study, hirudin was associated with a 50% reduction in composite event rate (new thrombosis, limb amputation, death) in patients with serologically confirmed HIT compared with historical controls (10% vs. 23% at 1 week, 25% vs, 52% at 1 month).[154] Argatroban improved clinical outcomes in 304 patients with HIT, significantly reducing a composite primary endpoint of all-cause death, amputation, and new thrombosis and new thrombosis and death due to thrombosis without increased bleeding risk.[155] Further clinical trials are necessary to determine whether early treatment with such therapies is safe and effective when HIT is suspected.

Thrombin Inhibitors and Heparin

Comparison trials have not shown sufficient promise to replace unfractionated heparin with hirudin, a direct antithrombin, in the management of acute ischemic syndromes. In OASIS-1 (a multicenter, randomized, and partially blinded dose-finding pilot study that compared low and medium doses of hirudin with heparin for 3 days), 6.5% of patients in the heparin group, 4.4% in the low-dose hirudin group, and 3.0% in the medium-dose hirudin group suffered the composite endpoint of death, myocardial infarction, or refractory angina (p = 0.047 for heparin vs. medium-dose hirudin).[156] OASIS-2, a multicenter, randomized trial including over 10,000 patients, used medium-dose hirudin or heparin for 72 hours. The primary endpoints of death and new myocardial infarction were lower in the hirudin group by 16%; the composite endpoint of death, myocardial infarction, and refractory angina was 18%. When both trials were combined, there was an initial reduction in combined events at 3 days (p = 0.0002) but a loss of effect by 35 days (p = 0.57).[157] In addition, the rate of ischemic stroke was higher for hirudin than for heparin (0.7% vs. 0.3%, p = 0.007), as were the rates for non–life-threatening bleeding (0.8% vs. 0.3%, p = 0.001) and fatal bleeding (60 patients vs. 34 patients, p = 0.024). While approved for HIT, the Cardio-Renal Drugs Advisory Committee of the Food and Drug Administration has not yet approved hirudin for use in acute coronary syndromes.

Heparin Dosing

Higher aPTTs have been associated with worse clinical outcomes in acute coronary syndromes. Granger et al. reviewed aPTT data from the 29,656 patients treated in the GUSTO-1 trial.[134] Thrombolytics were given with intravenous heparin, which was administered as a 5000-unit bolus followed by an initial infusion of 1000 units/hour, with dose adjustments to achieve a target aPTT of 60–85 seconds. An aPTT of 50–70 seconds was associated with the greatest benefit and the lowest risk of bleeding. An aPTT above 70 seconds was associated with a greater likelihood of death, stroke, bleeding, and reinfarction, even after adjusting for patient characteristics (e.g., lighter weight, female sex, older age). A review of TIMI-3 showed no increased benefit when the aPTT was greater than 60 seconds.[158]

The clinical benefit of heparin is reduced when the aPTT is subtherapeutic. The relative risk of mural thrombosis in acute myocardial infarction, recurrent ischemia after streptokinase therapy, and coronary artery reocclusion after tissue plasminogen activator is increased when the heparin dose is subtherapeutic.[159–161] Lidon et al. found that the aPTT was lower in patients with a recurrent ischemic event.[162] Melandri et al. found that failure to reach an activated clotting time of 1.5 times control was associated with a significantly higher rate of recurrent ischemia.[163]

The use of a standard nomogram minimizes the variability in dosing adjustments and improves the achievement of a target aPTT.[41,164,165] Previous nomograms have concentrated on the avoidance of underanticoagulation in patients with a large clot burden due to venous thromboembolism. This approach may be inappropriate for patients with acute ischemic syndromes, who have a relatively minute clot burden.[166] No caveats have been published about adverse events if the aPTT overshoots target levels, and it is unclear whether heparin levels considered therapeutic for thromboembolic disorders are appropriate for acute coronary syndromes. Heparin levels correspond to a wide range of aPTTs.[167] Becker et al. were unable to find an advantage to direct plasma heparin concentrations vs. titration of heparin therapy by routine monitoring of aPTT.[158] Volles et al. measured ex vivo samples from patients who had been on heparin for more than 24 hours. "Therapeutic" concentrations corresponded to an aPTT of 64–106 seconds, or 2.3–3.9 times control, well above the traditionally defined therapeutic range of 1.5–2.5 times control.[168]

Based on emerging data, the 1999 update to the ACC/AHA Guideline for the Management of Acute Myocardial Infarction recommends a lower dose of heparin: bolus of 60 units/kg (maximum = 4000 U) and an initial infusion of 12 units/kg/hour (maximum = 1000 units/hour) for patients receiving thrombolysis with tissue plasminogen activator and for high-risk patients requiring heparin.[169] Heparin doses are adjusted primarily to an aPTT that is 1.5–2.5 times control or a therapeutic range of 50–70 seconds, based on a baseline aPTT of 26–36 seconds, rather than to drug levels. Earlier guidelines for unstable angina published in 1994 recommended an 80-unit/kg bolus followed by an 18-unit/kg/hour infusion, but these recommendations predated many of the clinical trials that correlated outcome with aPTT.[80] Hochman et al. compared three different heparin regimens in patients with unstable angina and non–Q-wave myocardial infarction: (1) a fixed dose of a 5000-unit bolus followed by 1000 units/hour; (2) a higher-dose, weight-based regimen of a 70-unit/kg bolus followed by a 15-unit/kg/hour infusion; and (3) a lower-dose, weight-based nomogram of 60 units/kg (maximum = 4000 units), with an infusion of 12 units/kg/hour (maximum = 1000 units/hour). They found that the lower-dose, weight-based protocol was superior in achieving early therapeutic levels of anticoagulation and reduced the need for dose adjustments.

Table 1 provides guidelines, based on available data, for weight-based dosing for deep venous thrombosis vs. acute coronary syndromes, with or without thrombolysis with tissue plasminogen activator. Table 2 is a modified nomogram for continued administration. Specific heparin protocols, however, must be standardized and validated for each institution, based on thromboplastin reagent, control aPTT levels, and patient population.

Conclusion

Heparin has been a valuable adjunct in the therapeutic armamentarium for acute coronary syndromes. Within the century of its discovery, however,

Table 1. Recommended Doses of Unfractionated Heparin Based on Published Nomograms

	DVT/PE	ACS/Thrombolysis with tPA
Heparin bolus	80 U/kg	60 U/kg with maximum of 4000-U bolus for patients > 70 kg
Infusion rate	18 U/kg/hr	12 U/kg/hr with maximum of 1000 U/kg/min for patients > 70 kg
Target aPTT	50–75 seconds*	50–70 seconds

DVT = deep venous thrombosis, PE = pulmonary embolism, ACS = acute coronary syndrome, tPA = recombinant tissue plasminogen activator, aPTT = activated partial thromboplastin time.
* Based on heparin levels of 0.2–0.4 U/ml by protamine titration or an anti-factor Xa level of 0.35–0.7 U/ml.
DVT/PE data from Raschke RA, Reilly BM, Guidry JR, et al: The weight-based heparin dosing nomogram compared with a "standard care" nomogram. Ann Intern Med 119:875–881, 1993; ACS data from Ryan TJ, Anderson JL, Antman EM, et al: 1999 Update: ACC/AHA Guidelines for the Management of Patients with Acute Myocardial Infarction: Executive Summary and Recommendations: A Report of the American College of Cardiology/American Heart Association Task Force on Practice Guidelines (Committee on Management of Acute Myocardial Infarction). Circulation 100:1016–1030, 1999.

research is focusing on newer agents, such as low-molecular-weight heparins, glycoprotein IIb/IIIa antagonists, and thrombin inhibitors, to replace heparin because of concerns about efficacy, thrombotic rebound, and heparin-induced thrombocytopenia. In addition, better understanding of the role of platelets and thrombin generation in the pathophysiology of these syndromes has led to the targeting of specific molecules (e.g., adhesion proteins, glycoprotein receptors, thrombin) for inhibition. In addition to improvements in efficacy, newer agents must have fewer adverse reactions; they also should be easier to administer, at least as safe, and, hopefully, less expensive. The newer agents are most likely to benefit patients with previous heparin-induced thrombocytopenia or aspirin resistance and patients at high risk for myocardial infarction (i.e., patients with abnormal electrocardiographic findings, release of cardiac enzymes, or markers such as troponin). At present, heparin appears to remain the drug of choice for infarct angioplasty and acute ischemic syndromes when the need for reversal of antithrombotic therapy may be required. Despite heparin's key role in the development of therapy for acute coronary syndromes, it is quite likely that its use will decline to the level of historical interest in the twenty-first century.

Table 2. Heparin Adjustment Nomogram for Standard Laboratory Reagents
(Mean Control aPTT = 26–36 Seconds)

aPTT(sec)	Bolus Dose (U)	Stop Infusion (min)	Rate Change (U/hr)	Repeat aPTT
< 49	3000	0	+100	6 hr
40–49	0	0	+50	6 hr
50–70	0	0	No change	Next morning*
71–85	0	0	−50	Next morning
86–100	0	30	−100	6 hr
101–150	0	60	−150	6 hr
> 150	0	60	−300	6 hr

aPTT = activated partial thromboplastin time.
* Pending two consecutive therapeutic aPTTs 6 hours apart.
Note: For aPTTs obtained within 12 hr after initiation of tissue plasminogen activator, do not decrease infusion unless bleeding is significant or aPTT > 150 sec. Infusion may be increased if aPTT < 50 sec. For aPTTs obtained ≥ 12 hr after initiation of thrombolytic therapy, use entire nomogram.

References

1. McLean J: The thromboplastic action of cephalin. Am J Physiol 41:250–257, 1916.
2. McLean J: The discovery of heparin. Circulation 19:75–78, 1959.
3. Ancalmo N, Ochsner J: Heparin, the miracle drug: A brief history of its discovery. J La State Med Soc 142:22–24, 1990.
4. Marcum JA: William Henry Howell and Jay McLean: The experimental context for the discovery of heparin. Perspect Biol Med 33:214–230, 1990.
5. Jay McLean (1890–1957) discoverer of heparin. JAMA 201:770, 1967.
6. Couch NP: About heparin, or … whatever happened to Jay McLean. J Vasc Surg 10:1–8, 1989.
7. Lam CR: The strange story of Jay McLean, the discoverer of heparin. Henry Ford Hosp Med J 33:18–23, 1985.
8. Howell WH, Holt E: Two new factors in blood coagulation—heparin and proantithrombin. Am J Physiol 47:328–341, 1918.
9. Charles AF, Scott DA: Studies on heparin. IV: Observations on the chemistry of heparin. Biochem J 30:1927–1933, 1936.
10. Best CH: Preparation of heparin and its use in the first clinical cases. Circulation 19:79–86, 1959.
11. Rodén L, Ananth S, Campbell P, et al: Heparin: An introduction. In Lame DA et al (eds): Heparin and Related Polysaccharides. New York, Plenum Press, 1992, pp 1–20.
12. Craaford C: Preliminary report on post-operative treatment with heparin as a preventive of thrombosis. Acta Chir Scand 79:407–426, 1937.
13. Murray GDW, Best CH: The use of heparin in thrombosis. Ann Surg 108:163–173, 1938.
14. Wright IS: Experience with anticoagulants. Circulation 29:110–113, 1959.
15. Davies MK, Hollman A: Heparin. JAMA 80:120, 1994.
16. Frye WB: Acute myocardial infarction: A historical summary. In Gersh BJ, Rahimtoola SH (eds): Acute Myocardial Infarction. New York, Chapman & Hall, 1997, pp 1–15.
17. Solandt DY, Best CH: Heparin and coronary thrombosis in experimental animals. Lancet ii:130–132, 1938.
18. Nichol ES: Personal experiences with anticoagulants for coronary atherosclerosis. Circulation 29:129–134, 1959.
19. Nichol ES, Phillips WC, Casten GG: Virtue of prompt anticoagulant therapy in impending myocardial infarction: Experiences with 318 patients during a 10-year period. Ann Intern Med 50:1158–1173, 1959.
20. Mitchell JRA: Anticoagulants in coronary heart disease-retrospect and prospect. Lancet 257–262, 1981.
21. Theroux P, Ouimet H, McCans J, et al: Aspirin, heparin or both to treat unstable angina. N Engl J Med 319:1105–1111, 1988.
22. Falk E, Shah PK, Fuster V: Coronary plaque disruption. Circulation 92:657–671, 1995.
23. Weitz JI, Bates SM: Beyond heparin and aspirin: New treatments for unstable angina and non–Q-wave myocardial infarction. Arch Intern Med 160:749–758, 2000.
24. Mann KG: The coagulation explosion. Ann N Y Acad Sci 714:265–269, 1994.
25. Marmur JD, Thiruvikraman SV, Fyfe BS, et al: Identification of active tissue factor in human coronary atheroma. Circulation 94:1226–1232, 1996.
26. Annex BH, Denning SM, Channon KM, et al: Differential expression of tissue factor protein in directional atherectomy specimens from patients with stable and unstable coronary syndromes. Circulation 91:619–622, 1995.
27. Toschi V, Gallo R, Lettino M, et al: Tissue factor modulates the thrombogenicity of human atherosclerotic plaques. Circulation 95:594–599, 1997.
28. Broze GJ Jr: The tissue factor pathway of coagulation. In Loscalzo J, Schafer AI (eds): Thrombosis and Hemorrhage. Boston, Blackwell Scientific Publications, 1994, pp 57–86.
29. Furie B, Furie BC: Molecular and cellular biology of blood coagulation. N Engl J Med 326:800–806, 1992.
30. Antman EM, Handin R: Low-molecular-weight heparins: An intriguing new twist with profound implications. Circulation 98:287–289, 1998.
31. Eidr JH, Allison P, Noble S, et al: Thrombin is an important mediator of platelet aggregation in stenosed canine coronary arteries with endothelial injury. J Clin Invest 84:18–27, 1989.
32. Gast A, Tschopp TB, Baumgartner HR: Thrombin plays a key role in late platelet thrombus growth and/or stability: Effect of a specific thrombin inhibitor on thrombogenesis induced by aortic subendothelium exposed to flowing rabbit blood. Arterioscler Thromb 14:1466–1474, 1994.
33. Rho R,Tracy RP, Bovill EG, et al: Plasma markers of procoagulant activity among individuals with coronary artery disease. J Thromb Thrombolysis 2:239–243, 1995.

34. Merlini PA, Bauer KA, Oltrona L, et al: Persistent activation of coagulation mechanism in unstable angina and myocardial infarction. Circulation 90:61–68, 1994.

35. Biasucci LM, Liuzzo G, Caligiuri G, et al: Temporal relation between ischemic episodes and activation of the coagulation system in unstable angina. Circulation 93:2121–2127, 1996.

36. Becker RC, Tracy RP, Bovill EG, et al, for the TIMI III Thrombosis and Coagulation Study Group: Surface 12-lead electrocardiographic findings and plasma markers of thrombin activity and generation in patients with myocardial ischemia at rest. J Thromb Thrombolysis 1:101–107, 1994.

37. Green D, Hirsh J, Heit J, et al: Low molecular weight heparin: A critical analysis of clinical trials. Pharmacol Rev 46:89–109, 1994.

38. Abildgaard U: Highly purified antithrombin III with heparin cofactor activity prepared by disc electrophoresis. Scan J Clin Lab Invest 21:89–91, 1968.

39. Danielsson A, Raub E, Lindahl U, Bjork I: Role of ternary complexes, in which heparin binds both antithrombin and proteinase, in the acceleration of the reactions between antithrombin and thrombin or factor Xa. J Biol Chem 261:15467–15473, 1986.

40. Anderson LO, Barrowcliffe TW, Holmer E, et al: Anticoagulant properties of heparin fractionated by affinity chromatography on matrix bound antithrombin III and by gel filtration. Thromb Res 9:574–583, 1976.

41. Hirsch J: Heparin. N Eng J Med 324:1565–1564, 1991.

42. Turpie AG: Low-molecular-weight heparins in acute unstable coronary artery disease: An update. Haemostasis 29(Suppl 1):72–75, 1999.

43. Small BM: Update in thrombosis and coagulation in the long-term care setting. Clin Geriatr 8:66–78, 2000.

44. Blajchman MA, Young E, Ofosu FA: Effects of unfractionated heparin, dermatan sulfate and low molecular weight heparin on vessel wall permeability in rabbits. Ann NY Acad Sci 556:245–254, 1989.

45. Castellot JJ Jr, Favreau LV, Karnovsky MJ, Rosenberg RD: Inhibition of vascular smooth muscle cell growth by endothelial cell-derived heparin: Possible role of a platelet endoglycosidase. J Biol Chem 257:11256–11260, 1982.

46. Becker RC, Spencer FA, Li Y, et al: Thrombin generation after the abrupt cessation of intravenous unfractionated heparin among patients with acute coronary syndromes: Potential mechanisms for heightened prothrombotic potential. J Am Coll Cardiol 34:1020–1027, 1999.

47. Lindahl AK, Abildgaard U, Staalesen R: The anticoagulant effect in heparinized blood and plasma resulting from interactions with extrinsic pathway inhibitor. Thromb Res 64:155–168, 1991.

48. Hoppensteadt DA, Jeske W, Fareed J, Bermes EW Jr: The role of tissue factor pathway inhibitor in the mediation of the antithrombotic actions of heparin and low-molecular-weight heparin. Blood Coagul Fibrinol 6:S57–S64, 1995.

49. Sandset PM, Abildgaard U, Larsen ML: Heparin induces release of extrinsic coagulation pathway inhibitor. Thromb Res 50:803–813, 1988.

50. Harenberg J, Siegele M, Dempfle CE, et al: Protamine neutralization of the release of tissue factor pathway inhibitor activity by heparins. Thromb Haemost 6:942–945, 1993.

51. Valentin S, Lamkjar A, Ostergaard P, et al: Characterization of the binding between tissue factor pathway inhibitor and glycosaminoglycans. Thromb Res 75:173–183, 1994.

52. Lindahl AK, Sandset PM, Abildgaard U: The present status of tissue factor pathway inhibitor (TFPI) is restricted to its free form in human plasma [abstract]. Thromb Haemost 73:1260, 1995.

53. Valentin S, Ostergaard P, Kristensen H, Norfang O: Synergism between full length TFPI and heparin: Evidence for TFPI as an important factor for the antithrombotic activity of heparin. Blood Coag Fibrinol 3:221–222, 1992.

54. Sandset PM: Tissue factor pathway inhibitor (TFPI): An update. Haemostasis 26(Suppl 4):154–165, 1996.

55. Hanson JB, Sandset PM, Huseby KR, Huseby NE: Depletion of intravascular pools of tissue factor pathway inhibitor (TFPI) during repeated or continuous intravenous infusion of heparin in man. Thromb Haemost 76;703–309, 1996.

56. Hull RD, Raskob GE, Hirsh J, et al: Continuous intravenous heparin compared with intermittent subcutaneous heparin in the initial treatment of proximal-vein thrombosis. N Engl J Med 315:1109–1114, 1986.

57. Pini M, Pattachini C, Quintavalla R, et al: Subcutaneous vs intravenous heparin in the treatment of deep venous thrombosis: A randomized clinical trial. Thromb Haemost 64:222–226, 1990.

58. de Swart CA, Nijmeyer B, Roelofs JM, Sixma JJ: Kinetics of intravenously administered heparin in normal humans. Blood 60:1251–1258, 1982.

59. Olsson P, Lagergren H, Ek S: The elimination from plasma of intravenous heparin: An experimental study on dogs and humans. Acta Med Scand 173:619–630, 1963.
60. Brill-Edwards P, Ginsberg JS, Johnston M, Hirsh J: Establishing a therapeutic range for heparin therapy. Ann Intern Med 119:104–109, 1993.
61. Hirsh J, Fuster V: Guide to anticoagulant therapy. Part 1: Heparin. Circulation 89:1449–1468, 1994.
62. Meyer D, Girma JP: VonWillebrand factor: Structure and function. Thromb Haemost 70:99–104, 1993.
63. Sobel M, McNeill PM, Carlson P, et al: Heparin inhibition of von Willebrand factor in vitro and in vivo. J Clin Invest 87:1787–1793, 1991.
64. Sobel M, Bird KE, Tyler-Cross R, et al: Heparins designed to specifically inhibit platelet interactions with von Willebrand factor. Circulation 93:992–999, 1996.
65. Montalescot G, Philippe F, Ankri A, et al: Early increase of von Willebrand factor predicts adverse outcome in unstable coronary artery disease. Beneficial effects of enoxaparin. Circulation 98:294–299, 1998.
66. Wood P: Acute and subacute coronary insufficiency. BMJ 1:1779–1782, 1961.
67. Vakil RJ: Preinfarction syndrome-management and follow-up. Am J Cardiol 14:55–63, 1954.
68. Davies MJ, Thomas AC: Plaque fissuring-the cause of acute myocardial infarction, sudden ischaemic death, and crescendo angina. Br Heart J 53:363–373, 1985.
69. DeWood MA, Spores J, Notske R, et al: Prevalence of total coronary occlusion during the early hours of transmural myocardial infarction. N Engl J Med 303:897–902, 1980.
70. Telford AM, Wilson C: Trial of heparin versus atenolol in prevention of myocardial infarction in intermediate coronary syndrome. Lancet i:1225–1228, 1981.
71. Yusef S, Sleight: Atenolol, heparin and the intermediate coronary syndrome. Lancet 2:46, 1981.
72. Theroux P, Ouimet H, McCans J, et al: Aspirin, heparin or both to treat unstable angina. N Engl J Med 319:1105–1111, 1988.
73. RISC Group: Risk of myocardial infarction and death during treatment with low dose aspirin and intravenous heparin in men with unstable coronary artery disease. Lancet 336:827–830, 1990.
74. Theroux P, Waters D Qiu S, et al: Aspirin versus heparin to prevent myocardial infarction during the acute phase of unstable angina. Circulation 88:2045–2048, 1993.
75. Neri Serneri GG, Gensini GF, Poggesi L, et al: Effect of heparin, aspirin, or alteplase in reduction of myocardial ischaemia in refractory unstable angina. Lancet 335:615–618, 1990.
76. Cohen M, Adams PC, Parry G, et al: Combination antithrombotic therapy in unstable rest angina and non-Q-wave infarction in nonprior aspirin users. Primary end points analysis from the ATACS trial. Antithrombotic Therapy in Acute Coronary Syndromes Research Group. Circulation 89:81–88, 1994
77. Oler A, Whooley MA, Oler J, Grady D: Adding heparin to aspirin reduces the incidence of myocardial infarction and death in patients with unstable angina. A meta-analysis. JAMA 276:811–815, 1996.
78. Wallentin LC: Aspirin (75 mg/day) after an episode of unstable coronary artery disease: Long-term effects on the risk for myocardial infarction, occurrence of severe angina and the need for revascularization. Research Group on Instability in Coronary Artery Disease in Southeast Sweden. J Am Coll Cardiol 18:1587–1593, 1991.
79. Cairns JA, Theroux P, Lewis D Jr, et al: Antithrombotic agents in coronary artery disease. Chest 114:611S–633S, 1998.
80. Braunwald E, Mark DB, Jones RH, et al: Unstable angina: Diagnosis and management. Clinical Practice Guideline No. 10 (amended). Rockville, MD, Public Health Service, Agency for Health Care Policy and Research, National Heart, Lung, and Blood Institute. AHCPR Publication No. 94-0602, 1994.
81. Cornelli U, Fareed: Human pharmacokinetics of low molecular weight heparins. Semin Throm Hemost 25(Suppl 3):57–61, 1999.
82. Fareed J, Jeske W, Hoppensteadt D, et al: Are the available low molecular-weight heparin preparations the same? Semin Thromb Hemost 22:77–91, 1996.
83. Gurfinkel EP, Manos EJ, Mejail RI, et al: Low molecular weight heparin versus regular heparin or aspirin in the treatment of unstable angina and silent ischemia. J Am Coll Cardiol 26:313–318, 1995.
84. Fragmin During Instability in Coronary Artery Disease (FRISC) Study Group: Low molecular weight heparin during instability in coronary artery disease. Lancet 347:561–568, 1996.
85. FRAXIS Study Group: Comparison of two treatment durations (6 days and 14 days) of a low molecular weight heparin with a 6-day treatment of unfractionated heparin in the initial management of unstable angina or non–Q-wave myocardial infarction: FRAXIS (Fraxiparine in Ischaemic Syndrome). Eur Heart J 20:1553–1562, 1999.

86. Klein W, Buchwald A, Hillis WS, et al (FRIC Investigators): Comparison of low molecular weight heparin with unfractionated heparin acutely and a placebo for six weeks in the management of unstable coronary disease. Circulation 96:61–68, 1997.
87. Cohen M, Demers C, Gurfinkel EP, et al: A comparison of low molecular weight heparin with unfractionated heparin for unstable coronary artery disease. N Engl J Med 337:447–452, 1997.
88. Goodman S, Langer A, Demers C, et al (for the ESSENCE Group): One year follow-up of the ESSENCE trial (enoxaparin vs. heparin in unstable angina/non-Q wave myocardial infarction): Sustained clinical benefit. Can J Cardiol 14:122F, 1998.
89. Antman EM, McCabe C, Gurfinkel EP, et al, for the TIMI 11B Investigators: Enoxaparin prevents death and cardiac ischemic events in unstable angina/non–q-wave myocardial infarction: Results of the Thrombolysis In Myocardial Infarction (TIMI) 11B trial Circulation 100:1602–1608, 1999.
90. Antman EM, Cohen M, Radley D, et al, for the TIMI 11B and ESSENCE Investigator: Assessment of the treatment effect of enoxaparin for unstable angina/non–Q-wave myocardial infarction: TIMI 11B-ESSENCE meta-analysis. Circulation 100:1602–1608, 1999.
91. Kaul S, Cercek B, Shah PK: Low-molecular-weight heparin in acute coronary syndrome: Evidence for superior or equivalent efficacy compared to unfractionated heparin? J Am Coll Cardiol 35:344A, 2000.
92. Kereiakes DJ, Fry E, Matthai W, et al: Combination enoxaparin and abciximab therapy during percutaneous coronary intervention: "NICE guys finish first." J Invas Cardiol 12(Suppl A):1A–5A, 2000.
93. Helgason CM, Bolin KM, Hoff JA, et al: Development of aspirin resistance in persons with previous ischemic stroke. Stroke 25:2331–2336, 1994.
94. Schrör K: Aspirin and platelets: The antiplatelet action of aspirin and its role in thrombosis treatment and prophylaxis. Semin Thromb Hemost 23:349–356, 1997.
95. Lancaster GI, Lancaster CJ, Radley D, et al: Prior aspirin use in unstable coronary syndromes results in a lower incidence of non–Q-wave MI but a higher rate of medical therapy failure with unfractionated heparin: The aspirin paradox. Circulation 100(Suppl 1):3271, 1999.
96. Collins R, MacMahon S, Flather JM, et al: Clinical effects of anticoagulant therapy in suspected acute myocardial infarction: Systematic overview of randomized trials. BMJ 313:652–659, 1996.
97. Collins R, Peto R, Baigent C, et al: Aspirin, heparin, and fibrinolytic therapy in suspected acute myocardial infarction. N Engl J Med 336:847–860, 1997.
98. ISIS-2 (Second International Study of Infarct Survival) Collaborative Group: Randomized trial of intravenous streptokinase, oral aspirin, both, or neither among 17,187 cases of suspected acute myocardial infarction: ISIS-2. Lancet 2:349–360, 1988.
99. Gruppo Italiano per lo Studio della Sopravvivenza nellíinfarto Miocardico: GISSI-2: A factorial randomized trial of alteplase and heparin versus no heparin among 12,490 patients with acute myocardial infarction. Lancet 336:65–71, 1990.
100. GUSTO Investigators: An international randomized trial comparing four thrombolytic strategies for acute myocardial infarction. N Engl J Med 329:673–682, 1993.
101. International Study Group: In-hospital mortality and clinical course of 20,891 patients with suspected acute myocardial infarction randomized between alteplase and streptokinase with or without heparin. Lancet 336:71, 1990.
102. ISIS-3 Collaborative Group Collaborative Group: ISIS-3: A randomized comparison of streptokinase vs. tissue plasminogen activator vs. anistreplase and of aspirin plus heparin vs. aspirin alone among 41,299 cases of suspected acute myocardial infarction. Lancet 339:753–770, 1992.
103. O'Connor CM, Meese R, Camey R, et al: A randomized trial of intravenous heparin in conjunction with anistreplase (anisoylated plasminogen streptokinase activator complex) in acute myocardial infarction: The Duke University Clinical Cardiological Study (DUCCS) 1. J Am Coll Cardiol 23:11–18, 1994.
104. Cairns JA, Kennedy JW, Fuster V: Coronary thrombolysis. Chest 114:634S–657S, 1998.
105. GUSTO Angiographic Investigators: The effects of tissue plasminogen activators, streptokinase, or both on coronary-artery patency, ventricular function, and survival after acute myocardial infarction. N Engl J Med 329:1615–1622, 1993.
106. Hsia J, Hamilton WP, Keiman N, et al, for the Heparin-Aspirin Reperfusion Trial (HART) Investigators: A comparison between heparin and low-dose aspirin as adjunctive therapy with tissue plasminogen activator for acute myocardial infarction. N Engl J Med 323:1433–1437, 1990.
107. Bleich SD, Nichols T, Schumbacher RR, et al: Effect of heparin on coronary patency after thrombolysis with tissue plasminogen activator in acute myocardial infarction. Am J Cardiol 66:1412–1417, 1990.

108. De Bono DP, Simoons MI, Tijssen J, et al, for the European Cooperative Study Group: Effect of early intravenous heparin on coronary patency, infarct size, and bleeding complications after alteplase thrombolysis: Results of a randomized double-blind European Cooperative Study Group trial. Br Heart J 67:122–128, 1992.

109. Hsia J, Kleiman N, Aquirre F, et al: Heparin-induced prolongation of partial thromboplastin time after thrombolysis: Relation to coronary artery patency. HART Investigators. J Am Coll Cardiol 20:31–35, 1992.

110. Thompson PL, Aylward PE, Federma J, et al: A randomized comparison of intravenous heparin with oral aspirin and dipyridamole 24 hours after recombinant tissue-type plasminogen activator for acute myocardial infarction. Circulation 83:1534–1542, 1991.

111. Weaver WD, Simes RJ, Betriu A, et al: Comparison of primary coronary angioplasty and intravenous thrombolytic therapy for acute myocardial infarction: A quantitative review. JAMA 278:2093–2098, 1997.

112. Doucet S, Malekianpour M, Theroux P, et al: Randomized trial comparing intravenous nitroglycerin and heparin for treatment of unstable angina secondary to restenosis after coronary artery angioplasty. Circulation 101:955–961, 2000.

113. Hirsh J, Levine MN: Low molecular weight heparin. Blood 79:1–17, 1992.

114. Melandri G, Semprini F, Cervi V, et al: Comparison of efficacy of low molecular weight heparin (parnaparin) with that of unfractionated heparin in the presence of activated platelets in healthy subjects. Am J Cardiol 72:450–454, 1993.

115. Okuno R, Crockatt D: Platelet factor 4 activity and thromboembolic episodes. Am J Clin Pathol 167:351–355, 1977.

116. Prager NA, Abendschein DR, McKenzie CR, Eisenberg PR: Role of thrombin compared with factor Xa in the procoagulant activity of whole blood clots. Circulation 92:962–967, 1995.

117. Weitz JI, Hudoba M, Massel D, et al: Clot-bound thrombin is protected from inhibition by heparin-antithrombin III but is susceptible to inactivation by antithrombin-III independent inhibitors. J Clin Invest 86:385–391, 1990.

118. Kumar R, Beguin S, Hemker HC: The effect of fibrin clots and clot-bound thrombin on the development of platelet procoagulant activity. Thromb Haemost 74:962–968, 1995.

119. Kumar R, Beguin S, Hemker HC: The influence of fibrinogen and fibrinogen thrombin generation: Evidence for feedback activation of the clotting system by clot-bound thrombin. Thromb Haemost 72:713–721, 1994.

120. Gallo R, Webster MWI, Fuster V, Chesebro J: Antithrombotic therapy in acute myocardial infarction: Enhancement of thrombolysis, reduction of reocclusion, and prevention of thromboembolism. In Gersh BJ, Rahimtoola SH (eds): Acute Myocardial Infarction. New York, Chapman & Hall, 1997, pp 472–501.

121. Dehmer GJ, Melton LG, Thompson CM, et al: Standard tests to assess heparin efficacy may not accurately reflect anticoagulation. J Am Coll Cardiol 35:344A, 2000.

122. Rosenberg RD: Heparin, antithrombin, and abnormal clotting. Annu Rev Med 29:367–378, 1978.

123. Ofosu FA, Gray E: Mechanisms of action of heparin: Applications to the development of derivatives of heparin and heparinoids with antithrombin properties. Semin Thromb Hemost 14:9–17, 1988.

124. Gallino A, Haeberli A, Hess T, et al: Fibrin formation and platelet aggregation in patients with acute myocardial infarction: Effects of intravenous and subcutaneous low dose heparin. Am Heart J 12:285–290, 1986.

125. Becker RC, Spencer FA, Li Y, et al: Thrombin generation after the abrupt cessation of intravenous unfractionated heparin among patients with acute coronary syndromes: Potential mechanisms for heightened prothrombotic potential. J Am Coll Cardiol 34:1020–1027, 1999.

126. Theroux P, Waters D, Lam J, et al: Reactivation of unstable angina after the discontinuation of heparin. N Eng J Med 327:141–145, 1992.

127. Conrad-Smith AJ, Holt RE, Fitzpatrick K, et al: Transient thrombotic state after abrupt discontinuation of heparin in percutaneous coronary angioplasty. Am Heart J 131:434–439, 1996.

128. Smith AJ, Holt RE, Fitzpatrick K, et al: Transient thrombotic state after abrupt discontinuation of heparin in percutaneous coronary angioplasty. Am Heart J 131:434–439, 1996.

129. Oltrona L, Eisenberg PR, Lasala JM, et al: Association of heparin resistant thrombin activity with acute ischemic complications of coronary interventions. Circulation 94:2064–2071, 1996.

130. Granger CB, Miller JM, Bovill EG, et al: Rebound increase in thrombin generation and activity after cessation of intravenous heparin in patients with acute coronary syndromes. Circulation 91:1929–1935, 1995.

131. Van't Veer C, Hackeng TM, Delahaye C, et al: Activated factor X and thrombin formation triggered by tissue factor on endothelial cell matrix in a flow model: Effect of the tissue factor pathway inhibitor. Blood 84:1132–1139, 1994.

132. Kaiser B, Hoppensteadt DA, Jeske W, et al: Inhibitory effects of TFPI of thrombin and factor Xa generation in vitro-modulatory action of glycosaminoglycans. Thromb Res 75:609–619, 1994.
133. DeCrisofaro R, DeCandia E, Landolfi R: Effect of high- and low-molecular weight heparins on thrombin-thrombomodulin interaction and protein C activation. Circulation 98:1297–1301, 1998.
134. Granger CB, Hirsh J, Califf RM, et al, for the GUSTO-1 Trial Investigators: Activated partial thromboplastin time and outcome after thrombolytic therapy for acute myocardial infarction: Results from the GUSTO-1 Trial. Circulation 93:870–878, 1996.
135. ACC/AHA Committee on Management of Acute MI: ACC/AHA Guidelines for the Management of Patients with Acute MI. J Am Coll Cardiol 28:1328–1428, 1996.
136. Hirsh J, Rascke R, Warkentin TE, et al: Heparin: Mechanism of action, pharmacokinetics, dosing considerations, monitoring efficacy and safety. Chest 108(Suppl):248S–275S, 1995.
137. Warkentin TE, Hayward CPM, Boshkov LK, et al: Sera from patients with heparin-induced thrombocytopenia generate platelet-derived microparticles with procoagulant activity: An explanation for the thrombotic complications of heparin-induced thrombocytopenia. Blood 84:3691–3699, 1994.
138. Cines D, Tomaski A, Tannenbaum S: Immune endothelial-cell injury in heparin-associated thrombocytopenia. N Engl J Med 316:581–589, 1987.
139. Chong BH: Heparin-induced thrombocytopenia. Br J Haematol 89:431–439, 1995.
140. Warkentin TE, Levine MN, Hirsh J, et al: Heparin-induced thrombocytopenia in patients treated with low-molecular-weight heparin or unfractionated heparin. N Engl J Med 332:1330–1335, 1995.
141. Brieger DB, Mak K, Kottke-Marchant K, Topol EJ: Heparin-induced thrombocytopenia. J Am Coll Cardiol 31:1449–1459, 1998.
142. Warkentin TE, Kelton JG: Heparin-induced thrombocytopenia. Prog Hemost Thromb 10:1–34, 1991.
143. Warkentin TE, Kelton JG: A fourteen year study of heparin-induced thrombocytopenia. Am J Med 101:502–507, 1996.
144. Wallis DE, Workman DL, Lewis BE, et al: Failure of early heparin cessation as treatment for heparin-induced thrombocytopenia. Am J Med 106:629–635, 1999.
145. Janssens U, Khanduja R, Lorenz N, et al: The immunologic form of heparin induced thrombocytopenia: Incidence and outcome in 1000 consecutive patients. J Am Coll Cardiol 35:319a, 2000.
146. Greinacher A, Amiral J, Dummel V, et al: Laboratory diagnosis of heparin-associated thrombocytopenia and comparison of platelet aggregation test, heparin-induced platelet activation test, and platelet factor 4/heparin enzyme-linked immunosorbent assay. Transfusion 83:3232–3239, 1994.
147. Kelton JG, Warkentin T: Diagnosis of heparin-induced thrombocytopenia: Still a journey, not a destination. Am J Clin Pathol 104:611–613, 1995.
148. Chong BH: Heparin-induced thrombocytopenia. Aust N Z J Med 22:145–152, 1992.
149. Bauer TL, Arepally G, Konkle BA, et al: Prevalence of heparin-associated antibodies without thrombosis in patients undergoing cardiopulmonary bypass surgery. Circulation 95:1242–1246, 1997.
150. Laster J, Cikrit D, Walker N, Silver D: The heparin-induced thrombocytopenia syndrome: An update. Surgery 102:763–770, 1987.
151. Almeida JI, Coats R, Liem TK, Silver D: Reduced morbidity and mortality rates of the heparin-induced thrombocytopenia syndrome. J Vasc Surg 27:309–314, 1998.
152. Hirsh J, Warkentin TE, Raschke R, et al: Heparin and low-molecular-weight heparin: Mechanisms of action, pharmacokinetics, dosing considerations, monitoring, efficacy and safety. Chest 114(Suppl):489S–551S, 1998.
153. Lewis BE, Walenga JM, Wallis DE: Anticoagulation with Novastan (argatroban) in patients with heparin-induced thrombocytopenia and heparin-induced thrombocytopenia and thrombosis syndrome. Semin Thromb Haemost 23:197–202, 1997.
154. Greinacher A, Völpel H, Janssens U, et al: Recombinant hiruden (lepirudin) provides safe and effective anticoagulation in patients with heparin-induced thrombocytopenia: A prospective study. Circulation 99:73–80, 1999.
155. Lewis BE, Wallis DE, Matthai WM: Argatroban provides effective and safe anticoagulation in patients with heparin-induced thrombocytopenia: A prospective, historical controlled study [abstract]. J Am Coll Cardiol 35:266A, 2000.
156. Organization to Assess Strategies for Ischemic Syndromes (OASIS) Investigators: Comparison of the effects of two doses of recombinant hirudin compared with heparin in patients with acute myocardial ischemia without ST elevation: A pilot study. Circulation 96: 769–777, 1997.

157. Organization to Assess Strategies for Ischemic Syndromes (OASIS-2) Investigators: Effects of recombinant hirudin (lepirudin) compared with heparin on death, myocardial infarction, refractory angina, and revascularization procedures in patients with acute myocardial ischemia without ST elevation: A randomized trial. Lancet 353:429–438, 1999.

158. Becker RC, Cannon CP, Tracy RP, et al: Relation between systemic anticoagulaton as determined by activated partial thromboplastin time and heparin measurements and in-hospital clinical events in unstable angina and non–Q-wave myocardial infarction. Thrombolysis in Myocardial Ischemia II B Investigators. Am Heart J 131:421–433, 1996.

159. Turpie AG, Robinson JG, Doyle DJ, et al: Comparison of high-dose with low-dose subcutaneous heparin to prevent left ventricular mural thrombosis in patients with acute transmural anterior myocardial infarction. N Engl J Med 320:352–357, 1989.

160. Kaplan K, Davison R, Parker M, et al: Role of heparin after intravenous thrombolytic therapy for acute myocardial infarction. Am J Cardiol 59:241–244, 1987.

161. Arnout J, Simoons M, deBono D, et al: Correlation between level of heparinization and patency of the infarct-related coronary artery after treatment of acute myocardial infarction with alteplase (rt-PA). J Am Coll Cardiol 20:513–519, 1992.

162. Lidon RM, Theroux P, Juneau M, et al: The partial thromboplastin time during episodes of recurrent ischemic pain in unstable angina patients treated with heparin. Circulation 86:1857, 1992.

163. Melandri G, Branzi A, Traini AM, et al: A prospective study of the value of monitoring heparin treatment after thrombolysis with the activated clotting time. J Am Coll Cardiol 57A, 1994 [special issue].

164. Flaker GC, Bartolozzi J, Davis V, et al: Use of a standardized nomogram to achieve therapeutic anticoagulation after thrombolytic therapy in myocardial infarction. Arch Intern Med 154:1492–1496, 1994.

165. Raschke RA, Reilly BM, Guidry JR, et al: The weight-based heparin dosing nomogram compared with a "standard care" nomogram. Ann Intern Med 119:875–881, 1993.

166. Hochman JS, Wali AU, Gavrila D, et al: A new regimen for heparin use in acute coronary syndromes. Am Heart J 138:313–318, 1999.

167. Brill-Edwards P, Ginsberg JS, Johnston M, Hirsh J: Establishing a therapeutic range for heparin therapy. Ann Intern Med 119:104–109, 1993.

168. Volles DF, Ancell CJ, Michael KA, et al: Establishing an institution-specific therapeutic range for heparin. Am J Health Syst Pharm 55:2002–2006, 1998.

169. Ryan TJ, Anderson JL, Antman EM, et al: 1999 Update: ACC/AHA Guidelines for the Management of Patients with Acute Myocardial Infarction: Executive Summary and Recommendations: A Report of the American College of Cardiology/American Heart Association Task Force on Practice Guidelines (Committee on Management of Acute Myocardial Infarction). Circulation 100:1016–1030, 1999.

Low-molecular-weight Heparins in Acute Coronary Syndromes

ERIC D. GRASSMAN, MD, PhD

Acute coronary syndromes are broadly defined as two ischemic coronary conditions: (1) unstable angina and non–Q-wave myocardial infarction and (2) Q-wave myocardial infarction. Pathophysiologically, both conditions result from disruption of coronary artery atherosclerotic plaque with consequent thrombin generation, platelet activation, and thrombus formation.[1,2] From a clinical standpoint, non–Q-wave myocardial infarction consists of mild elevation of cardiac enzymes without the development of Q waves on the electrocardiogram. Patients with unstable angina have been described clinically as patients whose presentations did not result in the elevation of cardiac enzymes. Unstable angina has three possible presentations:

1. Symptoms of angina at rest (usually prolonged > 20 minutes)
2. New onset (< 2 months) of exertional angina of at least Canadian Cardiovascular Society Classification (CCSC) class III in severity or recent (less than 2 months) acceleration of angina as reflected by an increase in severity of at least one CCSC class to at least CCSC class III
3. Postinfarction angina

Evidence that both platelet activation and thrombin generation are involved in the thrombotic process provides the rationale for the use of both aspirin and unfractionated heparin (UFH) in the management of acute coronary syndromes. The past decade has seen much research and debate about the value of these agents alone or in combination. UFH and aspirin have become the standard treatment of patients presenting with acute coronary syndromes.[3] Administration of UFH, however, has several disadvantages. The anticoagulant response varies significantly among patients. This variation is thought to be due to individual differences in concentrations of heparin neutralizing plasma proteins as well as variable elevations in factor VIII as part of the acute-phase response to ischemia. Bleeding is another common complication of UFH, which can induce bleeding by inhibiting blood coagulation, impairing platelet function, and increasing capillary permeability. Finally, heparin-induced thrombocytopenia occurs in approximately 3–4% of heparin-treated patients. The pathogenic antibody, usually immunoglobulin G, recognizes a complex of heparin and platelet factor 4. This adverse drug reaction is associated with a high risk of thrombotic complications.

The disadvantages of UFH triggered interest in low-molecular-weight (LMW) heparins as an alternative treatment for acute coronary syndromes. It is thought that the enhanced ratio of anti-Xa to anti-IIa and reduced platelet interactions of LMW heparins may provide significant advantages over UFH. LMW heparins also have greater bioavailability and possibly cause fewer bleeding problems. The efficacy and safety of three LMW heparins—enoxaparin, dalteparin, and nadroparin—have been investigated in six large clinical trials of acute coronary syndromes. This chapter reviews the data from evidence-based trials of LMW heparins in the treatment of acute coronary syndromes by comparing some LMW heparins with others and with UFH.

LMW heparins are produced by enzymatic or chemical depolymerization of UFH to yield chains of molecular weights ranging from 4,000 to 6,500 daltons[4-6] (Table 1). LMW heparins have a reduced ability to catalyze the inactivation of thrombin relative to their ability to catalyze the inactivation of factor Xa, probably because of their small molecular size. Thus, compared with UFH, LMW heparins have a ratio of antifactor Xa to antifactor IIa between 4:1 and 2:1 (see Table 1). The relative importance of inhibition of factor Xa and thrombin in mediating the antithrombotic effect of UFH and LMW heparin is unclear, but evidence indicates that both are necessary. In addition, the reduced protein binding of LMW heparins improves their pharmokinetic properties. Their minimal interaction with platelets may be responsible for the reduced microvascular bleeding and lower incidence of heparin-induced thrombocytopenia.[4,5] The bioavailability of LMW heparins after subcutaneous injections is approximately 90% compared with 30% for UFH.[6] This higher bioavailability is probably due to the lower rate of protein binding of LMW heparin compared with UFH and may explain the more predictable anticoagulant response that can be obtained at a given dose of LMW heparins. Their half life of 2–4 hours after intravenous administration and 3–6 hours after subcutaneous injection is longer than that of UFH.[7-9]

Overall, the combination of the predictable anticoagulant response, high bioavailability, and long half-life of LMW heparins means that an adequate and predictable anticoagulant response can be achieved with 1 or 2 daily subcutaneous injections. In addition, because LMW heparins do not affect activated partial thromboplastin time (aPTT), routine monitoring to assess the anticoagulant effect is not necessary. An antifactor Xa assay is available, but it is not routinely used because of lack of a clinically defined therapeutic range and expense. Table 2 summarizes the comparison of UFH and LMW heparins.

Table 1.   Characteristics of Low-molecular-weight Heparins

LMW Heparin	Mean Molecular Weight (Daltons)	Anti-Xa/ Anti-IIa Ratio	Half-life (hr)	North America Availability
Nadroparin (Fraxiparine)	4500	3.6:1	2.2–3.5	Canada
Ardeparin (Normiflo)	6000	1.9:1	3	United States
Tinzaparin (Innohep)	4500	1.9:1	1.4–1.9	Canada
Dalteparin (Fragmin)	6000	2.7:1	2.0–5.0	Canada/U.S.
Enoxaparin (Lovenox)	4200	3.8:1	2.2–5.0	Canada/U.S.

Table 2. Comparison of Unfractionated Heparin and Low-molecular-weight Heparins

Unfractionated Heparin	Low-molecular-weight Heparins
Unpredictable anticoagulant response	More predictable anticoagulant response
Requires aPTT monitoring	No laboratory monitoring required
Poor bioavailability	Better bioavailability at lower doses
Short half-life	Longer half-life
Risk of bleeding complications	Slightly lower risk of major bleeding complications
Risk of thrombocytopenia	Lower risk of thrombocytopenia

aPTT = activated partial thromboplastin time.

Treatment with LMW heparins in animal models seems to result in less bleeding than treatment with UFH. This finding may be explained by the following factors:

1. LMW heparins have a lower affinity for platelets and thus inhibit them less than UFH.

2. Unlike UFH, LMW heparins do not increase microvascular permeability.

3. The low affinity of LMW heparins for endothelial cells, von Willebrand factor and platelets makes them less likely to interfere with the prothrombotic interaction between platelets and vessel walls. Because of lesser interaction with platelets, heparin-induced thrombocytopenia seems to be less common with LMW heparins.

The reduction in risk of bleeding observed in early experimental animal models does not seem to be as obvious in clinical human studies, as detailed in a review of evidence-based studies later in this chapter.

The efficacy of aspirin in the treatment in unstable angina has been demonstrated in a number of randomized, controlled trials.[10-13] The addition of UFH to aspirin may further improve survival rates and prevent progression to nonfatal myocardial infarction (MI).[10-16] Oler[17] conducted a meta-analysis of 6 randomized trials involving 1,353 patients. Patients given aspirin plus UFH were compared with patients given aspirin alone. At 30 days, the addition of UFH to aspirin was associated with a 33% reduction in death or myocardial infarction. The event rate in the aspirin-treated group was 10.4% compared with 7.9% in the group treated with aspirin plus UFH. The confidence intervals were wide in these statistically marginal events. Lack of benefit may have resulted from limitations of UFH rather than lack of importance of thrombin inhibition in reducing ischemic events.

No published trials have assessed the role of LMW heparins in the treatment of acute Q-wave MI. The Heparin and Aspirin Reperfusion Therapy (HART) II trial was presented at the American College of Cardiology Scientific Session in March, 2000. Patients with acute ST-elevation MI were randomized to subcutaneous enoxaparin or intravenous UFH for 72 hours. Rates of total patency at 90 minutes, which was the principal end-point, showed a trend in favor of enoxaparin (80.1% vs. 75.1%). Hemorrhagic complications were comparable for the two agents. The direct thrombin inhibitor hirudin was used as adjunct therapy in two randomized trials of thrombolysis for acute Q-wave MI.

This chapter reviews six prospective, randomized, controlled clinical trials that evaluated the use of LMW heparin in patients with unstable angina and non–Q-wave MI. The LMW heparins used in the studies were enoxaparin, nadroparin, and dalteparin. Table 3 summarizes the six clinical trials reviewed below.

Table 3. Summary of Controlled Trials Using Low-molecular-weight Heparins in Acute Coronary Syndromes

Trial	Drug	Duration of Unstable Angina	Duration of Non-Q MI	Cath/PTCA	End-point	Acute Treatment	Chronic Treatment	Patients Enrolled	Results
TIMI-IIB	Enoxaparin	Chest pain > 5 min, history of CAD, or ST deviation	Chest pain > 5 min, positive enzymes, no Q-wave MI	Physician's discretion	MI, R, or D at 8 d and 43 d	ASA + UFH vs. ASA + enoxaparin 1 mg/kg (100 anti-Xa U/kg) bid 2–8 d	ASA + placebo vs. enoxaparin 43 d (40 mg for < 65 kg, 60 mg for > 65 kg	3910	8 d, p = 0.03 / 43 d, p = 0.061
ESSENCE	Enoxaparin	Chest pain > 10 min, history of CAD, or ST deviation	None	Not discussed	MI, R, D, or A at 14 d	ASA + UFH vs. ASA + enoxaparin 1mg/kg (100 anti-XA U/kg) bid 2–8 d		3171	p = 0.02
FRISC	Dalteparin	Chest pain and ST deviation	None	Disabling angina or positive ETT	MI, D, or R at 6 d, 40 d, and 150 d	ASA + dalteparin 120 U/kg bid in hospital vs. ASA + placebo	ASA + dalteparin 7500 U qd for 40 vs. ASA + placebo	1499	6 d, p < 0.001 / 40 d, p = 0.005 / 150 d, p = 0.18
FRIC	Dalteparin	Modified Braunwald + ST or T-wave changes	Chest pain and positive enzymes	Refractory angina or positive ETT	MI, D, or A at 6 d and 45 d	ASA + dalteparin 120 120 IU/kg bid vs. ASA + UFH 1–6 d	ASA + dalteparin 7500 IU qd vs. ASA + placebo for 45 d	1482	6 d, p = NS / 48 d, p = NS
FRAXIS	Nadroparin	Chest pain + ST deviation or T-wave inversion	Chest pain and positive enzymes	Not discussed	MI, D, or A at 14 d	86 anti-Xa/kg bid for 6 d vs. same for 14 d vs. UFH for 6 d		3468	p = NS
Gurfinkel	Nadroparin	Recent onset or prolonged (> 10 min), spontaneous rest chest pain; and objective evidence of CAD	Excluded	Local institutional practice	R, MI, A, D, or major bleeding 5–7 d	ASA vs. ASA + UFH vs. nadroparin 214 U; institute Choay/kg anti-Xa bid		219	Nadroparin vs. ASA, p = 0.00001 / Nadroparin vs. UHF, p = 0.00001

CAD = coronary artery disease, MI = myocardial infarction, R = revascularization, D = death, A = recurrent angina, ASA = aspirin, UFH = unfractionated heparin.

ESSENCE

The Efficacy and Safety of Subcutaneous Enoxaparin in Non–Q-Wave Coronary Events (ESSENCE) Trial[18] is a large study involving 3171 patients. It compared the efficacy of aspirin and UFH with the efficacy of aspirin and enoxaparin. The end-point, measured at 14 days, included death, MI, urgent revascularization, or recurrent angina. The enoxaparin dose was 100 U/kg administered twice a day. At 14 days, the composite end-point was lower in the enoxaparin-treated group with a p value of 0.02. Safety analysis found no difference in the rate of major hemorrhage in the UFH (7%) and enoxaparin (6.5%) groups. The incidence of minor hemorrhage was increased significantly in the enoxaparin group (11.9%) compared with the UFH group (7.2%). The most frequent type of minor hemorrhage was injection ecchymoses. The authors discussed the differences between their results and those of the FRIC study (see below), which found no difference in effect between LMW heparins and UFH. The authors speculate that this difference may be due to the fact that enoxaparin has a ratio of anti-Xa to anti-IIa of 3 :1 compared with 2:1 for dalteparin.

TIMI-IIB

The Thrombolysis In Myocardial Infarction (TIMI-IIB) Trial[19] is similar to the ESSENCE Trial, but it followed patients for 43 days. Acute treatment with aspirin and UFH or aspirin and enoxaparin showed the same results as in the ESSENCE Trial. The dose of enoxaparin used in TIMI-IIB was obtained from the TIMI-II A Trial, which was a dose-ranging study. It was found that subcutaneous injections of 1 mg/kg every 12 hours was associated with a major hemorrhage rate of 1.9%, whereas a higher dose of 1.25 mg/kg every 12 hours was associated with a major hemorrhage rate of 6.5%. The rate of myocardial ischemia was similar in the two groups. Thus it was believed that a dose of 1.0 mg/kg was associated with a lower risk of major hemorrhage with no apparent loss of efficacy. The combined end-point of death, MI, or urgent revascularization was compared at 8 days and 43 days. At 8 days, as in the ESSENCE Trial, the combined end-point was lower for the LMW heparin group (p = 0.03). This benefit was sustained at 43 days, despite a borderline p value of 0.061. The major hemorrhage rate during hospitalization was the same for enoxaparin and UFH. Enoxaparin was associated with a higher rate of minor hemorrhage, usually ecchymosis at the injection site or hematoma at the site of a sheath inserted for cardiac catheterization. During the chronic phase, there was a significant increase in the number of major and minor hemorrhages with enoxaparin compared with placebo. This finding is probably not surprising.

FRISC

The Fragmin during Instability in Coronary Artery Disease (FRISC) Trial[21] compared dalteparin with placebo in 1499 patients. The combined end-point was death, MI, or urgent revascularization at 6 days, 40 days, and 150 days. Treatment was continued for 40 days. The combined end-point was significantly lower in the LMW heparin group at 6 days and 40 days, but the benefit was not sustained at 150 days (p = 0.18). There were few major hemorrhages, no cerebral bleeding, and no overall differences between the two treatment groups in terms of hemorrhage. Minor bleeding, mainly subcutaneous hematoma at injection sites, was more common in the actively treated group. The FRISC Trial was followed by the FRISC-II Trial,[22] which compared early invasive vs. conservative strategy and dalteparin for treatment of unstable coronary artery disease. At both 45 and 90 days, the study found no significant difference in the primary end-point of death or MI in patients treated with dalteparin compared with those treated with placebo. At 6 months, patients randomized to either dalteparin or placebo had similar rates of death or MI, suggesting no significant advantage of dalteparin in outcome.

FRIC

The Fragmin in Unstable Coronary Artery Disease (FRIC) Trial[23] included 1482 patients. The combined end-point of death, MI, or recurrent angina was measured at 6 days and 45 days. During the acute phase, patients were treated with aspirin and dalteparin if they had initially been randomized to LMW heparin vs. aspirin and UFH. The acute phase lasted from 1–6 days. In the chronic phase, the LMW heparin group was treated with aspirin and dalteparin or aspirin and placebo for 45 days. At neither 6 days nor 45 days was the combined end-point lower in the LMW heparin group. There was no difference in the incidence of major bleeding during the acute or chronic phase. There was a higher incidence of minor bleeding (28% vs. 15%) for dalteparin compared with placebo.

FRAXIS

The Fraxiparin in Ischaemic Syndrome (FRAXIS) Trial[24] involved 3486 patients. The combined end-point of death, MI, or recurrent angina was measured at 14 days. Patients were randomized to receive UFH for 6 days, nadroparin for 6 days, or nadroparin for 14 days. At 14 days there was no significant reduction in the combined end-point in the LMW heparin group. During the first 6 days of treatment there were marginal differences in the incidences of major hemorrhages in the three groups (1% for UFH, 0.7% for 6 days of nadroparin, and 1.3% for 14 days of nadroparin). At day 14 the risk of major hemorrhage, after prolonged treatment with nadroparin was 3.5% compared with 1.6% (p = 0.0035) after 6 days of UFH treatment and 1.5% after 6 days of nadroparin treatment. Nadroparin was not associated with an increased risk of major bleeding compared with aspirin alone or aspirin and UFH.

GURFINKEL

In the trial reported by Gurfinkel,[25] nadroparin was evaluated in the setting of unstable angina; patients with MI were excluded. The combined end-point was urgent revascularization, MI, recurrent angina, death, or measured bleeding noted at 5–7 days. The study included 219 patients, who were randomized to receive aspirin alone, aspirin and UFH, or aspirin and nadroparin. A relatively high dose of nadroparin was used. In the relatively short follow-up, nadroparin was superior to UFH in reducing the composite major end-point.

TIMI-IIB–ESSENCE Meta-analysis

A meta-analysis of the TIMI-IIB and ESSENCE Trials[26] extracted from the two studies the following data:

- Event rates of death
- Composite end-points of death and nonfatal MI
- Composite end-points of death, nonfatal MI, and urgent revascularization
- Rates of major hemorrhage

All heterogeneity tests for efficacy end-points were negative, which suggests that the findings of the two trials are comparable. Compared with treatment with UFH, enoxaparin was associated with a 20% reduction in death and serious cardiac ischemic events that appeared within the first few days of treatment. This benefit was sustained through 43 days.

Discussion

LMW heparin appears to be superior to placebo and UFH in reducing ischemic events or death in the acute phase of unstable angina or non–Q-wave MI. Major bleeding complications are similar for LMW heparins and UFH, but minor bleeding complications are more common with LMW heparins, primarily because of injection site hematomas. Enoxaparin has a beneficial effect in both acute and chronic phases in the two studies. Studies of dalteparin and nadroparin failed to show significant long-term benefit with either agent. It appears that enoxaparin is the preferred LMW heparin for patients with unstable angina and non–Q-wave MI. At a dose of 1 mg/kg subcutaneously twice daily, enoxaparin appears effective for 72 hours but probably is not necessary beyond the hospital phase.

The possibility of clinical differences between the LMW heparins raises the question of which drug characteristics contribute to variation in performance. The importance of anti-Xa activity in the treatment of unstable angina is yet to be defined. Monitoring and comparison of anti-Xa activities with dalteparin and enoxaparin in the FRIC and TIMI-IIA Trials revealed higher trough values for anti-Xa in enoxaparin-treated patients compared with patients receiving dalteparin. This difference may indicate a suboptimal anticoagulant effect in the FRIC Trial, possibly contributing to failure to demonstrate superiority over UFH. Of note, the higher sustained anti-Xa levels in enoxaparin-treated patients were not associated with increased risk of major bleeding compared with UFH. These data may provide important guidelines for target anti-Xa levels in future studies.

Another biochemical parameter that recently has received attention is von Willebrand factor. A substudy of the ESSENCE Trial revealed that early elevation in von Willebrand factor in patients with unstable angina or non–Q-wave MI was associated with an adverse outcome. Enoxaparin, but not UFH, blunted this early increase. The effect on levels of von Willebrand factor may stem from more efficient binding of exonaparin to the heparin-binding site of von Willebrand factor compared with UFH, causing increased inhibition of von Willebrand binding to platelets. Platelet adhesion thus would be reduced.

The potential role of tissue factor pathway inhibitor (TFPI) also has been studied. TFPI inactivates tissue factor VIIIa:Xa complex, thereby contributing to the antithrombotic effect. LMWH is different from UFH, and the various

LMW heparins differ in their propensity to release TFPI in a manner that is independent of anti-Xa activity, possibly explaining, at least in part, the variation in clinical performance.

Conclusion

Randomized clinical studies have compared unfractionated heparin and low-molecular-weight heparins in the acute and long-term management of patients with unstable angina and non–Q-wave myocardial infarction. Enoxaparin was found to be superior to unfractionated heparin without increasing the risk of major hemorrhagic events. The improvement in clinical outcome was maintained for 1 year. Other low-molecular-weight heparins (nadroparin and dalteparin) have not demonstrated clinical superiority over UFH. Low-molecular-weight heparins have not been systematically studied in patients with Q-wave myocardial infarction. Only preliminary, unpublished results have been reported.

References

1. Fuster V, Badimon L, Cohen M, et al: Insights into the pathogenesis of acute ischemic syndromes. Circulation 77:1213–1220, 1998.
2. Davies MJ, Thomas A: Plaque fissuring: The cause of acute myocardial infarction, sudden ischemic death, and crescendo angina. Br Heart J 53:363–373, 1985.
3. Cairns JA, Lewis HD, Meade TW, et al: Antithrombotic agents in coronary artery disease. Fourth ACCP Consensus Conference on Antithrombotic Therapy. Chest 108 (Suppl4):380S–400S, 1995.
4. Hirsh J, Levine MN: Low molecular weight heparin. Blood 79:1–17, 1992.
5. Weitz JI: Low-molecular-weight heparins. N Engl J Med 337:688–698, 1997.
6. Turpie AGG: Pharmacology of the low-molecular-weight heparins. Am Heart J 135:S329–S335, 1998.
7. Martineau P, Tawil N: Low-molecular-weight heparins in the treatment of deep-vein thrombosis. Ann Pharmacother 32:588–601, 1998.
8. Harenberg J: Pharmacology of low molecular weight heparins. Semin Thromb Hemost 16(Suppl):12–18, 1990.
9. Matzsch T, Bergquist D, Hedner U, Ostergaard P: Effects of an enzymatically depolymerized heparin as compared with conventional heparin in healthy volunteers. Thromb Haemost 57:97–101, 1987.
10. Theroux P, Ouimet H, McCans J, et al: Aspirin, heparin, or both to treat acute unstable angina. N Engl J Med 219:1105–1111, 1988.
11. RISC Group: Risk of myocardial infarction and death during treatment with low-dose aspirin and intravenous heparin in men with unstable coronary artery disease. Lancet 336:827–830, 1990.
12. Cairns JA, Gent M, Singer J, et al: Aspirin, sulfinpyrazone, or both in unstable angina: Results of a Canadian multicenter trial. N Engl J Med 313:1369–1375, 1985.
13. Lewis H Jr, Davis JW, Archibald DG, et al: Protective effects of aspirin against acute myocardial infarction and death in men with unstable angina: Results of a Veterans Administration Cooperative Study. N Engl J Med 309:396–403, 1983.
14. Theroux P, Waters D, Qiu S, et al: Aspirin versus heparin to prevent myocardial infarction during the acute phase of unstable angina. Circulation 88:2045–2048, 1993.
15. Theroux P, Waters D, Lam J, et al: Reactivation of unstable angina after the discontinuation of heparin. N Engl J Med 327:141–145, 1992.
16. Holdright D, Patel D, Cunningham D, et al: Comparison of the effect of heparin and aspirin versus aspirin alone on transient myocardial ischemia and in-hospital prognosis in patients with unstable angina. J Am Coll Cardiol 24:39–45, 1994.
17. Oler A, Whooley MA, Oler J, Grady D: Adding heparin to aspirin reduces the incidence of myocardial infarction and death in patients with unstable angina: A meta-analysis. JAMA 276:811–815, 1996.
18. Cohen M, Demers C, Gurfinkel EP, et al: A comparison of low-molecular-weight heparin with unfractionated heparin for unstable coronary artery disease. N Engl J Med 337:447–452, 1997.

19. Antmann EM, et al: Enoxaparin prevents death and cardiac ischemic events in unstable angina/non-q-wave myocardial infarction: Results of thrombolysis in myocardial infarction (TIMI) IIB trial. Circulation 100:1593–1601, 1999.
20. Thrombolysis In Myocardial Infarction (TIMI) IIA investigators: Dose ranging trial of enoxaparin for unstable angina: Results of TIMI II A. J Am Coll Cardiol 29:1474–1482, 1997.
21. Fragmin during Instability in Coronary Artery Disease (FRISC) Study Group: Low-molecular-weight heparin during instability in coronary artery disease. Lancet 347:561–568, 1996.
22. Presented at the 48th Annual Scientific Session of the American College of Cardiology, New Orleans, 1999.
23. Klein W, Buchwald A, Hillis SE, et al: Comparison of low-molecular-weight heparin with unfractionated heparin acutely and with placebo for 6 weeks in the management of unstable coronary artery disease: Fragmin in Unstable Coronary Artery Disease Study (FRIC). Circulation 96:61–68, 1997.
24. Leizorovicz A: The FRAXIS study: Optimal duration of treatment of unstable angina in the acute phase—preliminary results [abstract]. Presented at the 20th Congress of the European Society of Cardiology, August 22–26, 1998, Vienna, Austria.
25. Gurfinkel EP, Manos EJ, Mejail RI, et al: Low molecular weight heparin versus regular heparin or aspirin in the treatment of unstable angina and silent ischemia. J Am Coll Cardiol 26:313–318, 1995.
26. Antonon EM, et al: Assessment of the treatment effect of enoxaparin for unstable angina/non–Q-wave myocardial infarction: TIMI IIB-ESSENCE meta-analysis. Circulation 100:1600–1608, 1999.

Antithrombin Agents: The New Class of Antithrombotic Drugs

JAWED FAREED, PhD

DEBRA A. HOPPENSTEADT, PhD

PETER BACHER, MD

HARRY L. MESSMORE, MD

The central role of thrombin in coagulation and platelet activation is now well established. Thus it provides an important target for control of thrombogenesis. Thrombin inhibitors such as recombinant hirudin, hirulog, and argatroban are currently under development for various clinical indications. These drugs produce a direct anticoagulant response by targeting thrombin. In addition to amplifying the coagulation cascade by activating factors V and VIII, mediating stabilization of fibrin by activating factor XIII, and activating platelets, thrombin exerts several regulatory activities to maintain hemostatic balance. However, it is capable of activating protein C, which is an anticoagulant and profibrinolytic enzyme.[20] Furthermore, thrombin is a potent stimulator of secretion of tissue-type plasminogen activator (tPA) from endothelial cells.[19,21] Although plasminogen is activated to plasmin directly by endogenous enzymes, such as urokinase-type plasminogen activator (uPA)[60] and tPA,[40] other enzymes, such as kallikrein,[18] factor XIIa,[35] and activated protein C[20,62] also promote the activation of plasminogen. Some of the synthetic thrombin inhibitors also can inhibit these enzymes.[8,15,32] Thus, both physiologic and pharmacologic fibrinolysis can be compromised. Thrombin inhibitors, therefore, exert a complex effect on the coagulation network and are under careful evaluation in various clinical trials.

In the absence of heparin, thrombin is marginally neutralized by endogenous inhibitors such as heparin cofactor II (HCII) and antithrombin III (ATIII). Because of their mass, these inhibitors are not capable of effectively neutralizing clot-bound thrombin. On the other hand, the lower mass of thrombin inhibitors allows them to penetrate the thrombus, to inhibit the thrombin contained within, and to control further enlargement of the thrombus. Thus, smaller-molecular-weight thrombin inhibitors can inhibit clot-bound thrombin and may be more effective than heparin.

OVERVIEW OF THROMBIN INHIBITORS

Direct inhibitors of thrombin may be classified according to source, structure, and type of interaction as endogenous inhibitors, analogs of natural substrates, or recombinant and synthetic inhibitors. Some of these agents are directed against the catalytic site of thrombin, whereas others bind to the exosites of thrombin (Fig. 1). In addition, some are reversible inhibitors, whereas others are irreversible. Table 1 lists the currently available site-directed thrombin inhibitors, and Figure 2 depicts diagrammatic representations.

Among the natural thrombin inhibitors, hirudin, which is found in the saliva of the leech *Hirudo medicinalis*, is one of the most potent. It is a single polypeptide chain of 65 amino acid residues, stabilized in a characteristic conformation by three disulfide bridges.[63] Hirudin and its variants have been produced by recombinant technology.[14,24,29,36] Point mutations have been used to develop variant forms of hirudin.[63] Recently polyethylene glycol (PEG) coupling of recombinant hirudin has been used to develop longer-lasting agents.[29,82] Several experimental and clinical trials have shown that polyethylene glycol coupling of hirudin increases its efficacy. Various derivatives of hirudin are under aggressive development for several clinical indications.

Coupling of peptides that mimic the carboxy terminal of hirudin to peptides that are specific for inhibition of the catalytic site of thrombin (D-Phe-Pro-Arg) has led to the development of a series of chimeric molecules termed *hirulogs*. The amino terminus consists of the catalytic site-directed peptides, whereas the carboxy terminus consists of the 12 terminal residues of hirudin. The two moieties are linked together by a bridge of glycine residues of variable length.[23,51] Thus, hirulogs inhibit thrombin by binding to both its catalytic site and its anion-binding exosite, thus conferring specificity for thrombin. Hirulog-1 has been developed aggressively for several cardiovascular indications.[16,72,73] However, its superiority over heparin has not been established.

A novel synthetic thrombin inhibitor, CVS#995, is composed of 19 amino acids, in which recognition sequences for the catalytic and primary exosite binding domains of thrombin have been linked by a transition-state analog.[77] The K_i value for thrombin is in the pM range for this slow and tight-binding inhibitor. Compared with hirulog-1, CVS#995[77] is superior at inhibiting platelet aggregation and venous thrombosis in rats.[77]

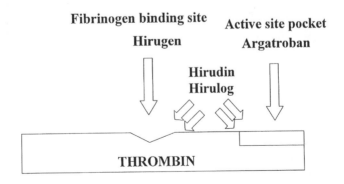

Figure 1. Sites of action of different antithrombin agents.

Table 1. Developmental Status of Site-directed Thrombin Inhibitors

Agents	Chemical Nature	Developmental Status
Hirudin, PEG hirudin, and related variants	Recombinant analogs of natural hirudin and their derivatives	Various clinical phases of-development; additional-derivatives are being. developed One product is-available in Europe.
Hirulogs	Synthetic bifunctional oligopeptides	Phase II and III clinical studies are completed. Additional studies are currently under way.
Peptidomimetics	Synthetic heterocyclic derivatives	Phase II and III clinical develop-ment in the U.S. Argatroban (reversible) is used in Japan.
Peptides and their derivatives	Peptide arginals and boronic acid peptide derivatives	Various products are in phase II clinical development.
Aptamers	DNA- and RNA-derived oligo-nucleotides with thrombin-binding domains	Preclinical stage. Limited animal data available.

PEG = polyethylene glycol.

One of the building blocks used to develop synthetic inhibitors is arginine with optimal C and/or N-terminal modifications. Many of these agents have been found to be highly toxic because of inhibition of butyl cholinesterase.[39] The introduction of a COOH group on the carboxy terminal results in decreased affinity for butyl cholinesterase and therefore less toxicity. After further modifi-cations an isomer called argatroban (MD805 or MCI9038) has been generated as a selective inhibitor of thrombin (K_i =0.019 µM).[31] This compound also has a

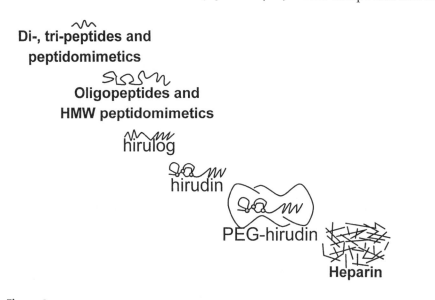

Di-, tri-peptides and peptidomimetics

Oligopeptides and HMW peptidomimetics

hirulog

hirudin

PEG-hirudin

Heparin

Figure 2. Diagrammatic representation of various antithrombin drugs. All of these agents except heparin produce a direct antithrombin effect and are in various phases of clinical development. Heparin is used for comparison.

sizeable affinity for trypsin (K_i = 5.0 µM).[39] It inhibits thrombin directly and prevents it from acting in the coagulation and fibrinolytic systems.[52,67,68] Argatroban is effective in preventing thrombus formation in various animal models at low concentrations (> 1 µM).[39,52] It is being tested clinically for several indications.[53,58,81]

With the knowledge of the primary structure of serine proteases and the identification of their proteolytic activation cleavage sites, specific chromogenic substrates for thrombin have been developed by synthesis of peptides mimicking the amino acid sequence adjacent to the substrate's cleavage site and attaching a para-nitroaniline (pNA) group on the carboxy terminus.[8] A comprehensive survey of the effects of many peptide inhibitors belonging to various classes has been completed by Fareed and colleagues on a spectrum of serine proteases, using clotting and novel amidolytic systems.[28]

Several tripeptide aldehydes containing arginine have been developed as the first reversible peptide thrombin inhibitors. The prototype compound to be synthesized is D-Phe-Pro-Arg-H (GYKI-14166).[7] Although it is a highly selective and potent inhibitor of thrombin, it is quite unstable in neutral aqueous solution, where it cyclizes and becomes inactivated. To prevent cyclization, a derivative has been synthesized with a protective amino terminal t-butyloxycarbonyl (Boc) group: Boc-D-Phe-Pro-Arg-H (GYKI 14451).[5] This compound is more stable than its parent but not as specific for thrombin because it inhibits plasmin as well. To achieve compounds that are both stable and specific for thrombin, a series of N-alkyl derivatives has been synthesized (a basic amino terminus promotes thrombin specificity). From this series the methyl derivative D-MePhe-Pro-Arg-H (GYKI 14766)[3,4,6] has been found to be as potent and as selective a reversible inhibitor of thrombin as the prototype aldehyde. The K_i for the aldehyde derivatives is around 0.1 µM. All three aldehydes are effective antithrombotics in various animal models. One of these agents, efegatran (D-MePhe-Pro-Arg-H), is currently undergoing clinical trials for prevention of reocclusion during interventional cardiovascular procedures.

Peptides of arginine chloromethyl ketones correspond to the primary structure of physiologic substrates of target proteases.[46] These agents are used in biochemical studies of thrombin and hemostasis as well as in pharmacologic studies. The toxicity of the tripeptide chloromethyl ketone D-Phe-Pro-ArgCH$_2$Cl (PPACK) is species-dependent. Its antithrombotic effects also have been examined extensively in various animal models (rats, dogs, and rabbits); all studies indicate that it is an effective antithrombotic after both intravenous and subcutaneous administration.

Tripeptide derivatives with α-nitrile groups have been synthesized as competitive inhibitors of thrombin. The peptide derivative D-Phe-Pro-Arg-CN[63] has proved to be a strong competitive inhibitor of thrombin with a K_i = 0.7 µM. It is also an effective antithrombotic in various rat models of thrombosis.

The search for selective and potent inhibitors of thrombin has led to the development of three more classes of reversible tripeptide inhibitors:

1. Trifluoromethyl ketones. The representative compound D-Phe-Pro-Arg-CF$_3$[55] has a K_i in the nM range.

2. Alpha-aminophosphonic acid tripeptide derivatives with K_is in the nM range.[17] These compounds form a new group of thrombin inhibitors because they have only neutral side chains.

3. Alpha-aminoboronic acid derivatives.[45] The boronic acid derivatives were first developed as inhibitors of elastase and chymotrypsin. To develop a compound that is specific for thrombin, the arginine in the sequence D-Phe-Pro-Arg has been substituted with its boronic acid derivative. This substitution led to the synthesis of Ac-(D)-Phe-Pro-boroArg (K_i = 41 pM), Boc-(D)-Phe-Pro-boroArg (K_i = 3.6 pM), and H-(D)-Phe-Pro-boroArg (K_i < 1 pM). Ac-D-Phe-Pro-boroArg also possesses antithrombotic effects as demonstrated by two thrombosis models. H-(D)-Phe-Pro-boroArg demonstrates antithrombotic effects in a baboon model of thrombosis.

Inhibitors derived from boronic acid lack specificity for thrombin. In an attempt to overcome this limitation, the C terminal of the tripeptides has been extended.[45] However, the resulting compounds still lack specificity for thrombin. Tapparelli et al.[69] replaced the boroArg in the third position (corresponding to the S1 pocket site of thrombin) with a neutral boron-containing moiety. The resulting compound, Z-D-Phe-Pro-boroMpgC$_{10}$H$_{16}$, has a lower K_i for thrombin (8.9 nM) than its predecessors, but the specificity for thrombin is improved.[69] However, it is a weak anticoagulant in global clotting tests and does not inhibit thrombin-induced platelet aggregation in vitro or in vivo.

Although all of these agents are potent thrombin inhibitors, little attention is paid to their mode of inhibition, which may be important to the efficacy of their anticoagulant and antithrombotic effects. Because the new thrombin inhibitors vary in their mechanism of action, it is likely that they also differ in their effects on the coagulation cascade and the feedback mechanisms involved. Despite the fact that nonspecific thrombin inhibitors such as Ac-D-Phe-Pro-boroArg-OH and D-MePhe-Pro-Arg-H are known to inhibit several of the fibrinolytic enzymes, systematic studies of their in vivo effects on the fibrinolytic/thrombolytic processes are limited. Although the majority of published experimental studies suggest no interference or even enhancement of thrombolysis by thrombin inhibitors, recent reports from clinical investigations suggest that some of these agents produce a fibrinolytic deficit.[15] Such observations are supported by studies exploring the antifibrinolytic effects of several thrombin inhibitors both in vitro and in vivo.[15]

Aptamers are oligonucleotides (double- or single-stranded DNA or single-stranded RNA) that act directly on thrombin. Thirty-two such aptamers have been recently isolated as inhibitors of thrombin with binding affinities in the range of 20–200 nM.[10] One of the most potent thrombin aptamers interacts with the anion-binding exosite of thrombin and thus competes with substrates that interact with this specific site, such as fibrinogen and thrombin platelet receptors.[50,59] This aptamer recently was shown to reduce arterial platelet thrombus formation in an animal model and to inhibit clot-bound thrombin in an in vitro system.[49] Recently, a second pool of aptamers was isolated. They have a different sequence composition, incorporate modified bases, and show promising anticoagulant activities.[47] Another recent development in the area of oligonucleotide inhibitors of thrombin is the isolation of two RNAs that bind thrombin with high affinity (K_d in the nM range). These oligonucleotides have been shown to inhibit fibrinogen clotting in an in vitro test.[47]

The development of oral thrombin inhibitors is somewhat slow because of their limited bioavailability. Currently several of these agents are in various phases of clinical trials. Most of the oral thrombin agents are peptidomimetic types of inhibitors. Their bioavailability varies from 5–20%. Unlike the orally active glycoprotein (GP) IIb/IIIa inhibitors, which for the most part are pro-drugs, the oral antithrombin drugs are active thrombin inhibitors and do not require metabolic transformation after absorption. Their relative inhibitory potency is also variable; however, their antithrombin effects are comparable to those observed with intravenously active antithrombin agents.

It has been suggested that the oral antithrombin agents may be of use in out-patient/extended management of both arterial and venous thrombosis. Some investigators have equated these agents with oral anticoagulant therapy. However, the mechanisms of the two types of drugs are quite different. Although the oral thrombin inhibitors offer an attractive approach in the management of thrombotic disorders, several problems are associated with their development:

1. Marked intraindividual variability in absorption, dependent on such factors as age, gender, and circadian rhythm
2. Influence of food and drug intake on absorption
3. Physiologic factors that influence gastrointestinal function
4. Potential metabolic transformation during gastrointestinal passage

All of the above factors contribute significantly to the pharmacodynamic profile of oral thrombin inhibitors. In addition, drug interactions markedly influence their overall pharmacodynamics. It is likely that specific formulations may help to alleviate some of these problems. However, because of the narrow therapeutic index, careful dosing will be needed.

The preclinical development of thrombin inhibitors has been based primarily on the use of heparin as an anticoagulant for various indications. The various thrombin inhibitors represent a diverse variety of synthetic and recombinant agents, whose biochemical and pharmacologic profiles differ significantly from those of heparin. A systematic approach to investigation on the basis of chemical structure and projected pharmacologic properties, using structure-activity relationship concepts, has not been made. Furthermore, the antithrombin and cumulative anticoagulant properties of these agents are taken into consideration regardless of other expected vascular and pharmacologic effects.

Currently, hirudin, hirulog-1, inogatran, napsagatran, melagatran, and argatroban are under development for various indications in vascular and cardiovascular areas. Efegatran initially was intended for interventional cardiovascular indications; however, its development is currently on hold. The only consideration for dosage and pharmacologic effects is the anticoagulant response as measured by the activated clotting time (ACT) or the activated partial thromboplastin time (aPTT). Because of a lack of pharmacologic data, additional effects on other components of the hemostatic system are not taken into account. To address some of these issues, a series of experiments have been designed to profile some of the available thrombin inhibitors and to determine their non–thrombin-mediated effects.

Clinical Applications of Antithrombin Drugs

Considering the crucial role of thrombin in both thrombotic and cardiovascular events, it was initially thought that the inhibition of thrombin would be an efficient way to control all of the thrombin-mediated processes. In addition, several limitations of heparin and low-molecular-weight heparin were considered, including the following:

1. Narrow therapeutic window (wide variation in pharmacologic results)
2. Endogenous modulation by proteins and platelet factor 4
3. Inability to inhibit clot-bound thrombin and factor Xa
4. Heparin-induced thrombocytopenia (HIT) with bleeding or thrombosis
5. Requirement for antithrombin III
6. Osteoporosis

For the above reasons, thrombin inhibitors such as hirudin, PEG hirudin, hirulog, and argatroban were developed for various clinical indications. Several other thrombin inhibitors, such as efegatran, napsagatran, inogatran, and melanogatran, were evaluated in limited clinical trials.[75,76] Currently, however, a strong thrust in the clinical development of hirudin, PEG hirudin, and argatroban is evident. These developments have been reviewed recently.[1,2,37,75,76] A recombinant hirudin preparation (Lepirudin, HBW 023) is currently approved in some European countries and the U.S. for use as an alternate anticoagulant in patients with HIT. It was developed for this indication by Hoechst and is sold as Refludan. Another recombinant hirudin (desirudin) initially was developed for various coronary syndromes by the former Ciba Geigy; currently it is managed by the newly formed company, Novartis, under the trade name of Revasc. Although argatroban is available in Japan for various indications, it has undergone an extensive clinical trial in the management of HIT. Currently argatroban is under development by Texas Biotechnology under the trade name Novastan. Recently argatroban was approved for prophylaxis and treatment of thrombosis in patients with HIT.

Antithrombin Agents in Acute Coronary Syndrome

To validate the hypothesis that direct thrombin inhibitors are superior to heparin in acute ischemic syndromes, several clinical trials have been completed recently.[1,2,70,71] The GUSTO-2a and TIMI-9a trials compared hirudin with heparin for treatment of acute myocardial infarction. Both reported a 14% reduction in re-infarction rates at 30 days, but neither demonstrated the superior efficacy of hirudin in terms of mortality rate or combined endpoint (death or nonfatal myocardial infarction). Event rates were 10.8% for hirudin and 10.0% for heparin. A higher bleeding rate was observed with hirudin than with heparin. The cumulative outcome of the trials was rather disappointing and failed to validate the hypothesis that thrombin inhibitors result in a better clinical outcome. The GUSTO-2b trial, in contrast, showed a reduced rate of bleeding with a lower dose of hirudin and a reduction in the 24- and 48-hour risk of death.[72] Table 2 shows the results of the clinical trials using direct thrombin inhibitors in the management of acute myocardial infarction. These drugs are used in conjunction with tPA and streptokinase. In most trials, bleeding is a major complication—and may be due in part to interactions among these agents.

OASIS-1 studied the use of desirudin (another hirudin) in patients with non–ST-elevation acute ischemia.[41] The investigators used a different hirudin and a slightly modified dosage. A significant reduction in the combined incidence of death, myocardial infarction, and revascularization was noted at 7 days. However, bleeding was still more common with desirudin. OASIS-2, a larger randomized trial with a longer follow-up, was completed recently.[57] This trial compared the benefit of moderate-dose hirudin in patients with unstable angina and non–ST-segment myocardial infarction. A total of 10,141 patients were randomly assigned to heparin or hirudin for 72 hours. The incidences of cardiovascular death and myocardial infarction at 7 days were 4.2% and 3.2%,

Table 2.   Clinical Trials of Direct Thrombin Inhibitors for Thrombolytic Therapy
in Patients with Acute Myocardial Infarction

Trial	Drug/Procedure	Major Endpoints	Results
TIMI-5	IV heparin and hirudin + front-loaded tPA and aspirin; dose escalation study	TIMI grade 3 flow at 90 min and 18–36 hr without death or re-infarction	TIMI grade 3 flow at 90 min: 64.8% hirudin vs. 57.1% heparin
TIMI-6	Hirudin vs. heparin + IV SK and aspirin	Major hemorrhage, death, nonfatal reinfarction, heart failure, cardiogenic shock	Major hemorrhage is similar; no significant differences between treatment groups
TIMI-9A	IV heparin vs. IV hirudin after TT (SK or r-tPA); all patients received aspirin	Clinical safety and efficacy	Similar rates of hemorrhage; no superiority of hirudin over heparin
TIMI-9B	IV heparin vs. IV hirudin after TT (SK or r-tPA); all patients received aspirin	Rate of hemorrhage, composite of death, myocardial infarction, severe heart failure, cardiogenic shock	Rate of hemorrhage was similar (5.3% vs. 4.6%)' no difference in efficacy (11.9% vs. 12.9%)
GUSTO-2B (substudy)	Hirudin + SK or hirudin + tPA	Mortality, nonfatal re-infarction	Beneficial interaction with SK but not with tPA
HIT-3	tPA + hirudin vs. heparin	30-day death, reinfarction	Early termination due to un-acceptable bleeding rate
HIT-4	SK + hirudin vs. heparin	30-day death, reinfarction	No significant difference
HERO-1	Hirulog vs. heparin + SK and aspirin	TIMI grade 3 flow at 90 min	34% relative benefit, less minor bleeding with hirulog

TIMI = Thrombolysis in Myocardial Infarction, GUSTO = Global Utilization of Streptokinase and Tissue plasminogen activator for Occluded coronary arteries, HIT = r-Hirudin for Improvement of Thrombolysis, HERO = Hirulog Early Reperfusion/Occlusion, SK = streptokinase, tPA = tissue plasminogen activator, r-tPA = recombinant tPA, TT = thrombolytic therapy.

respectively. The greatest difference between treatments was observed during the first 72 hours, when hirudin led to a reduction in death and myocardial infarction. Excessive major bleeding required transfusion in the hirudin-treated patients. A recent advisory committee meeting of the Food and Drug Administration rejected the use of recombinant hirudin in acute coronary syndrome because of safety concerns in the OASIS studies.

As discussed earlier, hirulog is a 20-amino acid synthetic peptide that directly inhibits clot-bound thrombin. It was developed by Biogen under the name of bivalirudin. The Hirulog Early Reperfusion (HERO) trial tested the efficacy of two hirulog protocols for early and complete flow in the infarct-related artery and their relative safety compared with heparin.[79] Hirulog showed an increase in the TIMI grade 3 patency at 90 minutes after the administration of streptokinase. Additional studies are planned in a large mortality trial. The Food and Drug Administration has issued an approvable letter for hirulog (Angiomax) for patients with unstable angina and patients undergoing percutaneous transluminal coronary angioplasty (PTCA). Thrombin inhibitors also have been used for the management of post-PTCA restenosis. The HELVETICA trial was one of the earlier clinical trials that compared heparin and hirudin for the prevention of restenosis after coronary angioplasty.[64] Hirudin resulted in a significant reduction in early cardiac events; at 6 months, however, there was no difference in angiographic restenosis rates. Similar results were obtained with hirulog.[9]

A phase 1 trial of argatroban (Novastan) was carried out in patients with unstable angina or non–Q-wave myocardial infarction.[34] The results showed that thrombin–antithrombin III complexes were not suppressed and that unstable angina recurred rapidly when the drug was stopped at 4 hours. Argatroban also was developed as an adjunct anticoagulant with thrombolytic agents (ALTEPLASE Study) in 112 patients with acute myocardial infarction.[74] No significant differences were noted between argatroban and heparin. Recently argatroban was used in PTCA.[37,48] Figure 3 depicts the clinical use of argatroban as an example of the use of antithrombin agents in various clinical conditions. Argatroban has been tested in various clinical trials as an anticoagulant for PTCA, stenting and other percutaneous interventions.[48] In addition, it has been used in the management of thrombotic stroke in Japan. Continuous infusion of argatroban has been used to provide therapeutic anticoagulation in heparin-compromised patients.

Thrombin inhibitors also have been used for the management of postoperative venous thrombosis after hip or knee surgery[11,26,33] and in the management of HIT.[48]

Despite major developments in the use of antithrombin agents, several issues remain unresolved, including dosing for various indications, monitoring of anticoagulant effects, rebound thrombin-induced thrombosis, and drug interactions. The bleeding complications discussed in some of the earlier trials may be due to the interaction of antithrombin agents with aspirin, but aspirin appears to prevent rebound thrombin-induced thrombosis.[80]

Synthetic thrombin inhibitors and hirudin have a short half-life of about 30–45 minutes. Hence, it may not be necessary to require an antagonist to neutralize their effects. It has been proposed that in normal people with no hemostatic deficit, hirudin at therapeutic levels should not produce bleeding.[27] However, considering drug interactions and risks for bleeding from associated

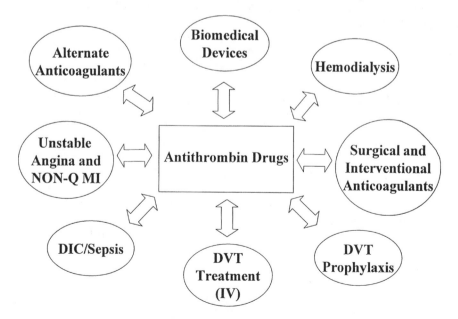

Figure 3.   Potential clinical uses of antithrombin agents.

problems, antagonists may be necessary. An antithrombin antidote may be essential in case of accidental overdose or in patients with renal disease. Potential candidates under investigation as possible hirudin antagonists include di-iso-propyl-phosphoryl-thrombin (DIP-thrombin[70]), recombinant factor VIIa, 1-des-amino-8-arginine vasopressin (DDAVP), factor VIII,[13] bazotroxobin, ecarin-induced formation of meizothrombin, and activated prothrombin complexes, such as factor VIII bypass inhibitor (FEIBA; Autoplex).[13,22,30,31,42,43,44,56,66] Further studies are needed to evaluate these antidotes for argatroban and related drugs.

Molecular engineering of prothrombin molecules has resulted in the development of a number of variants that lack procoagulant actions but can complex with hirudin to neutralize its anticoagulant effects.[13] These recombinant proteins have been found to be effective in the neutralization of the anticoagulant activity of hirudin.

Monitoring of Thrombin Inhibitors

Thrombin inhibitors are of natural, recombinant, and synthetic origin and produce a reversible or nonreversible effect on thrombin. They can be directed against the catalytic site of thrombin or bind to the exosites of thrombin. The mechanism and kinetics of their activity can be readily studied with biochemical methods. However, biochemical methods are not practical for clinical monitoring.

All antithrombin agents produce an anticoagulant effect in such global tests as PT and aPTT. In these assays hirudin is the most potent anticoagulant. Efegatran, argatroban, and hirulog have similar profiles in PT and aPTT assays. In the Heptest assay, however, argatroban is a stronger anticoagulant than the other two agents. Although each of these agents is capable of inhibiting thrombin, the mechanism of their actions is different; therefore, differences in prolongation of the clot-based assays may not be an indication of their anticoagulant or antithrombotic potency. The aPTT test has been recommended for monitoring Refludan therapy in patients with HIT or heparin-induced thrombocytopenia and thrombosis in the United States.

Recently a new clot-based assay known as the ecarin clotting time (ECT) was developed for the specific monitoring of antithrombin agents.[14] Ecarin, the venom of the snake *Echis carinatus*, converts prothrombin to meizothrombin and eventually produces a clotting endpoint in citrated whole blood and plasma. Each thrombin inhibitor has its own distinct anticoagulant effect in this assay. Hirulog produces the weakest effect, whereas hirudin shows the strongest effect in whole blood. ECT is sensitive to antithrombin agents and can be used to monitor their effect in whole blood. It must be stressed that ECT measures primarily the absolute concentration of thrombin inhibitors. Its relevance to physiologic effects is rather limited.

Clot-based assays and the chromogenic substrate-based anti-IIa assay also can be used to monitor the effects of antithrombin drugs. At low concentrations, however, the anti-IIa assay cannot measure the absolute concentration of some antithrombin agents. Thus, it has a limited sensitivity and in clinical settings may not be practical for monitoring the anticoagulant actions of antithrombin agents.

Some of the enzyme-linked immunosorbent assays (ELISAs), such as prothrombin fragment F1.2 , thrombin–antithrombin complex, and fibrinopeptide A (FPA), can measure the effect of antithrombin agents on thrombin at different stages of its activation. These assays may assist in the monitoring of the effect of antithrombin agents. In addition, ELISAs using monoclonal antibodies have been developed to measure absolute drug concentration of hirudin and several other antithrombin agents. Several assays for hirudin are commercially available (Stago, Paris; American Diagnostica, Greenwich, CT).

Cost Considerations

Information about the cost of thrombin inhibitors is limited. In the case of recombinant hirudin, cost considerations have been taken into account only for specific indications, and a very limited database is available. Currently, most of the indications for hirudin are the same as for unfractionated heparin or low-molecular-weight heparins. Cost analysis, therefore, must be based on site-specific indications, such as surgical anticoagulation, prophylaxis and treatment of deep venous thrombosis, and cardiovascular use.

From the standpoint of production cost, recombinant hirudin is certainly more expensive than the heparins. However, for each of the specific indications, a comprehensive pharmacoeconomic analysis involving dosage, nursing care, monitoring, incidence of adverse reactions, and clinical outcome must be taken into account. Such a comprehensive analysis may provide different cost values for hirudin and related drugs.

In conjunction with the GUSTO-2b study, a cost analysis from a pharmacoeconomic substudy was reported recently.[73] Reimbursement was received from 50% of the treated patients. Considering that recombinant hirudin (r-hirudin) prevented 2 deaths and 7 myocardial infarctions per 1000 study patients, it was computed that if the drug was priced at $500, the cost per year of life saved would be around $16,000. If the price of r-hirudin was $1000, the cost would be $32,000; if the price was $1500, the estimated cost would be around $48,000. This information suggests that a cost below $1500 would be considered cost-effective. The projected cost, however, is much higher than the cost for heparin and other synthetic antithrombin agents. Whether the cost calculated on the basis of survival estimate is valid for such comparisons is questionable. If mortality rates alone were used, the drug would have to be priced at a much lower level to be cost-effective. A price of $500 would give a cost per year of life saved of $31,250. The cost-effective analysis based on nonsignificant results, such as the one reported in the GUSTO-2b substudy, may not be accurate. Additional data are needed.

Future Trends

The development of thrombin inhibitors has added a new dimension to the management of thrombotic and vascular disorders. Although the major clinical indications include interventional cardiovascular procedures and deep venous thrombosis prophylaxis, limited information is available about their use for surgical and therapeutic anticoagulation. It is expected that many of the newer thrombin inhibitors, such as hirudin and argatroban, will be developed as anticoagulants and will be used as a substitute for heparin in clinically validated indications. Synthetic tripeptides, which have a broader serine protease inhibitory spectrum, offer unique opportunities to control thrombogenesis at different levels and may prove to be more useful in chronic indications, including prophylaxis. They also can be developed for potential oral anticoagulation. The usefulness of various thrombin inhibitors in a given medical or surgical indication can be proved only in properly designed clinical trials. Several clinical trials are currently ongoing and have provided useful data to optimize the use of new antithrombin drugs.

In the coming years, newer antithrombin agents with varying degrees of specificity for thrombin and other serine proteases will become available. Beside the inhibition of serine proteases, they also produce effects on blood, vascular, and cellular targets, including several receptor sites. Furthermore, the newer antithrombin agents also may have some direct interactions with plasmatic proteins and cellular sites. Such interaction may influence their pharmacologic profile and clinical outcome. The endogenous transformation of antithrombin agents also may play an important role, and observed clinical effects can be strongly influenced by this process. Thus, the consequences resulting in endogenous transformations and interactions may have to be taken into account in the optimal development of antithrombin agents. Each of the thrombin inhibitors should be considered a distinct drug, and the results of thrombin inhibition should not be the sole determinant of their actions. Another unresolved issue is related to metabolic conversion. To date, no information is available about the metabolites and their contribution to overall antithrombotic effects.

Because of the defined chemical nature of the thrombin inhibitors, they have been coupled with other pharmacologic agents to develop hybrid multiple effects. Thus, a bifunctional hybrid to target desired activation sites can be developed. Many antithrombin agents also can be conjugated with inert linker or carrier molecules to obtain desired biologic half-life and site specificity. PEG-hirudin, which is currently under clinical development, has an extended half-life and is more potent then hirudin at equivalent antithrombin levels. Biotechnology, organic synthesis, and knowledge of natural products may lead to the development of many molecularly developed "designer" antithrombin agents. Despite the development of a desirable molecule with prolonged pharmacodynamics, the coupling groups, such as the PEG moieties, also may have strong effects. Such effects clearly should be investigated.

Because of multiple sites of action, thrombin inhibitors may exhibit strong drug interactions, which must be considered a crucial factor in clinical development. A systematic investigation of potential interactions of antithrombin agents with commonly used drugs in specific indications is highly desirable because many patients already are taking antiplatelet drugs such as aspirin. These agents also may exhibit significant interaction with other drugs, such as oral anticoagulants and thrombolytic agents.

Although several agents exhibiting thrombin inhibitory properties will be developed under the classification of antithrombin drugs, thrombin inhibition may be only one of their many actions. Besides modulating thrombin-mediated functions, these agents also exhibit secondary and tertiary pharmacologic effects, which will influence significantly their clinical profile. Although a new class of anticoagulant drugs known as antithrombin agents will emerge, thrombin inhibition will be one of many pharmacologic actions. Thrombin inhibitors also exhibit significant interactions with antiplatelet drugs. In cardiovascular indications, such interactions may play an important role.

Beside systemic administration, the newer thrombin inhibitors also can be developed for oral, nonparenteral, and on-site delivery. Furthermore, they can be incorporated with biomaterials and formulated for depot delivery. Iontophoresis, phonophoresis, and other delivery modalities can be used.

Table 3.   Development of Antithrombin Drugs

Agent	Company	Developmental Status
Revasc	Novartis	Antithrombotic/DVT prophylaxis
Desirudin (Refludan)	Aventis*	Antithrombotic/cardiovascular
PEG-hirudin	Knoll	Cardiovascular
Novastan	Texas Biotechnology/Smith Kline/ Mitsubishi Sanofi	Anticoagulant

DVT = deep venous thrombosis.
* Aventis was formed by the merger of Hoechst and Rhone-Poulenc Rorer.

Thrombin inhibitors, therefore, provide a wide spectrum of newer anticoagulant and antithrombotic drugs that can be developed for multiple indications to control thrombosis and related pathophysiologic events. However, it must be understood that they are not heparin; each product is a distinct entity and must be developed as a new drug for a given indication. The safety and efficacy of each agent must be evaluated individually.

At present several pharmaceutical companies are in the process of developing thrombin inhibitors for various indications (Table 3). Revasc, the trade name of the recombinant hirudin from Novartis, has been developed for prophylaxis of deep venous thrombosis. Refludan, the trade name of the recombinant hirudin from Aventis, has been approved as an alternate anticoagulant in HIT syndrome. PEG-hirudin has been developed for various coronary indications by Knoll. Novastan is the only non–hirudin-related antithrombin agent with advanced clinical development in Europe and North America for several indications. It recently was approved in the U.S. for alternate anticoagulant management of heparin-compromised patients—in particular, HIT syndrome. However, Novastan is in clinical use in Japan for stroke and other indications. Other antithrombin agents, such as napsagatran and efegatran, are in clinical trials. Their developmental status is unclear.

Undoubtedly antithrombin agents such as hirudin will be useful in the management of anticoagulation and prophylaxis of deep venous thrombosis in heparin-compromised patients. Additional uses may include cardiovascular and cerebrovascular indications. However, because of their distinct mechanism of action and pharmacodynamic individuality, antithrombin agents may not be a true substitute for heparin. However, they will be quite useful as anticoagulants for medical and surgical indications. Optimization and monitoring considerations are important in the developmental stages. Use of antithrombin agents requires proper understanding of their activities and should be considered with extreme caution.

References

1. Antman EM, for the TIMI 9A Investigators: Hirudin in acute myocardial infarction: Safety report from the Thrombolysis and Thrombin Inhibition in Myocardial Infarction (TIMI) 9A trial. Circulation 90:1624–1630, 1994.
2. Antman EM: Antiplatelet/antithrombotic agents. Presented at the Plenary Seminar, Joint AHA/European Society of Cardiology Symposium: Contemporary Strategies for Acute Myocardial Infarction. American Heart Association, 68th Scientific Sessions, Anaheim, CA, November 1995 [unpublished].
3. Bagdy D, Barabás E, Bajusz S, Széll E: In vitro inhibition of blood coagulation by tripeptide aldehydes—a retrospective screening study focused on the stable D-MePhe-Pro-Arg-H•H_2SO_4. Thromb Haemost 67(3):325–330, 1992.

4. Bajusz S, Széll E, Bagdy D, Barabas E, Dioszegi M, Fittler Z, Josza F, Horvath G, Tomori E: US Patent No. 4,703,036, 1987.
5. Bajusz S, Barabás E, Tolnay P, et al: Inhibition of thrombin and trypsin by tripeptide aldehydes. Int J Peptide Protein Res 12:217–221, 1978.
6. Bajusz S, Széll E, Bagdy D, et al: Highly active and selective anticoagulants: D-Phe-Pro-Arg-H, a free tripeptide aldehyde prone to spontaneous inactivation, and its stable N-methyl derivative, D-MePhe-Pro-Arg-H. J Med Chem 33:1729–1735, 1990.
7. Bajusz S, Barabás E, Széll E, Bagdy D: Peptide aldehyde inhibitors of the fibrinogen-thrombin reaction. In Meienhofer J (ed): Peptides—Chemistry, Structure and Biology. Ann Arbor, MI, Ann Arbor Scientific Publications, 1975, pp 603–608.
8. Barabas E, Szell E, Bajusz S: Screening for fibrinolysis inhibitory effect of synthetic thrombin inhibitors. Blood Coagul Fibrinol 4:243–248, 1993.
9. Bittl A, et al for the Hirulog Angioplasty Study (HAS): Treatment with bivalirudin (hirulog) as compared with heparin during coronary angioplasty for unstable angina or postinfarction angina. N Engl J Med 333:764–769, 1995.
10. Bock LC, Griffin LC, Latham JA, et al: Selection of single-stranded DNA molecules that bind and inhibit human thrombin. Nature 355(6360):564–566, 1992.
11. Bounamex H, Ehringer H, Hulting J, et al: An exploratory trial of two dosages of a novel synthetic thrombin inhibitor (Napsagatran, Ro 46-6240) compared with unfractionated heparin for treatment of proximal deep-vein thrombosis. Thromb Haemost 78:997–1002, 1997.
12. Bruggener E, Walsmann P, Markwardt F: Neutralization of hirudin anticoagulant action by DIP-thrombin. Pharmazie 44:648–649, 1989.
13. Butler KD, Dolan SL, Talbot MD, et al: Factor VIII and DDAVP reverse the effect of recombinant desulfatohirudin (CGP-39393) on bleeding in the rat. Blood Coag Fibrinol 4:459–464, 1993.
14. Callas D, Fareed J: Comparative anticoagulant effects of various thrombin inhibitors, as determined in the ecarin clotting time method. Thromb Res 83:463–468, 1996.
15. Callas D, Bacher P, Iqbal O, et al: Fibrinolytic compromise by simultaneous administration of site-directed inhibitors of thrombin. Thromb Res 74(3):193–205, 1994.
16. Cannon CP, Maraganore JM, Loscalzo J: Anticoagulant effects of hirulog, a novel thrombin inhibitor, in patients with coronary artery disease. Am J Cardiol 71:778–782, 1993.
17. Cheng L, Scully MF, Goodwin CA, et al: Peptide α-aminophosphonic acids. A new type of thrombin inhibitor. Thromb Haemost 65:1289, 1991.
18. Coleman RW: Activation of plasminogen by human plasma kallikrein. Biochem Biophys Res Commun 35:273–279, 1968.
19. Collen D, Lijnen HR, Todd PA, Goa KL: Tissue-type plasminogen activator: A review of its pharmacology and therapeutic use as a thrombolytic agent. Drugs 38:346–388, 1989.
20. De Fouw NJ, van Hinsberg VW, de Jong YF, et al: The interaction of activated protein C and thrombin with the plasminogen activator inhibitor released from human endothelial cells. Thromb Haemost 57:176, 1987.
21. Dichek D, Quertermous T: Thrombin regulation of mRNA levels of tissue plasminogen activator inhibitor-1 in cultured human umbilical vein endothelial cells. Blood 74:222–228, 1989.
22. Diehl KH, Romisch B, Hein B, et al: Potential hirudin antidote: Investigation of an activated prothrombin complex concentrate in animal models. In Annals of Hematology: Proceedings of the 3rd Annual Meeting in Munich, February 16–19, 1994. The German Society of Thrombosis and Hemostasis 68(II): A86.
23. DiMaio J, Gibbs B, Munn D, et al: Bifunctional thrombin inhibitors based on the sequence of hirudin. J Biol Chem 265(35):21698–21703, 1990.
24. Dodt J, Kohler S, Schmitz T, Wilhelm B: Distinct binding sites of Ala 48-hirudin 1-47 and Ala 48-hirudin 48-65 on α thrombin. J Biol Chem 265:713–718, 1990.
25. Eriksson BI, Renberg L, Bredberg U, et al: Animal pharmacokinetics of inogatran, a low-molecular-weight thrombin inhibitor with potential use as an antithrombotic drug. Biopharm Drug Disp 19:55–64, 1998.
26. Eriksson BI: Recombinant hirudin, desirudin (REVASC®) for prophylaxis of thromboembolic complications in patients undergoing total hip replacement. Fourteenth International Congress of Thrombosis, Montpellier, VT, 1996.
27. Fareed J, Walenga JM, Iyer L, et al: An objective perspective on recombinant hirudin: A new anticoagulant and antithrombotic agent. Blood Coag Fibrinol 2:135–147, 1991.
28. Fareed J, Messmore HL, Kindel G, Balis JU: Inhibition of serine proteases by low molecular weight peptides and their derivatives. NY Acad Sci 370:765–784, 1981.
29. Fareed J, Callas D, Hoppensteadt D, et al: Recent developments in antithrombotic agents. Exp Opin Invest Drugs 4(5):389–412, 1995.
30. Fuster V, Verstraete M: Thrombosis in Cardiovascular Disorders. Philadelphia, W.B. Saunders, 1992.

31. Gibbs CS, Coutre SE, Tsiang M, et al: Conversion of thrombin into an anticoagulant by protein engineering. Nature 378:413–416, 1995.
32. Gilboa N, Villannueva, Fenton II JW: Inhibition of fibrinolytic enzymes by thrombin inhibitors. Enzyme 40:144–148, 1988.
33. Ginsberg JS, Nurmohamed MT, Gent M, et al: Use of hirulog in the prevention of venous thrombosis after major hip or knee surgery. Circulation 90:2385–2389, 1994.
34. Gold HK, Torres FW, Garabedian HD, et al: Evidence for a rebound coagulation phenomenon after cessation of a 4-hour infusion of a specific thrombin inhibitor in patients with unstable angina pectoris. J Am Coll Cardiol 21:1039–1047, 1993.
35. Goldsmith GH, Saito H, Ratnoff OD: The activation of plasminogen by Hageman factor fragments. J Clin Invest 62:54–60, 1978.
36. Harvey RP, Degryse E, Stefani L, et al: Cloning and expression of cDNA coding for the anticoagulant hirudin from the bloodsucking leech *Hirudo medicinalis.* Proc Natl Acad Sci USA 83:1084–1088, 1986.
37. Hermann JR, Kutryk MJ, Serruys PW: Clinical trials of direct thrombin inhibitors during invasive procedures. Thromb Haemost 78:367–376, 1997.
38. Herrman PR, Suryapranata H, den Heijer P, et al: Argatroban during percutaneous transluminal angioplasty; results of a dose verification study. J Thromb Thrombolysis 3:367–375, 1996.
39. Hijikata-Okunomiya A, Okamoto S: A strategy for a rational approach to designing synthetic selective inhibitors. Semin Thromb Hemost 18:135–149, 1992.
40. Hoylaerts M, Rijken D, Lijnen HR, Collen D: Kinetics of the activation of plasminogen by human tissue plasminogen activator, role of fibrin. J Biol Chem 257:2912–2919, 1982.
41. Investigators of the OASIS trial: Comparison of the effects of two doses of recombinant hirudin compared with heparin in patients with acute myocardial ischemia without ST elevation. Circulation 96:769, 1997.
42. Irani MS, White HJ, Sexon RN: Reversal of hirudin-induced bleeding diathesis by prothrombin complex concentrate. Am J Cardiol 75:422–423, 1995.
43. Kaiser B, Callas D, Hoppensteadt D, et al: Comparative studies on the inhibitory spectrum of recombinant hirudin, DuP 714 and heparin on the generation of thrombin and factor Xa generation in biochemically defined systems. Thromb Res 73(5):327–335, 1994.
44. Kaiser B, Fareed J, Hoppensteadt D, et al: Influence of recombinant hirudin and unfractionated heparin on thrombin and factor Xa generation in extrinsic and intrinsic activated systems. Thromb Res 65:157–164, 1992.
45. Kettner C, Mesinger L, Knabb R: The selective inhibition of thrombin by peptides of boroarginine. J Biol Chem 265:18289–18297, 1990.
46. Kettner C, Shaw E: The selective inactivation of thrombin by peptides of chloromethyl ketone, p129–144. In Lundblad RL, JW Fenton, KG Mann (eds): Chemistry and Biology of Thrombin. Ann Arbor , MI, Ann Arbor Scientific Publications, 1996.
47. Latham JA, Johnson R, Toole JJ: The application of a modified nucleotide in aptamer selection: Novel thrombin aptamers containing 5-(1-pentynyl)-2'-deoxyuridine. Nucl Acids Res 22(14):2817–2822, 1994.
48. Lewis B, Grassman E, Johnson S, et al: Pilot study of argatroban in patients with heparin allergy [abstract 2188]. In Abstracts from the 69th Scientific Sessions of the American Heart Association, New Orleans, 1996, p 1233.
49. Li WX, Kaplan AV, Grant GW, et al: A novel nucleotide-based thrombin inhibitor inhibits clot-bound thrombin and reduces arterial platelet thrombus formation. Blood 83:677–682, 1994.
50. Macaya RF, Schultze P, Smith FW, et al: Thrombin-binding DNA aptamer forms a unimolecular quadruplex structure in solution. Proc Natl Acad Sci USA 90:3745–3749, 1993.
51. Maraganore JM, Bourdon P, Jablonski J, et al: Design and characterization of hirulogs: A novel class of bivalent peptide inhibitors of thrombin. Biochemistry 29:7095–7101, 1990.
52. Maruyama I: Synthetic anticoagulants. Jpn J Clin Hematol 31:776–781, 1990.
53. Matsuo T, Kario K, Kodama K, Okamoto S: Clinical applications of the synthetic thrombin inhibitor, Argatroban (MD-805). Semin Thromb Hemost 18:155–160, 1992.
54. Mehta JL, Chen L, Nichols WW, et al: Melagatran, an oral active-site inhibitor, prevents or delays formation of electrically induced occlusive thrombus in the canine coronary artery. J Cardiovasc Pharm 31:345–351, 1998.
55. Neises B, Tarnus C: Thrombin inhibition by the tripeptide trifluoromethyl ketone D-Phe-Pro-Arg-F3 (MDL73756). Thromb Haemost 65:1290, 1991.
56. Nowak G, Bucha E: Ecarin-induced prothrombin intermediate formation: An effective antidote principle to antagonize toxic levels of hirudin. Proceedings of the 5th Annual Symposium on Advances in Anticoagulant, Antithrombotic and Thrombolytic Therapeutics, in Boston, October 24–25, 1994, by International Business Communications.

57. OASIS-2 Investigators: Effects of recombinant hirudin (lepirudin) compared with heparin on death, myocardial infarction, refractory angina and revascularization procedures in patients with acute myocaridal ischemia without ST elevation: A randomized trial. Lancet 3553: 429–438, 1999.

58. Oshiro T, Kanbayashi J, Kosaki G: Antithrombotic therapy of patient with peripheral arterial reconstruction-clinical study on MD805. Blood Vessel 14:216–218, 1983.

59. Paborsky LR, McCurdy SN, Griffin LC, et al: The single-stranded DNA aptamer binding site of human thrombin. J Biol Chem 268:20808, 1993.

60. Pannell R, Gurewich V: Pro-urokinase: A study of its stability in plasma and of a mechanism for its selective fibrinolytic effect. Blood 67:1215–1223, 1989.

61. Petersen TE, Roberts HR, Sottrup-Jensen L, Magnusson S: Primary structure of hirudin, a thrombin-specific inhibitor. In Peters H (ed): Peptides of the Biological Fluids. Oxford, Pergamon, 1976, pp 145–149.

62. Sakata Y, Curriden S, Lawrence D, et al: Activated protein C stimulates the fibrinolytic activity of cultured endothelial cells and decreases antiactivator activity. Proc Natl Acad Sci USA 82:1121–1125, 1985.

63. Scharf M, Engels J, Tripier D: Primary structures of new "isohirudins." FEBS Lett 225:105–110, 1989.

64. Serruys PW, Herrman J-PR, Simon R, et al: A comparison of hirudin with heparin in the prevention of restenosis after coronary angioplasty. N Engl J Med 995:333:757–763.

65. Stüber W, Kosina H, Heimburger N: Synthesis of a tripeptide with a C-terminal moiety and the inhibition of proteinases. Int J Peptide Protein Res 31:63–70, 1988.

66. Stuever TA, Fareed J, Hoppensteadt D, et al: Neutralization of recombinant hirudin by FEIBA®. In press.

67. Tamao Y, Yamamoto T, Hirata T, et al: Effect of argipidine (MD-805) on blood coagulation. Jpn Pharmacol Ther 14:869–874, 1986.

68. Tamao Y, Yamamoto T, Kimumoto R, et al: Effect of a selective thrombin-inhibitor MCI-9038 on fibrinolysis in vitro and in vivo. Thromb Haemost 562:28–34, 1986.

69. Tapparelli C, Metternich R, Ehrhardt C, et al: In vitro and in vivo characterization of a neutral boron-containing thrombin inhibitor. J Biol Chem 268:473–474, 1993.

70. The Global Use of Strategies to Open Occluded Coronary Arteries (GUSTO) IIa Investigators: Randomized trial of intravenous heparin versus recombinant hirudin for acute coronary syndromes. Circulation 90:1631–1637, 1994.

71. The Global Use of Strategies to Open Occluded Coronary Arteries (GUSTO) IIa Investigators: A comparison of recombinant hirudin with heparin for the treatment of acute coronary syndromes. N Engl J Med 335:775–782, 1996.

72. Theroux P, Lidon R: Anticoagulants and their use in acute ischemic syndromes. In Topol EJ (ed): Textbook of Interventional Cardiology. Philadelphia, W.B. Saunders, 1994, pp 23–45.

73. Topol EJ, Bonan R, Jewitt D, et al: Use of a direct antithrombin, hirulog, in place of heparin during coronary angioplasty. Circulation 87:1622–1629, 1993.

74. Vermeer F, Vahanian A, Fels PW, et al: Intravenous argatroban versus heparin as co-medication to alteplase in the treatment of acute myocardial infarction: Preliminary results of the ARGAMI pilot study. J Am Coll Cardiol 29:185–186, 1997.

75. Verstraete M: Direct thrombin inhibitors: Appraisal of the antithrombotic/hemorrhagic balance. Thromb Haemost 78:357–363, 1997.

76. Verstaete M, Zoldhelyi P, Willerson JT: Specific thrombin inhibitors. In Verstaete M, Fuster V, Topol EJ (eds): Cardiovascular Thrombosis: Thrombocardiology and Thromboneurology, 2nd ed. Philadelphia, Lippincott-Raven, 1998, pp 141–172.

77. Vlasuk G, Vallar PL, Weinhouse MI, et al: A novel inhibitor of thrombin containing multiple recognition sequences linked by α-keto amide transition state. Circulation 90(4 Pt 2):I-348, 1994.

78. White HD, Aylward PE, Frey M, et al: A randomized, double-blind comparison of hirulog versus heparin in patients receiving streptokinase and aspirin for acute myocardial infarction (HERO). Submitted for publication, 1997.

79. Willerson JT, Casscells W: Thrombin inhibition in unstable angina. Rebound or continuation of angina after argatroban withdrawal. J Am Coll Cardiol 21:1048, 1993.

80. Yonekawa Y, Handa H, Okamoto S, et al: Treatment of cerebral infarction in the acute stage with synthetic antithrombin MD805: Clinical study among multiple institutions. Arch Jpn Chir 55:711–726, 1986.

81. Zawilska K, Zozulinska M, Turowiecka Z, et al: The effect of a long-acting recombinant hirudin (PEG-hirudin) on experimental disseminated intravascular coagulation (DIC) in rabbits. Thromb Res 69:315–320, 1993.

Thrombolytic Therapy in Acute Coronary Syndrome

OMER IQBAL, MD

AHMET MUZAFFER DEMIR, MD

DEBRA A. HOPPENSTEADT, PhD

WILLIAM H. WEHRMACHER, MD

HARRY L. MESSMORE, JR., MD

JAWED FAREED, PhD

Coronary heart disease (CHD) is the most common cause of mortality not only in the United States (accounting for 481,287 deaths in 1995) but world-wide.[1,2] Annually an estimated 1.1 million Americans experience a new or recurrent acute myocardial infarction (AMI) due to CHD, and in one-third the event is fatal.[1] The age-adjusted mortality rate of CHD has declined dramatically from 2.8% per year in 1965 to 1.5% since 1990.[3] The reasons for the age-adjusted decline in incidence, case fatality, and CHD mortality rate are many:[4–6] the advent of the coronary care unit with intensive monitoring, aggressive treatment of complications, and reperfusion therapies such as thrombolysis, percutaneous transluminal coronary angioplasty (PTCA), and coronary artery bypass graft (CABG) surgery. The goal in the care of patients with AMI is to make these effective treatments available in a timely manner.

Table 1 lists the thrombolytic drugs currently in use and under development. Selection criteria are listed in Table 2. Distinctive features of the available thrombolytic agents are shown in Tables 3, 4, and 5. Selection of the specific drug for a particular patient must include prior use because antibody-mediated resistance may have developed (see Table 3, 4 and 5 for the immunogenicity of each drug). Cost factors also are important, as shown in the above tables. Other than these two factors, the real differences among the various products are insufficient to prompt choices based on patient factors such as age or sex. Cerebral hemorrhage is slightly more common with tissue plasminogen activator (tPA) in the elderly, but this disadvantage is offset by the effectiveness of tPA in elderly patients.

The time from AMI to reperfusion (thrombolytic) therapy is commonly divided into three periods.[7] The first period is the time from the onset of symptoms to the patient's action to seek treatment, such as going to the hospital or calling

Table 1. Three Generations of Thrombolytic Agents and Drugs under Development

First generation	Streptokinase
	Urokinase
Second generation	Recombinant tissue plasminogen activator (r-tPA, alteplase, duteplase)
	Anisoylated plasminogen streptokinase activator complex (APSAC, anistreplase)
	Single-chain urokinase-type plasminogen activator (scu-PA, prourokinase)
Third generation	Vampire bat salivary plasminogen activator
	Reteplase (rPA)
	TNK-Tpa
	Lanoteplase (n-PA)
	Tenecteplase
	Staphylokinase
	Recombinant glycosylated plasminogen activator
Thrombolytic drugs under development	Antibody-targeting thrombolytic agents
	Polyethylene glycol coupled thrombolytic agents
	Mutant and variants of plasminogen activator
	Recombinant chimeric plasminogen activator (Fibrolase)

emergency medical services (EMS). This delay constitutes 60-70% of the total time to starting reperfusion (thrombolytic) therapy. This delay may be shortened by primary prevention through the education of patients and their families about heart disease and the importance of early response to symptoms. Delay results in cardiac muscle loss. The second component of delay is the time to EMS response and transit time to an emergency care facility (3–8% of the total delay). The third delay is the time from arrival at the hospital to definitive treatment

Table 2. Selection Criteria for Thrombolytic Therapy

Indications
- Chest pain for >30 minutes and <12 hours
- ST elevation (0.1 mm) in two contiguous precordial leads in anatomically related limb leads or new left bundle branch block

Contraindications*
Acute
- Active internal bleeding
- Blood pressure $\geq$ 200/120 mmHg
- Suspected or known aortic dissection

Subacute or chronic
- Arteriovenous malformation
- Tumor involving spinal cord or cranial structures
- Hemorrhagic retinopathy
- Pregnancy
- Active peptic ulcer
- Warfarin use
- Bleeding diathesis

In the past 2 months
- Trauma or surgery in the past 2 weeks with a risk of bleeding into closed space
- Spinal or intracranial procedure in the previous 8 weeks
- Recent head trauma
- Prolonged or traumatic cardiopulmonary resuscitation
- Prior hemorrhagic stroke or any stroke within the prior year

* Advanced age is not a contraindication. Elderly patients have increased complications (especially intracranial hemorrhage) but also the highest absolute mortality reduction.

Table 3. Characteristics of First-generation Thrombolytic Drugs

	Streptokinase	Urokinase
Source	Group C streptococci	Recombinant, human fetal kidney
Molecular weight (kDa)	47	35–55
Immunogenicity	Yes	No
Mode of action	Forms an activator complex	Direct
Fibrin specificity	No	No
Plasma half-life (min)	18–23	14–20
Metabolism	Hepatic	Hepatic
Dose	1.5 million unit over 1 hr IV	3 million unit
Cost per dose	$300	$2000

(25–33% of the total delay). Factors contributing to effective, timely reperfusion therapy are patient education, EMS availability and proficiency, and reduced delay in the hospital.[1,2,8,9] Trials of prehospital thrombolytic therapy have resulted in reduced time to treatment and improvement in mortality rates.[3,10–14]

Pharmacology and Clinical Use

The characteristics and functional properties of thrombolytic agents commonly in current use are summarized in Tables 1, 3, 4, and 5. These drugs are either direct activators of plasminogen, such as tPA, urokinase, and anisoylated plasminogen-streptokinase activator complex (APSAC), or indirect activators, such as streptokinase. Average dosages are shown in Tables 3, 4, and 5. APSAC and tPA are "fibrin-specific" in that they bind to fibrin and activate plasminogen at the site, whereas streptokinase and urokinase are not fibrin-specific, lysing both fibrinogen and fibrin (Fig. 1). Streptokinase and APSAC (which contains streptokinase) cannot be reused because they are antigenic and give rise to

Table 4. Characteristics of Second-generation Thrombolytic Drugs

	APSAC	rtPA (Alteplase)	Scu-PA (Saruplase)
Source	Group C streptococci Plasminogen anisoylated (complex)	Recombinant, human	Prodrug from a naturally occurring physiologic protease
Molecular weight (kDa)	131	63–70	49
Immunogenicity	Yes	No	No
Mode of action	Direct	Direct	Direct
Fibrin specificity	–	++	+
Plasma half-life (min)	70–120	4–6	9
Metabolism	Hepatic	Hepatic	Hepatic
Dose	30 units IV over 2–5 minutes	5-mg bolus + 90-minute infusion up to 85 mg (accelerated protocol)	20-mg bolus + 60-mg infusion for 1 hr
Cost per dose	$2400	$2200	$2100

APSAC = anisoylated plasminogen streptokinase activator complex, scu-PA = single-chain urokinase plasminogen activator.

Table 5.   Characteristics of Third-generation Thrombolytic Drugs

	rPA (Reteplase)	n-PA (Lanoteplase)	TNK-tPA	Vampire Bat PA	Staphylokinase
Source	Recombinant, human mutant tissue-type PA	Chinese hamster ovary cells	Variant of tPA rearranging gene sequence	Saliva of *Desmodus rotundus*	PA of bacterial origin–strains of *S. aureus*
Molecular weight (kDa)	39	~39	~39	52	15.5
Immunogenicity	No	?	No	Yes	Yes
Mode of action	Direct	Direct	Direct	Indirect	Indirect
Fibrin specificity	Yes	+	+++	+++	+++
Plasma half-life (min)	14	37	20	170	6
Metabolism	Renal	Hepatic	Hepatic	Hepatic	Hepatic
Dose	20 million U single bolus	120,000 U/kg single bolus	+0.5 mg/kg single bolus	0.5 mg/kg single bolus	15 mg + 15 mg double bolus over 30 min

PA = plasminogen activator, *S* = *Staphylococcus*.

circulating antibodies. Because urokinase and tPA are of human origin, they do not induce antibodies. As a practical matter, urokinase is rarely used for AMI because of the necessity for intracoronary administration. The two commercially available recombinant forms of tPA, reteplase and alteplase, are given intravenously, as are streptokinase and APSAC. APSAC has not been studied in patients over 75 years of age and may be unsafe in this age group. Theoretically, the longer half-life of a single bolus of APSAC makes it ideal for prehospital therapy.[15] All thrombolytic drugs have the potential to cause more bleeding in elderly than in younger patients, and most manufacturers' warnings advise caution. This risk must be weighed against anticipated benefit. Table 6 summarizes the clinical trials of these drugs.

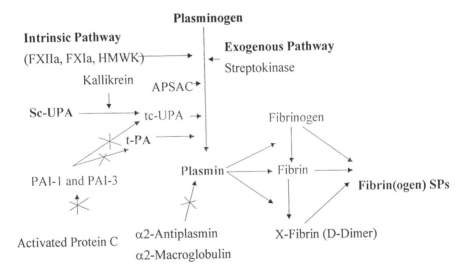

Figure 1.   Fibrinolytic mechanism. Intrinsic: direct action on plasminogen; exogenous: indirect action (via complex formation with plasminogen before formation of plasmin from plasminogen). X = inhibitory effect.

TABLE 6. Synopsis of Thrombolytic Therapy in AMI Trials

Trial Name (Ref. No.)	Design	Population n, years old	Drug/ Procedure	Major Endpoints	Results
GISSI-1 (56)	R, OL, PC, MCS	11,712; no age limit	IV SK vs. no thrombolytic therapy	Mortality benefits at 21 days and 1 year	Reduction in mortality of 10.7% at 21 days and of 17.2% at 1 year
GISSI-2 (57)	MCS, R, OL, 2×2 factorial	12,381; no age limit	IV SK vs. tPA	Mortality rate, rate of reinfarction, stroke rate, incidence of post-infarction angina	SK and tPA were equally effective within 6 hours of the onset of symptoms.
ISIS-2 (58)	MCS, PC, R, DB, 2×2 factorial	17,187; no age limit	IV SK + aspirin vs. placebo	Mortality and stroke risk	SK and aspirin independently reduced mortality in patients with AMI. The combination of two drugs had a synergistic effect on mortality without increase in rates of stroke.
ISAM (59)	P, R, DB, PC, MCS	1,741; ≤ 75 years	SK vs. placebo	21-day mortality rate	Nonsignificant reduction in 21-day mortality rate; significantly higher LVEF
White HD, et al. (60)	R, DB	219; no age limit	SK vs. placebo	LVEF; mortality rate	Increased LVEF and significantly lower mortality rate in SK group
TIMI-I (61)	R, DB, MCS	290; < 75 years	IV SK or placebo vs. IV rtPA or placebo	Coronary angiography to assess reperfusion at 90 min	Higher reperfusion rate with rtPA; no difference in mortality rate, bleeding complications, or LVF
ASSET (62)	R, MCS, DB, PC	5013; 18–75 years	tPA vs. placebo	Mortality rate	TPA treatment within 5 hr of onset of symptoms reduced mortality sustained to 1 yr, but not rates of recurrent infarction or development of heart failure compared with placebo.
TAMI-6 (63)	P, R, DB, PC, MCS	197; ≤ 75 years	tPA vs. placebo	Vessel patency at 6–24 hours	Better early patency with tPA but similar rate for late patency, in-hospital mortality rate, LVEF
LATE (64)	R, MCS, DB, PC	5711; > 18 years	r-tPA vs. placebo 6–24 hr from onset of symptoms	Mortality rate	Reduced 35-day mortality rate even if given up to 12 hr after onset of symptoms
GREAT (15)	P, R, DB, PG, MCS	311; no age limit	Anistreplase at home vs. in hospital	Mortality rate	52% lower 1-year mortality rate in home-treated group
TEAM-2 (65)	R, DB, MCS	370; < 76 years	Anistreplase (APSAC) or SK	Early patency and reocclusion rates	Both agents were equally effective and safe.

Table continued on following page

TABLE 6.   Synopsis of Thrombolytic Therapy in AMI Trials *(Continued)*

Trial Name (Ref. No.)	Design	Population n, years old	Drug/ Procedure	Major Endpoints	Results
AIMS (66)	R, MCS, DB, PC	1004; ≤ 70 years	APSAC or placebo	Mortality	IV APSAC within 6 hr of onset of symptoms reduced mortality in AMI
Meinertz T, et al (67)	R	313; no age limit	APSAC vs. heparin	28-day mortality rate	Less cardiogenic shock and 56% lower 28-day moratlity rate in APSAC group
ISIS-3 (68)	MCS, PC, R, DB, OL, 3×2 factorial	41,299; no age limit	IV SK, APSAC, r-tPA	Mortality and reinfarction rate at 35-days and 6 months	No difference in 35-day or 6-month mortality rates
TIMI-4 (69)	R, DB, MCS	382; < 80 years	Front-loaded r-tPA or APSAC or combination of r-tPA and APSAC	Coronary angiographic estimation of infarct-related artery patency and TIMI grade 3 flow at 90 min	TIMI grade 3 flow at 90 min; r-tPA 60.2%, APSAC 42.9%, combination 44.8%
GUSTO-I (16)	R, OL, MCS	41,021; no age limit	IV SK + SC heparin, IV SK + IV heparin, accelerated tPA + IV heparin, SK + tPA + IV heparin	Mortality, hemorrhagic stroke	Reduced mortality rate in tPA + IV heparin group
GUSTO-III (17)	R, MCS, OL	15,059; no age limit	Alteplase vs. Reteplase	Mortality and stroke risk	Both agents were identical.
INJECT (70)	R, DB, MCS	6010; ≥ 18 years	Reteplase vs. SK	Mortality at 35 days and 6 months	Reteplase is safe and effective thrombolytic agent.
RAPID (71)	R, MCS, OL	606; 18–75 years	r-PA (reteplase bolus vs. infusion of standard-dose alteplase	Artery patency and LVF	r-PA given as double bolus of 10 MU + 10 MU 30 min apart resulted in more rapid and complete reperfusion than standard-dose tPA and was associated with improved global and regional LV function at discharge.
RAPID-II (72)	R, MCS, PG, OL	324; ≥ 18 years	Double bolus reteplase or front-loaded accelerated alteplase	Artery patency and TIMI grade 3 flow at 90 min	Double bolus dose of reteplase was associated with higher rates of reperfusion at 60 and 90 min after initiation of therapy than front-loaded alteplase infusion, without increase in risk of complications.
COBALT (73)	R, MCS, OL	7169; no age limit	Accelerated infusion of alteplase or double bolus of alteplase	Mortality and stroke risk	Accelerated infusion alteplase remains preferred regimen.

Table continued on following page

TABLE 6. Synopsis of Thrombolytic Therapy in AMI Trials *(Continued)*

Trial Name (Ref. No.)	Design	Population n, years old	Drug/ Procedure	Major Endpoints	Results
TAMI-7 (74)	R, MCS	219; 18–76 years	5 different regimens of tPA	Patency rate, re-occlusion rate, LVEF, death, bleeding	Accelerated tPA administration according to protocol 3 is relatively safe, achieving high 90-min patency rate and low rates of reocclusion and complications.
Carney RJ, et al (75)	R, OL	281; no age limit	Standard vs. accelerated tPA regimen	TIMI grade 3 flow at 60 min and 90 min	Better patency at 60 min but not at 90 min. Similar rates of recurrent ischemia, reinfarction, stroke, and bleeding
COMPASS (76)	R, MCS, DB	3089; > 20 years	Saruplase or SK	Efficacy, safety, and mortality	Similar mortality rate, but more hemorrhagic stroke in saruplase group
PERM (77)	Retrospective	481; no age limit	SK vs. tPA	TIMI grade 3 flow at 90 min	SK, but not tPA, was found to be less effective when administered after 3 hr, regardless of whether TIMI flow grades 2 and 3 were pooled or grade 3 flow was considered alone.
In TIME-I (78)	R, MCS, DB DP	602	Lanoleptase or alteplase	TIMI grade 3 at 60 and 90 min	Increased coronary patency in lanoleptase group
PACT (79)	R	606; no age limit	Precatheterization tPA or placebo	Predischarge EF	No significant difference between two groups in predischarge EF
GUSTO Angiographic Investigators (80)	P, R, MCS, OL	2,431; no age limit	IV SK + SC heprin, IV SK + IV heparin, accelerated tPA + IV heparin, SK + tPA + IV heparin	TIMI grade 3 flow at 90 min	Highest patency at 90 min with tPA and IV heparin: 81% vs. 54% with SK and SC heparin; 73% combination
In TIME-II (81)	R, MCS, DB	15,078; no age limit	Lanoteplase vs. tPA	30-day mortality rate	Similar 30-day mortality rate; higher incidence of intracranial hemorrhage in tPA group
TIMI-10A (82)	Phase 1, dose-ranging pilot trial	113; no age limit	Dose ranging of TNK-tPA	Coronary angiography at 90 min and hemorrhage	TIMI grade 3 flow at 90 min in 64% of patients; major hemorrhage 6.2%
TIMI-10B (83)	R, MCS	886; no age limit	Single bolus of TNK-tPA vs. front-loaded tPA	Coronary angiography at 90 min and hemorrhage	TIMI grade 3 flow is similar.
ASSENT-2 (84)	P,R, DB, OL, MCS	16,949; no age limit	TNK-tPA (tenecteplase) vs. front-loaded alteplase	All-cause mortality at 30 days	Nearly identical all-cause mortality rate at 30 days and similar intracranial hemorrhage rate

Table continued on following page

TABLE 6.   Synopsis of Thrombolytic Therapy in AMI Trials *(Continued)*

Trial Name (Ref. No.)	Design	Population n, years old	Drug/ Procedure	Major Endpoints	Results
TAPS (85)	R	421; no age limit	APSAC vs. front-loaded r-tPA	TIMI grades 2 and 3 at 90 min	Higher 90-min patency (TIMI grade 2 or 3 flow) was achieved with r-tPA (84% vs. 70%; p = 0.0007), as were fewer in-hospital deaths (2.4% vs. 8.1%; p < 0.01)
TEAM-3 (86)	R	325; no age limit	Anistreplase vs. alteplase	LVF, morbidity, 1-day patency	Higher EF before discharge and at 1 month in r-tPA group; similar patency rate; no differences in mortality rate
PATENT (87)	R, OL	1011; no age limit	Sequential combination of r-tPA and prourokinase	TIMI grade 3 flow at 90 min; mortality rate	60% TIMI grade 3 flow at 90 min; 1 in-hospital death
STAR (88)	R, OL	100	Staphylokinase vs. r-tPA	TIMI grade 3 flow at 90 min	Similar TIMI grade 3 flow at 90 min
DUCCS-II (89)	R	162	Front-loaded tPA + IV heparin; anistreplase without heparin	Patency, reinfarction, heart failure, shock, stroke, death	Similar patency rate; 19% fewer end-points in tPA group
TIMI-IIB (90)	R, OL, MCS	2948, < 76 years	Immediate IV beta blockade (metoprolol) vs. beta blockade after r-tPA	Ventricular function, mortality	No difference in clinical outcome at 6 weeks or 1 year
GISSI-3 (91)	MCS, OL, R, 2×2 factorial	18,895; no age limit	Lisinopril or open control Nitrate or placebo 72% of patients received thrombolytic therapy	Effect of ACE inhibitor (lisinopril), transdermal nitrate, or combination on survival and LVF after MI	ACE inhibitor reduced mortality (6.3% vs. 7.1% for no ACE inhibitor or nitrate) at at 6 weeks
ISIS-4 (92)	R, DB, PC, OC, MCS	58,050; no age limit	Captopril or placebo, mononitrate or placebo, IV magnesium or placebo 70% of patients received thrombolytic therapy	Mortality benefit	Magnesium and oral nitrates had no mortality benefit, but captopril reduced 5-week mortality by 7%

AMI = acute myocardial infarction, OL = open label, P = prospective, R = randomized, PC = placebo-controlled, DB = double-blind, MCS = multicenter study, SK = streptokinase, tPA = tissue plasminogen activator, ACE = angiotensin-converting enzyme, LVF = left ventricular function, EF = ejection fraction, APSAC = anisoylated plasminogen-streptokinase activator complex, PG = parallel group, GISSI = Gruppo Italiano per lo Studio della Streptochinasi nell'Infarto Miocardio, ISIS = International Study of Infarct Survival, GUSTO = Global Utilization of Streptokinase and Tissue Plasminogen Activator for Occluded Coronary Arteries, ASSET = Anglo-Scandinavian Study of Early Thrombolysis, COMPASS = Comparison Trial of Saruplase and Streptokinase, LATE = Late Assessment of Thrombolytic Efficacy, AIMS = APSAC Intervention Mortality Study, InTIME = Intravenous nPA for Treatment of Infarcting Myocardium Early, TEAM = Thrombolytic Trial of Eminase in AMI, RAPID = Reteplase Angiographic Phase II International Dose-Ranging Study, INJECT = International Joint Efficacy Comparison of Thrombolytics, COBALT = Continuous Infusion versus Double Bolus Administration of Alteplase, SESAM = Study in Europe with Saruplase and Alteplase in AMI, TAMI = Thrombolysis and Angioplasty in Myocardial Infarction, ISAM = Intravenous Streptokinase in Acute MI, GREAT = Grampian Region Early Anistreplase Trial, PERM = Prospective Evaluation of Reperfusion Markers Study Group, PACT = Plasminogen Activator-Angioplasty Compatibility Trial, DUCCS = Duke University Clinical Cardiology Group Study, PATENT = Prourokinase and t-PA Enhancement of Thrombolysis, TAPS = rt-PA-APSAC Patency Study, ASSENT = Assessment of the Safety and Efficacy of a New Thrombolytic: TNK-tPA.

Table 7. Thrombolytic Agents Approved by the Food and Drug Administration

Streptokinase (Steptase)	APSAC (Eminase)
Urokinase (Abbokinase)	Reteplase (Retevasc)
Alteplase (Activase)	TNKase (Tenecteplase)*

• Recently approved.

Choice of Agent

The type of thrombolytic drug is not as critical and important as the delay to administration. The GUSTO-I trial showed that accelerated tPA was better than streptokinase for most patients with AMI.[16] The GUSTO-III trial showed no mortality benefit of reteplase over alteplase. Both lanoteplase and TNK-tPA (Tenecteplase) can be administered as a single bolus. TNK-t-PA was recently approved by the Food and Drug Administration[17] (Table 7).

Prehospital Thrombolysis

Several prehospital thrombolytic therapy trials were designed to evaluate time-saving, left ventricular function, infarct size, and differences in mortality rates (Table 8).[11–15,18–21] The largest trial, the European Myocardial Infarction Project (EMIP),[13] was carried out in 15 European countries and Canada. Administration of anistreplase as a bolus in the prehospital setting in 2750 patients was compared with hospital treatment in 2719 patients. The 30-day mortality rate was 9.7% vs. 11.1% in the prehospital and hospital groups, respectively (risk reduction = 13%, 95% CI = 1–26%, p = 0.08). The cardiac mortality rate was 8.3% vs. 9.8%, respectively (risk reduction = 16%, 95% CI = 0–29%, p = 0.049). There was no obvious correlation between the reduction in mortality at 30 days and the interval between the onset of symptoms and the first injection. There were no differences between the groups in the incidence of bleeding, overall incidence of stroke, ventricular fibrillation, or shock during the hospital period. The Grampian Region Early Anistreplase Trial (GREAT) compared prehospital thrombolytic therapy given by the practitioner in patients' homes with treatment after hospital arrival in 311 patients.[15] The average time to treatment was 101 vs. 240 minutes, respectively. Patients treated in their home had fewer Q-wave myocardial infarctions and improved left ventricular

Table 8. Prehopsital Administration of Thrombolytic Therapy

Trial Name (Ref. No.)	Design	Population (n, age)	Drug/Procedure	Major Endpoints	Results
EMIP (13)	R, MCS, DB	5469, no age limit	Prehospital anistreplase + placebo after admission; prehospital placebo + anistreplase after admission	Efficacy, safety, reduction of risk	Reduced cardiac mortality; prehospital administration is feasible and safe
MITI-1 (105)	R, C, MCS	2472, ≤ 75 years	Prehospital or in-hospital alteplase	Clinical outcome	No improvement in clinical outcome
MITI-2 (106)	R, C, MCS	360, ≤ 75 years	Prehospital or in-hospital alteplase	Clinical outcome	No improvement in

R = randomized, MCS = multicenter study, DB = double-blinded, EMIP = European Myocardial Infarction Project Group, MITI = Myocardial Infarction Triage and Intervention Trial.

function compared with the group treated in the hospital.[15] The Myocardial Infarction Triage and Intervention (MITI) trial was the largest randomized trial of prehospital thrombolysis in the U.S. The MITI trial evaluated 360 patients who were initially screened by paramedics using a checklist and electrocardiograms. Because the trial included only patients with a short delay to treatment in both prehospital and hospital settings (92 minutes in prehospital-treated vs. 120 minutes in hospital-treated patients), prehospital treatment provided only a modest time saving of 33 minutes.[22]

Adjuvant Therapy

Each of the thrombolytic agents is more likely to cause more minor bleeding when antiplatelet and anticoagulant drugs are given simultaneously or later. The studies in the tables list major hemorrhage as an end-point, prompting cessation of infusion of the thrombolytic agent as well as the adjuvant drug. Aspirin and anticoagulants have been used in conjunction with thrombolytic drugs for increased efficacy but always with the warning that the risk of bleeding is increased. It is routine to use both aspirin and heparin with recombinant tPA drugs. Trials of hirudin and glycoprotein (GP) IIb/IIIa inhibitors (abciximab-murine monoclonal antibodies, 7E3) as adjuvants are shown in Tables 9 and 10, respectively. The TIMI 14 trial and the Strategies for Patency Enhancement in Emergency Department (SPEED) trial showed significant benefit in terms of TIMI grade 3 flow at 60–90 minutes. Based on these results, the GUSTO-IV trial (Global Utilization of Streptokinase and tissue Plasminogen Activator for Occluded Coronary Arteries) will evaluate 30-day mortality in 17,000 patients with AMI randomized to treatment with reteplase vs. full- dose abciximab plus reteplase at half the usual dose.[23]

The optimal regimen of an antiplatelet drug with or without an anticoagulant drug administered in conjunction with thrombolytic drugs of various types will be determined by future trials.

Adjuvant Percutaneous Transluminal Coronary Angioplasty

Studies have shown that immediate PTCA may be superior to streptokinase in terms of recurrent ischemia, reinfarction, and stroke rates as well as in patients with cardiogenic shock (Tables 11 and 12).[24–28] The 4% risk of intracerebral hemorrhage in elderly patients receiving thrombolytic therapy can be greatly reduced or eliminated with primary PTCA, and insertion of a stent may add to the advantages of angioplasty.[29]

Because the efficacy of angioplasty depends more on operator skill and availability of suitable facilities and support personnel than does thrombolytic therapy and because of the significant delay in starting the procedure, PTCA cannot replace conventional thrombolytic therapy for most patients. It has been suggested, however, that thrombolytic therapy should be given in reduced dosage, even in the prehospital setting, and followed by PTCA in the hospital. The addition of abciximab or a similar antiplatelet agent and a stent in appropriate cases may optimize the treatment of AMI.[29,30,119]

Rescue PTCA for failed thrombolysis may be a valuable procedure, particularly in patients with anterior MI. GP IIb/IIIa inhibitors and stenting may be useful as well.[30,119]

Table 9. Direct Thrombin Inhibitors with Thrombolytic Therapy Trials in Acute Myocardial Infarction

Trial Name (Ref. No.)	Design	Population (n, age)	Drug/Procedure	Major Endpoints	Results
TIMI-5 (93)	R, MCS	246, no age limit	IV heparin and hirudin + front-loaded tPA and aspirin, dose escalation study	TIMI grade 3 flow at 90 min and 18 hr without death or reinfarction	64.8% of hirudin vs. 57.1% of heparin at 90 min TIMI grade 3 flow
TIMI-6 (94)	R, MCS	193, no age limit	Hirudin vs. heparin + IV SK and aspirin	Major hemorrhage, death, nonfatal reinfarction, heart failure, cardiogenic shock	Major hemorrhage is similar, no significant difference between any treatment groups
TIMI-9A (95)	R, DB, MCS	757, no age limit	IV heparin vs. IV hirudin after SK or r-tPA All received aspirin	Clinical safety and efficacy	Similar rates of hemorrhage; no superiority of hirudin over heparin
TIMI-9B (96)	R, DB, MCS	3002, no age limit	IV heparin vs. IV hirudin after SK or r-tPA All received aspirin	Rate of hemorrhage, composite of death, MI, severe heart failure, and cardiogenic shock	Rate of hemorrhage was similar (5.3% vs. 4.6%), no difference (11.9% vs. 12.9%) in efficacy
GUSTO-2B (Substudy) (97)	R, MCS	3289, no age limit	Hirudin + SK or hirudin + tPA	Mortality, nonfatal reinfarction	Beneficial interaction with SK but not with tPA
HIT-3 (98)	R, DB, MCS	7000	tPA + hirudin vs. heparin	30-day death, reinfarction	Early termination due to unacceptable bleeding rate
HIT-4 (99)	R, DB, MCS	1211	SK + hirudin vs. heparin	30-day death, reinfarction	No significant difference
HERO-1 (100)	P, R, DB, MCS	412	Hirulog vs. heparin + SK and aspirin	TIMI grade 3 flow flow at 90 min	34% relative benefit

TIMI = Thrombolysis in Myocardial Infarction, GUSTO = Global Utilization of Streptokinase and Tissue Plasminogen Activator for Occluded Coronary Arteries, HIT = r-Hirudin for Improvement of Thrombolysis Study, HERO = Hirulog Early Perfusion/Occlusion Trial, R = randomized, DB= double-blinded, MCS = multicenter study, P = prospective, SK = streptokinase, tPA = tissue plasminogen activator.

Thrombolytic Therapy in Elderly Patients with Acute Myocardial Infarction

Advanced age is the most important risk factor predictive of mortality in AMI. Although thrombolytic therapy has increased since the 1990s, it is still underused in elderly patients.[31,32] In patients 65–74 years of age, thrombolytic therapy has the greatest margin of benefit in absolute risk reduction.[33] Despite concern of increased risk of bleeding in patients older than 75 years, the absolute net benefit is striking, with 18 lives saved per 1000 patients treated. To combat the risk of hemorrhage, direct percutaneous revascularization procedures may be considered in this age group.

Thrombolytic Therapy in Diabetic Patients with Acute Myocardial Infarction

Diabetes is associated with a poor outcome after AMI.[34] Mak et al.[35] have shown that in the GUSTO-I trial diabetic patients were older and more likely to

Table 10. Glycoprotein IIb/IIIa Inhibitors with Thrombolytic Therapy Trials
in Acute Myocardial Infarction

Trial Name (Ref. No.)	Design	Population (n, age)	Drug/Procedure	Major Endpoints	Results
TIMI-12 (101)	R, DB, dose ranging trial	329, no age limit	Oral sibrafiban vs. aspirin	Safety, tolerability	Effective long-term platelet inhibition with sibrafiban; high incidence of minor bleeding; no difference in major hemorrhage
TIMI-14 (102)	R, OL, dose finding and dose confirmation phases	888, 18–75 years	Accelerated-dose alteplase Abciximab + reduced-dose SK Abciximab + reduced-dose alteplase Abciximab alone	TIMI grade 3 flow at 90 min	52% in r-tPA–only arm; 32% in abciximab-only arm; 53%, 63%, and 61% in r-tPA + abciximab; 42%, 38%, and 48% in SK + abciximab
PARADIGM (103)	Part A: OL Part B: R, DB Part C: R, DB	353, no age limit	Lamifiban + tPA or SK	Rate of bleeding	More rapid perfusion but higher incidence of bleeding
GUSTO IV (SPEED) (23)	R, MCS, dose escalating	305 (phase 1) 225 (phase 2)	Abciximab or abciximab + reteplase	TIMI grade 3 flow at 60 min, efficacy	Improved perfusion rate with sustained fibrinolytic therapy during abciximab infusion
IMPACT-AMI (104)	PC, MCS, dose ranging	180, 18–75 years	Integrilin or placebo + accelerated alteplase	TIMI grade 3 flow at 90 min	Reperfusion speed improved but not in-hospital outcome

TIMI = Thrombolysis in Myocardial Infarction, GUSTO = Global Utilization of Streptokinase and Tissue Plasminogen Activator for Occluded Coronary Arteries, PARADIGM = Platelet Aggregation Receptor Antagonist Dose Investigation and Reperfusion Gain in Myocardial Infarction, IMPACT-AMI = Integrilin to Manage Platelet Aggregation to Prevent Coronary Thrombosis in Acute Myocardial Infarction, R = randomized, DB= double-blinded, OL = open-labeled, MCS = multicenter study, tPA = tissue plasminogen activator.

be female, to present with anterior MI, to receive thrombolytics later, and to have triple-vessel disease. The 30-day mortality rate was higher in this group (12.5 and 9.7% for insulin- and non–insulin-treated patients, respectively) than in nondiabetic patients (6.2%). Diabetics, like other higher-risk groups, derive a greater benefit from thrombolytic therapy, as shown by the GUSTO-I trial. The concerns about higher bleeding risks associated with thrombolytic therapy are not clearly supported by large clinical trials. The GISSI-2/International Study Group Trial showed a similar incidence of stroke and major bleeding in diabetic and nondiabetic patients.[36] The GUSTO-II trial did show a higher incidence of these events in diabetics.[37] Hasdai et al.[38] compared the outcomes of 177 diabetics with the outcomes of 961 nondiabetics who were randomized between primary angioplasty and thrombolysis in the GUSTO-II angioplasty substudy. They showed that diabetics had worse baseline clinical and angiographic profiles than nondiabetics. Despite more severe stenosis and poorer flow in the culprit arteries in diabetics, there was no difference in procedural success rates between the two groups. The 30-day outcome was better for

Table 11. Synopsis of Primary Angioplasty with Thrombolytic Therapy Trials in Acute Myocardial Infarction

Trial Name (Ref. No.)	Design	Population (n, age)	Drug/Procedure	Major Endpoints	Results
TIMI-IIA (107)	R, OL, MCS	586, < 76 years	Immediate PTCA or delayed PTCA or CABG + IV r-tPA	Predischarge LVEF	No advantage of immediate revascularization following r-tPA
GUSTO-IIB (97)	R, MCS	1138, no age limit	Primary angioplasty or accelerated tPA	Mortality, nonfatal reinfarction, stroke risk	Angioplasty has small-to-moderate short-term clinical advantage over tPA
TAMI-5 (108)	R, MCS, OL, 3×2 factorial	575, < 76 years	UK vs. tPA vs. UK + tPA; + angioplasty	Early patency rates, predischarge patency, LVEF	Combination therapy is more effective and has better clinical outcome
PAMI (109)	P, R, OL, MCS	395, no age limit	Immediate PTCA vs. tPA	In-hospital death, reinfarction, intracranial bleeding, and LVEF at 6 wk	Lower in-hospital mortality rate, significant reduction in reinfarction, less intracranial bleeding with PTCA
Riebeiro EE, et al (110)	R	100	SK vs. immediate PTCA	Mortality rate, LVEF, patency	No significant difference between two groups
O'Neil W, et al (111)	First R trial	56, < 75 years	SK vs. PTCA	Residual stenosis, LVEF	Decreased residual stenosis and significant improvement in LVEF in PTCA group
Ziljstra F, et al (24)	R	142	SK vs. immediate PTCA	Reinfarction rate, LVEF	Lower reinfarction rate and higher LVEF in PTCA group
MITI (105)	Retrospective	3145	Thrombolysis with altepase (65%), SK (32%), or UK vs. PTCA	In-hospital or 3-year mortality rate	No significant difference
Schömig A, et al (119)	R	140	Stent + abciximab vs. thrombolysis	Myocardial salvage, death, reinfarction, CVA at 6 mo	Better outcome with stent and abciximab

TIMI = Thrombolysis in Myocardial Infarction, GUSTO = Global Utilization of Streptokinase and Tissue Plasminogen Activator for Occluded Coronary Arteries, MITI = Myocardial Triage and Intervention Trial, TAMI = Thrombolysis and Angioplasty in Acute Myocardial Infarction, PAMI = Primary Angioplasty in Myocardial Infarction, R = randomized, DB= double-blinded, OL = open-labeled, MCS = multicenter study, UK = urokinase, SK = streptokinase, PTCA = percutaneous transluminal coronary angioplasty, CABG = coronary artery bypass graft, tPA = tissue plasminogen activator, LVEF = left ventricular ejection fraction, CVA = cerebrovascular accident.

nondiabetics randomized to angioplasty vs. alteplase, and a similar trend was found for diabetics. The authors concluded that primary angioplasty was similarly successful in diabetics and nondiabetics and appeared to be more effective than thrombolytic therapy among diabetics with AMI. In an editorial, King[39] commented that in the GUSTO-IIb study, the in-hospital mortality was

Table 12. Synopsis of Primary Angioplasty after Thrombolytic Therapy Trials in Acute Myocardial Infarction

Trial Name (Ref. No.)	Design	Population (n, age)	Drug/Procedure	Major Endpoints	Results
TAMI (112)	P, R, MCS	386, ≤ 75 years	Single-chain tPA followed by PTCA vs. immediate PTCA	Infarct-related vessel patency, LVEF	Similar reocclusion rate; no improvement in global LV function in either group
TIMI-IIA (107)	R, OL, MCS	586, < 76 years	Immediate PTCA or delayed PTCA or CABG + IV r-tPA	Predischarge LVEF	No advantage to immediate revascularization following r-tPA
Califf RM, et al (TAMI Study Group) (113)	P, R, OL, PC, MCS	575, ≤ 75 years	UK vs. r-tPA vs. combination therapy with PTCA	Global LVEF	Well-preserved and nearly identical global LVEF in PTCA group. Better results with fewer adverse outcomes in aggressive strategies
SWIFT (114)	P, R, MCS	800, < 70 years	Early appropriate intervention vs. conservative care + anistreplase	Mortality and reinfarction rates	No difference in 1-year mortality or reinfarction rate
DANAMI (115)	R, MCS	1008, < 69 years	Conservative therapy vs. PTCA or CABG	Death, reinfarction, unstable angina	Lower rates of death, reinfarction, and unstable angina in invasive therapy group
ECSG-4 (116)	R	367	Invasive vs. noninvasive strategy + tPA	Mortality and recurrent ischemia rates and bleeding complications	Lower mortality and recurrent ischemia rates, fewer bleeding complications with invasive strategy

TAMI = Thrombolysis and Angioplasty in Acute Myocardial Infarction, TIMI = Thrombolysis in Myocardial Infarction, SWIFT = Should We Intervene Following Thrombolysis Trial, DANAMI = Danish Trial in Acute Myocardial Infarction, ECSG = European Cooperative Study Group, P = prospective, R = randomized, MCS = multicenter study, OL = open-labeled, PC = placebo-controlled, tPA = tissue plasminogen activator, PTCA = percutaneous transluminal coronary angioplasty, CABG = coronary artery bypass graft, LVEF = left ventricular ejection fraction.

5.1% in the thrombolysis group but 9.1% in the angioplasty group (differences not significant). The EPISTENT investigators demonstrated a dramatic reduction in periprocedural MI in diabetic patients with use of GP IIb/IIIa inhibitors.[40]

Unstable Angina and Non–Q Wave Myocardial Infarction

Several studies have shown that thrombolytic therapy is not useful in unstable angina or non–Q-wave MI.[41,42] Furthermore, it is associated with increased bleeding and higher MI rates. Adjunctive intracoronary thrombolytic therapy showed no benefit during PTCA in the Thrombolysis and Angioplasty in Unstable Angina (TAUSA) Trial.[43]

Future Considerations

Despite several randomized trials proving that early thrombolytic therapy in patients with AMI reduces the mortality rate by approximately 30% and that reperfusion therapy provides better results when administered in the first 60–90 minutes after symptom onset, the median time from symptom onset to thrombolytic therapy is 2.5 hours, and the "door to thrombolytic injection" is still more than 50 minutes. Measures to reduce this period will improve outcomes. Another approach to improving the results of thrombolysis, regardless of timing, is to inhibit clot stabilization and thereby promote thrombolytic potential. Blocking factor XIIIa-mediated reactions in a controlled and selective manner that does not interfere with the primary clotting time may prevent a significant portion of the clot from progressing to the fully stabilized state.[44] Viscoelastic moduli of clots may be reduced by inhibitors of factor XIIIa,[45] which also enhance clot lysis.[46] One such agent is the protein isolated from a giant Amazon leech; its exact mechanism of action is not fully known.[47–49] Another approach is monoclonal antibody directed against the thrombin cleavage site of factor XIII. This approach blocks the activation of factor XIII by thrombin.[50] The factor XIIIa-catalyzed covalent attachment of $\alpha2$-plasmin inhibitor ($\alpha2$-PI) to fibrin, which contributes significantly to lytic resistance, can be blocked by a monoclonal antibody against $\alpha2$-PI.[51] The antibody to $\alpha2$-PI was shown to be effective in promoting clot lysis in vitro and thrombolysis in animal models.[51–53] Recent results from a mutant form of $\alpha2$-PI suggest more possibilities for enhancing the fibrinolytic susceptibilities of thrombi.[54] Inhibitors of clot stabilization may facilitate thrombolysis with much lower doses of plasminogen activators than are currently used without lengthening the clotting times and avoiding extra risk of hemorrhage. Blocking the action of factor XIII and of $\alpha2$-PI in conjunction with even low-dose thrombolytic therapy may cause excessive hemorrhage.[55]

Conclusion

Thrombolytic therapy for AMI is highly effective when applied early, preferably within 1 hour but not longer than 6 hours after the onset of symptoms.

A number of effective agents are available; newer ones are in the developmental stage. Combinations with antiplatelet and anticoagulant drugs have become standard, and newer adjuvants of this type are in development.

Some investigators have proposed the combination of PTCA, when feasible, with reduced-dosage thrombolytic therapy in the prehospital setting or early after the event.[29] Combination with GP IIb/IIIa inhibitors and PTCA with or without stent also may be useful.[29] However, a number of studies using a combination of thrombolysis followed by angioplasty, immediate or delayed, have shown no benefit or even reduced benefit when it is done on a routine basis.[30] The cost of combined therapy is much higher than thrombolytic therapy alone.[28] Nevertheless, assessment by angiography after thrombolytic therapy provides evidence of failed thrombolysis, which is an indication for angioplasty. Additional studies are needed to assess its value compared with conservative therapy.[117] The results may be influenced by the choice of adjuvant drugs and the use of stents.[118]

References

1. American Heart Association: 1998 Heart and Stroke Statistical Update. Dallas, American Heart Association,1997.
2. Murray CJ, Lopez AD: Mortality by cause for eight regions of the world. Global Burden of Disease Study. Lancet 349:1269, 1997.
3. National Institutes of Health, National Heart, Lung, and Blood Institute, Public Health Service of National Institutes of Health: Morbidity and Mortality: 1998 Chart Book on Cardiovascular, Lung and Blood Diseases. Washington, DC, U.S. Department of Health and Human Services, 1998.
4. Mc Govern PG, Pankow JS, Shahar E, et al, for the Minnesota Heart Survey Investigators: Recent trends in acute coronary heart disease, mortality, morbidity, medical care and risk factors. N Engl J Med 334:884–890, 1996.
5. Goldman L, Cook EF: The decline in ischemic heart disease mortality rates: An analysis of the comparative effects of medical interventions and changes in life style. Ann Intern Med 101:825–836, 1984.
6. Stern MP: The recent decline in ischemic heart disease mortality. Ann Intern Med 91:630–640, 1979.
7. Simons-Morton DG, Goff DC, Osganian S, et al, for the REACT Research Group: Rapid early action for coronary treatment: Rationale, design, and baseline characteristics. Acad Emerg Med 5:726–738, 1998.
8. Selker HP, Beshnsky JR, Griffith JL, et al: Use of the acute cardiac ischemia time-intensive predictive Instrument (ACI-TIPI) to assist with triage of patients with chest pain or other symptoms suggestive of acute cardiac ischemia: A multicenter, controlled clinical trial. Ann Intern Med 129:845–855, 1998.
9. Anfderheide TP, Rowlandson I, Lawrence SW, et al: Test of the acute cardiac ischemia time-insensitive predictive instrument (ACI-TIPI) for pre-hospital use. Ann Emerg Med 27:193–198, 1996.
10. Gilliam RF: Trends in acute myocardial infarction and coronary heart disease death in the United States. J Am Coll Cardiol 23:1273–1277, 1994.
11. Fine DG, Weiss AT, Sapoznikov D, et al: Importance of early initiation of intravenous streptokinase therapy for acute myocardial infarction. Am J Cardiol 58:411–417, 1986.
12. Koren G, Weiss AT, Hasin Y, et al: Prevention of myocardial damage in acute myocardial ischemia by early treatment with intravenous streptokinase. N Engl J Med 313:1384–1389, 1985.
13. European Myocardial Infarction Project Group: Pre-hospital thrombolytic therapy in patients with suspected acute myocardial infarction. N Engl J Med 329:383–389, 1993.
14. Roth A, Barbash GI, Hod H, et al: Should thrombolytic therapy be administered in the mobile intensive care unit in-patients with evolving myocardial infarction? A pilot study. J Am Coll Cardiol 15:932–936, 1990.
15. Rawles J: Halving of mortality at 1 year by domiciliary thrombolysis in the Grampian Region Early Anistreplase Trial (GREAT). J Am Coll Cardiol 23:1–5, 1994.
16. GUSTO Investigators: An International randomized trial comparing four thrombolytic strategies for acute myocardial infarction. N Engl J Med 329:673, 1993.
17. Global Use of Strategies to Open Occluded Arteries (GUSTO III) Investigators: A comparison of reteplase with alteplase for acute myocardial infarction. N Engl J Med 337:1118, 1997.
18. Bippus PH, Storch WH, Andersen D, et al: Thrombolysis started at home in acute myocardial infarction: Feasibility and time-gain [abstract]. Circulation 76(Suppl IV):IV-122, 1987.
19. Bossaert LL, Demey HE, Colemont LJ, et al: Pre-hospital thrombolytic treatment of acute myocardial infarction with anisoylated plasminogen streptokinase activator complex. Crit Care Med 16:823–830, 1988.
20. Castigne AD, Herve C, Duval-Moulin AM, et al: Pre-hospital use of APSAC: Results of a placebo-controlled study. Am J Cardiol 64:30A–33A, 1989.
21. Risenfors M, Gustavson G, Ekstrom L, et al: Pre-hospital thrombolysis in suspected acute myocardial infarction: Results from the TEAHAT Study. J Intern Med (Suppl) 734:3–10, 1991.
22. Ralf Z, Schiele R, Seidl K, et al: Acute myocardial infarction occurring in versus out of the hospital: Patient characteristics and clinical outcome. J Am Coll Cardiol 35:1820–1826, 2000.
23. Ohman EM, Lincoff AM, Bode C, et al: Enhanced early reperfusion at 60 minutes with low dose reteplase combined with full-dose abciximab in acute myocardial infarction: Preliminary results for the GUSTO-4 pilot (SPEED) dose ranging trial [abstract]. Circulation 98 (Suppl 1):504, 1998.
24. Zijlsta F, Hoorntje JC, de Boer MJ, et al: Long-term benefit of primary angioplasty as compared with thrombolytic therapy for acute myocardial infarction. N Engl J Med 341:1413–1439, 1999.
25. Every NR, Parsms LS, Hlatky M, et al: A comparison of thrombolytic therapy with primary coronary angioplasty for acute myocardial infarction. N Engl J Med 335:1253–1260, 1996.
26. Lange RA, Hillis LD, Grines CL: Should thrombolysis or primary angioplasty be treatment of choice for acute myocardial infarction? N Engl J Med 335:1311–1317, 1996.

27. Weaver WD, Simes RJ, Betrin A, et al: Comparison of primary angioplasty and intravenous thrombolytic therapy acute myocardial infarction. JAMA 278:2093–2098, 1997 [erratum: JAMA 279:1876, 1998].

28. de Boer MJ, van Hout BA, Leim AL, et al: A cost-effective analysis of primary coronary angioplasty versus thrombolytic therapy for acute myocardial infarction. Am J Cardiol 76:830–833, 1995.

29. Bates ER: Commentary: Zijlsta et al. N Eng J Med 341:1413–1439, 1999. ACP Journal Club 132:81, 2000.

30. Goldman LE, Eisenberg MJ: Identification and management of patients with failed thrombolysis after acute myocardial infarction Ann Intern Med 132:556–565, 2000.

31. Lambrew CT, Bowlby LJ, Rogers WJ, et al: Factors influencing the time to thrombolysis in acute myocardial infarction. Time to thrombolysis sub-study of the National Registry of Myocardial infarction-1. Arch Intern Med 157:2277, 1997.

32. Sommerai SB, McLaughlin TJ, Gurwitz JH, et al: Effect of local medical opinion leaders on quality of care for acute myocardial infarction: A randomized controlled trial. JAMA 279:1358, 1998.

33. Lauer MA, Topol EJ: Taking the fibrinolytic era into the new millennium. Cardiol Rev 16(10):10–23, 1999.

34. Garcia MJ, McNamara PM, Gordon T, et al: Morbidity and mortality in diabetes in the Framingham population: Sixteen-year follow-up study. Diabetes 23:105–111, 1974.

35. Mak KM, Moliterno DJ, Granger CB, et al: Influence of diabetes mellitus on clinical outcome in the thrombolytic era of acute myocardial infarction. J Am Coll Cardiol 30:170–179, 1997.

36. International Study Group: In hospital mortality and clinical course of 20,891 patients with suspected acute myocardial infarction randomized between alteplase and streptokinase with or without heparin. Lancet 336:71–75, 1990.

37. Lee KL, Woodlief LH, Topol EJ, et al: Predictors of 30-day mortality in the era of reperfusion for acute myocardial infarction: Results from an international trial of 41,021 patients. Circulation 91:1659–1968.

38. Hasdai D, Granger CB, Srivatsa SS, et al: Diabetes mellitus and outcome after primary coronary angioplasty for acute myocardial infarction: Lessons from the GUSTO-IIb Angioplasty substudy. J Am Coll Cardiol 35:1502–1512, 2000.

39. King SB III: Acute myocardial infarction: Are diabetics different? [editorial comment]. J Am Coll Cardiol 35:1513–1515, 2000.

40. EPISTENT Investigators: Randomized placebo-controlled and balloon-angioplasty-controlled trial to assess safety of coronary stenting, the use of platelet glycoprotein IIb/IIIa blockade. Lancet 352:87–92, 1998.

41. Bar FW, Verheugt FW, Col J et al: Unstable Angina Study Using Eminase (UNASEM). Thrombolysis in patients with unstable angina improves the angiographic but not the clinical outcome: Results of UNASEM, a multicenter, randomized, placebo-controlled, clinical trial with anistreplase. Circulation 86:131–137, 1992.

42. Early effects of tissue type plasminogen activator added to conventional therapy on the culprit coronary lesion in patients presenting with ischemic cardiac pain at rest: Results of the thrombolysis in myocardial ischemia (TIMI IIIA) Trial. Circualation 87:38–52, 1993.

43. Ambrosa JA, Almeida OD, Sharma S, et al: Adjunctive thrombolytic therapy during angioplasty for ischemic rest angina: Results of the TAUSA trial. Circulation 90:69–77, 1994.

44. Lorand L: Research on clot stabilization provides clues for improving thrombolytic therapies. Sol Sherry Lecture in Thrombosis. Arterioscler Thromb Vasc Biol 20:2–9, 2000.

45. Ryan Ek, Mockro LF, Weisel JW, et al: Structural origins of fibrin clot rheology. Biophys J 77:2813–2826, 1999.

46. Freund KF, Doshi KP, Gaul SL, et al: Transglutaminase inhibition by 2-[(2-oxypropyl) thiol] imadazolium derivatives. Mechanism of factor XIIIa inactivation. Biochemistry 33:10109–10119, 1994.

47. Seale L, Finney S, Sawyer RT, et al: Triadegin, a novel peptide inhibitor of factor XIIIa from the leech, *Haementeria ghilianii*, enhances fibrinolysis in vitro. Thromb Haemost 77:959–963, 1997.

48. Wallis RB, Seale L, Finney S, et al: Reduction of plasma clot stability by a novel factor XIIIa inhibitor from the giant Amazon leech, *Haementeria ghilianii*. Blood Coagul Fibrinolysis 8:291–295, 1997.

49. Finney S, Seale L, Sawyer RT, et al: Tridegina, new peptide inhibitor of factor XIIIa from the blood sucking leech, *Haementeria ghilianii*. Biochem J 324:797–805, 1997.

50. Reed GL III, Lukacova D: Generation and mechanism of action of a potent inhibitor of factor XIII function. Thromb Haemost 74:680–685, 1995.

51. Reed GL III, Matsueda GR, Haber E: Synergistic fibrinolysis: Combined effects of plasminogen activators and an antibody that inhibits alpha 2-antiplasmin. Proc Nat Acad Sci USA 87:1114–1118, 1990.

52. Reed GL III, Matsueda GR, Haber E: Inhibition of clot bound alpha2-antiplasmin enhances in vivo thrombolysis. Circulation 82:164–168, 1990.

53. Buttl AN, Houng AK, Jang I-Kyung, et al: Alpha2-antiplasmin causes thrombi to resist fibrinolysis induced by tissue plasminogen activator in experimental pulmonary embolism. Circulation 95:1886–1891, 1997.

54. Reed GL, Houng AK: The contribution of activated factor XIII to fibrinolytic resistance in experimental pulmonary embolism. Circulation 99:299–304, 1999.

55. Lee KN, Tae WC, Jackson KW, et al: Characterization of wild type and mutant alpha2 antiplasmin: Fibrinolysis enhancement by reactive site mutant. Blood 94:164–171, 1999.

56. Gruppo Italiano per lo studio della streptokinasi nell'Infarto Miocardico (GISSI): Effectiveness of intravenous thrombolytic treatment in acute myocardial infarction. Lancet 1:397, 1986.

57. Gruppo Italiano per lo studio della streptokinasi nell'Infarto Miocardico (GISSI-2): A factorial randomized trial of alteplase vs. streptokinase and heparin vs. no heparin among 12,490 patients with acute MI. Lancet 336:65–71, 1990.

58. ISIS-2 (Second International Study of Infarct Survival) Collaborative Group: Randomized trial of intravenous streptokinase, oral aspirin, both, or neither among 17,187 cases of suspected acute myocardial infarction: ISIS-2. Lancet 2:349, 1988.

59. ISAM Study Group: A prospective trial of intravenous streptokinase in acute myocardial infarction (ISAM): Mortality, morbidity and infarct size at 21 days. N Engl J Med 314:1465, 1986.

60. White HD, Norris RM, Brown MA, et al: Effect of intravenous streptokinase on left ventricular function and early survival after acute MI. N Engl J Med 317:850–855, 1987.

61. Chesbero JH, Knatterud G, Roberts R et al: Thrombolysis in Myocardial Infarction (TIMI) Trial, phase I: A comparison between intravenous tissue plasminogen activator and intravenous streptokinase. Clinical findings through hospital discharge. Circulation 76:142–154, 1987.

62. ASSET: Trial of tissue plasminogen activator for mortality reduction in acute myocardial infarction. Angio-Scandinavian Study of Early Thrombolysis. Lancet I: 525–530, 1988.

63. Topol EJ, Califf RM, Vandermeal M, et al: A randomized trial of late reperfusion therapy for acute MI. Circulation 85:2090–2099, 1992.

64. Late Study Group: Late assessment of thrombolytic efficacy (LATE) study with alteplase 6–24 h after onset of acute myocardial infarction. Lancet 342:759–766, 1993.

65. Anderson JL, Sorenson SG, Moreno FL, et al: Multicenter patency trial of intravenous anistreplase compared with streptokinase in acute myocardial infarction (TEAM-2). Circulation 83:126–140, 1991.

66. AIMS Trial Study Group: Long-term effects of intravenous anistreplase in acute myocardial infarction: Final report of the AIMS study. Lancet 335:427–431, 1990.

67. Meinertz T, Kasper W, Schumacher M, et al: The German Multicenter Trial of anisoylated plasminogen streptokinase activator complex versus heparin for acute MI. Am J Cardiol 62: 347–351, 1988.

68. ISIS-3 Collaborative Group: A randomized comparison of streptokinase vs tissue plasminogen activator vs anistreplase and of aspirin plus heparin vs aspirin alone among 41,299 cases of suspected acute myocardial infarction. Lancet 339:753–770, 1992.

69. Cannon CP, McCabe CH, Diver DJ, et al: Comparison of front loaded recombinant tissue type plasminogen activator, anistreplase, and combination thrombolytic therapy for acute myocardial infarction: Results of the Thrombolysis in Myocardial Infarction (TIMI) 4 Trial. J Am Coll Cardiol 24:1602–1610, 1994.

70. International Joint Efficacy Comparison Thrombolytics: Randomized, double-blind comparison of reteplase double bolus administration with streptokinase in acute myocardial infarction (INJECT): Trial to investigate equivalence. Lancet 346:329–336, 1995.

71. Smalling RW, Bode C, Kalbfleisch J, et al: More rapid, complete, and stable coronary thrombolysis with bolus administration of reteplase compared with alteplase infusion in acute myocardial infarction. Circulation 91:2725–2732, 1995.

72. Bode C, Smalling RW, Berg G, et al: Randomized comparison of coronary thrombolysis achieved with double bolus reteplase (recombinant plasminogen activator) and front loaded, accelerated alteplase (recombinant tissue plasminogen activator) in patients with acute myocardial infarction. Circulation 94:891–898, 1996.

73. Continuous Infusion vs. Double Bolus Administration of Alteplase (COBALT) Investigators: A comparison of continuous infusion alteplase with double bolus administration for acute myocardial infarction. N Engl J Med 337:1124–1130, 1997.

74. Wall TC, Califf RM, George BS, et al: Accelerated plasminogen activator dose regimens for coronary thrombolysis. J Am Coll Cardiol 19:482–489, 1992.

75. Carney RJ, Murhy GA, Brandt TR, et al: Randomized angiographic trial of recombinant tissue-type plasminogen activator (alteplase) in MI. J Am Coll Cardiol 20:17–23, 1992.

76. Tebbe U, Michels R, Adgey J, et al: Randomized, double blind study comparing saruplase with streptokinase therapy in acute myocardial infarction the COMPASS equivalence trial. J Am Coll Cardiol 31:487–493, 1998.

77. Steg PG, Lapreche T, Golmard JL, et al: Perspective Evaluation of Reperfusion Markers (PERM) Study Group. Efficacy of streptokinase, but not tissue-type plasminogen activator, in achieving 90-minute patency after thrombolysis for acute MI decreases with time to treatment. J Am Coll Cardiol 31:776–779, 1998.

78. Heijer PD, Vermeer E, Ambrosioni E, et al: Evaluation of a weight adjusted single bolus plasminogen activator in patients with myocardial infarction. A double blind, randomized angiographic trial of lanoteplase vs alteplase. Circulation 98:2117–2125, 1998.

79. Ross AM: Plasminogen Activator Angioplasty Compatibility Trial (PACT). Intern Med News 4:1, 1998.

80. GUSTO Angiographic Investigators: The effects of tissue plasminogen activator, streptokinase, or both on coronary artery patency, ventricular function and survival after acute MI. N Engl J Med 329:1615–1622, 1993.

81. InTIME-II: Intravenous nPA for Treatment of Infarcting Myocardium Early 2. Presented at the 48th Annual Scientific Session of the American College of Cardiology, New Orleans, March, 1999.

82. Cannon CP, McCabe CH, Gibson M, et al: TNK-tissue plasminogen activator in acute myocardial infarction of the thrombolysis in myocardial infarction (TIMI) 10A dose ranging trial. Circulation 95:351–356, 1997.

83. Cannon CP, McCabe CH, Gibson M, et al: TNK-Tissue plasminogen activator compared with front loaded alteplase in acute myocardial infarction. Results of the TIMI 10B Trial. Circulation 98:2805–2814, 1998.

84. ASSENT-II: Assessment of the Safety and Efficacy of a New Thrombolytic: TNK-tPA. Presented at the 48th Annual Scientific Session of the American College of Cardiology, New Orleans, March, 1999.

85. Neuhaus KL, von Essen R, Tebbe U, et al: Improved thrombolysis in acute MI with front-loaded administration of alteplase. Results of the rt-PA-APSAC Patency Study (TAPS). J Am Coll Cardiol 19:885–891,1992.

86. Anderson JL, Sorenson SG, Moreno FL, et al: Anistreplase vs alteplase in acute myocardial infarction: comparative effects on left ventricular function, morbidity and one-day coronary patency (TEAM-3). J Am Coll Cardiol 20:753–766, 1992.

87. Zarich SW, Kowalchuk GJ, Weaver WD, et al: Pro-urokinase and t-PA Enhancement of Thrombolysis (PATENT). Sequential combination thrombolytic therapy for acute MI: results of PATENT trial. J Am Coll Cardiol 26:374–379, 1995.

88. Vanderschueren S, Barrious S, Kerdsinchai P, et al: A randomized trial of recombinant staphylokinase vs alteplase for coronary artery patency in acute MI. STAR Trial Group: Circulation 92:2044–2049, 1995.

89. O'Connor CM, Meeses RB, McNulty S, et al: The Duke University Clinical Cardiology Group Study (DUCCS) II Investigators: A randomized factorial trial of reperfusion strategies and aspirin dosing in acute MI. Am J Cardiol 77:791–797, 1996.

90. Roberts R, Rodger WJ, Mueller HS, et al: Immediate vs. deferred beta blockade following thrombolytic therapy in patients with acute myocardial infarction: Results of the thrombolysis in myocardial infarction (TIMI) II-B Study. Circulation 83:422–437, 1991.

91. Zuanetti G, Latini R, Maggioni AP, et al: Effect of lisinopril and transdermal glyceryl trinitrate singly and together on 6-week mortality and ventricular function after acute MI. Lancet 343:1115–1122, 1994.

92. ISIS-4 (4th International Study of Infarct Survival) Collaborative Group: ISIS-4: A randomized factorial trial assessing early oral captopril, oral mononitrate, and intravenous magnesium sulphate in 58,050 patients with suspected acute myocardial infarction. Lancet 345:669–685, 1995.

93. Canon CP, McCabe CH, Henry TD, et al: A pilot trial recombinant desulfohirudin compared with heparin in conjunction with tissue type plasminogen activator and aspirin for acute myocardial infarction: Results of the thrombolysis in myocardial Infarction (TIMI) 5 Trial. J Am Coll Cardiol 23:993–1003,1994.

94. Lee LV, for the TIMI 6 Investigators: Initial experience with hirudin and streptokinase in acute myocardial infarction: Results of the Thrombolysis in Myocardial Infarction (TIMI) 6 Trial. Am J Cardiol 75:7–13, 1995.

95. Antman EM, for the TIMI 9A Investigators: Hirudin in acute myocardial infarction: Safety report from Thrombolysis in Myocardial Infarction (TIMI) 9A Trial. Circulation 90:1624–1630, 1994.

96. Antman EM, for the TIMI 9B Investigators: Hirudin in acute myocardial infarction: Thrombolysis and Thrombin inhibition in Myocardial Infarction (TIMI) 9A Trial. Circulation 94:911–921, 1994.

97. Metz BK, White HD, Granger CB, et al: Randomized comparison of direct thrombin inhibitor vs. heparin in conjunction with fibrinolytic therapy for acute myocardial infarction: Results from the GUSTO IIb Trial. J Am Coll Cardiol 31:1493–1498, 1998.

98. Neuhaus KL, von Essen R, Tebbe U, et al: Safety observation from the pilot phase of the randomized r-Hirudin for Improvement of the Thrombolysis (HIT-3) study. Circulation 90:1638–1642, 1994.

99. Neuhaus KL, Molhoek GP, Zeymer U, et al: Recombinant Hirudin (Lepirudin) for Improvement of the Thrombolysis with streptokinase in patients with acute myocardial infarction: Results of the HIT-4 Trial. J Am Coll Cardiol 34:966–973, 1999.

100. White HD, Aylward PE, Frey MJ, et al, on behalf of the HERO Trial Investigators: A randomized, double-blind comparison of hirulog versus heparin in patients receiving streptokinase and aspirin for acute myocardial infarction. Circulation 96:2155–2166, 1996.

101. Canon CP, McCabe CH, Borzak S, et al: Randomized trial of an oral platelet glycoprotein IIb/IIIa antagonist, sibrafiban, in patients after acute myocardial syndrome: Results of the TIMI 12 Trial. Circulation 97:340–349, 1998.

102. Antman EM, Giuglianio RP, Gibson M, et al: Abciximab facilitates the rate and extent of thrombolysis: Results of the Thrombolysis in Myocardial Infarction (TIMI) 14 Trial. Circulation 99:2720–2732, 1999.

103. PARADIGM Investigators: Combining thrombolysis with the platelet glycoprotein IIb/IIIa inhibitor lamifiban: Results of the platelet aggregation receptor antagonist dose investigation and reperfusion gain in myocardial infarction (PARADIGM) trial. J Am Coll Cardiol 32:2003–2010, 1998.

104. Ohman EM, Kleiman NS, Gacioch G, et al: Combined accelerated tissue-plasminogen activator and platelet glycoprotein IIb/IIIa receptor blockade with integrilin in acute myocardial infarction: Results of a randomized, placebo controlled, dose ranging trial. Circulation 95:846–854, 1997.

105. Weaver WD, Eisenberg MS, Martin JS, et al: MI Triage and Intervention project phase I (MITI-1): Patient characteristics and feasibilty of prehospital initiation of thrombolytic therapy. J Am Coll Cardiol 15:925–931, 1990.

106. Weaver WD, Cerqueria M, Hallstrom AD, et al: MI Triage and Intervention (MITI-2). Prehospital versus hospital-initiated thrombolytic therapy. JAMA 270:1211–1216, 1993.

107. Rogers WJ, Baim DS, Gore JM, et al: Comparison of immediate invasive, delayed invasive, and conservative strategies after tissue-type plasminogen activator: Results of the Thrombolysis in Myocardial Infarction (TIMI) Phase 2A trial. Circulation 81:1457–1476, 1990.

108. Califf RM, Topol EJ, Stack RS, et al: Evaluation of combination thrombolytic therapy and timing of cardiac catheterization in acute myocardial infarction: Results of Thrombolysis and Angioplasty in myocardial infarction—Phase 5 randomized trial. Circulation 83:1543–1556, 1991.

109. Gringes CL, Browne KF, Marco J, et al: A comparison of immediate angioplasty with thrombolytic therapy for acute myocardial infarction. N Engl J Med 328:673–679, 1993.

110. Rieberio EE, Silva LA, Carnerio R, et al: Randomized trial of direct coronary angioplasty versus intravenous streptokinase in acute MI. J Am Coll Cardiol 22:376–380, 1993.

111. O'Neil W, et al: A prospective randomized clinical trial of intracoronary streptokinase versus coronary angioplasty for acute MI. N Engl J Med 314:812–818, 1986.

112. Topol EJ, Califf RM, George BS, et al: A randomized trial of immediate vs delayed elective angioplasty after intravenous tissue plasminogen activator in acute myocardial infarction. N Engl J Med 317:581–588, 1987.

113. Califf RM, Topol EJ, Stack RS, et al: Evaluation of combination thrombolytic therapy and timing of cardiac catheterization in acute MI: Results of TAMI Study Group. Circulation 83:1543–1556, 1991.

114. SWIFT Trial Group: SWIFT trial of delayed elective intervention vs. conservative treatment after thrombolysis with anistreplase in acute myocardial infarction. BMJ 302:555–560, 1991.

115. Madsen JK, Grande P, Saunamaki K, et al: Danish multicenter randomized study of invasive vs conservative treatment in patients with inducible ischemia after thrombolysis in acute myocardial infarction (DANAMI). Circulation 96:748–755, 1997.

116. Simmons ML, Arnold AE, Betriu A, et al: Eurepean Cooperative Study Group. Thrombolysis with tissue plasminogen activator in acute MI: No additional benefit from immediate percutaneous coronary angioplasty. Lancet 331:197–202, 1988.

117. Iqbal O, Messmore H, Hoppensteadt D, et al: Thrombolytic drugs in acute myocardial infarction. Clin Appl Thromb Hemost 6:1–13, 2000.

118. Iqbal O, Ahsan A, Messmore H Jr, et al: Bovine lung heparin vs porcine intestinal mucosa heparin: clinical implications. In Pifarré R (ed): Management of Bleeding in Cardiovascular Surgery. Philadelphia, Hanley & Belfus, 2000, pp 193–214.

119. Schömig A, Kastrati A, Dirschinger J, et al: Coronary stenting plus platelet glycoprotein IIb/IIIa blockade compared with tissue plasminogen activator in acute myocardial infarction. N Engl J Med 343:385–391, 2000.

Oral Anticoagulation in Acute Coronary Syndromes

G. STEINAR GUDMUNDSSON, MD
PATRICK SCANLON, MD

With constant evolution of knowledge about the pathophysiology of coronary artery disease, approaches to management also have evolved. This chapter discusses the evolution of oral anticoagulation since it was first used for coronary artery disease and the data that support its use. Specific topics include the pharmacology, adverse effects and monitoring of available oral anticoagulants; data from randomized clinical studies of oral anticoagulation in primary prevention of coronary artery disease; and the role of oral anticoagulation in treatment of acute coronary syndromes.

Available Oral Anticoagulants

Two main groups of oral anticoagulants are available. One group is chemically related to 4-hydroxycoumarin (warfarin, phenprocoumon, dicumarol) and the other to indanedione (diphenadione, phenindione, anisindione).[1] Because of their association with several life-threatening adverse reactions, including agranulocytosis, hyperpyrexia, hepatitis, and exfoliative dermatitis, compounds in the latter group are inappropriate for therapeutic use.[2-5]

Pharmacology

All of the oral anticoagulants have a similar mechanism of action. They interfere with the cyclic interconversion of vitamin K and its 2,3 epoxide, which is a necessary cofactor in the activation of the vitamin K-dependent coagulation factors II (prothrombin), VII, IX, and X. Vitamin K is an essential cofactor for the posttranslational carboxylation of glutamate residues to γ-carboxyglutamates on the N-terminal regions of vitamin K-dependent proteins. The carboxylation is necessary for the proteins to become active and is catalyzed by a carboxylase that is dependent on the reduced form of vitamin K (vitamin KH_2). Vitamin KH_2 is oxidized to vitamin K epoxide (KO) during this process and then is recycled by vitamin K epoxide reductase to vitamin K and back to the reduced form vitamin KH_2 by vitamin K reductase. The oral anticoagulants exert their antagonistic effect on vitamin K by inhibiting vitamin K epoxide reductase and possibly

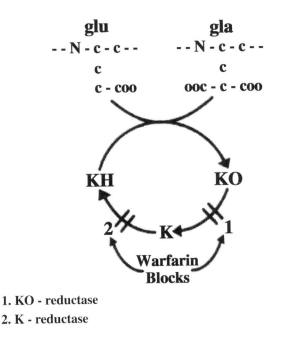

1. KO - reductase

2. K - reductase

Figure 1. Vitamin KH$_2$ is oxidized to vitamin K epoxide (KO) and recycled by vitamin K epoxide reductase (1) to vitamin K (K) and back to the reduced form vitamin KH$_2$ by vitamin K reductase (2). (Adapted from Hrish J, Dalen JE, Anderson DR, et al: Mechanism of action, clinical effectiveness, and optimal therapeutic range. Chest 114:445S–469S, 1998.)

vitamin K reductase (Fig. 1). This inhibition leads to the depletion of vitamin KH$_2$ and limits the γ-carboxylation of the coagulant factors as well as carboxylation of the regulatory proteins C and S. As a result, the liver produces and secretes dysfunctional coagulation factors II, VII, IX, and X and dysfunctional anticoagulation regulatory proteins C and S.[6]

Monitoring of Oral Anticoagulant Therapy

The prothrombin time (PT) is the most commonly used method for monitoring oral anticoagulant therapy. It is performed by adding a mixture of calcium and thromboplastin to citrated plasma. The PT increases with depression of factors II, VII, and X. Initially PT reflects primarily the depression of factor VII, which has the shortest half-life.

Thromboplastin responsiveness varies markedly and depends on the method of preparation and tissue of origin. This variation made standardization of PT difficult and led to erratic dosing. To improve the monitoring of oral anticoagulant therapy a calibration system was developed known as the international normalized ratio (INR). It is based on the assumption of a linear relationship between the logarithm of the PT obtained with reference and test thomboplastins.[7,8] The PT ratio observed with the local thromboplastin is converted into an INR, which is the patient's PT divided by plasma control PT (median normal-range PT) times a value (C) that represents the international sensitivity index (ISI) (Fig. 2). It is a measurement of the responsiveness of a given thromboplastin to reduction of the vitamin K-dependent coagulation factors. The lower the

$$INR = \left(\frac{\textbf{Patient PT}}{\textbf{Mean Normal PT}} \right)^{ISI}$$

i.e., log INR = ISI × log observed PT ratio

Figure 2. The international normalized ratio (INR) is the patient's prothrombin time (PT) divided by mean normal-range PT multiplied by the international sensitivity index (ISI). (Adapted from Hrish J, Dalen JE, Anderson DR, et al: Mechanism of action, clinical effectiveness, and optimal therapeutic range. Chest 114:445S–469S, 1998.)

ISI, the more responsive the reagent and the closer the derived INR will be to the observed PT ratio.[8] A specially designed nomogram provides INR values from the PT ratio value obtained with a thromboplastin reagent and its ISI without the need for calculations.[9]

In addition to the variability of the PT due to the difference in responsiveness of the thromboplastins, the results can be influenced by two technical factors: the equipment used for clot detection and the magnitude of difference in ISI values between the test thromboplastin and the international reference preparation, which has an ISI of 1.0.[10] The range of ISI used in North America has been reported in two studies as 2.0–2.6 and 1.8–2.8, respectively.[7,11]

Currently, two levels of intensity are recommended for the optimal therapeutic range for laboratory evaluation of oral anticoagulant therapy: (1) less intense therapy with an INR of 2.0–3.0 and (2) a more intense regimen corresponding to an INR of 2.5–3.5.[12]

Despite the fact that oral anticoagulants generally are absorbed rapidly, their anticoagulant effect is not observed until decarboxylated, inactive vitamin K-dependent clotting factors replace the normal ones. The delay may range from 2 to 7 or more days. The anticoagulants also suppress the synthesis of proteins S and C, natural anticoagulant proteins. Protein C has a short half-life, and early deficiency of active protein C after initiation of oral anticoagulant therapy produces the potential risk of prothrombotic effect for the first 24–48 hours. If heparin is administered with an oral anticoagulant, therefore, it should be discontinued only when the INR is in the therapeutic range for two consecutive days.[13]

Adverse Effects

The most common adverse reaction of the oral anticoagulants is hemorrhage.[14] The most common sites of major bleeding complications are the gastrointestinal tract and the cranium. Cranial hemorrhages, predominantly subdural hematomas, are the most common fatal form of hemorrhage.[15] Minor hemorrhage is also common from the genitourinary tract, mucous membranes, and skin. Overall, the risk of bleeding is related to the intensity of the anticoagulant therapy. Risk of oral anticoagulant bleeding also is increased with concomitant use of high doses of aspirin, age over 65 years, history of stroke, gastrointestinal tract bleeding, renal insufficiency, or anemia.[16–18]

Skin necrosis, the most important nonhemorrhagic complication, is seen most frequently in women with decreased or absent protein C. This adverse reaction can be fatal if severe.[19] Intrahepatic cholestasis and hypersensitiviy reaction also have been noted.

Oral anticoagulant therapy during pregnancy can lead to perinatal loss due to either hemorrhage or teratogenic effects. The oral anticoagulants easily pass the maternal-placenta barrier and can cause cleft palate, digestive tract abnormalities, and retardation. Their use also has been associated with occlusion of outlets of the fourth cerebral ventricle, leading to displaced cerebellar hemispheres and development of posterior fossa cysts (Dandy-Walker syndrome).[20]

Primary Prevention of Coronary Artery Disease

The Northwick Park Heart Study examined the relationship between hemostatic factors and subsequent coronary heart disease in middle-aged men. A highly significant positive association, independent of serum cholesterol, was found between plasma factor VII coagulant activity and individual risk of primary myocardial infarction.[21] Based on this information, the Thrombosis Prevention Trial evaluated low-intensity oral anticoagulation with warfarin and low-dose aspirin for primary prevention of ischemic heart disease.[22] Patients were recruited through general practices in the United Kingdom. Within each practice, men in the top 20% of a risk score distribution based on smoking, family history, body mass index, blood pressure, serum cholesterol, plasma fibrinogen, and factor VII activity or, in regions with particularly high mortality rates due to ischemic heart disease, men in the top 25% were considered eligible for the trial. Of 10,557 men considered to be at high risk and eligible for the trial, a total of 5499 (52%) entered the study. They were randomized to four treatment groups: (1) warfarin and aspirin, (2) warfarin and placebo, (3) placebo and aspirin, or (4) placebo and placebo. The mean INR of men receiving warfarin was 1.47 with a mean warfarin dose of 4.1 mg/day. There were 410 ischemic events (142 fatal, 268 nonfatal).

The main effect of warfarin with or without aspirin in comparison with aspirin alone or placebo was a 21% reduction ($p = 0.003$) in all ischemic heart disease, due mainly to a 39% reduction in fatal events ($p = 0.02$). Warfarin also reduced the death rate from all causes by 17% ($p = 0.04$). For all ischemic heart disease, the absolute reduction due to warfarin was 2.6 per 1000 person years. Compared with placebo warfarin reduced all ischemic heart disease by 24% ($p = 0.006$). It also increased hemorrhagic and fatal stroke. Ruptured aortic or dissecting aneurysms occurred in 15 men receiving warfarin compared with only three men in the groups that had not received warfarin ($p = 0.01$)[23] (Table 1).

Oral Anticoagulation in Unstable Angina and Suspected Non–Q-Wave Infarction

Unstable angina pectoris ranges over a broad spectrum from progressive or accelerating angina to the higher-risk subset of resting angina with reversible electrocardiographic changes.[24] The goals of therapy are to block the growth of thrombus and to stop the progression to myocardial infarction with endogenous lysis of the intracoronary thrombus. Both aspirin and heparin are effective in reducing the incidence of thrombotic events in patients with unstable angina.[25–27] Early reports of the effectiveness of oral anticoagulants were enthusiastic. However, the earlier studies were not blinded or randomized and often lacked good controls.[28,29] Studies performed before the introduction of British

Table 1.　Randomized Trials of Oral Anticoagulation

Trial (ref.no.)	Design	Number/ Age (yr)	Drug/Procedure	Major Endpoints	Results
Primary prevention					
TPT (23)	R, DB, MCS	5499 45–69	Warfarin and aspirin, warfarin and placebo, placebo and aspirin, placebo and placebo	IHD as coronary death and fatal or nonfatal MI	21% reduction in all IHD with warfarin compared with aspirin and placebo. Increased strokes and vascular complications with warfarin
Unstable angina or suspected non–Q-wave myocardial infarction					
Williams (30)	R, OL	102 No age limit	Warfarin vs. conventional treatment	Recurrent USA, MI, or death	12% in treatment group vs. 34% had events at 6 mo
ATACS (31)	R, OL, MCS	214, > 21	Aspirin vs. aspirin and heparin followed by aspirin and warfarin	Recurrent angina with ECG changes, MI, and/or death	No significant difference at 12 weeks
OASIS (32)	R, OL, MCS	Phase 1, 309 Phase 2, 197 No age limit	Phase 1: warfarin (FD) vs. standard therapy Phase 2: warfarin (AD) vs. standard therapy	Death, MI, refractory angina, readmission for USA, major bleed, and stroke	Phase 1: no difference except for increase in minor bleed in warfarin Phase 2: reduced rate of recurrent ischemic events with warfarin; excess of minor bleed with warfarin

TPT = Thrombosis Prevention Trial, ATACS = Antithrombotic Therapy in Acute Coronary Syndromes, OASIS = Organization to Assess Strategies for Ischemic Syndromes, R = randomized, DB = double-blinded, MCS = multicenter study, OL = open label, FD = fixed dose, AD = adjusted dose, IHD = ischemic heart disease, MI = myocardial infarction, USA = unstable angina, ECG = electrocardiographic.

standardized thromboplastin in the early 1970s used inadequate doses and may have underestimated the effectiveness of oral anticoagulants.

A randomized, prospective, nonblinded trial of anticoagulant therapy in 102 patients with unstable angina was reported in 1986. Fifty-one patients received 10,000 units of intravenous heparin every 6 hours along with 10 mg of warfarin, beginning on the day of admission to hospital. The warfarin therapy was adjusted after 3 days to maintain a patient-to-control prothrombin ratio > 2. The control group received only antianginal therapy as indicated. At 6-month follow-up, 17 patients (34%) in the control group had recurrent unstable angina, myocardial infarction, or death compared with only six (12%) in the treatment group (p < 0.05).[30]

Cohen and colleagues randomized 214 patients with unstable angina at rest or non–Q-wave infarction, none of whom were prior users of aspirin, to either aspirin alone or a combination of aspirin with heparin followed by daily aspirin and warfarin. At 14-day follow-up, 10.5% of the 105 patients in the combination group had recurrent angina with electrocardiographic changes, myocardial infarction, or death compared with 27% of the control group. However, despite a large reduction in adverse events in the combination arm, the difference between the two groups was no longer statistically significant at 12-week follow-up (13% vs. 25%, p = 0.06). The frequency of minor and major bleeding was slightly higher in the combination group.[31]

A Canadian trial in patients with unstable angina or suspected non–Q-wave my-ocardial infarction compared the effects of long-term warfarin at two intensities in two consecutive controlled studies. In the first study, 309 patients were random-ized either to fixed low doses (3 mg/day) of warfarin for 6 months, producing a mean INR of 1.5 ± 0.6, or to standard therapy. Most patients also received aspirin. The rates of cardiovascular death, new myocardial infarction, and refractory angina were not significantly different in the two groups. Nor was there a differ-ence in terms of rehospitalization for unstable angina or major bleeding. However, a significant excess of minor bleeding was found in the warfarin group.

The second study was based on a modified protocol in which 197 patients were randomized either to adjusted-dose warfarin, producing a mean INR of 2.3 ± 0.6 , or to standard therapy for 3 months. No significant difference in rates of cardiovascular death, new myocardial infarction, and refractory angina was found in the two groups. However, rates of all-cause mortality, new myocardial infarction, and stroke were only 5.1% in the warfarin group compared with 13.1% in the standard group (p = 0.05) (Fig. 3). Significant reduction was found in rates of rehospitalization for unstable angina in the warfarin group com-pared with the standard therapy group (p =0 .03). Again, there was an excess of minor bleeding in the warfarin group. The administration of the anticoagulant was not exactly the same in the two phases of the trial. In the fixed-dose phase, warfarin was not started until 5–7 days after intravenous heparin or hirudin had been stopped because of concerns about potential hazards of combining the two drugs. In the later phase, adjusted-dose warfarin was started 12–24 hours after initiation of intravenous anticoagulation, and the drugs were given simultaneously for up to 3 days[32] (see Table 1).

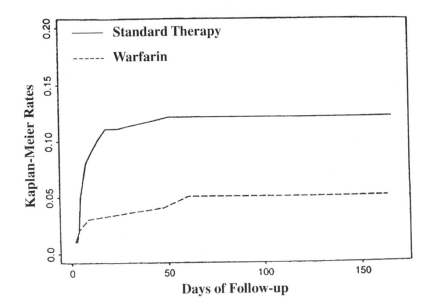

Figure 3. Cumulative Kaplan-Meier rates of cardiovascular death, myocardial infarction, and re-fractory angina in phase two of the OASIS study. (From Anand SS, Yusuf S, Pogue J, et al, for the OASIS Pilot Study Investigators: Long-term oral anticoagulant therapy in patients with unstable angina or sus-pected non-Q-wave myocardial infarction. Circulation 98:1064–1070, 1998, with permission.)

Myocardial Infarction

As a result of early trials, it was widely accepted in the late 1940s and 1950s that oral anticoagulation effectively decreased the risk of reinfarction and post-infarction death. Later these trials were criticized for methodologic flaws, and their results were challenged in subsequent studies. As a result, the use of anti-coagulants after infarction declined.[33–35]

In 1980 the results of the Sixty Plus Reinfarction Study, a well-designed, mul-ticenter trial, were reported. A total of 912 postinfarction patients were random-ized to continuous oral anticoagulation or placebo. The two-year total mortality rate was 13.4% in the placebo group compared with 7.6% in the treated group (relative risk = 43%, p = 0.0017). The incidence of recurrent infarction also was significantly lower in the treated group, with a relative risk reduction of 64%. Episodes of major hemorrhage were more frequent in the treated group.[36] Because participants already had been treated with anticoagulants at entry into the study for an average of more than 6 years, it has been argued that the study tested the effect of random discontinuance rather than initiation of treatment.[37]

The Warfarin Reinfarction Study (WARIS) randomized 1214 men after acute myocardial infarction to warfarin or placebo for an average of 37 months. The relative risk reduction with warfarin was 24% (p = 0.0267) for all-cause mortal-ity, 35% (p = 0.0007) for reinfarction, and 55% (p = 0.0015) for stroke. Serious bleeding episodes were reported in 0.6% of the warfarin-treated patients each year[38] (Table 2).

Another large trial, Anticoagulants in the Secondary Prevention of Events in Coronary Thrombosis (ASPECT), studied the effect of the anticoagulants nicoumalone and phenprocoumon on patients who had sustained a recent acute infarction. Target PT was 2.8–4.8. Follow-up of 3404 patients randomized to treatment or placebo showed a risk reduction of 10% in all-cause mortality, 53% in reinfarction, and 40% in stroke. Again, the incidence of major bleeding was higher in the treatment group (1.4% vs. 0.4% per year).[39]

Oral anticoagulation has not been shown to provide any clinical benefit beyond aspirin in trials comparing the two regimens. The EPSIM trial com-pared 500 mg of aspirin with oral anticoagulation adjusted for a PT within the range of 25–35% of normal. Differences in deaths, reinfarction, or bleeding episodes were not statistically different after a mean follow-up of 29 months.[40] Another German-Austrian trial that compared 946 patients treated with

Table 2.   Distribution of Adverse Events According to Treatment Group in the WARIS Trial

Type of Analysis and Event	Warfarin (n = 607)	Placebo (n = 607)	Risk Reduction (95% CI)	p Value
Intention to treat				
Death	94	123	24 (4–44)	0.0267
Reinfarction	82	124	34 (19–54)	0.0007
Cerebrovascular accident	20	44	55 (30–77)	0.0015
On treatment				
Death	60	92	35 (17–57)	0.0050
Reinfarction	70	122	43 (29–61)	0.0001
Cerebrovascular accident	16	41	61 (38–81)	0.0003

From Smith P, Arnesen H, Holme I: The effect of warfarin on mortality and reinfarction after myocardial infarction. N Engl J Med 323:147–152, 1990, with permission.

phenprocoumarin, aspirin, or placebo detected no difference among the three groups.[41] The Coumadin Aspirin Reinfarction Study (CARS) randomly assigned 8803 postinfarction patients to treatment with 160 mg aspirin, 3 mg warfarin with 80 mg aspirin, or 1 mg warfarin with 80 mg aspirin. Fixed-dose warfarin combined with aspirin did not improve the outcome compared with 160 mg of aspirin alone.[42]

In summary, long-term anticoagulation after acute myocardial infarction has been proved to improve survival and reduce reinfarction rates.[36,38] Survivors of acute myocardial infarction have a lower risk of recurrent infarction, stroke, and all-cause mortality with either aspirin or oral anticoagulation compared with placebo. However, warfarin or a combination of low fixed doses of warfarin and aspirin has not been shown to be more effective than aspirin alone in decreasing mortality and infarction.[40,42] The complicated dosing of warfarin, its increased cost, and the higher risk of bleeding make aspirin the preferable agent.[43,45] Warfarin should be considered for infarct patients at risk of developing or with documented mural thrombi, venous thrombosis and pulmonary embolization and for patients unable to take aspirin[13] (Table 3).

Table 3.   Randomized Trials of Oral Anticoagulation in Patients with Myocardial Infarction

Trial (ref.no.)	Design	Number/ Age (yr)	Drug/Procedure	Major Endpoints	Results
Sixty Plus (36)	R, DB, MCS	912 > 60	Continued anticoagulation after MI vs. placebo	Death, recurrent MI	Reduced mortality and recurrent MI in warfarin group vs. group taken off warfarin
WARIS (38)	R,DB, MCS	1214 < 75	Warfarin vs. placebo	Death and reinfarction	24% risk reduction and 33% relative risk in warfarin group 55% reduction in stroke in warfarin group
ASPECT (39)	R, DB, MCS	3404 No age limit	Nicoumalone or phenprocoumon vs. placebo	Death, recurrent MI, CVA, major bleed	10% reduction in mortality, 53% in reinfarction, 40% in stroke in warfarin group Higher incidence of major bleeding with warfarin
EPSIM (40)	R, MCS	1303 30–70	Aspirin vs. warfarin (AD)	Death, reinfarction	No difference in major endpoints
Breddin et al. (41)	R, DB, MCS	946 45–70	Phenprocoumarin vs. aspirin vs. placebo	Total mortality, coronary death, nonfatal recurrent MI	No difference among groups
CARS (42)	R, DB, MCS	8803 21–85	160 mg aspirin vs. 3 mg warfarin and 80 mg aspirin vs. 1 mg warfarin and 80 mg aspirin	Nonfatal MI, nonfatal ischemic stroke, CV death	No difference among groups

WARIS = Warfarin Reinfarction Study, ASPECT = Anticoagulants in the Secondary Prevention of Events in Coronary Thrombosis, EPSIM = Enquête de Prévention Secondaire de 1' Infarctus du Myocarde, CARS = Coumadin Aspirin Reinfarction Study, R = randomized, DB = double-blinded, MCS = multicenter study, MI = myocardial infarction, AD = adjusted dose, CVA = cerebrovascular accident, CV = cerebrovascular.

Systemic Embolization after Myocardial Infarction

Systemic embolization after myocardial infarction usually presents with a stroke. The presence of mural thrombus after infarction increases the risk of systemic embolism. According to echocardiographic studies, left ventricular thrombus is rare after inferior myocardial infarction but found in up to 40% of patients with anterior myocardial infarction. Higher-risk patients have extensive left ventricular dysfunction and congestive heart failure, a history of embolism, or atrial fibrillation. Mural thrombi tend to form early after acute myocardial infarction (within the first 24 hours) but may appear 1–2 weeks later. Most systemic emboli occur within the first few weeks after acute infarction. The risk appears to decrease after 2–3 months.[46,47] Oral anticoagulants significantly reduced the incidence of stroke in the WARIS and ASPECT trials.[38,39] Again, no difference was found in the incidence of stroke after myocardial infarction in the EPSIM and the CARS trials, which compared aspirin with oral anticoagulants.[40,42]

A small randomized, unblinded two-dimensional echocardiographic trial found that oral anticoagulants were effective in the resolution of left ventricular thrombosis.[48] Another small randomized study in survivors of acute anterior myocardial infarction with mural thrombus on two-dimensional echocardiography examined the effect of aspirin, anticoagulation, or no therapy. Anticoagulants and aspirin were equally effective (p < 0.01) compared with no treatment in terms of resolving left ventricular thrombosis and reducing the incidence of emboli. Spontaneous resolution was seen in few patients.[49] A meta-analysis of several small trials concluded that anticoagulation reduces the risk of embolization after anterior myocardial infarction and can prevent mural thrombus formation. Thrombolytic therapy may prevent mural thrombus formation, but evidence was not found to support a similar benefit with antiplatelet therapy.[50] In higher-risk patients with extensive left ventricular dysfunction and congestive heart failure, a history of embolism, or atrial fibrillation and in patients with transmural anterior myocardial infarction, evidence indicates the benefit of full oral anticoagulation for 3 months.[51]

Despite the common association of thrombus with chronic left ventricular aneurysm, systemic emboli are infrequent. A retrospective study of 89 patients, 20 of whom had received anticoagulants for 40 patient-years and 69 of whom had not been treated for 288 patient-years, found the incidence of systemic emboli to be very low (0.35/100 patients years). Based on this information, anticoagulant therapy has not been recommended in patients with left ventricular aneurysm, even when thrombus is present.[51,52]

Venous Thromboembolism

The incidence of deep venous thromboembolism in patients with acute myocardial infarction is high. Studies using ^{125}I fibrinogen leg scanning and autopsy data have shown that anticoagulation reduces the incidence of both pulmonary embolism and deep venous thrombosis in patients with myocardial infarction.[51,53]

Oral Anticoagulation after Thrombolysis

Most of the data about oral anticoagulation in postinfarction patients are from clinical trials conducted in the prethrombolytic era. To determine whether antithrombotic therapy reduces the risk for reocclusion after successful coronary thrombolysis in acute myocardial infarction, 300 patients were randomized to three antithrombotic regimens. Eligible patients had a patent infarct-related artery on angiography less than 48 after intravenous thrombolytic therapy. They were randomized to treatment with daily aspirin, placebo with discontinuation of heparin, or warfarin with continuation of heparin until oral anticoagulation was established (INR = 2.8–4.0). Vessel patency was reevaluated by angiogram at 3 months in 248 patients. Other end-points were recurrent myocardial infarction, coronary revascularization, change in left ventricular ejection fraction and event-free clinical course. The mean reocclusion rate at 3 months was 29% and did not differ significantly among the three groups. However, the study demonstrated a statistically significant reduction in reinfarction and revascularization in patients taking aspirin compared with patients receiving placebo. The aspirin group had better overall outcome with a lower combined rate of revascularization, reinfarction, and death than the placebo and warfarin groups. Patients in the warfarin group did no better on any endpoint than patients in the aspirin group, but the study reported trends toward better efficacy with warfarin than with placebo.[54]

In another trial comparing the risk of cardiac death and reinfarction in patients who had received anistreplase thrombolysis for myocardial infarction, 1036 patients were randomized to aspirin or intravenous heparin followed by an oral anticoagulant. At 30-day and 3-month follow-up no significant difference was found between the treatment groups except that the anticoagulation group was more likely to have had major bleeding or stroke (3.9% vs. 1.7%, p = 0.04)[55] (Table 4).

Oral Anticoagulation after Coronary Stenting

To reduce the risk of subacute thrombosis after angioplasty and stent placement, earlier anticoagulant regimens were aggressive and led to a high incidence of bleeding and vascular complications. Initially aspirin, dipyridamole, intravenous low-molecular-weight heparin, intravenous heparin, and warfarin often were used in combination. However, improved stenting methods and less aggressive anticoagulation reduced the risk of complications. A study of 517 patients treated with stents after acute myocardial infarction compared aspirin and ticlopidine with aspirin and intravenous heparin followed by phenprocoumon. The antiplatelet group had reduced risks of cardiac death, myocardial infarction, coronary bypass surgery, repeat angioplasty, hemorrhagic complications, and peripheral vascular events compared with the anticoagulation group.[56]

The Stent Anticoagulation Restenosis Study (STARS) involved 1653 patients undergoing stent placement. Patients were divided into three groups receiving aspirin, a combination of aspirin and ticlopidine, or aspirin and warfarin. At 30-day follow-up, the incidence of death, target lesion revascularization, angiographic thrombosis, and myocardial infarction was significantly lower in the group treated with aspirin and ticlopidine compared with the other two groups.[57] Therefore, oral anticoagulation is not recommended after stent implantation unless indications such as left ventricular dysfunction, atrial fibrillation, or mechanical heart valves are also present[58] (see Table 4).

Table 4. Randomized Trials of Oral Anticoagulation After Thrombolysis and Stenting

Trial (ref.no.)	Design	Number/ Age (yr)	Drug/Procedure	Major Endpoints	Results
After thrombolysis					
APRICOT (54)	R, DB	300 < 75	Aspirin vs. placebo vs. warfarin (AD)	Patency of infarct-related artery at follow-up angiography Recurrent MI, coronary surgery, or angioplasty	No significant difference in reocclusion rate No difference in revascularization and reinfarction rates with warfarin vs. placebo No difference in mortality
AFTER (55)	R, OL, MCS	1036 No age limit	Aspirin vs. anticoagulation	Cardiac death and recurrent infarction	No difference in major endpoints Higher incidence of severe bleeding and strokes with anticoagulation
After coronary stenting					
Schömig et al. (56)	R, OL	517 No age limit	Ticlopidine and aspirin vs. phenprocoumon and aspirin vs. aspirin	Cardiac death, reinfarction, revascularization	Aspirin and ticlopidine group had lower rate of stent thrombosis Higher incidence of bleeding than aspirin alone
STARS (57)	R, OL, MCS	1653 No age limit	Aspirin vs. aspirin and warfarin vs. aspirin and ticlopidine	Stent thrombosis on angiography within 30 days	Antiplatelet therapy superior to anticoagulation and aspirin in reducing cardiac events and hemorrhagic and vascular complications

APRICOT = Antithrombotics in the Prevention of Reocclusion In Coronary Thrombolysis, AFTER = Aspirin/Anticoagulant Following Thrombolysis with Eminase in Recurrent Infarction, STARS = Stent Anticoagulation Restenosis Study, R = randomized, DB = double-blinded, OL = open label, MCS = multicenter study, AD = adjusted dose, MI = myocardial infarction.

Conclusion

The oral anticoagulants inhibit vitamin K epoxide reductase and possibly vitamin K reductase, leading to the depletion of vitamin KH_2, which is essential for the activation of clotting factors II,VII, IX, and X. The most common adverse event is hemorrhage. Major bleeding complications usually originate in the gastrointestinal tract and cranium; the cranium is the most common site of fatal hemorrhage. The PT or the INR is used for monitoring of therapy.

The data from randomized studies in patients with unstable angina or suspected non–ST-elevation myocardial infarction and in patients with proven myocardial infarction suggest improved outcomes with oral anticoagulation compared with placebo. However, oral anticoagulation has not been shown to be more effective than aspirin alone in decreasing mortality and infarction in such patients. In addition, oral anticoagulation did not seem to improve outcome in patients with infarction who were treated with thrombolysis or coronary intervention. The complicated dosing of warfarin, its increased cost, and the higher risk of bleeding make aspirin the preferable agent. Oral anticoagulants may be used in patients with coronary artery disease; patients at risk of developing or with documented mural thrombi, venous thrombosis, pulmonary embolization, or atrial fibrillation; and patients who are not able to take aspirin.

References

1. Freedman MD: Oral anticoagulants: Pharmacodynamics, clinical indications and adverse effects. J Clin Pharmacol 32:196–209, 1992.
2. Tashjian AH, Leddy JP: Agranulocytosis associated with phenindione. Arch Intern Med 015:121–125, 1960.
3. Bingle J, Shine I: Phenindione sensitivity. Lancet 2:377–379, 1959.
4. Jones NL: Hepatitis due to phenindione sensitivity. BMJ 2:504–506, 1960.
5. Payne RW: Side-effects of phenindione. BMJ 2:667, 1960.
6. Choonara IA, Malia RG, Haynes BP, et al: The relationship between inhibition of vitamin K1 2,3-epoxide reductase and reduction of clotting factor activity with warfarin. Br J Clin Pharmacol 25:1–7, 1988.
7. Poller L: Progress in standardization in anticoagulant control. Hematol Rev 1:225–241, 1987.
8. Kirkwood TBL: Calibration of reference thromboplastins and standardization of the prothrombin time ratio. Thromb Heamost 49:238–244, 1983.
9. Poller L: A simple nomogram for the derivation of international normalized ratios for the standardization of prothrombin time. Thromb Haemost 60:18–20, 1988.
10. Poller L, Taberner DA, Thomson JM, Darby KV: Survey of prothrombin time in National External Quality Assessment Scheme exercises (1980–1987). J Clin Pathol 41:361–364, 1988.
11. Bussey HI, Force RW, Bianco TM, Leonard AD: Reliance on prothrombin time ratios causes significant errors in anticoagulation therapy. Arch Intern Med 152:278–282, 1992.
12. Hrish J, Dalen JE, Anderson DR, et al: Mechanism of action, clinical effectiveness, and optimal therapeutic range. Chest 114:445S–469S, 1998.
13. Smith SC Jr, Blair SN, Criqui MH, et al for the Secondary Prevention Panel: AHA medical/scientific statement: Preventing heart attack and death in patients with coronary disease. Circulation 92:2–4, 1995.
14. Coon WW, Willis PW: Hemorrhagic complications of anticoagulant treatment. Arch Intern Med 133:386–392, 1974.
15. Askey JM: Hemorrhage during long-term anticoagulant drug therapy. I. Intracranial hemorrhage. Calif Med 140:6–10, 1966.
16. Dale J, Myhre E, Loew D: Bleeding during acetylsalicylic acid and anticoagulant therapy in patients with reduced platelet reactivity after aortic valve replacement. Am Heart J 99:746–752, 1980.
17. Chesebro JH, Fuster V, Elveback LR, et al: Trial of combined warfarin plus dipyridamole or aspirin therapy in prosthetic heart valve replacement: Danger of aspirin compared with dipyridamole. Am J Cardiol 51:1537–1541.
18. Levine MN, Raskob G, Landefeld S, Kearon C: Hemorrhagic complications of anticoagulant treatment. Chest 114:511S–523S, 1998.
19. Rose VL, Kwaan HC, Williamson K, et al: Protein C antigen deficiency and warfarin necrosis. Am J Clin Pathol 86:653–655, 1986.
20. Kaplan LC: Congenital Dandy Walker malformation associated with first trimester warfarin: A case report and literature review. Teratology 32:333–337, 1985.
21. Meade TW, Mellows S, Brozovic M, et al: Haemostatic function and ischaemic heart disease: Principal results of the Northwick Park Heart Study. Lancet 2:533–537,1986.
22. Miller GJ: Antithrombotic therapy in the primary prevention of acute myocardial infarction. Am J Cardiol 64:29B–32B, 1989.
23. Medical Research Council's General Practice Research Framework: Thrombosis prevention trial: Randomized trial of low intensity oral anticoagulation with warfarin and low-dose aspirin in the primary prevention of ischemic heart disease in men at increased risk. Lancet 351:233–241, 1998.
24. Fahri JI, Cohen M, Fuster V: The broad spectrum of unstable angina pectoris and its implications for future controlled trials. Am J Cardiol 58:547–550, 1986.
25. Théroux P, et al: Aspirin, heparin, or both to treat acute unstable angina. N Engl J Med 319:11-5–11-11, 1988.
26. Lewis HD, et al: Protective effects of aspirin against acute myocardial infarction and death in men with unstable angina. N Engl J Med 309:396–403, 1983.
27. Théroux P, Waters D, Lam J, et al: Reactivation of unstable angina after the discontinuation of heparin. N Engl J Med 327:141–145, 1992.
28. Wood P: Acute and subacute coronary insufficiency. BMJ 1:1779–1782, 1961.
29. Nichol ES, Phillips WC, Casten GG: Virtue of prompt anticoagulant therapy in impending myocardial infarction: Experiences with 318 patients during a 10-year period. Ann Intern Med 50:1158–1173, 1959.
30. Williams DO, Kirby MG, McPherson K, Phear DN: Anticoagulant treatment in unstable angina. Br J Clin Pract 40:114–116, 1986.

31. Cohen M, Adams PC, Parry G, and the Antithrombotic Therapy in Acute Coronary Syndromes Research Group: Combination antithrombotic therapy in unstable rest angina and non-Q-wave infarction in nonprior aspirin users. Circulation 89:81–88, 1994.
32. Anand SS, Yusuf S, Pogue J, et al, for the OASIS Pilot Study Investigators: Long-term oral anticoagulant therapy in patients with unstable angina or suspected non-Q-wave myocardial infarction. Circulation 98:1064–1070, 1998.
33. Ebert RV: Use of anticoagulants in acute myocardial infarction. Circulation 45:903–910, 1972.
34. Ebert RV: Long-term anticoagulation therapy after myocardial infarction. Final report of the Veterans Administration Cooperative Study. JAMA 207:2263–2267, 1969.
35. Medical Research Council Working Party: An assessment of long-term anticoagulant administration after cardiac infarction. BMJ 2:837–843, 1964.
36. Sixty Plus Reinfarction Study Research Group: A double-blind trial to assess long-term anticoagulant therapy in elderly patients after myocardial infarction. Lancet 2:989–994, 1980.
37. Graham I, Mulcahy R, Hickey N: Anticoagulants after myocardial infarction. Lancet 1:717, 1981.
38. Smith P, Arnesen H, Holme I: The effect of warfarin on mortality and reinfarction after myocardial infarction. N Engl J Med 323:147–152, 1990.
39. ASPECT Research Group: Effect of long-term anticoagulant treatment on mortality and cardiovascular morbidity after myocardial infarction. Lancet 343:499–503, 1994.
40. EPSIM Research Group: A controlled comparison of aspirin and oral anticoagulants in prevention of death after myocardial infarction. N Engl J Med 307:701–708, 1982.
41. Breddin K, Loew D, Leckner K, et al: Secondary prevention of myocardial reinfarction: A comparison of acetylsalicylic acid, placebo and phenprocoumon. Haemostasis 9:325–344, 1980.
42. Coumadin Aspirin Reinfarction Study (CARS) Investigators: Randomized double-blind trial of fixed low-dose warfarin with aspirin after myocardial infarction. Lancet 350:389–396, 1997.
43. Prentice CRM: Antithrombotic therapy in the secondary prevention of myocardial infarction. Am J Cardiol 72:175G–180G, 1993.
44. Van Bergen PFMM, Jonker JJC, van Hout BA, et al: Costs and effects of long-term oral anticoagulant treatment after myocardial infarction. JAMA 273:925–928, 1995.
45. Cairns JA: Oral anticoagulants or aspirin after myocardial infarction? Lancet 343:497–498, 1994.
46. Asinger RW, Mikell FI, Elsperger J, et al: Incidence of left-ventricular thrombosis after acute transmural myocardial infarction: Serial evaluation by two-dimensional echocardiography. N Engl J Med 305:297–302, 1981.
47. Spirito P, Bellotti P, Chiarella F, et al: Prognostic significance and natural history of left ventricular thrombi in patients with acute anterior myocardial infarction: A two-dimensional echocardiographic study. Circulation 72:774–780, 1985.
48. Tramarin R, Pozzoli M, Poasich C, et al: Two-dimensional echocardiographic assessment of anticoagulant therapy in left ventricular thrombosis early after acute myocardial infarction. European Heart J 7:484–492, 1986.
49. Kouvaras G, Chronopoulos G, Soufras G, et al: The effects of long-term antithrombotic treatment on left ventricular thrombi in patients after an acute myocardial infarction. Am Heart J 111:73–78, 1990.
50. Vaitkus PT, Barnathan ES: Embolic potential, prevention and management of mural thrombus complicating anterior myocardial infarction: A meta-analysis. J Am Coll Cardiol 22:1004–1009, 1993.
51. Cairns JA, Theroux P, Lewis HD, et al: Antithrombotic agents in coronary artery disease. Chest 114:611S–633S, 1998.
52. Lapeyre AC III, Steele PM, Kazmier FV, et al: Systemic embolization in chronic left ventricular aneurysm: Incidence and the role of anticoagulation. J Am Coll Cardiol 6:534–538, 1985.
53. Wray R, Maurer B, Shillingford J: Prophylactic anticoagulant therapy in the prevention of calf-vein thrombosis after myocardial infarction. N Engl J Med 288:815–817, 1973.
54. Meijer A, Verheugt FWA, Werter CJPJ, et al: Aspirin versus coumadin in the prevention of reocclusion and recurrent ischemia after successful thrombolysis: A prospective placebo-controlled angiographic study. Results of the APRICOT study. Circulation 87:1524–1530, 1993.
55. Julian DG, Chamberlain DA, Pocock SJ, for the AFTER Study Group: A comparison of aspirin and anticoagulation following thrombolysis for myocardial infarction (the AFTER study): A multicentre unblinded randomised clinical trial. BMJ 313:1429–1431, 1996.
56. Schömig A, Neumann FJ, Kastrat A, et al: A randomized comparison of antiplatelet and anticoagulant therapy after the placement of coronary-artery stents. N Engl J Med 334:1084–1089, 1996.
57. Leon MB, Baim DS, Popma JJ, et al: A randomized trial comparing three drug regimens to prevent thrombosis following elective coronary stenting. N Engl J Med 339:1665–1671, 1998.
58. Popma JJ, Weitz J, Bittl JA, et al: Antithrombotic therapy in patients undergoing coronary angioplasty. Chest 114:728S–741S, 1998.

Beta Blockers in Acute Coronary Syndromes

SUDHAKAR B. CHENNAREDDY, MD

JOHN B. O'CONNELL, MD

Each year approximately 800,000 persons in the United States experience acute myocardial infarction (MI), and about 213,000 die as a result.[1] Several thousands more are admitted to the hospital with the diagnosis of unstable angina, non–Q-wave MI, worsening heart failure, or arrhythmias due to myocardial ischemia, further increasing the mortality and morbidity associated with ischemic heart disease. During the past two decades a constellation of therapies for patients with acute MI has been introduced, including aspirin, beta adrenoceptor-blocking agents, angiotensin-converting enzyme inhibitors, thrombolytic agents, and emergency revascularization with percutaneous transluminal coronary angioplasty (PTCA) or coronary artery bypass graft surgery. The combined use of these therapies has resulted in an impressive reduction in the early and 1-year mortality rates for patients with acute MI. Beta blockers are efficacious in managing patients not only with acute transmural MI but also with unstable angina, non–Q-wave MI, various arrhythmias, and congestive heart failure. Unfortunately, beta blockers are not widely prescribed during acute coronary syndromes despite their strong beneficial effects.[2] After a brief description of the beta adrenoreceptor, this chapter discusses the beneficial effects of beta blockers in acute coronary syndromes by reviewing the major randomized clinical trials.

Pharmacology of the Beta Receptor

In 1895 Oliver and Shaffer demonstrated that adrenal extracts contain chemical mediators that increase heart rate in cats.[3] Later it was discovered that sympathetic nerve stimulation, which has effects quite similar to those of adrenal extracts, also involves chemical mediators. Subsequently, norepinephrine was identified as the major sympathetic neurotransmitter. In 1948 Ahlquist suggested that catecholamines act via two principal receptors on smooth muscle, alpha and beta, which produce excitatory and inhibitory responses, respectively.[4] The order of potency at alpha-adrenergic receptors is as follows: epinephrine > norepinephrine >> isoproterenol. Beta-adrenergic receptors show the potency in series: isoproterenol > epinephrine > norepinephrine. Later beta-adrenergic receptors were divided into beta-1 (e.g., those in the myocardium) and beta-2 (smooth muscle and other sites). Epinephrine and norepinephrine are essentially equipotent at the beta-1 receptor, whereas epinephrine is 10- to 50-fold more potent than norepinephrine at the beta-2 receptor.[5] Recently a beta-3 receptor that plays a role in regulating lipolysis in adipose tissue has been identified; it is 10 times more sensitive to norepinephrine than to epinephrine.[6]

Structure of the Beta Receptor

Beta-adrenergic receptors are a family of closely related proteins containing seven hydrophobic membrane-spanning regions. In addition, the G protein heterotrimers (stimulatory [Gs] or inhibitory [Gi] proteins), which are made up of three subunits (Gα, Gβ, and Gγ), are closely associated with the beta-adrenergic receptor and play a role in sympathetic and parasympathetic signal transduction (Fig. 1). In basal states, beta-adrenergic receptors are bound to the nucleotide (guanosine triphosphate [GTP])-free stimulatory G protein complex (Gα, Gβ, Gγ), which increases the affinity of the receptor for its ligand—in this case, beta agonists. When an agonist binds to the receptor, it activates Gα protein, which binds to GTP, and Gα*GTP dissociates from its complex with Gβ and Gγ. It also separates from the beta-receptor complex. Activated Gα*GTP

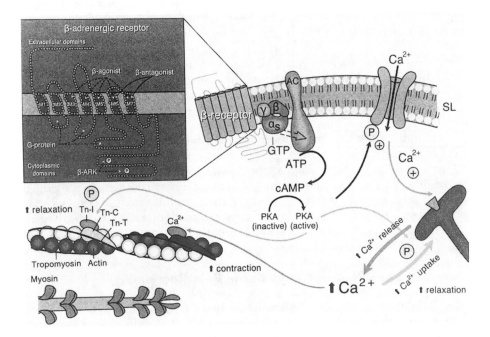

Figure 1. Beta-adrenergic signal systems. Catecholamines activate the beta-adrenergic receptor, which, through stimulatory G protein, activates adenylate cyclase (AC), resulting in increased production of cyclic adenosine monophosphate (cAMP) from adenosine triphosphate (ATP). In turn, cAMP activates protein kinases (PKA), leading to phosphorylation of the sarcolemmal calcium channel, increased calcium entry into the cell, calcium-induced calcium release, and increased rate of development of force and peak contraction. The inset shows the molecular structure of the beta-adrenergic receptor. The transmembrane domains (M1–M7) act as ligand-binding pocket. Domains M6 and M7 are more specific for beta antagonists. Beta agonist-binding is more diffuse. β-ARK = beta-adrenergic receptor kinase, GTP = guanosine triphosphate, SL = sarcolemma, Tn-C = troponin-C, Tn-I = troponin I, Tn-T = troponin T. (From Murphy JG: Mayo Clinic Cardiology Review, 2nd ed. Philadelphia, Lippincott Williams & Wilkins, 2000, with permission.)

stimulates adenylyl cyclase, which leads to increased synthesis of cyclic adeno-sisn monophosphate (AMP). Later Gα*GTP is dephosphorylated; the Gα dissociates from the resulting guanosine diphosphate (GDP) and reassociates with Gβ and Gγ units, which rebind to the beta receptor.

Cyclic AMP is the major second messenger of beta-receptor stimulation, leading to a cascade of events that increases influx of calcium into the cell and activates glycogen phosphorylase. Table 1 summarizes the effects of cyclic AMP-mediated beta-adrenergic stimulation of the heart. Increased calcium entry through plasmalemmal calcium channels and accelerated cross-bridge cycling favor myocardial contraction, whereas decreased calcium affinity of troponin and increased calcium uptake by the sarcoplasmic reticulum after phosphorylation of phospholamban favor relaxation. This integrated response to beta-adrenergic stimulation facilitates myocardial contraction and relaxation.[7]

Rationale for Beta Blockade

Beta-adrenoreceptor blockers are competitive inhibitors of catecholamines at the beta receptor, whose affinity for beta-1 and beta-2 receptors varies. Most of these drugs are pure antagonists; that is, they reduce the receptor occupancy of beta agonists without activating the receptor. Beta blockers such as pindolol and acebutolol are partial agonists and cause mild activation of the receptor (Table 2).

Acute MI causes sympathetic stimulation, increased levels of circulating catecholamines, and release of catecholamines from the storage depots in the ventricle, with consequent exposure of injured myocardial cells to relatively high concentrations of catecholamines during the transitional period of progressive

Table 1. Effects of Beta-adrenergic Stimulation of the Heart

1. Energy production	
Accelerated glycogenolysis	Increased availability of adenosine triphosphate
2. Plasma membrane	
Phosphorylation of calcium channels	
Increased calcium entry	
Atria and ventricles	Increased contractility
Sinoatrial node	Increased heart rate
Atrioventricular node	Accelerated atrioventricular conduction
Phosphorylation of sodium pump	
Increased sodium efflux	Increased calcium efflux via sodium–calcium exchange (lusiotropy)
3. Sarcoplasmic reticulum	
Phosphorylation of phospholamban	
Increased calcium pump turnover	Increased calcium uptake (lusiotropy)
Increased calcium sensitivity of pump	Increased calcium uptake (lusiotropy)
Increased calcium stores	Increased calcium release (inotropy)
4. Contractile proteins	
Troponin	
Phosphorylation of troponin 1	
Decreased calcium sensitivity of troponin complex	Decreased calcium binding (lusiotropy and inotropy)
Actinomyosin	
Increased calcium cross-bridge cycling	Increased shortening velocity (inotropy)

From Katz AM: Physiology of the Heart, 2nd ed. New York, Raven Press, 1992, with permission.

Table 2.   Properties of Beta Blockers

	Selectivity	ISA	Local Anesthetic Action	Lipid Solubility	Elimination Half-life	Bioavailability
Acebutolol	β1	Yes	Yes	Moderate	3–4 hr	50
Atenolol	β1	No	No	Low	6–9 hr	40
Betaxolol	β1	No	Slight	Moderate	14–22 hr	90
Bisoprolol	β1	No	No	Low	9–12 hr	80
Bucindolol*	None	Low	No	Low	2–7 hr	30
Carvedilol*	None	No	No	Low	7–10 hr	25–35
Esmolol	β1	No	No	Low	10 min	(100 IV)
Labetalol*	None	Yes, of β2	Yes	Moderate	5 hr	30
Metoprolol	β1	No	Yes	Moderate	3–4 hr	50
Nadolol	None	No	No	Low	14–24 hr	33
Pindolol	None	Yes	Yes	Moderate	3–4 hr	90
Propranolol	None	No	Yes	High	3–6 hr	30†
Sotalol	None	No	No	Low	12 hr	90
Timolol	None	No	No	Moderate	4–5 hr	50

ISA = intrinsic stimulating activity.
* Also causes alpha-1 adrenergic blockade.
† Dose-dependent.

myocyte injury. In experimental animals, beta-receptor density is acutely increased in the ischemic myocardium within 15–30 minutes of coronary occlusion as a result of externalization. With increased stimulation of adenylate cyclase, cyclic AMP levels are significantly increased. The metabolic effects of cyclic AMP, including calcium overloading, high-energy phosphate depletion, oxygen wastage by increased free fatty acid metabolism, and increased arrhythmogenicity, appear to play a role in catecholamine-induced ischemic cell injury.[8] Sympathetic hyperstimulation during acute MI also affects myocardial oxygen supply and demand. In ischemic myocardium, beta-adrenoreceptor stimulation leads to increases in heart rate, isometric force, and velocity of ventricular contraction, which cause an increase in myocardial work and oxygen consumption. Sympathetic-mediated vasoconstriction further increases systolic blood pressure and myocardial oxygen consumption. In the presence of coronary occlusion, blood flow to the ischemic area may be reduced further by diversion of flow to the nonischemic myocardium by a "steal" phenomenon due to increased metabolic demand. Sympathetic stimulation also leads to increases in tissue lipolysis and utilization of free fatty acids by the myocardium, which also increase myocardial oxygen consumption and may worsen ischemic damage. Beta blockers reduce the mortality rate in acute coronary syndromes by essentially antagonizing the metabolic effects of sympathetic hyperstimulation (Table 3).

Clinical Application

In 1963, one year after Black described the pharmacology of the beta-receptor blocker nathalide,[9,10] Alleyne and colleagues established the efficacy of pronethalol as an antianginal agent in a small series of patients. In 1965 Snow described the effects of propranolol in acute MI.[12] Subsequently several new

Table 3.   Beneficial Effects of Beta Blockers in Acute Coronary Syndromes

Anti-ischemic benefits
- Decreased oxygen utilization
- Decreased oxygen wastage
- Increased oxygen supply (increase in diastolic perfusion)
- Limiting of infarct size and reinfarction rate
- Reduction in silent ischemia
- Elimination of morning peak of myocardial infarction

Antiarrhythmogenic benefits
- Decreases in automaticity, membrane excitability, and conduction and electrical heterogeneity
- Increase in ventricular fibrillation threshold
- Decrease in other tachyarrhythmias
- Reduction in sudden cardiac death rate

Other benefits
- Positive effects on cardiac remodeling
- Prevention of cardiac rupture

Adapted from Murphy JG: Mayo Clinic Cardiology Review, 2nd ed. Philadelphia, Lippincott Williams & Wilkins, 2000.

beta blockers were developed, and their effects in the setting of acute coronary syndromes have been studied extensively. Several small studies conducted before 1980 showed inconclusive results. In the next decade, several large randomized trials confirmed a significant reduction in mortality due to acute MI with the use of beta blockers. In the Goteborg Metoprolol Trial,[13] International Study of Infarct survival (ISIS 1),[17] and Metoprolol in Acute Myocardial Infarction Trial (MIAMI),[19] beta blockade was used in the early hours of acute MI, whereas in the American Beta-Blocker Heart Attack Trial (BHAT)[20] and Norwegian Timolol Trial[25] it was started a few days later. These trials were conducted in the prethrombolytic era. In the Thrombolysis in Myocardial Infarction trial (TIMI II) the role of beta blockers was evaluated together with thrombolytics and angioplasty.[27]

The Goteborg Metoprolol Trial was a randomized, placebo-controlled study designed to assess the primary end-point of 3-month mortality reduction with metoprolol after MI.[13] Secondary end-points were infarct size, arrhythmias, and tolerability of the drug. The inclusion criteria were chest pain of acute onset and 30 minutes' duration or electrocardiographic signs of acute MI. There were 697 patients in the placebo group and 698 in the metoprolol group. As soon as possible after admission, treatment was initiated with intravenous metoprolol, 5 mg, or placebo, given in 3 doses separated by 2 minutes. Fifteen minutes after the IV boluses, depending on heart rate and blood pressure, metoprolol was administered orally to maximal dose of 200 mg/day in divided doses for at least 90 days. After 90 days, all patients in both groups with confirmed MI or angina were to continue metoprolol, 100 mg twice daily for 2 years. At 90 days the cumulative mortality rate for the metoprolol group was 5.7%; for the placebo group, 8.9%. The total reduction in mortality with metoprolol was 30% (p < 0.03). After 2 years, despite similar treatment for all patients the mortality benefit persisted (metoprolol = 13.2%; placebo = 17.2%; p = 0.043). Metoprolol reduced all causes of death, including sudden death due to arrhythmias and myocardial rupture. Patients with a heart rate above 70 beats/min, history of diabetes, or signs or treatment of heart failure[14,15] at entry responded particularly well; metoprolol resulted in a 50% reduction in mortality (Fig. 2). Metoprolol

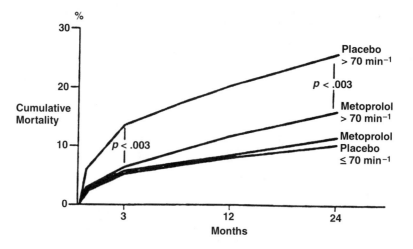

Figure 2. Cumulative mortality in patients with entry heart rate > 70 beats/min (median) or ≤ 70 beats/min during 2 years of the Goteborg Metoprolol Trial. (From Nash IS, Fuster V: Efficacy of Myocardial Infarction Therapy. New York, Marcel Dekker, 1999, with permission.)

significantly reduced the likelihood of completion of MI in a subset of patients treated within 12 hours and with a median heart rate above 70 beats/min (60.8% in the metoprolol group, 70.3% in the placebo group; p = 0.046); reduced infarct size, particularly among patients with a heart rate above 70 beats/min; decreased the incidence of ventricular fibrillation and other tachyarrhythmias; and reduced duration of chest pain and need for analgesic injections.[16]

In ISIS-1, 16,027 patients were randomized between mid 1981 and January 1, 1985 at a mean of 5 hours after onset of suspected acute MI to either the control group or to atenolol, 5 mg IV, administered immediately over 5 minutes, followed first by another 5-mg injection 10 minutes later if no bradycardia occurred and then by oral atenolol, 50 mg twice daily or 100 mg/day for 7 days.[17] Vascular mortality during the 7-day treatment period was significantly lower in the atenolol group: 313 deaths among 8037 patients (3.89%) vs. 365 deaths among 7990 patients (4.57%) in the control group. The overall reduction in mortality was 15% (p < 0.04). The mortality benefit in the atenolol group was maintained beyond 1 year (Fig. 3). The maximal benefit was seen in the first 24–36 hours (121 deaths in the atenolol group vs. 171 deaths in the control group; p < 0.003). Immediate beta blockade increased the extent of inotropic drug use by a small margin (1.6%), chiefly on days 0–1, when most of the improvement in vascular mortality was seen. A significant increase in complete heart block was not seen. This study demonstrated a highly significant (p < 0.0002) effect on the combined end-point of death, arrest, or infarction, suggesting that treatment of about 200 patients would lead to the avoidance of one reinfarction, one arrest, and one death during the first 24 hours. Retrospective analysis of early deaths in the British, Irish, and Scandinavian patients of ISIS-1 study were published in 1988.[18] Of the 193 records reviewed, 79 deaths were in the atenolol group and 114 in the control group; treatment with atenolol reduced cardiac rupture and sudden death.

In the MIAMI Trial the effect of metoprolol on mortality and morbidity after 15 days was compared with placebo in a double-blind, randomized international

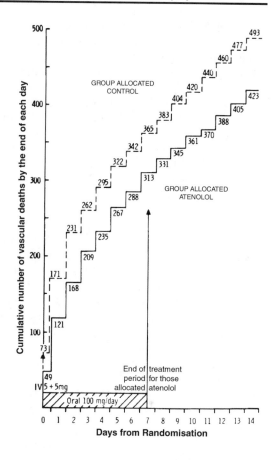

Figure 3. ISIS-1. Vascular mortality during scheduled treatment period (days 0–7) and immediately after (to day 14). (From International Study of Infarct Survival (ISIS-1) collaborative group: Randomized trial of intravenous atenolol among 16,027 cases of acute myocardial infarction. Lancet ii:57–66, 1986, with permission.)

trial of patients with definite or suspected acute MI.[19] During the recruitment phase, 26,439 patients were screened; of these, 5778 were randomized and 20,661 were excluded by various criteria. Treatment was initiated with intravenous metoprolol (total of 15 mg in 3 doses) or placebo shortly after the patient's arrival at the hospital within 24 hours of onset of symptoms. Oral treatment was continued with a total dose of 100 mg twice daily of metoprolol or placebo for 15 days. Definite MI was confirmed in 4127 patients. There were 142 deaths in the placebo group (4.9%) and 123 deaths in the metoprolol group (4.3%) (p = NS). The recruitment of more low-risk patients compared with other beta-blocker trials may explain the lack of a detectable difference. In a retrospective analysis, patients were divided into low-risk (< 2 risk factors) and high-risk groups (> 2 risk factors), depending on the following eight risk predictors:

1. Age > 60 years
2. Abnormal electrocardiogram at entry
3. History of MI
4. Angina pectoris
5. Congestive heart failure
6. Hypertension
7. Diabetes
8. Chronic or acute treatment with diuretics and/or cardiac glycosides before randomization

The placebo mortality rate increased from 0% in patients with no risk predictors to 11.6% in patients with five or more risk factors. Metoprolol demonstrated an increased effect among patients with more risk factors. Metoprolol had no effect in the low-risk group but decreased the mortality rate significantly in the high risk group by 29% (p = 0.033) (Figs. 4 and 5). Completion of MI was studied at days 0–3 and as late, first, or recurrent infarctions during days 4–15. More patients had definite MI in the placebo group than in the metoprolol group (72.5% vs. 70.5%) during 0–3 days. Patients with heart rates above the median of 80 beats/min who received metoprolol within 6 hours showed the greatest reduction in development of MI (70.7% in the metoprolol group vs. 77.6% in the placebo group). Metoprolol also reduced development of recurrent MI (3.0% vs. 3.9%, p = 0.08) and limited infarct size if started early, particularly in patients with heart rates above 80 beats/min. No significant effect on ventricular fibrillation was detected, but the number of episodes tended to be lower in the metoprolol group during days 6–15 days (24 vs. 54 episodes). The incidence of supraventricular arrhythmias, the use of cardiac glycosides and other antiarrhythmics, and the need for chest pain-relieving treatment were significantly diminished by metoprolol among all randomized patients. Adverse events associated with the use of metoprolol were infrequent, expected, and relatively mild.

In the multicenter BHAT study, sponsored by the National Heart, Lung, and Blood Institute, a total of 3,837 patients were randomized to either propranolol (180–240 mg/day in 3 divided doses) or placebo 5–21 days after MI.[20,21] The trial was stopped 9 months early because the total mortality rate was 7.2% in the propranolol and 9.8% in the placebo group (26% reduction, p = 0.004). More than 90% of the deaths were due to cardiovascular causes, and one-half were sudden. Sudden cardiac death was significantly reduced in the propranolol group

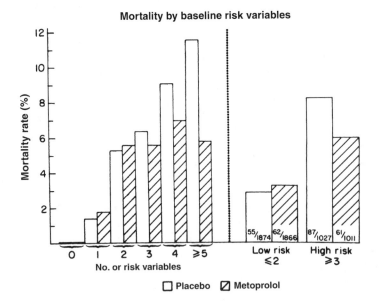

Figure 4. MIAMI trial research group. Total mortality in all patients in various mortality risk groups defined from baseline risk predictors. Number of deaths in the pooled low- and high-risk groups is indicated in bars. (From MIAMI Trial research group: Metoprolol in acute myocardial infarction: A randomized placebo-controlled trial. Eur Heart J 6:199–226, 1985, with permission.)

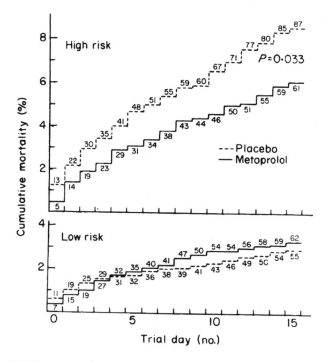

Figure 5. MIAMI trial research group. Cumulative mortality rate and number of deaths in low- and high-risk subgroups. (From MIAMI Trial research group: Metoprolol in acute myocardial infarction: A randomized placebo-controlled trial. Eur Heart J 6:199–226, 1985, with permission.)

(3.3% vs. 4.6% in the placebo group). Propranolol remained relatively effective in both low- and high-risk subgroups, although the absolute reduction was greater in the high risk group. The incidence of congestive heart failure was greater in the subset of propranolol-treated patients with a history of heart failure. However, propranolol showed its greatest relative and absolute benefit in patients with congestive heart failure, including a 47% reduction in sudden death.[22] BHAT data suggest that propranolol reduces the incidence of ventricular arrhythmias and blunts the midmorning rise in the occurrence of sudden cardiac death.[23,24]

The Norwegian Timolol Study, a multicenter, double-blind, randomized trial, compared the effects of timolol (5 mg twice daily for 2 days followed by 10 mg twice daily) to placebo in patients surviving acute MI.[25] Treatment was started 7–28 days after MI in 1884 patients (945 in the timolol group, 939 in the placebo group). Patients were followed for 12–33 months. There were 152 deaths in the placebo group and 98 deaths in the timolol group. The cumulative sudden-death rate over 33 months was 13.9% in the placebo group and 7.7% in the timolol group—a reduction of 44.6% (p = 0.0001) (Fig. 6). The cumulative reinfarction rate was 20.1% in the placebo group and 14.4% in the timolol group (p = 0.0006). The mortality benefit was consistent across all subgroups, and patients with large infarctions or signs of cardiac failure or other high-risk factors showed the greatest benefit. Survival benefit was due mainly to prevention of ventricular fibrillation. In a 6-year extended follow-up study of all-cause mortality, mortality curves between placebo and timolol groups remained parallel after 2 years without signs of convergence, indicating continued protection with timolol.[26]

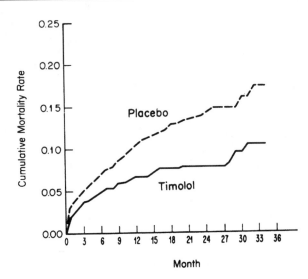

Figure 6. Life-table cumulated rates of sudden cardiac death during administration of medication or within 28 days of the last dose. Timolol after myocardial infarction—Norwegian study group. (From Norwegian Multicenter Study Group: Timolol-induced reduction in mortality and reinfarction in patients surviving acute myocardial infarction. N Engl J Med 304:801–807, 1981, with permission.)

TIMI-II was designed to compare (1) routine coronary angiography performed 18–48 hours after administration of recombinant tissue-type plasminogen activator (rt-PA), followed by prophylactic PTCA if angiography demonstrated suitable anatomy, and (2) conservative care without angiography and PTCA during the 6 weeks after random assignment to treatment (except in patients with evidence of spontaneous or exercise-induced ischemia).[27] Results showed that in patients with acute MI who were treated with rt-PA, heparin, and aspirin, an invasive strategy with prophylactic PTCA offered no reduction in mortality or reinfarction over a more conservative strategy. A group of 1390 patients eligible for a beta-blocker substudy were randomized to receive either immediate intravenous metoprolol (total 15 mg IV, followed by 100 mg twice daily) or delayed oral metoprolol (50 mg twice daily for 1 day, followed by 100 mg twice daily thereafter) started on day 6. These patients also were randomized equally to invasive and conservative strategies. The primary end-point was left ventricular ejection fraction; secondary end-points included total mortality, nonfatal reinfarction, and recurrent ischemic events at 6 days and 6 weeks. No differences in the resting and exercise left ventricular ejection fraction could be detected at hospital discharge or at 6 weeks between immediate and delayed treatment (short duration). The effects of immediate beta blockade on ventricular function were similar in the invasive and conservative groups.

The TIMI-II study was underpowered to detect an effect of immediate intravenous administration of beta blockers on mortality rate, and no mortality benefit was observed at 6 days or 6 weeks. However, immediate metoprolol administration reduced the incidence of recurrent ischemia during the first 6 days (15% in the group with immediate treatment vs. 21% in the group with delayed treatment; p = 0.005). Immediate administration of metoprolol also significantly reduced the reinfarction rate (16 patients in the immediate group vs. 31 in delayed group; p = 0.02), resulting in a 40% relative reduction. This effect was maintained at 6 weeks. Analysis of prespecified subgroups revealed that, among patients treated within 2 hours of onset of symptoms, death or recurrent infarction occurred within 6 weeks in 9 of 181 patients (5.0%) compared with 23 of 190 patients (2%) in whom metoprolol therapy was delayed (p = 0.01). In the complementary group treated 2–4 hours after onset of symptoms, one of the end-points occurred in 42 of 515 patients (8.2%) compared with 43 of 504 patients (8.5%) in the delayed group.

Underutilization of Beta Blockers

Despite the strong evidence, accumulated over more than two decades, of their beneficial effects in acute coronary syndromes, beta blockers are not prescribed to many eligible patients; they are used even less frequently in patients with risk factors who are most likely to benefit. Many patients for whom beta blockers are prescribed do not receive effective doses, as prescribed in the above clinical studies. One retrospective study of 606 consecutive survivors of MI at four university hospitals in three countries found that roughly 50% of infarct survivors with no contraindications to their use were discharged without beta blockers. Only 6% of infarct survivors received the effective dosages.[28]

The investigators of the Cooperative Cardiovascular Project reviewed the records of more than 200,000 Medicare patients (most older than 65 years) discharged home with a diagnosis of MI between February 1994 and July 1995.[29] Only 34% received beta blockers, and the rate was even lower among the very elderly, African Americans, and patients with lowest ejection fractions, heart failure, chronic obstructive pulmonary disease, elevated creatinine, or type 1 diabetes mellitus. Yet the benefits of beta blockers were evident in every subgroup (Figs. 7, 8, and 9). It also was reported that the use of beta blockers varied

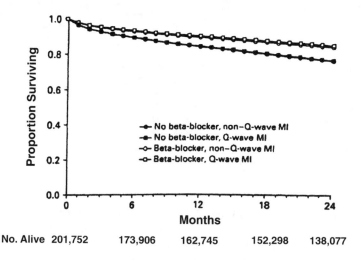

Figure 7. Adjusted probability of survival among patients with Q-wave and non–Q-wave myocardial infarction who received or did not receive beta blockers. Patients with Q-wave infarction or non–Q-wave myocardial infarction received similar benefit with beta blockade. (From Gottlieb S, McCarter RJ, Vogel RA: Effect of beta-blockade on mortality among high-risk and low-risk patients after myocardial infarction. N Engl J Med 339:489–497, 1998, with permission.)

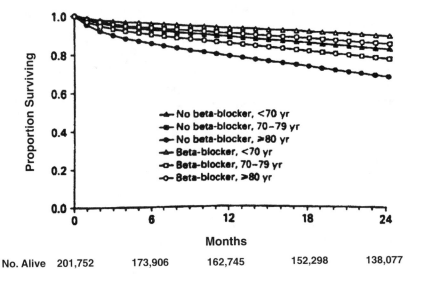

Figure 8. Adjusted probability of survival according to age among patients who received or did not receive beta-blocker treatment. The oldest patients had a smaller relative benefit (32% reduction in risk of death) but a larger absolute benefit than younger patients. The curve for patients not receiving beta blockers who were 70–79 years old overlaps the curve for patients receiving beta-blockers who were ≥ 80 years old. (From Gottlieb S, McCarter RJ, Vogel RA: Effect of beta-blockade on mortality among high-risk and low-risk patients after myocardial infarction. N Engl J Med 339:489–497, 1998, with permission.)

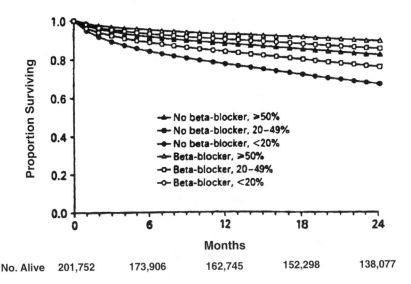

Figure 9. Adjusted probability of survival according to left ventricular ejection fraction among patients who received or did not receive beta blockers. Patients with ejection fractions under 20% had a smaller relative benefit but a larger absolute benefit than patients with normal ejection fractions. The curve for patients not receiving beta blockers who had ejection fractions of 20–49% is similar to the curve for patients receiving beta-blockers who had ejection fractions below 20%. (From Gottlieb S, McCarter RJ, Vogel RA: Effect of beta-blockade on mortality among high-risk and low-risk patients after myocardial infarction. N Engl J Med 339:489–497, 1998, with permission.)

by state of residence, ranging from 30% to 77% and that prescribed use of calcium blockers at discharge had a strong negative association with use of beta blockers.[30]

The Gruppo Italiano di Studio sulla Sopravvivenza nell'Infarto Miocardico (GISSI) investigators retrospectively analyzed beta-blocker prescriptions for the 36,817 patients with acute MI included in the GISSI-1–3 trials.[31] The prescription of beta blockers increased gradually from 8.5% in the GISS-1 trial (1984–1985) to only 25% in the GISSI-3 trial (1991–1993). The strongest positive predictors of beta-blocker use was the presence of postinfarction angina and a history of hypertension. However, even in the presence of these factors only 1 patient in 4 in the GISSI-2 trial and 1 in 3 in the GISSI-3 trial were prescribed beta blockers. Use of calcium channel blockers or angiotensin-converting enzyme inhibitors was a strong predictor of nonprescription of beta blockers. High-risk factors—advanced age, transitory cardiac failure, and arrhythmias—were important predictors of nonprescription, despite the fact that such patients derived the greatest benefit in beta-blocker trials (Fig. 10).

Guidelines to Increase Utilization

The American College of Cardiology (ACC) and American Heart Association (AHA) published practice guidelines that stress the importance of beta blockers in the management of patients with acute MI.[32] For **early therapy** in acute MI, recommendations are as follows:

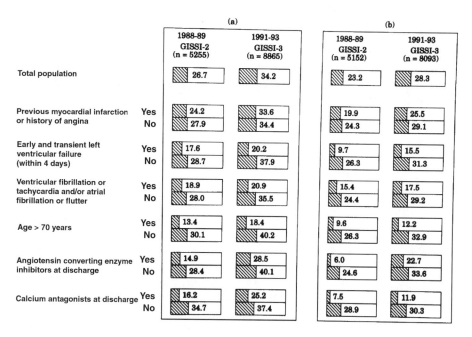

Figure 10. GISSI 2 and 3. Prescription of beta blockers at discharge in patients with (a) and without (b) clinical indications (history of hypertension, postmyocardial infarction angina, or positive exercise test) in GISSI 2 and 3 studies, according to clinical characteristics. Hatched box indicates percentage of patients receiving beta blockers in presence (yes) or absence (no) of each condition. (From Avanzini F, Zuanetti G, Latini R, et al: Use of beta-blocking agents in secondary prevention after myocardial infarction: A case for evidence-based medicine? Eur Heart J 18:1447–1456, 1997, with permission.)

Class I (conditions for which evidence and/or general agreement supports a given procedure or treatment as beneficial, useful, and effective)
- Patients with no contraindication to beta-blocker therapy who can be treated within 12 hours of onset of infarction, regardless of administration of concomitant thrombolytic therapy or performance of primary angioplasty
- Patients with continuing or recurrent ischemic pain
- Patients with tachyarrhythmias, such as atrial fibrillation, with a rapid ventricular response
- Non–ST-elevation MI

Class IIb (usefulness and efficacy are less well established by evidence or opinion)
- Patients with moderate left ventricular failure (presence of bibasilar rales without evidence of low cardiac output or other contraindications to beta-blocker therapy), provided that they can be monitored closely

Class III (conditions for which evidence and/or general agreement indicates that a procedure or treatment is not useful or effective and, in some cases, may be harmful)
- Patients with severe left ventricular failure

Recommendations for **long-term therapy** with beta blockers in survivors of MI are as follows:

Class I
- All patients without a clear contraindication except those at lowest risk. Treatment should begin within a few days of the event (if not initiated acutely) and continue indefinitely.

Class IIa (weight of evidence or opinion is in favor of usefulness or efficacy)
- Low-risk patients without a clear contraindication to beta-blocker therapy.
- Survivors of non–ST-elevation MI

Class IIb
- Patients with moderate or severe left ventricular failure or other relative contraindication to beta-blocker therapy, provided they can be monitored closely.

Class III
- None

Conclusion

The available data provide compelling evidence that use of beta blockers after acute MI decreases the rates of cardiovascular mortality and reinfarction and increase the probability of long-term survival. The degree of benefit in patients with unstable angina and non–Q-wave myocardial is less clear, but a 25% decrease in mortality and reinfarction rates has been observed in an overview of all trials.[32–35] The important predictors of death in patients with acute coronary syndromes without persistent ST-segment elevation are increasing age, heart rates above 70 beats/min, low systolic blood pressure, signs of heart failure, ST-segment depression, and elevated cardiac enzymes.[36] Beta blockers are most beneficial in these patients. The benefits of beta blockers in reducing reinfarction and mortality rates may outweigh its risks, even in patients with asthma, insulin-dependent diabetes mellitus, chronic obstructive pulmonary disease, severe peripheral vascular disease, PR interval > 0.24 second, and moderate left ventricular failure. The use of beta blockers in such patients requires careful monitoring to avoid adverse events.[32]

The ACC/AHA Task Force on Acute MI Practice Guidelines conclude that the salutary effect of long-term beta-blocker therapy is greatest in high-risk patients (i.e., those with evidence of large or anterior infarction). Debate continues about whether low-risk patients (i.e., those without previous infarction, anterior infarction, advanced age, complex ventricular ectopy, or hemodynamic evidence of left ventricular systolic dysfunction) should be treated with beta blockers because their long-term prognosis is extremely favorable, regardless of such therapy. Although adverse effects of beta blockers, such as fatigue, depression, sexual dysfunction, nightmares, and difficulty with recognition of hypoglycemia in diabetics, do occur, their frequency and severity are sufficiently low to warrant use of beta blockers even in low-risk patients. Although no prospective study has determined whether long-term beta-blocker therapy should be administered to survivors of MI who subsequently undergo successful revascularization, evidence suggests that they are as effective in reducing mortality in elderly patients who have undergone coronary bypass surgery or coronary angioplasty as in nonrevascularized patients.[37] Consequently, except in the presence of an absolute contraindication, all patients with acute coronary syndromes should receive life-long beta blockade.

References

1. National Heart, Lung, and Blood Institute: Morbidity and Mortality: Chart Book on Cardiovascular, Lung, and Blood Diseases. Bethesda, MD, U.S. Department of Health and Human Services, Public Health Service, National Institutes of Health, 1992.
2. Soumerai SB, McLaughlin TJ, Spiegelman D, et al: Adverse outcomes of underuse of beta-blockers in elderly survivors of acute myocardial infarction. JAMA 277:115–121, 1997.
3. Oliver G, Schafer EA: The physiological action of extract of the suprarenal capsules. J Physiol (Lond) 18:230-276, 1895.
4. Ahlquist RP: A study of adrenotropic receptors. Am J Physiol 153:586–600, 1948.
5. Lands AM, Luduena FP, Buzzo HJ: Differentiation of receptors responsive to isoproterenol. Life Sci 6:2241–2249, 1967.
6. Lonnqvist F, Krief S, Strosberg AD, et al: Evidence for a functional b-3 adrenoreceptor in man. Br J Pharmacol 110:929–936, 1993.
7. Katz AM: Physiology of the Heart, 2nd ed. New York, Raven Press, 1992, pp 319–350.
8. Thandroyen FT, Muntz KH, Buja ML, Willerson JT: Alterations in b-adrenergic receptors, adenylate cyclase, and cyclic AMP concentrations during acute myocardial ischemia and reperfusion. Circulation 82(Suppl II):II30-II36, 1990.
9. Black JW, Stephenson JS: Pharmacology of a new adrenergic beta-receptor blocking compound (nethalide). Lancet 2: 311–314, 1962.
10. Black JW, Crowther AF, Shanks RG, et al: A new adrenergic beta-receptor antagonist. Lancet i:1080–1081, 1964.
11. Alleyne GAO, Dickinson CJ, Dornhorst AC: Effect of pronethalol in angina pectoris. BMJ 4:1226–1229, 1963.
12. Snow PJD: Treatment of acute myocardial infarction with propranolol. Lancet ii:551–553, 1965.
13. Hjalmarson A, Elmfeldt D, Herlitz J, et al: Effect on mortality of metoprolol in acute myocardial infarction. A double-blind randomized trial. Lancet 2:823–827, 1981.
14. Karlsson BW, Herlitz J, Hjalmarson A: Impact of clinical trials on the use of beta-blockers after acute myocardial infarction and its relation to other risk indicators for death and 1-year mortality rate. Clin Cardiol 17:311–316, 1994.
15. Herlitz J, Waagstein F, Lindquist J, et al: Effect of metoprolol on the prognosis for patients with suspected acute myocardial infarction and indirect signs of congestive heart failure. Am J Cardiol 80(9B):40j–44j, 1997.
16. Ryden L, Ariniego R, Hjalmarson A, et al: A double blind trial of metoprolol in acute myocardial infarction: Effects on ventricular tachyarrhythmias. N Engl J Med 308:614–618, 1983.
17. International Study of Infarct Survival (ISIS-1) collaborative group: Randomized trial of intravenous atenolol among 16,027 cases of acute myocardial infarction. Lancet ii:57–66, 1986.

18. ISIS-1 collaborative group: Mechanisms for early mortality reduction produced by beta-blockade started early in acute myocardial infarction. Lancet i:921-923, 1988.
19. MIAMI Trial research group: Metoprolol in acute myocardial infarction: A randomized placebo-controlled trial. Eur Heart J 6:199–226, 1985.
20. Beta-blocker Heart Attack Trial research group: A randomized trial of propranolol in patients with acute myocardial infarction. I: Mortality results. JAMA 247:1707–1714, 1982.
21. Beta-blocker Heart Attack Trial research group: A randomized trial of propranolol in patients with acute myocardial infarction. II: Morbidity results. JAMA 250:2814–2819, 1983.
22. Chadda K, Goldstein S, Byington R, Curb JD: Effect of propranolol after acute myocardial infarction in patients with congestive heart failure. Circulation 73: 503–510, 1986.
23. Muller JE, Ludmer PL, Willich SN, et al: Circadian variation in the frequency of sudden cardiac death. Circulation 75:131–138, 1987.
24. Peters RW, Muller JE, Goldstein S, et al: Propranolol and the morning increase in the frequency of sudden cardiac death (BHAT study). Am J Cardiol 63:1518–1520, 1989.
25. Norwegian Multicenter Study Group: Timolol-induced reduction in mortality and reinfarction in patients surviving acute myocardial infarction. N Engl J Med 304:801–807, 1981.
26. Pedersen TR: Six-year follow-up of the Norwegian Multicenter Study on timolol after acute myocardial infarction. N Engl J Med 313:1055–1058, 1985.
27. TIMI study group: Comparison of invasive and conservative strategies after treatment with intravenous tissue plasminogen activator in acute myocardial infarction. Results of TIMI phase II trial. N Engl J Med 320: 618–627, 1989.
28. Viskin S, Kitzis I, Lev E, et al: Treatment with beta-adrenergic blocking agents after myocardial infarction: From randomized trials to clinical practice. J Am Coll Cardiol 25:1327–1332, 1995.
29. Gottlieb S, McCarter RJ, Vogel RA: Effect of beta-blockade on mortality among high-risk and low-risk patients after myocardial infarction. N Engl J Med 339:489–497, 1998.
30. Krumholz H, Radford M, Wang Y, et al: National use and effectiveness of beta-blockers for the treatment of elderly patients after acute myocardial infarction. JAMA 280:623–629, 1998.
31. Avanzini F, Zuanetti G, Latini R, et al: Use of beta-blocking agents in secondary prevention after myocardial infarction: A case for evidence-based medicine? Eur Heart J 18:1447–1456, 1997.
32. American College of Cardiology/American Heart Association: 1999 update: ACC/AHA guidelines for management of patients with acute MI: Executive summary and recommendations. A report of ACC/AHA task force on practice guidelines. Circulation 100:1016–1030, 1999.
33. Yusuf S, Wittes J, Probstfield J: Evaluating effects of treatment in subgroups of patients within a clinical trial: The case of non–Q-wave myocardial infarction and beta-blockers. Am J Cardiol 66:220–223, 1990.
34. Holland Interuniversity Nifedipine/metoprolol Trial (HINT) research group: Early treatment of unstable angina in the coronary care unit: A randomized double-blind, placebo-controlled comparison of recurrent ischemia in patients treated with nifedipine or metoprolol or both. Br Heart J 56:400–413, 1986.
35. Yusuf S, Peto R, Lewis J, et al: Beta blockade during and after myocardial infarction: An overview of the randomized trials. Prog Cardiovasc Dis 27:335–371, 1985.
36. Boersma E, Pieper KS, Steyerberg EW, et al for the PURSUIT Investigators: Predictors of outcome in patients with acute coronary syndromes without persistent ST-segment elevation: Results from an international trial of 9461 patients. Circulation 101:2557–2567, 2000.
37. Chen J, Radford MJ, Wang Y, et al: Are β-blockers effective in elderly patients who undergo coronary revascularization after acute myocardial infarction? Arch Intern Med 160:947–952, 2000.

Calcium Antagonists for the Acute Coronary Syndromes

FUNDADOR L. ADAJAR, MD

FRED LEYA, MD

Calcium antagonists were first introduced into clinical medicine in the late 1970s. They are now the most frequently prescribed class of drugs for the treatment of cardiovascular disease.[1] Calcium antagonists share the common property of blocking the transmembrane flow of calcium ions through voltage-gated L-type channels.[2] Blockade of L-type calcium channels in vascular tissue leads to relaxation of vascular smooth muscle and in cardiac tissues results in a negative inotropic effect. Verapamil and diltiazem also slow atrioventricular conduction and cause sinus node depression. Therapeutic uses of calcium antagonists include control of hypertension and relief of angina and cardiac arrhythmias. They also may be beneficial in patients with Raynaud's phenomenon, migraine, preterm labor, esophageal spasm, and bipolar disorders.

Pharmacokinetics and Pharmacodynamics

The bioavailability of calcium antagonists varies depending on first-pass metabolism in the walls of the intestines and liver. All are metabolized into less active metabolites by the cytochrome P450 enzyme family in the liver. Hepatic biotransformation of verapamil may be greater in women than in men.[3]

Nifedipine is the most potent vasodilator among the different calcium antagonists. In vitro, several calcium antagonists (i.e., nifedipine, nisoldipine, and isradipine) bind with some selectivity to the vascular L-type calcium channel, whereas verapamil binds equally well to cardiac and vascular L-type calcium channels.[4,5] Only verapamil and diltiazem cause delay in atrioventricular conduction or sinus node depression at clinically used doses.[6]

Clinical Uses

In 1980, Antman et al.[7] reported the first clinical experience in the United States with the use of nifedipine in patients with coronary spasm. The authors used nifedipine capsules to treat 127 patients with Prinzmetal's angina. The average weekly occurrences of angina were reduced from 16 to 2; in addition, nifedipine reduced nitroglycerin requirements, completely controlled angina in 63% of patients, and reduced the frequency of angina by at least 50% in 87% of cases. Since that time, a number of trials with different calcium channel blockers, including nifedipine, diltiazem, verapamil, and amlodipine, have consistently shown that these agents are efficacious in reducing the morbidity of Prinzmetal's angina.[8]

Trials of Calcium Antagonists in Acute Coronary Syndromes

Myocardial Infarction

There have been at least 24 randomized controlled trials of calcium antagonist in the early phase or after acute myocardial infarction (Table 1). Most of the experiences have been with nifedipine, verapamil, and diltiazem, and most of the trials are small. Even the larger trials are too small in patient number to have enough statistical power to detect a moderately sized treatment effect (15–20% difference).

Nifedipine

Nifedipine, a dihydropyridine, is the most extensively studied agent. Overall, 9464 patients were included in 13 trials.[10–22] Most of the trials had a primary endpoint of infarct size or left ventricular function. Three of the trials were designed primarily to study mortality rates.[17,21,22] The doses of nifedipine varied between 40 and 120 mg/day divided into 3–6 doses. In the small studies, the duration of treatment varied from 2 days to 2 weeks and in the mortality trials from 1 to 6 months.

Table 1. Mortality Rates in Trials of Calcium Antagonists in Myocardial Infarction

Trial	Active Treatment	Control (Placebo)	Odds Ratio for Drug	Significance
Nifedipine				
Wilcox et al.[17]	150/2240	141/2251	1.07	NS
SPRINT-I[21]	65/1130	65/1146	1.02	NS
SPRINT-II[22]	105/680	90/678	1.19	NS
Nine small trials[10–15,16–20]	46/560	34/281	1.14	NS
Subtotal	365/4731	330/4733	1.13	NS
Diltiazem				
MDPIT[32]	166/1232	167/1234	0.99	NS
Four small trials[29–31,33]	14/342	14/343	1.00	NS
Subtotal	180/1574	181/1577	0.99	NS
Verapamil				
DAVIT-I[26]	149/1729	145/1718	1.02	NS
DAVIT-II[27]	84/878	107/897	0.78	NS
CRIS[28]	30/521	29/542	1.07	NS
Two small trials[24,25]	0/37	2/34	0.16	NS
Subtotal	263/3165	283/3191	0.93	NS
Lidoflazine				
Myocardial Infarction Study Group[34]	178/904	167/888	1.06	NS
Total	986/10,374	961/10,389	1.02	NS

SPRINT = Secondary Prevention of Reinfarction Israel Nifedipine Trial, MDPIT = Multicenter Diltiazem Postinfarction Trial, DAVIt = Danish Verapamil Infarction Trial, CRIS = Calcium Antagonist Italian Study, NS = not significant.
From Held PH, Yusuf S: Calcium antagonists in the treatment of ischemic heart disease: Myocardial infarction. Coron Artery Dis 5:21–26, 1994, with permission.

The nine trials that studied infarct size found no difference between treatment and control groups. The largest trial that studied the effects on mortality rate[17] randomly assigned 4491 patients with suspected myocardial infarction to 40 mg/day nifedipine vs. placebo. No difference was found in the number of patients developing infarction; 150 patients in the nifedipine group died compared with 141 patients in the placebo group (not sigificant) at the end of the 28-day period.

In the Secondary Prevention of Reinfarction Israeli Nifedipine Trial I (SPRINT-I),[21] 1–3 weeks after the acute phase of myocardial infarction 2276 patients were randomly assigned to 30 mg/day of nifedipine or placebo. After 10 months of follow-up the study was stopped by its safety committee because of absence of effect. Sixty-five patients died in each group (NS).

In the SPRINT-II trial, 1358 patients were randomly assigned as early as possible to 60 mg/day or placebo. Patients were considered to be at high risk (anterior or recurrent myocardial infarction, history of angina or hypertension, or enzymatically large infarcts). This study, like SPRINT-I, was terminated early, in this case because of a trend toward increased mortality in the nifedipine group during the early phase. One-hundred five patients died in the nifedipine group compared with 90 in the placebo group (NS).

In all of these nifedipine trials (13 total), 365 of 4731 patients (7.7%) in the nifedipine group died compared with 330 of 4733 (7.0%) in the placebo group. These results represents a 13% higher odds ratio of death in the nifedipine group with a 95% confidence interval (CI) of –3% to 32%. There was a strong trend toward higher mortality and reinfarction rates in the treatment group.

A recent meta-analysis by Furburg[23] showed that overall the use of nifedipine was associated with a significant adverse effect on mortality (risk ratio = 1.16, 95% CI = 1.01–1.33). For daily doses of nifedipine of 30–50 mg, 60 mg, and 80 mg, the risk ratios for total mortality were 1.06 (95% CI = 0.89–1.27), 1.18 (95% CI = 0.93–1.50), and 2.83 (95% CI = 1.35–5.93), respectively.

Diltiazem

Five randomized trials of diltiazem for treatment of acute myocardial infarction in a total of 3151 patients have been published.[29–33]

The Multicenter Diltiazem Postinfarction Trial (MDPIT),[32] by far the largest of the diltiazem studies, evaluated 2466 patients younger than 75 years with documented myocardial infarction (25% had non–Q-wave myocardial infarction). Patients were randomly assigned to receive 60 mg of diltiazem 4 times/day or placebo, starting 3–15 days after the onset of infarction. Treatment was continued for up to 52 months with a mean follow-up of 25 months. Approximately 54% of patients were on beta-blocker therapy. At the end of the study period, the mortality rates were no different: 166 deaths in 1232 patients in the diltiazem group compared with 167 deaths in 1234 placebo patients. There was a lower incidence of nonfatal reinfarction in the diltiazem group (99 vs. 116 patients; not significant).

The Diltiazem Reinfarction Study Group performed a double-blind, randomized trial to evaluate the effect of diltiazem on reinfarction after a non–Q-wave myocardial infarction. Diltiazem was given to 287 patients at a dose of 90 mg every 6 hours, beginning 24–72 hours after the onset of infarction and continuing for up to 14 days. Placebo was given to 289 patients. Reinfarction occurred in 15 patients in the diltiazem group (5.2%) and 27 patients in the placebo group

(9.3%)—a 51.2% reduction with diltiazem (p = 0.02). Diltiazem also reduced the frequency of refractory postinfarction angina by 49.7% (p = 0.035). Mortality was similar in the two groups. Diltiazem was well tolerated despite concurrent treatment with beta blockers in 61% of patients.

Overall the incidence of mortality in the five diltiazem trials was 180 of 1574 patients (11.4%) in the diltiazem group compared with 181 of 1577 patients (11.5%) in the placebo group.

Verapamil

More than 6300 patients were studied in the five randomized trials that evaluated verapamil[24–28] in patients with acute myocardial infarction. Two relatively large mortality trials have been reported: the Danish Verapamil Infarction Trials (DAVIT) I and II.

In DAVIT-I,[26] 3447 patients with suspected myocardial infarctions were randomized early to verapamil or placebo, and treatment was continued for 6 months. Patients taking beta blockers were excluded. There was no difference in mortality rate. Retrospective analysis revealed a trend toward lower mortality rates over 4 weeks of follow-up in the verapamil treatment group.

In DAVIT-II,[27] 1775 patients were randomly assigned to receive verapamil or placebo for an average of 16 months. Treatment was initiated between 1 and 3 weeks after the acute event. Ninety-five of the 878 patients in the verapamil group died compared with 119 of 897 in the placebo group (p = 0.15). There was also a parallel trend in the reduction of reinfarction. Of 2606 patients treated with verapamil, 138 had reinfarctions compared with 171 in 2624 patients in the placebo group.

In the Calcium Antagonist Reinfarction Italian Study (CRIS), 1073 low-risk patients receiving beta blockers were randomized to verapamil, 120 mg every 8 hours, or placebo.[28] After 2 years the number of deaths was similarly low: 30 of 531 patients in the verapamil group and 29 of 542 patients in the placebo group. As in the DAVIT trials, the authors found a statistically nonsignificant trend toward fewer nonfatal reinfarctions in the verapamil group (39/531) compared with placebo-treated patients (49/542).

Lidoflazine

Although lidoflazine was the first calcium antagonist to be studied in a randomized trial of acute myocardial infarction,[34] it is not readily available. The study included 1792 patients randomly assigned to receive 60 mg of lidoflazine 3 or 4 times/day or placebo. Treatment was started within 2 months of infarction and continued for up to 5 years. No benefit was found with mortality as the endpoint. Of 904 patients treated with lidoflazine, 178 died compared with 167 of 888 placebo-treated patients (not significant).

Unstable Angina

Although calcium antagonists have been used for the treatment of unstable angina since the late 1970s, relatively few randomized trials have evaluated their efficacy in this setting.

Nifedipine

Nifedipine, the first available calcium antagonist, is also the most vigorously studied. Genstenblith et al. assessed the efficacy of adding nifedipine to conventional treatment, which included beta blockers and nitrates, in a prospective, double-blind, randomized, placebo-controlled study of 138 patients with unstable angina.[35] Failure of medical treatment (sudden death, myocardial infarction, or coronary artery bypass grafting [CABG] within 4 months) occurred in 43 of 70 placebo-treated patients and 30 of 68 patients given nifedipine, revealing a significant benefit for nifedipine over placebo (p = 0.03). The benefit was particularly marked in patients with ST-segment elevation during angina.

Muller et al. conducted a blinded, randomly assigned, titrated schedule of conventional therapy (propranolol and isosorbide dinitrate) or nifedipine for 14 days in 126 patients with unstable angina.[36] They found no significant differences between treatment groups in regard to time of relief of pain, decrease in anginal attacks per 24 hour from day 0 to day 2, nitroglycerine usage, need for morphine, or percentage of patients who developed infarction (14% in both groups). In the subgroup of 67 patients who received propranolol before randomization, addition of nifedipine was more effective for pain control than an increase in conventional therapy (p = 0.026). In the subgroup not receiving prior propranolol, initiation of conventional therapy produced more rapid pain relief than initiation of nifedipine therapy alone (p < 0.001), which tended to increase heart rate. Thus, nifedipine appeared to be better used as a second-line agent after treatment first with propranolol.

Gottlieb et al. tested the hypothesis that a beta blocker would be of additive benefit to vasodilators in unstable angina.[37] They conducted a double-blind, randomized, placebo-controlled 4-week trial in 81 patients, 39 of whom were treated with placebo and 42 with propranolol in a dose of at least 160 mg/day. All patients were also treated with 80 mg/day of nifedipine and long-acting nitrates. The incidence of cardiac death, myocardial infarction, and need for CABG or angioplasty did not differ between the propranolol and placebo groups. The propranolol group reported significant lessening of angina (p = 0.013), and significantly fewer ischemic ST-segment changes were noted on continuous monitoring (p = 0.03), with a shorter duration of ischemia (p = 0.039). Thus, if nifedipine is to be used for unstable anigna, it is best used with a beta blocker.

The largest randomized trial of nifedipine for unstable angina was the Holland Interuniversity Nifedipine/Metoprolol Trial Research Group (HINT).[38] HINT was a double-blind, placebo-controlled, randomized trial of nifedipine, metoprolol, and nifedipine combined with metoprolol in 338 patients not pretreated with a beta blocker and of nifedipine in 177 patients pretreated with a beta blocker. The main outcome event was recurrent ischemia or myocardial infarction within 48 hours. In patients not pretreated with a beta blocker, the event rate ratios relative to placebo were 1.15 for nifedipine, 0.76 for metoprolol, and 0.80 for nifedipine plus metoprolol. In this group the nifedipine rate ratio for infarction only was 1.51. In patients already taking a beta blocker, the addition of nifedipine was beneficial (rate ratio = 0.68). The HINT group concluded that in patients not on prior beta blockade, metoprolol has a beneficial short-term effect on unstable angina and that nifedipine may be detrimental. On the other hand, the addition of nifedipine to existing beta blockade when the patient's condition is unstable seems beneficial.

The above trials strongly indicate that in patients with unstable angina nifedipine should not be used as a first-line agent but should be used only when beta-blocker and nitrate therapy are inadequate for control of ischemia.

Diltiazem

Göbel et al. conducted a randomized, double-blind trial comparing diltiazem with glyceryl trinitrate, both given intravenously, in 129 patients with unstable angina.[39] Endpoints were refractory angina or myocardial infarction. Refractory angina occurred significantly less often (10%) in the diltiazem group than in the nitrate group (28%; p = 0.02). Over 48 hours the combined endpoint of refractory angina and infarction occurred in 20% of patients treated with diltiazem vs. 41% treated with nitrate (relative risk = 0.49, p = 0.02). There were no significant complications with the use of either agent intravenously. The authors concluded that intravenous diltiazem, compared with intravenous glyceryl trinitrate, significantly reduces ischemic events and can be used safely in patients with unstable angina.

Andre-Fovet et al. compared the efficiency of oral diltiazem to oral propranolol in a single-blind randomized trial of 70 patients with spontaneous angina, selected according to ST-T changes during chest pain.[40] In the whole group and in subgroups of patients with and without ST-segment elevation at rest, response to diltiazem did not differ from that to propranolol. Among 24 patients with angina exclusively at rest, diltiazem was significantly more efficacious (9 of 13 improved with diltiazem, 1 of 11 improved with propranolol, and 8 of the 10 propranolol failures improved with diltiazem). The authors concluded that diltiazem is preferable to propranolol for unstable angina in patients with angina that is exclusively spontaneous.

Theroux et al. randomized 100 consecutive patients hospitalized with unstable angina to diltiazem or propranolol.[41] They excluded from the trial any patient with Prinzmetal's angina or prior coronary bypass surgery and patients receiving a beta blocker on admission. They found no significant difference between the two drugs in frequency of chest pain, myocardial infarction, death, or need for bypass surgery. They suggested that diltiazem can be used as an alternative to beta blockers for unstable angina.

Fang et al. evaluated 18 consecutive patients who were admitted with unstable angina and had 48-hour Holter monitoring after random assignment to aspirin plus intravenous nitroglycerin or aspirin plus intravenous diltiazem.[42] All of the patients treated with nitroglycerin still had ischemic episodes after 48 hours, but only 11% of the diltiazem group had ischemia, which was silent. During the 48 hours, the diltiazem group had significantly fewer ischemic episodes (17) than the nitroglycerin group (145).

In summary, oral diltiazem is generally safe in patients with unstable angina and is about as effective in controlling ischemia as beta blockers. In patients in whom vasospasm is suspected, it is preferable to beta blockers. Diltiazem has not been shown to reduce the incidence of infarction or death. Intravenous diltiazem has been shown to be safe and more effective than intravenous nitrates and should be used more often than it is at present.

Verapamil

Verapamil has been studied in several small randomized studies.[43-45] Generally it has been shown to be well tolerated and helpful in controlling ischemic symptoms. It compares favorably with beta blockers, especially when coronary spasm is suspected. It has not been shown to reduce the incidence of myocardial infarction or death during short-term follow-up.

Potentially Harmful Mechanisms

The principal mechanisms of action of the calcium antagonists are via peripheral and coronary vasodilatation. They also may reduce myocardial oxygen demand by lowering blood pressure, slowing heart rate, and decreasing myocardial contractility. The relative potency of these pharmacologic actions varies among the calcium antagonists; thus, their clinical effects may be different. These differences, however, are generally in degree rather than kind.

Proischemic Effect

Proischemia, according to Waters,[46] is "the potential of an antianginal drug to occasionally worsen ischemia in an unpredictable and dangerous manner." The most common form of proischemia is an increase in anginal symptoms. Jariwalla[47] first reported the link between nifedipine and increasing angina. Reporting on a cohort study, Stone et al. concluded that nifedipine was associated with an increase of anginal frequency in 13–29% of 716 patients. This increase was often observed in patients with no evidence of vasospasm.[48] In a double-blind, randomized crossover trial, Ergstrup and Andersen[49] found that the therapeutic effect of nifedipine in patients with stable angina depends on the presence or absence of collateral circulation. In patients with poor or no collateral circulation, nifedipine reduced the frequency and intensity of ischemic episodes. But in patients with good collateral flow, nifedipine could significantly increase the ischemic episodes. In certain instances, severe proischemia could precipitate major coronary events, the so-called coronary steal phenomenon.[50]

Negative Inotropic Effect

It is well established that the entire class of calcium antagonists has a negative inotropic effect and that this action varies among agents. Subgroup analysis in the Multicenter Diltiazem Post Infarction Trial (MDPIT) showed that a diltiazem-induced increase in the risk of new or worsening heart failure was closely related to ejection fraction.[32] This adverse effect was most apparent in patients with ejection fractions < 25% and 25–34%. In patients with ejection fractions < 40%, late congestive heart failure appeared in 12% of 326 placebo patients and 21% of 297 diltiazem-treated patients (p = 0.004).

Effect on Rhythm

Short-acting calcium antagonists not only increase sympathetic activation but also activate the renin-angiotensin system. Packer[50] suggested that activation of the renin-angiotensin system may predispose to the occurrence of complex ventricular tachyarrhythmias, either by potentiating the development of catecholamine-induced arrhythmias or by increasing production of mineralocorticoids, which may exacerbate diuretic-induced potassium depletion. This effect during a coronary event is highly unfavorable.

Prohemorrhagic Effects

Calcium antagonists have varying degrees of antiplatelet activity. They prevent the influx of calcium in response to several platelet activators. In the Thombolysis in Myocardial Infarction (TIMI) Phase II trial, which randomized patients to recombinant tissue-type plasminogen activator (tPA) or placebo, the incidence of intracerebral hemorrhage was almost 4 times higher in patients taking a calcium antagonist at study entry than in patients not taking these drugs.[51]

Hypotensive Effect

Sublingual nifedipine, a common therapy in the past, markedly reduces blood pressure in some patients with a hypertensive crisis. Hypoperfusion of the subendocardium, accompanied by major T-wave inversions on the electrocardiogram, is induced in about 25 % of such patients.[52] The development of myocardial infarction has been reported after administration of sublingual nifedipine.

Conclusion

In patients with acute myocardial infarction nifedipine appears to have an adverse effect on mortality and should not be used. Diltiazem has not been shown to be harmful. Its use has not resulted in a lessening of mortality in patients with infarction, but it may lower the incidence of postinfarction angina and reinfarction, especially in patients with non–Q-wave infarction. Verapamil also appears to be safe in patients with infarction, but it has not been shown to alter significantly mortality or reinfarction rates.

In patients with unstable angina, nifedipine is best used as a second-line agent after initial treatment with a beta blocker. The exception may be patients with ST-segment elevation during angina. Diltiazem is essentially equivalent to beta blockade for the relief of ischemia but is preferred in patients suspected of having significant coronary vasospasm. Verapamil has been less well studied in the early phase of unstable angina. It seems to be safe and effective in controlling ischemic episodes, particularly in patients with vasospasm. None of the calcium antagonists has been clearly shown to reduce the short-term incidence of myocardial infarction or death in patients with unstable angina.

References

1. Freher M, Challapalli S, Pinto JV, et al: Current status of calcium channel blockers in patients with cardiovascular disease. Curr Probl Cardiol 24:236–240, 1999.
2. Mcdonald TF, Pelzer S, Trautwein W, Pelzer DJ: Regulation and modulation of calcium channels in cardiac, skeletal, and smooth muscle cells. Physiol Rev 74:365–507, 1994.
3. Schwarts JB, Capili H, Daugherty J: Aging of women alters S-verapamil pharmacokinetics and pharmacodynamics. Clin Pharmacol Ther 55:509–517, 1994.
4. Morel N, Buryi V, Feron O, et al: The action of calcium channel blockers on recombinant L type calcium channel alpha 1-subunits. Br J Pharmacol 125:1005–1012, 1998.
5. Soldatov NM, Bouron A, Reuter H: Different voltage–dependent inhibition by dihydropyridines of human Ca^{2+} channel splice variants. J Biol Chem 270:10540–10543, 1995.
6. Abernethy DR, Schwartz JB, Wood AJ: Calcium antagonist drug. N Engl J Med 341:1447–1457, 1999.
7. Antman E, Muller J, Goldberg S, et al: Nifedipine therapy for coronary spasm: Experience in 127 patients. N Engl J Med 302:1269–1273, 1980.
8. Stone PH: Calcium antagonist for Prinzmetal's variant angina, unstable angina and silent myocardial ischemia: Therapeutic tool and probe for identification of pathophysiologic mechanisms. Am J Cardiol 59 101B–115B, 1987.
9. Held PH, Yusuf S: Calcium antagonist in the treatment of ischemic heart disease: Myocardial infarction. Coron Artery Dis 5:21–26, 1994.
10. Sirens PA, Overskeid K, Pederson TR, al: Evaluation of infarct size during the early use of nifedipine in patients with acute myocardial infarction. The Norwegian Nifedipine Multicenter Trial. Circulation 70:638–644, 1984.
11. Muller JE, Morrison J, Stone PH, et al: Nifedipine therapy for threatened and acute myocardial infarction: A randomized, double blind, placebo controlled comparison. Circulation 69:740–747, 1984.

12. Gordon GD, Mabin TA, Isaacs S, et al: Hemodynamic effect of sublingual nifedipine in acute myocardial infarction. Am J Cardiol 53:1228–1232, 1984.

13. Gottlieb SO, Becker L, Weiss JL, et al: Nifedipine in acute myocardial infarction: An assessment of left ventricular function, infarct size, and infarct expansion in a double blind randomized trial. Br Heart J 59:411–418, 1988.

14. Eisenber PR, Lee RG, Biello DR, et al: Chest pain after non transmural infarction: The absence of remediable coronary vasospasm. Am Heart J 110:515–521, 1985.

15. Branagan JP, Walsh K, Kelly P, et al: Effect of early treatment with nifedipine in suspected acute myocardial infarction. Eur Heart J 7:859–865, 1986.

16. Loogna E, Sylven C, Groth T, Mogensen L: Complexity of enzyme release during acute myocardial infarction in a controlled study with early nifedipine treatment. Eur Heart J 6:114–119, 1985.

17. Wilcox RG, Hampton JR, Banks DC, et al: Trial of early nifedipine in acute myocardial infarction: The TRENT study. BMJ 293:1204–1208, 1986.

18. Walker L, Mackenzie A, Adgey J: Effect of nifedipine on enzymatically estimated infarct size in the early phase of acute myocardial infarction. Br Heart J 39:403–410, 1988.

19. Jaffe AS, Biello DR, Sobel BE, GEltman EM: Enhancement of metabolism of jeopardized myocardium by nifedipine. Int J Cardiol 15:77–79, 1987.

20. Erbel R, Pop T, Meinertz T, et al : Combination calcium channel blocker and thrombolytic therapy in acute myocardial infarction. Am Heart J 115:529–538, 1988.

21. Israeli SPRINT Study Group (Secondary Prevention of Reinfarction Israeli Nifedipine Trial): A randomized intervention trail of nifedipine in patients with acute myocardial infarction. Eur Heart J 9:354–364, 1988.

22. Goldbourt T, Behar S, Reicher-Reiss H, et al: Early administration of nifedipine in suspected acute myocardial infarction: The Secondary Prevention of Reinfarction Israeli Nifedipine Trial 2 Study. Arch Intern Med 153:345–353, 1993.

23. Furburg CD,Psaty B,Meyer J: Nifedipine dose-related increase in mortality in patients with coronary heart disease. Circulation 81:1326–1331, 1995.

24. Bussman WD, Ser W, Gruengrass M: Reduction of creatine kinase and creatine kinase MB indexes of infarct size by intravenous verapamil. Am J Cardiol 54:1224–1230, 1984.

25. Crea F, Deanfield J, Crean P, et al: Effect of Verapamil in preventing post infarction angina and reinfarction. Am J Cardiol 55:900–904, 1985.

26. Danish Study Group on Verapamil in Myocardial Infarction: Verapamil in acute myocardial infarction. Eur Heart J 5:516–528, 1984.

27. Danish Study Group on Verapamil in Myocardial Infarction: Effect of verapamil on mortality and major events after myocardial infarction (The Danish Verapamil Infarction Trail II–DAVIT II). Am J Cardiol 66:779–785, 1990.

28. Rengo F, Pierugo C, Pahor M, et al: A controlled trial of verapamil in patients after acute myocardial infarction: Results of the Calcium Antagonist Reinfarction Italian Study (CRIS). Am J Cardiol 77:365–369, 1986.

29. Gibson RS, Boden WE, Thereoux P, et al: Diltiazem and reinfarction in patients with non–Q-wave myocardial infarction. N Engl J Med 315:423–429, 1986.

30. Zannad F, Amor M, Karcher G, et al : Effect of diltiazem on infarct size estimated by enzyme release, serial thallium-201 single photon emission computed tomography and radionuclide angiography. Am J Cardiol 61:1172–1178, 1988.

31. Machecourt J, Cassagnes J, Andr-Fouet X, et al: Diltiazem infused within 6 hours after an acute anterior myocardial infarction in man. Significant reduction of ventricular arrhythmias: No significant reduction of infarct size. In Proceedings of the Tenth World Congress of Cardiology. Washington DC, American Heart Association, p 250A, 1986.

32. Multicenter Diltiazem Postinfarction Trial Research Group: The effect of diltiazem on mortality and reinfarction after myocardial infarction. N Engl J Med 319;385–392, 1988.

33. Bartels M, Remme W, Wiesfeld A, Vanderlaase A: High dose diltiazem increases infarct size in acute uncomplicated myocardial infarction: A placebo- controlled study. J Am Coll Cardiol 19:381A, 1992.

34. Myocardial Infarction Study Group: Secondary prevention of ischemic heart disease: A long-term controlled lidoflazine study. Acta Cardiol 34(Suppl 24):7–46, 1979.

35. Gerstenblith G, Ouyang P, Achuff SC, et al: Nifedipine in unstable angina. A double-blind randomized trial. N Engl J Med 306:885–889, 1982.

36. Muller JE, Turi ZG, Pearle DL, et al. Nifedipine and conventional therapy for unstable angina pectoris: A randomized, double-blind comparison. Circulation 69:728–739, 1984.

37. Gottlieb SO, Weisfeldt ML, Ouyang P, et al: Effect of the addition of propanolol to therapy with nifedipine for unstable angina pectoris: A randomized, double-blind, placebo-controlled trial. Circulation 73:331–337, 1986.

38. Holland Interuniversity Nifedipine/Metoprolol Trial (HINT) Research Group: Early treatment of unstable angina in the coronary care unit: A randomized double-blind placebo controlled comparison of recurrent ischemia in patients treated with nifedipine or metoprolol or both. Br Heart J 56:400–413, 1986.
39. Gobel E, Hautvast R, van Gilst W, et al: Randomized double-blind trial of intravenous diltiazem versus glyceryl trinitrate for unstable angina pectoris. Lancet 346;1653–1657, 1995.
40. Andre-Fovet K, Usdin JP, Gayet C, et al: Comparison of short-term efficacy of diltiazem and propranolol in unstable-angina at rest: A randomized trial in 70 patients. Eur Heart J 4:691–698, 1983.
41. Théroux P, Taeymans Y, Morisette D, et al: A randomized study comparing propranolol and diltiazem in the treatment of unstable angina. J Am Coll Cardiol 5:717–722, 1985.
42. Fang ZY, Picart N, Abramowicz M, et al: Intravenous diltiazem versus nitroglycerine for silent and symptomatic myocardial ischemia in unstable angina pectoris. Am J Cardiol 68:42C–46C, 1991.
43. Mavritson DR, Johnson SM, Winniford MD, et al: Verapamil for unstable angina at rest: A short-term randomized, double-blind study. Am Heart J 106:652–658, 1983.
44. Parodi O, Smonetti I, Michelassi C, et al: Comparison of verapamil and propranolol therapy for angina pectoris at rest: A randomized, multiple-crossover controlled trial in the coronary care unit. Am J Cardiol 57:899–906, 1986.
45. Singh N, Mironov D, Goodman S, et al: Treatment of silent ischemia in unstable angina: A randomized comparison of sustained-release verapamil versus metoprolol. Clin Cardiol 18:653–658, 1995.
46. Waters D: Proischemic complications of dihydropyridine calcium channel blockers. Circulation 84:2598–2600, 1991.
47. Jariwalla AG, Anderson AG: Production of ischemic cardiac pain by nifedipine. BMJ 1:1181–1182, 1978.
48. Stone PH, Muller JE, Turi ZG, et al: Effect of nifedipine therapy in patients with refractory angina pectoris: Significance of the presence of coronary spasm. Am Heart J 106:644–652, 1983.
49. Ergstrup K, Andersen PE: Transient myocardial ischemia during nifedipine therapy in stable angina and its relation to collateral flow and comparison with metoprolol. Am J Cardiol 71:170–183, 1991.
50. Packer M, for the PRAISE Trial (Prospective Randomized Amlodipine Survival Evaluation): Background and main result. Presented at the American College of Cardiology Annual Meeting, New Orleans, March 1995.
51. Gore JM, Sloan M, Price TR, et al. and the TIMI investigators: Intracerebral hemorrhage, cerebral infarction and subdural hematoma after acute myocardial infarction and thrombolytic therapy in the Thrombolysis in Myocardial Infarction. Phase II, Pilot and Clinical Trial. Circulation 83:448–459, 1991.
52. Phillips RA, Goldman ME, Ardeljan M, et al: Isolated T-wave abnormalities and evaluation of left ventricular wall motion after nifedipine for severe hypertension. Am J Hypertens 4:432–437, 1991.

Nitrates in the Acute Coronary Syndromes

12

KEVIN J. COCHRAN, MD
PATRICK J. SCANLON, MD

Nitrates have been used in the treatment of angina for over 120 years. They are used most commonly in the treatment of chronic stable angina.[1] In the early 1900s, nitroglycerin was considered to be contraindicated in evolving myocardial infarctions because the available oral and sublingual forms sometimes induced hypotension and reflex tachycardia. In the 1970s, intravenous glyceryl trinitrate was used with a suggested beneficial effect on ischemic myocardium. In October of 1981, intravenous nitroglycerin was approved in the United States for general clinical use in unstable angina and left ventricular failure complicating acute myocardial infarction.[2] In the following years, considerable research was conducted to determine the safety and efficacy of nitrates in the acute coronary syndromes of unstable angina and acute myocardial infarction. This chapter reviews the pertinent randomized trials of nitrates in the acute coronary syndromes.

Pharmacology

Nitrates and nitrites are simple nitric and nitrous acid esters of polyalcohols. They are prodrugs and undergo biotransformation in which nitrite ion (NO_2^-) is released and metabolized to nitric oxide (NO). Nitrates are absorbed rapidly through the skin, mucous membranes, and gastrointestinal tract. Organic nitrates taken orally may have a significant first-pass effect in the liver. Therefore, the bioavailability of oral nitrates is typically quite low (<10%).[3]

Once absorbed, unchanged nitrate compounds have a half-life of 2–8 minutes. Partially denitrated metabolites have a longer half-life of about 1–3 hours. The 5-mononitrate metabolite of isosorbide dinitrate does not undergo first-pass metabolism and is almost 100% bioavailable. The differences are important to clinical use. The sublingual route is preferred for quickly achieving a therapeutic blood level. To avoid hypotension, dosage is limited, which shortens the duration of action. When a longer duration of action is needed, dinitrate or mononitrate preparations are available that contain an amount of drug sufficient to result in sustained systemic blood levels of drug or active metabolites.[3] Intravenous nitrates combine short half-life with the ability to titrate the dosage rapidly.

Mechanism of Action

Nitrates act through an endothelial-independent pathway to relax all types of vascular smooth muscle to varying degrees. Nitrates are converted to nitric oxide, which then activates guanylate cyclase. Guanylate cyclase, in turn, produces cyclic guanosine monophosphate (cGMP), which leads to increased levels of intracellular cGMP and vasodilation[3] (Fig. 1).

Nitrates are thought to be clinically effective through their vasodilatory effect, which leads to decreased venous return to the heart and thus decreased preload. Arterial pressure also decreases. The combined effect is a decrease in intraventricular pressure and volume, which leads to decreases in wall tension and myocardial oxygen requirement. Other benefits of nitroglycerin include dilation of epicardial coronary vessels, increase in collateral flow to endocardial regions, and relief of coronary spasm. However, the decrease in myocardial oxygen requirement is thought to be the primary therapeutic effect in anginal syndromes.

Side Effects and Tolerance

Side effects of nitroglycerin include (1) headache, (2) hypotension, (3) dermal erythema (with patches), (4) methemoglobinemia (after prolonged use) due to oxidation of hemoglobin to methemoglobin by nitrate ions, (5) pulmonary hypoxemia due to ventilation-perfusion mismatch, and (6) rebound ischemia (with sudden withdrawal).

Tachyphylaxis (tolerance) to nitrates is a problem with prolonged exposure. The mechanism of tolerance is unknown, but it is unrelated to drug pharmakinetics. Proposed theories include the following:

- Depletion of sulfhydryl groups necessary for biotransformation of nitrate to nitric oxide
- Neurohormonal effects (long-term nitrate use is associated with increases in catecholamines, renin, endothelin, and other vasoactive hormones that lead to reflex vasoconstriction)

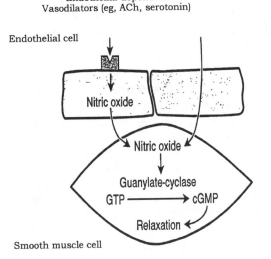

Figure 1.   Mechanism of action of nitrates on vascular smooth muscle cells. ACh = acetylcholine.

- Plasma volume expansion with chronic use
- Formation of superoxide anions that inactivate nitric oxide
- Downregulation of high-affinity receptors

All of these hypotheses are controversial, but it has been established that nitrate-free intervals are effective in preventing or reducing tolerance.[4]

Clinical Use of Nitrates in the Acute Coronary Syndromes

Unstable Angina

Karlberg et al. performed a randomized, double-blind, placebo-controlled study involving 162 patients with unstable angina. Patients received either intravenous nitroglycerin (Perlinguanit, 1 mg/ml, Orion Pharma, Sweden) or placebo. Sublingual nitroglycerin was available to both groups. Fewer patients treated with intravenous nitroglycerin had more than two new attacks of chest pain lasting < 20 minutes or one new attack of chest pain lasting > 20 minutes, despite sublingual nitroglycerin. In addition, fewer patients in the intravenous nitroglycerin group required more than two sublingual tablets.[5] Thus, fewer patients in the intravenous nitroglycerin group had ischemic events compared with placebo.

Intravenous nitroglycerin is particularly well suited to unstable angina because of its short half-life and the feasibility of rapid dose titration. However, other forms of nitroglycerin have been used safely in the treatment of unstable angina. Buccal administration was shown to be as safe and as well tolerated as intravenous administration in a small, randomized study involving 29 patients.[6]

Intravenous glyceryl trinitrate was compared with intravenous diltiazem in a randomized, double-blind trial involving 129 patients with unstable angina. The clinical end-points were development of refractory angina or myocardial infarction. Refractory angina, alone or in combination with myocardial infarction, occurred in significantly fewer patients treated with diltiazem. Refractory angina developed in 6 (10%) of the diltiazem group compared with 17 (28%) of the glyceryl trinitrate group. Refractory angina and myocardial infarction occurred in 9 (15%) vs. 23 (38%) of the diltiazem and glyceryl trinitrate groups, respectively. Over 48 hours, 8 (13%) of the diltiazem group and 18 (30%) of the glyceryl trinitrate group developed refractory angina. Likewise, refractory angina and myocardial infarction were less common in the diltiazem group (12 [20%]) compared with the glyceryl trinitrate group (25 [41%]). The incidence of bradyarrythmias did not differ. Atrioventricular conduction disturbances were more frequent in the diltiazem group but responded to dose reduction or cessation of the infusion.[7] At 1-year follow up, event-free survival was significantly better in the diltiazem group (45%) than the glyceryl trinitrate group (34.4%).[8]

Intravenous nitroglycerin also may be beneficial in the treatment of unstable angina due to restenosis after angioplasty. Doucet et al. randomized 200 patients hospitalized for unstable angina within 6 months after angioplasty (excluding intracoronary stents) and found that refractory angina occurred less often in the nitroglycerin groups than in the placebo and heparin-only groups.[9]

Intravenous nitroglycerin should be considered one of the drugs of choice for the acute phase of unstable angina. Tolerance may develop after 24 hours with recurrence of chest pain. Such patients usually respond to dose increases. Once the patient has been stabilized, intravenous nitroglycerin can be tapered gradually, and intermittent therapy with a longer-acting nitrate can be started about 1–2 hours before discontinuation of the nitrate infusion.[10]

Acute Myocardial Infarction

Many studies of nitrates in patients with acute myocardial infarction have been done over the years, but only a few have been randomized. Nonetheless, nitrates appear to have some beneficial effects.

Symptom Relief

Intravenous nitrates are probably helpful in reducing pain due to myocardial infarction. Lis et al. found that only 22% of patients receiving intravenous nitroglycerin required morphine for pain control compared with 54% of patients receiving placebo.[11] Similarly, Bussman et al. found that 39% of patients receiving intravenous nitroglycerin required morphine for pain control compared with 66% of the placebo group.[12] Jaffe et al, in contrast, found no difference in morphine requirements between the two groups.[1]

Infarct Size

Intravenous nitroglycerin also appears to have favorable effects on infarct size. Three randomized studies demonstrated a reduction in infarct size, as evidenced by the magnitude of creatine kinase (CK) and CK-MB release and/or ST-segment mapping, in patients receiving nitroglycerin.[11–13] Jaffe et al. showed significant reduction in infarct size in patients with inferior myocardial infarctions. A similar but statistically insignificant trend was noted in subendocardial myocardial infarctions. No difference was seen for anterior myocardial infarctions.[1] Flaherty et al. found no overall difference in infarct size, but retrospective analysis revealed a significant reduction in the subgroup of patients with small-to-moderate sized infarctions who were treated within 10 hours of symptom onset.[14]

Ventricular Performance and Remodeling

Nitrates are well known for reducing preload and, to a lesser extent, afterload. Seven randomized studies before 1989 demonstrated that left ventricular filling pressures are reduced with nitrates.[1,11–16] This reduction is thought to decrease left ventricular volume and thereby left ventricular wall stress and oxygen consumption. This effect was particularly beneficial for patients with significantly elevated filling pressures. Transdermal nitroglycerin also was shown to be safe and effective at reducing left ventricular filling pressures in patients with acute myocardial infarction and signs of left ventricular failure.[17] Similarly, transdermal patches were shown to prevent left ventricular dilation in survivors of acute infarction. The beneficial effects were limited to patients with depressed left ventricular function and were seen only at the lowest dose (0.4 mg/hr). Furthermore, continued administration was necessary to maintain efficacy.[18] In a study of 310 patients, Jugdutt and Warnica demonstrated that low-dose intravenous nitroglycerin decreased left ventricular diastolic and systolic dimensions and volumes in anterior and inferior infarctions for up to 1 year. Left ventricular ejection fraction was improved; infarct size, infarct expansion, and left ventricular thinning were limited; and a decrease was seen in cardiogenic shock, congestive heart failure, incidence of left ventricular thrombus, and in-hospital mortality.[15]

Mortality Rates

The effect of nitrates on long-term mortality after myocardial infarction is controversial. Yusuf et al. conducted a meta-analysis of several randomized, placebo-controlled trials involving nitrates for the treatment of acute myocardial infarction before the advent of thrombolytics. Two trials[12,13] showed statistically significant reduction in mortality in patients treated with nitrates. The other trials showed a trend in favor of treatment with nitrates but lacked the power to establish a statistically significant difference. When the trials were combined (over 1,000 patients), a statistically significant reduction in mortality was noted for patients treated with nitrates (20.5% in the control group vs. 12% in the nitrate group). In a prospective, randomized, double-blind, placebo-controlled study of 310 patients, Jugdutt and Warnica demonstrated a reduction in mortality for patients treated with nitrates.[15] This was the largest study of its type prior to the Gruppo Italiano per lo Studio della Streptochinasi nell'Infarto Miocardio (GISSI-3) and International Study of Infarct Survival (ISIS-4).

GISSI-3 involved 19,394 patients with acute myocardial infarction who were randomized within 24 hours of symptom onset. Patients received 6 weeks of oral lisinopril (5-mg initial dose, followed by 10 mg daily) or open control as well as nitrates (intravenously for the first 24 hours followed by transdermal nitroglycerin, 10 mg/day) or open control. Primary outcomes were all-cause mortality and the combined end-point of death plus late clinical congestive heart failure or extensive left ventricular damage (ejection fraction < 35%) without clinical heart failure. Seventy-two percent of patients received thrombolysis, 31% beta blockade, and 84% aspirin. At 6 weeks, there was no statistically significant difference in mortality rate between the open control group and the nitroglycerin group.[19]

ISIS-4 involved 58,050 patients with suspected acute myocardial infarction who were randomized within 24 hours of symptom onset. Treatment comparisons were oral captopril, oral controlled-release mononitrate, and 24 hours of intravenous magnesium. The nitrate arm involved comparison of 1 month of oral controlled-release mononitrate (30 mg initial dose titrated to 60 mg/day) vs. placebo. Seventy percent of patients received thrombolytics and 94% received antiplatelet therapy. However, 60% of the placebo group had also received nitrates during initial hospitalization. Analysis revealed no statistically significant reduction in the overall 5-week mortality rate or in any subgroup receiving mononitrates. Likewise, at 1-year follow up, no statistically significant improvement in mortality rate was noted between nitrates and placebo. The results of GISSI-3 and ISIS-4, given their significant statistical power, do not support the routine use of nitrates in patients with acute myocardial infarction.

Sudden Death

At present, no randomized, placebo-controlled, double-blind trials have evaluated sudden death in patients treated with nitrates. One prospective clinical study involving 1002 patients with healed myocardial infarction demonstrated an increase in cardiac events in patients treated with long-term nitrates.[21] Patients who were admitted to the hospital for acute myocardial infarction and survived the first 7 days were randomly divided into two groups: treatment with nitrates or nontreatment. The mean observation period was 18 ± 19.9 months. Of 621 patients treated with nitrates, 41 (6.6%) experienced cardiac events during the observational period, whereas only 12 of 381 (3.1%) untreated patients had cardiac events (p < 0.05). The increased mortality rate associated with nitrates may have been related to nitrate tolerance, possible rebound, or neurohormonal effects. Limitations of the study include lack of a placebo control arm and the possibility for introducing population selection bias by excluding patients who expired within 7 days of acute myocardial infarction.

Conclusion

Nitrates appear to have a role in the acute coronary syndromes. In patients with unstable angina they can reduce the severity and frequency of angina, but have not been clearly shown to reduce the risks of developing infarction or death. They can reduce ischemic pain as well as decrease left ventricular filling pressures in acute myocardial infarction complicated by congestive heart failure. They also appear to reduce infarct size and to alter favorably left ventricular remodeling. However, the two largest randomized, double-blind, placebo-controlled trials involving nitrates (GISSI-3 and ISIS-4) failed to show a survival benefit compared with placebo in patients treated with nitrates. Thus, current data do not support their routine use in patients with acute myocardial infarction.

References

1. Jaffe AS, et al: Reduction of infarct size in patients with inferior infarction with intravenous glyceryl trinitrate. A randomised study. Br Heart J 49:452–460, 1983.
2. Flaherty JT: Role of nitroglycerin in acute myocardial infarction. Cardiology 76:122–131, 1989.
3. Katzung BG, Chatterjee K: Vasodilators and the treatment of angina pectoris. In Katzung BG (ed): Basic and Clinical Pharmacology. Norwalk, CT, Appleton & Lange, 1989, pp 141–145.
4. Brady PA: Nitrates. In Murphy JG (ed): Mayo Clinic Cardiology Review. Philadelphia, Lippincott Williams, & Wilkins, 2000, pp 1227–1230.
5. Karlberg KE, et al: Intravenous nitroglycerin reduces ischaemia in unstable angina pectoris: A double-blind placebo-controlled study. J Intern Med 243:25–31, 1998.
6. Dellborg M, Gustafsson G, Swedberg K: Buccal versus intravenous nitroglycerin in unstable angina pectoris. Eur J Clin Pharmacol 41:5–9, 1991.
7. Gobel EJ, et al: Randomised, double-blind trial of intravenous diltiazem versus glyceryl trinitrate for unstable angina pectoris. Lancet 346:1653–1657, 1995.
8. Gobel EJ, et al: Long-term follow-up after early intervention with intravenous diltiazem or intravenous nitroglycerin for unstable angina pectoris. Eur Heart J 19:1208–1213, 1998.
9. Doucet S, et al: Randomized trial comparing intravenous nitroglycerin and heparin for treatment of unstable angina secondary to restenosis after coronary artery angioplasty. Circulation 101:955–961, 2000.
10. Thadani U, Opie LH: Nitrates for unstable angina. Cardiovasc Drugs Ther 8:719–726, 1994.
11. Lis Y, et al: A preliminary double-blind study of intravenous nitroglycerin in acute myocardial infarction. Intens Care Med 10:179–184, 1984.
12. Bussmann WD, et al: Reduction of CK and CK-MB indexes of infarct size by intravenous nitroglycerin. Circulation. 63:615–622, 1981.
13. Jugdutt BI, et al: Persistent reduction in left ventricular asynergy in patients with acute myocardial infarction by intravenous infusion of nitroglycerin. Circulation 68:1264–1273, 1983.
14. Flaherty JT, et al: A randomized prospective trial of intravenous nitroglycerin in patients with acute myocardial infarction. Circulation 68:576–588, 1983.
15. Jugdutt BI, Warnica JW: Intravenous nitroglycerin therapy to limit myocardial infarct size, expansion, and complications: Effect of timing, dosage, and infarct location. Circulation 78:906–919, 1988 [published erratum appears in Circulation 79:1151, 1989].
16. Nelson GI, et al: Haemodynamic advantages of isosorbide dinitrate over frusemide in acute heart-failure following myocardial infarction. Lancet i:730–733, 1983.
17. Melandri G, et al: Comparative haemodynamic effects of transdermal vs intravenous nitroglycerin in acute myocardial infarction with elevated pulmonary artery wedge pressure. Eur Heart J 11:649–655, 1990.
18. Mahmarian JJ, et al: Transdermal nitroglycerin patch therapy improves left ventricular function and prevents remodeling after acute myocardial infarction: Results of a multicenter prospective randomized, double-blind, placebo-controlled trial. Circulation 97:2017–2024, 1998.
19. GISSI-3: Effects of lisinopril and transdermal glyceryl trinitrate singly and together on 6-week mortality and ventricular function after acute myocardial infarction. Gruppo Italiano per lo Studio della Sopravvivenza nell'Infarto Miocardico. Lancet 343:1115–1122, 1994.
20. ISIS-4: A randomised factorial trial assessing early oral captopril, oral mononitrate, and intravenous magnesium sulphate in 58,050 patients with suspected acute myocardial infarction. ISIS-4 (Fourth International Study of Infarct Survival) Collaborative Group. Lancet 345:669–685, 1995.
21. Ishikawa K, et al: Long-term nitrate treatment increases cardiac events in patients with healed myocardial infarction. Secondary Prevention Group. Jpn Circ J 60:779–788, 1996.

Antiarrhythmic Therapy in the Management of Acute Coronary Syndromes

MARTIN C. BURKE, DO

MORTON F. ARNSDORF, MD

Sudden cardiac death is the major cause of death in the economically developed world. Cardiac arrest is a persistent clinical problem because of three factors: (1) the inability to predict arrhythmic events, (2) inefficient measurement and maintenance of antiarrhythmic drug levels in the field, and (3) the evolving metabolic substrate of the myocardium. These factors make the immediate and prolonged application of antiarrhythmic medicines a complicated task. Aggressive risk stratification of patients has been attempted to improve survival, but such strategies have been stymied by the transient nature of the acute coronary syndromes. Improving survival in patients with out-of-hospital cardiac arrest requires alternative approaches that improve public response to resuscitation and measures to prevent unstable coronary lesions. This chapter describes up-to-date applications of the available antiarrhythmic armamentarium and defibrillation science in the management of malignant arrhythmia during acute coronary syndromes.

Antiarrhythmic Drug Classification and Pharmacology

Pharmacologic intervention to prevent as well as treat dysrhythmia related to acute coronary syndromes evolved from pharmacologic and device-based therapy or a combination of both by the end of the CAST Trial.[1] Certainly, the conventional antiarrhythmic drugs reduce the probability of hemodynamically compromising ventricular arrhythmias, but they often lead to proarrhythmic effects and, unfortunately, an increase in mortality.[1,2] Investigations during the past 20 years have outlined the efficacy and tolerance of various classes of anti-arrhythmic therapies in the primary and secondary prevention of death and have found less-than-adequate results, even in revascularized patients.[1–10] The poor effects when a drug is taken alone for prophylaxis may indicate that the initial improvements in survival in the peri-infarct/ischemic period may be attributed to the early recognition of dysrhythmia in a critical care unit and application of defibrillation and, often, drug therapy simultaneously.[2,11]

   Contributing to an occasional misapplication of antiarrhythmic drugs is the difficulty in classification encountered by clinical and basic cellular scientists investigating their properties and efficacy. The incongruent and overlapping pharmacologic effects of these medicines invite broad interpretation of their use and benefit. Two classification systems have been widely accepted to accommodate the needs of clinicians and basic researchers. Most clinicians utilize the Singh-Vaughan Williams Classification (Table 1), which evolved in the early 1970s in response to the burgeoning number of antiarrhythmic drugs available for patient use.[12] This classification describes the pharmacologic influences of a medicine on maximal rate (V_{max}) of voltage charge during the cardiac action potential and action potential duration. It also allows a descriptive mechanism that physicians can apply clinically.

   Recently this approach to classification has come under scrutiny, and a large-scale cellular evaluation of individual antiarrhythmic drugs has been developed. The more descriptive Sicilian Gambit Classification system[13] (Fig. 1) allows better delineation of the cell and ion channel properties of each drug, thereby providing a mechanism by which cellular electrophysiologists may conduct more direct ion channel research. This chapter discusses the antiarrhythmic drugs using the Singh-Vaughan Williams system, which is more clinically salient.

Table 1.   Clinical Classifications of Antiarrhythmic Drugs

	Hoffman & Bigger (1971)	Singh & Vaughan Williams (1970)	Singh & Hausworth (1974)	Harrison (1981)	Current Classification
Group I	$\downarrow \dot{V}_{max}$, $\uparrow$ APD (Q, Pa)				
Group II	$0 (\downarrow)\dot{V}_{max}$, $\downarrow$ APD (L, DPH)				
Class I		$\downarrow \dot{V}_{max}$	$\downarrow \dot{V}_{max}$		
Class Ia			$\downarrow \dot{V}_{max}$, $\downarrow$ APD (Q, Pa)		$\downarrow \dot{V}_{max}$ (intermediate time constant) $\uparrow$ APD
Class Ib			$\downarrow \dot{V}_{max}$, $\downarrow$ APD (L, DPH)		$\downarrow \dot{V}_{max}$ (short time constant), $\uparrow$ APD
Class Ic				$\downarrow\downarrow \dot{V}_{max}$	$\downarrow\downarrow \dot{V}_{max}$ (long time constant, little Δ APD
Class II		Antisympathetic	Beta blockers		Beta blockers
Class III		$\uparrow$ APD	$\uparrow$ APD		$\uparrow$ APD
Class IV		Calcium channel blockers	Calcium channel blockers		Calcium channel blockers

V_{max} = maximal rate of voltage of charge during phase of the action potential, APD = action potential duration, Q = quinidine, Pa = procainamide, L = lidocaine, DPH = diphenylhydantoin.
Adapted from Nattel S, Singh BN, Dzau VJ, et al: Antiarrhythmic agents: Mechanisms and classification. In Singh BN, Dzau VJ, Vanhoutte PM (eds): Cardiovascular Pharmacology and Therapeutics. New York, Churchill Livingstone, 1994, pp 249–266.

ANTIARRHYTHMIC DRUG ACTIONS

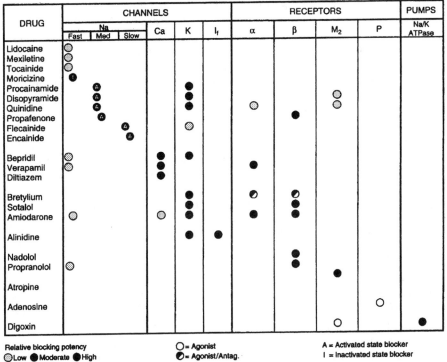

Figure 1.   Sicilian Gambit classification of common antiarrhythmic drugs. (From Task Force of the Working Group on Arrhythmias of the European Society of Cardiology: The Sicilian gambit: A new approach to the classification of antiarrhythmic drugs based on their actions on arrhythmogenic mechanisms. Circulation 84:1831, 1991. Reproduced with permission of the American Heart Association.)

A basic intellectual framework is useful. One of the authors (MFA) has developed the concept of "electrophysiologic matrix" for clinicians. The interested reader is directed to a recent detailed review.[14] In brief, the fundamental premises, based on experimental evidence, are as follows:

1. An electrophysiologic matrix of interacting active and passive cellular properties determines normal cardiac excitability.

2. The normal matrix may be altered by arrhythmogenic influences that affect one or more determinants of excitability, giving rise to a new matrix that may be proarrhythmic and lead to reentrant, automatic, and triggered arrhythmias.

3. The normal matrix deformed by arrhythmogenic influences interacts with antiarrhythmic drugs, forming yet another matrix that may be antiarrhythmic, antifibrillatory, or proarrhythmic. Each of these matrices represents an equilibrium of electrophysiologic properties that is maintained by complex feedback mechanisms.

The electrophysiologic actions of the so-called antiarrhythmic drugs are also complicated. The Sicilian Gambit classification system underscores the multiple effects exerted by the antiarrhythmic drugs, but it has proved to be of little clinical value because of its complexity. Consideration of experimental data in the context of the electrophysiologic matrix, however, has shown that, although a drug usually exerts several effects, the predominant effect depends on the characteristics of the clinical matrix. A given drug may have one predominant effect in a matrix established by the events of ischemia and quite another in a matrix established by hypokalemia.

The arrhythmogenic matrices may be fixed, as in the case of an anatomic substrate, or transient, as with ischemia, autonomic surges, and drug toxicity. A likely explanation of the results of the CAST study is that an underlying fixed anatomic matrix caused by myocardial infarction was responsible for the chronic premature ventricular beats. A new proarrhythmic matrix was established by the introduction of antiarrhythmic drugs into this electrophysiologic event, even though the drugs had suppressed premature ventricular beats during the control period. This new proarrhythmic matrix, in turn, awaited only an additional transient event, such as ischemia or an autonomic surge, to allow initiation of a malignant arrhythmia.[14]

A paradox that, for complicated reasons, one of the authors (MFA) has claimed as his own is that the multiplicities, discontinuities, dynamic interactions, and other complexities in and among the determinants of cardiac excitability should result in unpredictably complex behavior. Yet electrophysiologic events usually are coordinated sufficiently to produce predictable outcomes.[14,15] Order and self-organization can be found in this seeming chaos. The resolution to this paradox lies in the realization that the transition from one matrix or electrophysiologic equilibrium to another moves as a system. Ischemia, for example, causes a rather predictable electrophysiologic matrix in a common clinical setting and results in a rather predictable change when exposed to an antiarrhythmic drug. Thus the Singh-Vaughan Williams system is useful because it reflects the rather reproducible effect of an antiarrhythmic drug on a common and rather reproducible arrhythmogenic matrix.

The antiarrhythmic matrices created by the so-called antiarrhythmic drugs, however, are quite similar to the arrhythmogenic matrices caused by ischemia and other influences.[1,2] The proarrhythmic potential of the antiarrhythmic drugs is thus to be expected.

The multiple electrophysiologic equilibria can be conceptualized as different matrices. One equilibrium changes to another, often explosively, under the influence of pathophysiologic factors. The so-called antiarrhythmic drugs have complicated actions, and the predominant action depends on the electrophysiologic matrix. There is some degree of reproducibility and predictability in the sequence of electrophysiologic events because the electrophysiologic universe moves as a system, which, in turn, makes some drug classification system (such as that of Singh and Vaughan Williams) useful. Although there is self-ordering, it is not perfect. As the CAST study demonstrates, in reality antiarrhythmic drugs that suppressed the index arrhythmias increase the likelihood for sudden death by sensitizing patients to malignant arrhythmias triggered, perhaps, by other transient influences that were not present during the control period. The concept of electrophysiologic matrices helps to explain these highly complicated events.

Antiarrhythmic treatment of patients with life-threatening dysrhythmia in acute as well as chronic coronary syndromes requires obtaining and maintaining effective and safe serum concentrations of a drug. Understanding the drug's route of absorption, bioavailability, and distribution as it relates to the patient's clinical profile and concomitant medications is essential to minimize toxicity and proarrhythmia. In clinical terms, pharmacodynamics or the interaction of a drug with specific patient conditions factors heavily in the choice of antiarrhythmic drug. The patient's age, gender, body mass, volume of distribution, renal and hepatic function, and family and past medical history are part and parcel of everyday pharmacologic management. In other words, the pharmacokinetic properties of a drug are clinically meaningless if one does not account for the pharmacodynamic effects in the individual patient. For instance, the addition of a macrolide antibiotic to a patient already taking a class III antiarrhythmic such as sotalol may result in a markedly prolonged QT interval and torsade de pointes.[16] Oral therapy is quite different and intuitively slower to obtain and maintain effective drug levels in comparison with intravenous delivery. Thus immediate or nearly immediate serum drug concentrations require intravenous bolus and, depending on pharmacokinetics, repeat bolus and maintenance dose infusions.

Two models of distribution are generally considered in determining doses to obtain and maintain adequate serum levels. The one-compartment model is a simple description that matches the dosing amount to the accepting compartment size, taking into account a linear ratio; in other words, as the dose increases, so do the absorption and distribution without consideration, for instance, of first-pass kinetics (Fig. 2). In addition, a one-compartment model does not take into account time of distribution. The two-compartment model allows distribution over time and is therefore a more complicated model. A two-compartment model accounts for an initial central distribution that is

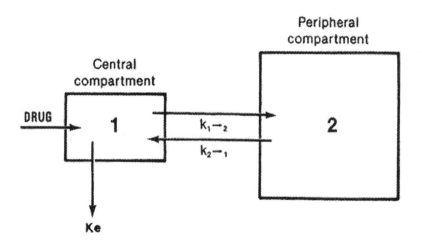

Figure 2. Two-compartment open model of drug distribution and elimination. The smaller central compartment, where the drug is administered and then eliminated, is connected in dynamic equilibrium with the larger peripheral compartment. (From Zipes D: Management of cardiac arrhythmias: Pharmacological, electrical and surgical techniques. In Braunwald's Heart Disease: A Textbook of Cardiovascular Medicine, 4th ed. Philadelphia, W.B. Saunders, 1992, with permission.)

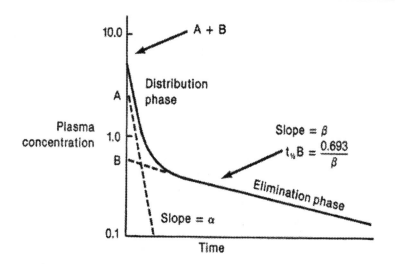

Figure 3. Semilogarithmic plot of drug plasma concentration in a two-compartment open model as a function of time after rapid intravenous injection. (From Zipes DP: Management of cardiac arrhythmias: Pharmacological, electrical and surgical techniques. In Braunwald's Heart Disease: A Textbook of Cardiovascular Medicine, 4th ed. Philadelphia, W.B. Saunders, 1992, with permission.)

either transferred to a peripheral compartment or excreted (Fig. 3). This model separates more efficiently the differences between oral and parenteral intake to predict an expected concentration.[17] Theoretically, either model could be used to deliver antiarrhythmic medicines via a closed-loop infusion device as the clinician computationally enters critical patient data and simultaneously receives serum drug levels at the bedside.

The Case for Antiarrhythmic Prophylaxis

Ventricular fibrillation (VF) in acute transmural myocardial infarction (MI) and the acute coronary syndromes is a sudden arrhythmia (Table 2) that contributes to the majority of sudden cardiac deaths from the earliest onset of symptoms to reperfusion[18] or any time after formation of a remodeled scar.[19] Three categories of VF (20) are generally accepted:

1. Primary VF associated with MI or ischemia in the absence of shock or severe end-stage heart failure
2. Primary VF not associated with MI (poor ejection fraction + coronary disease)
3. Secondary VF in patients in shock or severe end-stage heart failure

Table 2. Potential Cardiac Arrhythmias during Acute Coronary Syndromes

Electrical Instability	Excessive Sympathetic Stimulation	Conduction Disturbances
Ventricular premature beats	Sinus tachycardia	Sinus bradycardia
Ventricular tachycardia	Atrial fibrillation and/or	Junctional escape rhythm
Ventricular fibrillation	atrial flutter	Atrioventricular block and
Accelerated idioventricular rhythm	Paroxysmal supraventricular	intraventricular block
Nonparoxysmal atrioventricular	tachycardia	
junctional tachycardia		

The first category of primary VF has evolved broadly and may be expanded to the ST-segment elevation syndromes of Prinzmetal's variant angina and possibly Brugada syndrome (theorized to be sodium channel-mediated, although a nonepicardial coronary vascular abnormality may contribute to its etiology).[21-23] Why certain patients have a predilection for VF in MI or ST-segment elevation and others with similar clinical presentation do not is largely a mystery. The explanation is probably multifactorial, with infarction and ischemia providing a common denominator.

The true incidence of sustained ventricular tachycardia (VT) in acute coronary syndromes is difficult to pinpoint, although VF is certainly the most common ultimate rhythm in sudden cardiac death associated with MI.[24] Whether monomorphic VT is the initiating arrhythmia is the subject of considerable debate and speculation. VT has been reported as the instigating arrhythmic substrate in 62% of patients with recent or remote MI (n=157).[24] Certainly the outcome in hemodynamically compromising VT is as life-threatening. Reentrant VT is not beyond the pathologic scope of the acutely infarcting myocardium, depending on the timing and amount of tissue damage.[25] Rapid idioventricular rhythm also can result from reperfusion and often indicates a positive effect during the infusion of thrombolytics.[18,26]

Bradyarrhythmia as a result of MI is not uncommon, particularly in patients with inferior and posterior wall involvement.[27,28] Mechanisms of bradycardia in acute MI may involve the conduction bundles directly or abnormally exaggerated neurocardiogenic reflexes (ie., Bezold-Jarisch reflex).[29,30] Acute or acute on chronic infarction of the atrioventricular node or His–Purkinje system is associated with a higher 21-day mortality rate but has not been correlated with the progression of heart block to malignant ventricular arrhythmias.[31] Complete heart block or acute bifascicular block during MI implies a more extensive infarct zone and inadequate collateral blood flow and is a poor prognostic sign; either may signify a greater predisposition to pump failure.[32] The Bezold-Jarisch reflex can be seen in response to acute MI as well as reperfusion of a coronary artery after thrombolytic therapy or coronary intervention.[18] The advent of bradycardia and hypotension in patients suffering an MI often prevents the administration of antiarrhythmic drugs, especially beta blockers.

Predicting Ventricular Fibrillation

Unfortunately, VF is not predictable, although many attempts at correlation with warning signs have been investigated.[33] Frequent ectopy, described and categorized by Lown et al.,[34] was viewed as a harbinger of poor prognosis and ultimately fatal arrhythmia. Over the years, subsequent study has found simple and complex ectopy in a majority of patients suffering MI if they were monitored long enough; certainly it did not correlate with patients who necessarily progressed to ventricular arrhythmia.[35] Signal-averaged electrocardiography (SAEKG), heart rate variability, and, more recently, T-wave alternans technology have been tested for their ability to predict sudden cardiac death but have low sensitivity and specificity in peri-MI patients.[36-38] The best predictors of potential VF in MI are basically related to clinical factors (ST-segment elevation, ejection fraction), time from an index event (first 6 hours), dynamic triggers (ischemia, electrolyte imbalance), and genetic predisposition.[33] Most antiarrhythmic prophylactic regimens take into account the electrocardiographic findings and the onset of infarct symptoms. Timing from the onset of myocardial cell death to remodeling influences the prognosis of peri- and post-MI patients. Early revascularization and reperfusion appear to have a positive influence in decreasing mortality in short- and long-term follow-up through preservation of myocardial muscle mass and function. Nonetheless, predictability remains poor, and frequent arrhythmic deaths have led to many studies to evaluate the effect of the implantable cardioverter defibrillator on mortality (e.g., CABG Patch Trial).

Mechanisms of Fibrillation and Defibrillation

The many mechanisms triggering ventricular fibrillation and ventricular tachycardia are often transient and affected by circulating catecholamines and the autonomic nervous system[39,40] (Table 3). The transient influence of these triggers[39-43] (catecholamines, increased heart rate and oxygen demand, electrolyte imbalance, drug effects, low ejection fraction, and myocardial dilatation) shortens the effective refractory period (ERP) and in the face of ischemia or infarction promotes the development of VF.[40,43,44] The shorter ERP of myocardial cells and tissue is the cellular environment necessary to initiate the arrhythmic reentrant mechanism of VF/VT. The inclusion of genetic predisposition as a potential trigger of VT/VF in coronary artery disease is currently an active area of research and may provide insight into the discrepancy in sudden cardiac death among ischemic patients.[45,46] Pharmacologic and direct-current defibrillatory therapies intervene to prevent and treat VF by prolonging the ERP.[42,43,47]

Marked advances have been seen in defibrillation technology in the past 20 years. The development of better capacitors, shock waveforms, and internal device implantation has decreased mortality due to malignant ventricular arrhythmia in selected populations with coronary and noncoronary artery disease.[48-52] The internal cardioverter defibrillator (ICD) has proved highly effective in the termination of VT/VF with both high- and low-energy defibrillation (10–40 Joules) as well as antitachycardia pacing.[51,52] The engineering advances that have improved defibrillation have used biphasic and low-tilt waveforms with extended trailing edges of energy decay rather than the standard damped sinusoidal or monophasic waveforms during delivery[53-55] (Figs. 4 and 5). These types of waveforms hypothetically increase action-potential ERP

Table 3.   Mechanism of Arrhythmogenesis

Disorders of impulse formation	Disorders of impulse conduction
Automaticity	Block
Normal	Bi- or unidirectional without reentry
Abnormal	Unidirectional with reentry
Triggered activity	Reflection
Early after depolarizations	
Delayed after depolarizations	

Combined disorders
Interactions
Between automatic foci
Between automaticity and conduction

Adapted from Zipes DP: Management of cardiac arrhythmias: Pharmacological, electrical and surgical techniques. In Braunwald's Heart Disease: A Textbook of Cardiovascular Medicine, 4th ed. Philadelphia, W.B. Saunders, 1992, with permission.

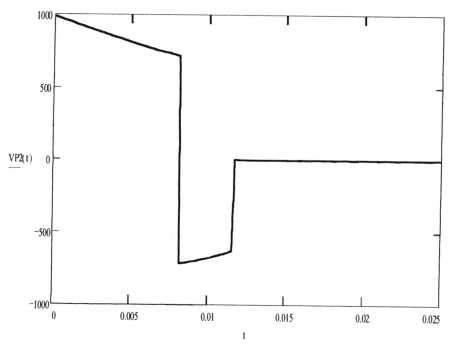

Biphasic Pulse 150 Joules 50 Ohms

Figure 4. Biphasic defibrillation waveform used in both internal and external defibrillators.

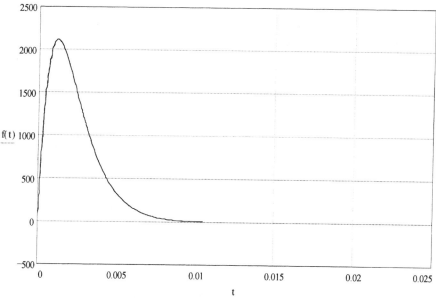

Hewlett-Packard 200 Joule Edmark Waveform

Figure 5. Damped sinusoidal monophasic defibrillation waveform commonly used in external defibrillators.

to a critical mass of ventricular tissue. This effect translates into termination of fibrillation with lower energy and less proarrhythmia.[56,57] Prolongation of ventricular refractoriness is also a common action of most but not all antiarrhythmic drugs. In VF, the application of a transthoracic shock often terminates the arrhythmia and leads to a more viable heart rhythm. The rapid application of defibrillation to the myocardium does not have as reliant an effect on pharmacokinetics, drug distribution, or laws of steady-state chronic delivery as its pharmacologic partner, although the direct cellular effects of defibrillation remain unclear. Some postulates suggest that the late benefits of defibrillation are due to a massive cellular potassium leak after shock delivery, which stabilizes the myocardial cell. Facilitating defibrillation and stabilizing myocardial cells may depend on early interventions and cellular preservation measures (i.e., cryogenics); trials are on the horizon. Automatic external defibrillators (AEDs), using similar sensing algorithms[58] as the internal devices to identify VT/VF, have shown first-shock success rates of defibrillation ranging from 76–93% of out-of-hospital cardiac arrest patients; rates of survival to hospital discharge approach 33%.[59] The external and internal automatic device waveforms have become highly efficacious in terminating VF or cardiac arrest, and survival to hospital discharge certainly will improve with expanded training of first responders and identification of high-risk patients. Clinical trials of defibrillation therapy with ICDs and AEDs, reported and currently on-going, are expanding and defining the communities of patients with acute and chronic coronary syndromes who are most likely to benefit from aggressive technology in both primary and secondary prevention.[60–63]

Managing Acute Coronary Syndromes (ST-segment Elevation, Non–Q-wave Myocardial Infarction, Unstable Angina)

Death from VT/VF occurs in approximately 50% of patients with acute MI before they arrive at a hospital.[64] The risk of primary VF in MI is about 4–18% within the first 4 hours of plaque rupture.[65-66] The problem, especially in larger urban areas, has been that the prolonged time to first shock has resulted in dismal mortality rates in sufferers of acute coronary syndromes and sudden cardiac death.[68,69] New paradigms of intervention in the management of out-of-hospital VT/VF are evolving. Strategies including early response to the detection of symptoms, rapid revascularization, public education about cardiopulmonary resuscitation (CPR), and automatic external defibrillation (AED) are improving survival rates.[70,74] These strategies are applied to reduce the incidence of VF and shorten the time to defibrillation and thus decrease the extent of anoxic encephalopathy. Potent antiarrhythmic therapies have an important role in the creation of efficient and effective delivery (Fig. 6) of these interventions to patients with out-of-hospital or in-hospital MIs.

Out-of-hospital Electrocardiography

Recognition of prehospital symptoms of MI is essential to activate an emergency response. Identifying the arrhythmic substrate of ST-segment elevation (MI, spasm, or Brugada syndrome) in a monitored environment generally leads to nearly immediate reactions with intravenous antiarrhythmic drugs and external cardioversion/defibrillation. Public education has been part of the American Heart Association's mission to improve the chain of survival.[70] Out-of-hospital

Primary ABCD Survey
Focus: Basic CPR and Defibrillation

Check responsiveness
Activate emergency response system
Call for a defibrillator

CHECK   a) **Airway**   b) **Breathing**   c) **Circulation**

DEFIBRILLATION: assess and shock VF/pulseless VT, up to 3 times (200J, 300J, 360J, or equivalent biphasic energy) if indicated.

↓

Assess Rhythm after shocks

↓

VF/pulselessVT Persists

↓

Secondary ABCD Survey
Focus: More advanced assessments and treatments

Place airway device
Confirm airway control
Secure device
Assess and confirm adequate oxygenation and ventilation

Establish IV access
Identify rhythm via monitor
Administer appropriate drugs (Epinephrine 1mg q 3-5 minutes or Vasopressin 40 U IV, single dose, 1 time only)

Search for and treat reversible causes

↓

Resume attempts to defibrillate 360J or biphasic equivalent within 30 – 60 seconds

↓

Consider anti-arrhythmics and buffers
Amiodarone, lidocaine, procainamide, magnesium

↓

Resume attempts to defibrillate

Figure 6. American Hospital Association ACLS Algorithm for Ventricular Fibrillation/Pulseless Ventricular Tachycardia.

12-lead electrocardiographic (EKG) transmission during chest pain to an emergency department by the paramedic on the scene has decreased the time to antiarrhythmic intervention, thrombolytic therapy, primary angioplasty, coronary bypass grafting, and reperfusion,[71–74] which in turn decreases the incidence of primary VF.[74] Canto et al. reported a higher rate of survival to discharge in patients receiving an out-of-hospital EKG compared with patients who did not (92% vs. 88%, p < .001).[74] The recent American Heart Association 2000 guidelines for cardiopulmonary resuscitation and emergency cardiovascular care make the implementation of out-of-hospital EKG diagnostic programs in paramedic systems a class I recommendation.[70]

Automatic External Defibrillation

Training nontraditional emergency responders to apply CPR and AED technology expands public access and responsibility as well as improves the survival rate of patients with out-of-hospital acute coronary syndromes through early defibrillation.[70,75] The AED can be used safely and effectively to resuscitate patients with VF by first responders with minimal training.[70] The Public Access to Defibrillation Trial (PAD Trial)[76] is currently enrolling participants in Canada and the United States. This trial should provide insight into out-of-hospital survival in diverse communities through the use of AEDs by trained nontraditional community responders. The premise for this trial has been the superb outcomes of nontraditional programs (e.g., at airlines and airports) in early defibrillation of patients with primary and secondary VF.[77] Once the patient is resuscitated, application of advanced cardiac life support algorithms[70] and pharmacologic interventions (thrombolytics, beta blockers, lidocaine, and/or amiodarone according to protocol) by traditional emergency medical personnel provides essential stabilizing links during transport to the hospital.

Vaughn Williams Class I Antiarrhythmic Drugs

Historically, prophylactic antiarrhythmic drug administration during acute coronary syndromes has decreased the incidence of VF but has had little effect on mortality.[78,79] The target arrhythmias in these prophylactic deliveries were largely premature ventricular contractions (PVCs) and nonsustained ventricular tachycardia (NSVT) due to acute ischemia/infarction, which results more often from a reentry mechanism and less often from an automaticity mechanism.[80] The mechanism of arrhythmia should affect the selection of antiarrhythmic drug. Lidocaine, an intravenous sodium channel blocker that slows conduction in the ventricular myocardium, diminishes automaticity and may not be the best prophylactic drug during the early stages of acute MI.[81] The prophylactic treatment of PVCs or NSVT in acute MI with lidocaine has been studied extensively in large populations and has been determined to be a nonviable strategy.[82–85] In fact, the preventive use of lidocaine in multivariate analysis is more harmful than beneficial because of proarrhythmic effects.[85] The therapeutic use of lidocaine in acute coronary syndromes should be reserved for patients with sustained, symptomatic, and life-threatening ventricular arrhythmia.[79] The use of lidocaine in reperfusion arrhythmias is not well delineated because of their transient nature and relative hemodynamic tolerance.

The other class Ia antiarrhythmic drugs (procainamide, disopyramide) have not been extensively studied in MI and acute coronary syndromes as either prophylactic or secondary preventive therapy.[79] Procainamide's tolerance in acute MI has been reported, and its suppression of PVCs is well documented.[86] Disopyramide cannot be delivered intravenously and has not been randomly studied as a prophylactic drug during acute MI or unstable angina. In addition, disopyramide is a strong vagolytic with negative inotropic effects that lead to vasoconstriction and poses a problem for patients with congestive heart failure and peripheral vascular disease. The intravenous administration of procainamide should be reserved for patients who have suffered a hemodynamically compromising ventricular arrhythmia, patients in whom lidocaine is contraindicated, or patients who suffer hemodynamically intolerant atrial arrhythmia (i.e., atrial fibrillation) during an acute coronary syndrome. The distribution and pharmacologic properties of procainamide affect both atrial and ventricular cellular function with sodium blockade as well as by increasing the effective refractory period (prolonging the QT interval).[12] Care should be taken in administering procainamide because of its vagolytic and negative inotropic effects with simultaneous vasodilation. The ability to obtain steady-state serum drug levels rather rapidly makes procainamide a useful addition to the pharmacologic management of acute coronary syndromes. Its use should be reserved for patients with clinically serious arrhythmias due to the proarrhythmic side effects, such as torsades de pointes, that occur in up to 4% of patients who are given procainamide.

The CAST Trial[1] attempted to eliminate ectopy in nonrevascularized patients after transmural MI with Vaughan Williams class I drugs, specifically encainide, flecainide, and moricizine. The primary intent was the prophylactic prevention of sudden cardiac death. However, the results of the CAST trial found a significant increase in mortality rate (Fig. 7) in the antiarrhythmic arm compared with the placebo arm in the immediate post-MI period. There has been no significant difference in the effects of the class Ic drugs when given to patients with non–Q-wave or Q-wave MI.[1,87] The outcome was always poor. Obviously class I drugs

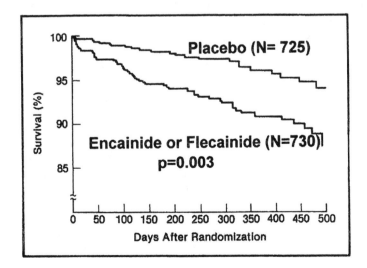

Figure 7. Kaplan-Meier survival curve derived from the CAST Trial. Survival within 1 year of randomization was significantly poor in patients administered the class Ic antiarrhythmic drugs, flecainide and encainide.

exert a detrimental effect on ischemic myocardium and should be avoided at all cost in patients with acute coronary syndrome.[88] Encainide has been removed from the market, and the use of class I antiarrhythmic drugs for prevention of sudden cardiac death or treatment of asymptomatic, benign ectopy is prohibited in patients with coronary artery disease. The results have been so poor for prophylactic antiarrhythmic therapy that the risk profile of the CAST trial has been applied to all patients with structural heart disease. Again, the class I drugs that have been studied were highly effective at suppressing ambient ectopy but also proved extremely proarrhythmic and deadly.

Vaughn Williams Class II Antiarrhythmic Drugs: Beta Blockade

PVCs and NSVT during the onset of the acute coronary syndromes often occur against the background of sinus tachycardia and an increase in catecholamine output.[89,90] This high sympathetic drive naturally led to the administration of beta-adrenergic blockers during the acute phase of evolving infarction/ischemia with impressive results in the suppression of sustained ventricular arrhythmias. However, the clinical power of earlier studies fails to show a significant difference in mortality rate because of the variance in cardiac substrate of the studied populations. Ongoing trials (BEST+ICD, MADIT II, DINIMIT, SCD-HeFT) are designed to compare directly the best medical therapy (beta blockers, angiotensin-converting enzyme [ACE] inhibitors, diuretics, and digoxin) with prophylactic ICDs. These studies include high-risk patients with prior MI and ejection fractions < 0.35 ; the primary endpoint is all-cause mortality. Amiodarone is mandatory or optional in some of these trials (MADIT II, SCD-HeFT and DINIMIT). The primary endpoint of all-cause mortality probably will provide the necessary power in these homogenous populations with coronary artery disease to advance clinical ability to apply the most efficacious therapy in the era of internal defibrillation.

Many randomized beta-blocker trials have demonstrated reduction in mortality rates, improvement in exercise capacity, decrease in infarct size, and overall tolerance in patients with heart failure.[89–92] Recent reports randomly and prospectively compared the effect on mortality of beta blockers and placebo with power and population homogeneity. The first and second International Study of Infarct Survival (ISIS-1 and ISIS-2)[93,94] trials randomized patients with acute MI (ST-segment elevation) within a mean of 5 hours of onset of symptoms to either atenolol or placebo and found a clear benefit in the atenolol group during transmural wall MI. The ISIS-2 trial demonstrated a 15% decrease in mortality rate at 1 week and 1 year. One reinfarction, one cardiac arrest, and one death have been avoided for every 200 patients receiving atenolol during the ISIS-2 trial. The mortality benefit of the beta blocker propranolol in patients with non–Q-wave MI (enzyme-positive, ST depression) is less convincing in the Beta-Blocker Heart Attack Trial (BHAT).[95] Despite a decrease in the incidence of angina in the propranolol group, there was neither a significant lowering of mortality risk nor a decrease in reinfarction rate. Symptomatic relief of angina with beta blockers has been well described in patients with preserved left ventricular function. Intuitively, beta-blocker therapy, when tolerated, has some benefit in all acute coronary syndromes as an antiarrhythmic therapy because of its effect on the extreme catecholamine state (an accepted trigger) with simultaneous decreases in platelet aggregation, myocardial oxygen demand, heart rate, and basal metabolic rate. A beta blocker should be administered (intravenously or orally) as soon as an acute coronary syndrome has been identified, unless it is contraindicated by cardiogenic shock, asthma, impending/present heart block, or hypersensitivity.

Vaughn Williams Class III Antiarrhythmic Drugs

The failure of class I drugs to improve outcome after infarction and ischemia[1] has led to the investigation of antiarrhythmic drugs that effectively block the potassium channels. Most trials have compared the safety and survival benefit of these drugs (usually amiodarone) with the implantation of internal cardioverter defibrillators. The comparison of medical therapy and device therapy has definitively demonstrated benefits to the ICD when the primary and secondary endpoint is mortality.[3,4,61,96] The question of beta blockers in comparison with ICDs is soon to be answered. Of interest, the Survival With ORal D-sotalol (SWORD) Trial[97] compared the pure class III pharmacologic effects of d-sotalol (without the beta blocker effect of d,l-sotalol) with placebo. The patients enrolled had previous MI (Q-wave or non–Q-wave) of either recent or remote occurrence with an ejection fraction of 0.40 or less. The investigators originally planned to randomize 6300 patients but closed the trial at 3121 patients (1549 received d-sotalol; 1572 received placebo) because of a significantly higher mortality in the d-sotalol group (Fig. 8). The patients were evenly matched, and most had a remote history of MI. The high expectations of the pure class III, potassium channel blocker were thwarted by the results of the SWORD trial, which have led to extensive investigations of amiodarone in the primary prevention of sudden cardiac death in patients with coronary artery disease. These results have supported the use of amiodarone in primary prevention trials despite its potential for serious side effects.

The European Myocardial Infarct Amiodarone Trial (EMIAT)[98] and Canadian Amiodarone Myocardial Infarction Arrhythmia Trial (CAMIAT)[9] have studied,

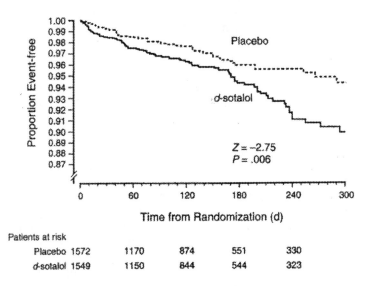

Figure 8. Kaplan-Meier arrhythmic event curve obtained from the SWORD Trial. As is clearly indicated, a significant (p = 0.006) higher event rate occurred in the d-sotalol arm of the trial compared with placebo. Most patients in this study had coronary artery disease.

prospectively and randomly, the primary prevention of mortality in postinfarction patients treated with amiodarone or placebo. EMIAT enrolled post-MI patients with an ejection fraction of no more than 0.40 and no PVCs or NSVT as prerequisites. The primary endpoint was all-cause mortality with secondary endpoints of cardiac death, arrhythmic death, and arrhythmic death plus resuscitated death. Of the original 23,493 evaluated, 1486 patients were randomized. The clinical characteristics were similar between the groups with a mean ejection fraction of 0.30. The primary endpoint of all-cause mortality found no difference between the groups and, therefore, no benefit to amiodarone therapy. The secondary endpoints demonstrated a significant reduction in arrhythmic death plus resuscitated cardiac arrest in the amiodarone group but no significance in arrhythmic death between amiodarone and placebo. Amiodarone failed to demonstrate survival benefit in this large, randomly prospective trial of primary prevention in high-risk patients.

CAMIAT[9] investigated a similar group of patients and compared amiodarone with placebo. However, the statistical setting differed from EMIAT, and CAMIAT investigated different primary and secondary endpoints. The primary endpoint in CAMIAT was resuscitated VF or arrhythmic death. The patients had to have ambient ectopy or nonsustained VT for entry into the trial. The trial reported a one-sided test and significant reduction of resuscitated VF or arrhythmic death in the amiodarone group. Like EMIAT, CAMIAT found no significant difference in the cumulative risk of mortality. There are, however, many weaknesses to the CAMIAT study. The one-sided test of significance assumes that amiodarone can be only neutral or beneficial. Only 56% of the patients in the study had a truly documented Q-wave or non–Q-wave infarct, diagnostic cardiac enzymes, and typical chest pain lasting 20 minutes. Most patients (97%) met the entry requirement of typical chest pain symptoms for longer than 20 minutes. The lack of demonstrable myocardial necrosis may explain the low event rate compared with the EMIAT population. The arrhythmic event rate was especially important because it was the primary endpoint. Finally, differentiating arrhythmic from nonarrhythmic death is extremely difficult, and in the case of CAMIAT the distinction was made weaker by the statistical premise and the low event rate, which suggests a less sick study population. Amiodarone has failed to demonstrate an overall survival benefit even if both EMIAT and CAMIAT are combined in meta-analysis.

Recently amiodarone was compared directly with the ICD in the Multicenter Automatic Defibrillator Implantation Trial (MADIT).[61] This trial enrolled a high-risk group to evaluate the best therapy for the primary prevention of all-cause mortality in a coronary artery disease population with ejection fractions ≤ 0.35. Patients were required to have frequent ectopy or NSVT during ambulatory monitoring as well as inducible VT refractory to suppression with procainamide. Of the 196 randomized patients, 95 received an ICD and 101 were placed in the conventional arm (amiodarone was used in 79%). The safety monitoring board closed the study because of the significant reduction in mortality in the ICD group (Fig. 9). Criticisms of MADIT include the failure of the conventional therapy arm to reflect current conventional therapy; only about 50% in both groups received an ACE inhibitor, and the ICD group was administered more beta blockers than the group treated largely with amiodarone. Although the difference in the dosing of the ACE inhibitor was not significant, it was overall low for patients at this level of risk with heart failure. Moreover, amiodarone,

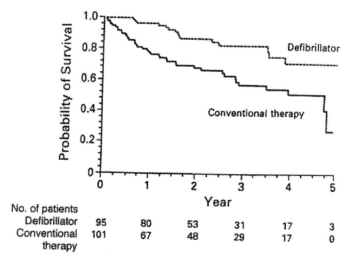

Figure 9. Kaplan-Meier survival curve obtained during the MADIT study demonstrates a significantly better actuarial survival for high-risk patients with inducible ventricular tachycardia and coronary artery disease who were treated with an automatic internal cardioverter defibrillator compared with those treated with conventional medical therapy.

which has never been proved to affect mortality, was substituted for the proven therapy of beta blockade, which has often been associated with better survival rates (see above discussion of Vaughn Williams class II drugs). This trial, although flawed, suggests that in a high-risk group of patients with inducible VT, ICDs improve survival. The clinical significance of MADIT is small because of the selection process in enrollment, but the study provided the lead-off for MADIT-II and SCD-HeFT, which involve a larger preventive population and better defined conventional medical therapy.

Amiodarone also has failed to render better results in secondary prevention trials. The Cardiac Arrest in Seattle: Conventional vs. Amiodarone Drug Evaluation (CASCADE) trial[99–101] enrolled 228 patients (82% with coronary disease) who survived an out-of-hospital resuscitation after VF. The endpoint was all-cause cardiac death, which included repeat out-of-hospital VF resuscitation, sudden arrhythmic death, and nonarrhythmic cardiac death. Patients were randomized to conventional antiarrhythmic drugs vs. amiodarone. If inducible ventricular arrhythmias were not suppressed at electrophysiology testing, crossover to the amiodarone arm of the study was permissible. ICDs were implanted in some patients, mostly after 1988, at the investigator's discretion but were not directly compared with amiodarone or conventional therapy. If patients with an ICD had syncope with shock, they were categorized as having a cardiac arrhythmic event (a primary endpoint). Compared with conventional antiarrhythmic therapy (mostly quinidine and procainamide), amiodarone showed an overall decrease in the primary endpoints: 9–23% at 1 year and 24–44% at 3 years. However, there was still a high event rate in the amiodarone-treated group, and a placebo comparison arm was not available. Amiodarone also demonstrated a high side effect profile, although it was based largely on subjective decision and poor diffusion capacity in routine pulmonary function tests with no clinical correlation.

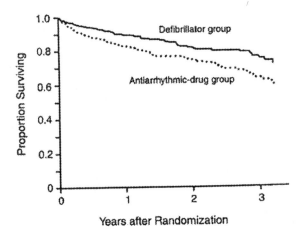

Figure 10.   Kaplan-Meier survival curve of the AVID Trial population demonstrates a significant survival benefit in patients who received an automatic internal cardioverter defibrillator vs. antiarrhythmic drugs, usually amiodarone. Patients presented with life-threatening ventricular arrhythmia before randomization.

The Antiarrhythmics Versus Implantable Device (AVID) trial[3] effectively shut the door on amiodarone and class III antiarrhythmic drugs as efficacious treatments for the secondary prevention of cardiac arrest and VF in a study population with a high rate (80%) of coronary disease and a mean ejection fraction of 0.32. Of 1016 randomized patients, 507 received an ICD and 509 received conventional antiarrhythmic therapy at entry. A class III drug was used in 85% (amiodarone in 70% and sotalol in 15%). The study was closed early because of a statistically significant benefit in survival with an ICD compared with antiarrhythmic drugs (Fig. 10). The study showed that an ICD afforded a relative reduction in mortality rates at 1, 2, and 3 years of actuarial follow up (39%, 27%, and 31%, respectively). AVID, which has withstood statistical criticism, indicates that in such high-risk patients, who present with an arrhythmic event, an ICD is the best therapy to prevent death from an almost inevitable recurrence.

Coronary Revascularization

Revascularization (direct coronary intervention, thrombolytic therapy, and coronary artery bypass surgery) within the initial 6 hours of MI onset decreases the size of the infarction and preserves left ventricular function, thereby affecting acute and remote incidences of sudden cardiac death.[93,94,102–104] The understanding of the pathophysiology of acute coronary syndromes has improved and advanced the therapeutic interventions that act to reverse myocardial cell necrosis. These procedures and pharmacologic applications have been well described throughout this book. Preserving myocardial left ventricular systolic function, as shown in multiple post-MI studies,[5,9,94,102–106] has been the most effective method to decrease arrhythmic events and mortality. The thrombolytic trials, without exception, revolutionized the care of patients with acute coronary syndromes with the addition of aspirin, systemic anticoagulation, and beta blockade.[94,102–104] These trials uniformly decreased mortality from acute MI, particularly larger infarcts, and rendered a better understanding of the natural history of MI. The survival benefits extend from acute hospitalization to more than 1 year after the initial coronary event. Similarly, direct coronary percutaneous transluminal coronary angioplasty (PTCA), when immediately available, produces more complete revascularization and less residual ischemia than thrombolytic therapy.[105-107] However, thrombolytic therapy remains a worldwide choice because of the huge resources necessary from the standpoint of operator availability and physical facilities. The mortality benefits have been as impressive with direct PTCA as with thrombolytic therapy, and PTCA may be the best intervention for acute coronary syndromes complicated by cardiogenic shock.[108]

The Coronary Artery Bypass Graft (CABG)-Patch Trial[109] is the best example of the true benefits of complete revascularization in terms of arrhythmic events and mortality. This trial investigated patients with no prior syncope or documented ventricular tachyarrhythmia, an ejection fraction ≤ 0.35, positive signal-averaged EKG, and need for CABG. The primary endpoint was all-cause mortality. Once meeting the inclusion criteria and consenting to and tolerating the bypass grafting, patients were randomized to receive epicardial defibrillation patches and an ICD or no device therapy (control group). Of the 1422 eligible patients, 1055 consented. After CABG (55% with multiple vessel disease), 900 were randomized. Most patients had suffered a previous MI (83%). The mean ejection fraction was 0.27. The use of a prophylactic ICD did not improve survival rates: 101 deaths had occurred in the ICD group and 95 deaths in the control group at about 3 years of follow–up. Once again, the use of conventional medical therapy, including ACE inhibitors (60%) and beta blockers (20%), was low, given the population's cardiac profile. The results of the CABG-Patch trial illustrate that not all cardiac deaths are due to arrhythmia and that revascularization may improve left ventricular systolic function with better tolerance or suppression of arrhythmia. The ICD group had a 57% incidence of shock within 2 years of implant. Uniform confirmation of arrhythmia was not possible because of the lack of stored electrograms in the earlier-generation devices (ICD group) and little EKG monitoring of the control group.

Conclusion

Survival and suppression of arrhythmia in acute coronary syndromes is best afforded by preventing rupture of the unstable plaque. This daunting task is best achieved by immediate intervention to stabilize the coronary artery, reestablish patency, and preserve left ventricular systolic function, thus reversing the substrate that initiates arrhythmia, specifically VT and VF. Immediately on presentation, the patient should receive beta blockade therapy, either intravenously or orally, if not contraindicated, because of its proven benefit in unstable angina, non–Q-wave MI and ST-segment elevation MI. More potent antiarrhythmic drugs, such as lidocaine, procainamide, and amiodarone, should be reserved for the management of symptomatic and sustained arrhythmias and not administered prophylactically. Remote risk of sudden arrhythmic death must be considered in the aftermath of myocardial necrosis and/or sustained, hemodynamically compromising ventricular arrhythmia. Such patients must be stratified based on the primary and secondary trials described above.

Public intervention, training, and access to automatic external defibrillation and CPR has expanded the community response and had limited success in controlled situations. This type of intervention may or may not have a dramatic impact since approximately 50% of acute coronary patients die before hospitalization. Many ongoing investigations will enlighten and direct our clinical response to the number-one cause of death in the industrial world. This unpredictable and deadly pathophysiology requires a combination of prevention, physician and public education, pharmacology, coronary interventions and device therapy over many years to produce markedly improved outcomes.

References

1. CAST Investigators: Special report: Effect of flecainide and encainide on mortality in the randomized trial of arrhythmia suppression after myocardial infarction. N Engl J Med 321: 406, 1989.
2. Hine LK, Laird N, Hewitt P et al: Meta-analytic evidence against prophylactic use of lidocaine in acute myocardial infarction. Arch Intern Med 321:2694, 1989.
3. AVID Investigators: A comparison of antiarrhythmic drug therapy with implantable defibrillators in patients resuscitated from near-fatal ventricular arrhythmias. N Engl J Med 337: 1576–1583, 1997.
4. Connolly SJ, Gent M, Roberts RS, et al: Canadian implantable defibrillator study (CIDS): A randomized trial of the implantable cardioverter defibrillator against amiodarone. Circulation 101:1297–1302, 2000.
5. ESVEM Investigators: Determinants of predicted efficacy of antiarrhythmic drugs in the electrophysiologic study versus electocardiographic monitoring trial. Circulation 87:323–329,1993.
6. Singh SN, Fletcher RD, Fisher SG, et al: Amiodarone in patients with congestive heart failure and asymptomatic ventricular arrhythmia. N Engl J Med 333: 77–82, 1995.
7. Doval HC, Nul DR, Grancelli HO, et al: Randomized trial of low dose amiodarone in severe heart failure. Lancet 344:493–498, 1994.
8. Amiodarone Trials Meta-analysis Investigators: Effect of prophylactic amiodarone on mortality after acute myocardial infarction and in congestive heart failure: meta-analysis of individual data from 6500 patients in randomized trials. Lancet 350:1417–1424, 1997.
9. Cairns JA, Connolly SJ, Roberts RS, and the CAMIAT Investigators: Randomized trial of outcome after myocardial infarction in patients with frequent or repetitive ventricular premature depolarizations: CAMIAT. Lancet 349:675–682, 1997.
10. Julian DG, Camm AJ, Frangin G, for the EMIAT Investigators: Randomized trial of effect of amiodarone on mortality in patients with left ventricular dysfunction after recent myocardial infarction: EMIAT. Lancet 349:667–674, 1997.
11. Lawrie DN, Higgins MR, Godman MJ, et al: Ventricular fibrillation complicating acute myocardial infarction. Lancet 2:523, 1968.
12. Singh BN, Hauswirth O: Comparative mechanisms of action of antiarrhythmic drugs. Am Heart J 87:367, 1974.
13. Task Force of the Working Group on Antiarrhythmics of the European Society of Cardiology: The Sicilian Gambit: A new approach to the classification of antiarrhythmic drugs based on their actions on arrhythmogenic mechanisms. Circulation 84:1831, 1991.
14. Arnsdorf MF, Makielski JC: Excitability and impulse propagation. In Sperekalis N, Kurachi Y, Terzac A, Cohen MV (eds): Physiology and Pathophysiology of the Heart. 4th edition, chapter 6. New York, Academic Press, 2000, pp 99–132.
15. Arnsdorf MF. Arnsdorf's paradox. J Cardiovascular Electrophysiol 1:42–52, 1990.
16. Jackman WM, Friday KJ, Anderson JL, et al: The long QT syndromes: A critical review, new clinical observations and a unifying hypothesis. Prog Cardiovasc Dis 31(2):115–172, 1988.
17. Zipes DP: Management of cardiac arrhythmias: Pharmacologic, electrical and surgical techniques. In Braunwald E (ed): Heart Disease: A Textbook of Cardiovascular Medicine, vol 1, 4th ed. Philadelphia, W.B. Saunders, 1992, pp 628–666.
18. Goldberg S, Greenspon AJ, Urban PL, et al: Reperfusion arrhythmia: A marker of restoration of antegrade flow during intracoronary thrombolysis for acute myocardial infarction. Am Heart J 105:26–32, 1983.
19. Adgey AAJ, Allen JD, Geddes JS, et al: Acute phase of myocardial infarction. Lancet 2:501–504, 1971.
20. Oliver MF, Julian DG, Donald KW: Problems in evaluating coronary care units: Their responsibility and their relation to the community. Am J Cardiol 20:465–474, 1967.
21. Tzivoni D, Keren A, Granot H, et al: Ventricular fibrillation caused by myocardial reperfusion in Prinzmetal's angina. Am Heart J 105: 323–325, 1983.

22. Brugada J, Brugada R, Brugada P: Right bundle branch block and ST segment elevation in leads V1 through V3: A marker for sudden death in patients without demonstrable structural heart disease. Circulation 97:457–460, 1998.
23. Nademanee K, Veerakul G, Nimmannit S, et al: Arrhythmogenic marker for the sudden unexplained death syndrome in Thai men. Circulation 96: 2595–2600, 1997.
24. Bayes de Luna A, Coumel P, Leclercq JF: Ambulatory sudden cardiac death: Mechanisms of production of fatal arrhythmia on the basis of data from 157 cases. Am Heart J 17:151–159, 1989.
25. Reimer KA, Jennings RB: The 'wavefront' phenomenon of myocardial ischemic cell death. II: Transmural progression of necrosis within the framework of ischemic bed size (myocardium at risk) and collateral flow. Lab Invest 65:161–171, 1980.
26. Balke CW, Kaplinsky E, Michelson EL, et al: Reperfusion ventricular tachyarrhythmias and duration of myocardial ischemia. Am Heart J 101:449–456, 1981.
27. Graner LE, Gershen BJ, Orlando MM, et al: Bradycardia and its complications in the pre-hospital phase of acute myocardial infarction. Am J Cardiol 32:607, 1973.
28. Adgey AA, Alley JD, Geddes JS, et al: Acute phase of myocardial infarction. Lancet 2:501, 1971.
29. Mark AL: The Bezold-Jarisch reflex revisited: Clinical implications of inhibitory reflexes originating in the heart. J Am Coll Cardiol 1:90, 1983.
30. Jarisch A, Zotterman Y: Depressor reflexes from the heart. Acta Physiol Scand 16:31, 1948.
31. Bassan R, Maia IG, Bozza A, et al: Atrioventricular block in acute inferior wall myocardial infarction: Harbinger of associated obstruction of the left anterior descending coronary artery. J Am Coll Cardiol 8:773, 1986.
32. Hindman MC, Wagner GS, JaRo M, et al: The clinical significance of bundle branch block, complicating acute myocardial infarction. I: Clinical characteristics, hospital mortality and one-year follow up. Circulation 58:679, 1978.
33. Myerburg RJ, Interian A Jr, Mitrani RM, et al: Frequency of sudden cardiac death and profiles of risk. Am J Cardiol 80(5B):10F–19F, 1997.
34. Lown B, Calvert AF, Armington R, et al: Monitoring for serious arrhythmias and high risk of sudden death. Circulation 55:189–198, 1975.
35. Gradman AH, Batsford WP, Rieur EC, et al: Ambulatory electrocardiographic correlates of ventricular inducibility during programmed electrical stimulation. J Am Coll Cardiol 5:1087–1093, 1985.
36. Turitto G, Fontaine JM, Ursell S, et al: Value of the signal-averaged electrocardiogram as a predictor of the results of programmed stimulation in the nonsustained ventricular tachycardia. Am J Cardiol 61:1272–1278, 1988.
37. Simson MB: Noninvasive identification of patients at high risk for sudden cardiac death. Circulation 85(Suppl I):I-145–I-151, 1992.
38. Ponikowski P, Anker SD, Chua TP, et al: Depressed heart rate variability as an independent predictor of death in chronic congestive heart failure secondary to ischemic or idiopathic dilated cardiomyopathy. Am J Cardiol 79:1645–1650, 1997.
39. Janse MJ, Wit AL: Electrophysiological mechanisms of ventricular arrhythmias resulting from myocardial ischemia and infarction. Physiol Rev 69:1049–1149, 1989.
40. Kasanuki H, Ohnishi S, Ohtuka M, et al: Idiopathic ventricular fibrillation induced with vagal activity in patients without obvious heart disease Circulation 95:2277–2285, 1997.
41. Schwartz PJ, Priori SG: Sympathetic nervous system and cardiac arrhythmias. In Zipes DP, Jalife J (eds): Cardiac Electrophysiology: From Cell to Bedside. Philadelphia, W.B. Saunders, 1999, pp 330–343.
42. De Ferrari GM, Salvati P, Grossoni M, et al: Pharmacologic modulation of the autonomic nervous system in the prevention of sudden cardiac death: A study with propranolol, methacholine, and oxotremorine in conscious dogs with a healed myocardial infarction. J Am Coll Cardiol 21: 283–290, 1993.
43. Stacy GP Jr, Jobe RL, Taylor K, et al: Stretch-induced depolarizations as a trigger of arrhythmias in isolated canine left ventricles. Am J Physiol 263: H613–H621, 1992.
44. Reiter MJ, Zetelaki Z, Kirchoff CJ, et al: Decrease in ventricular refractoriness due to dilatation is cycle length dependent. Circulation 90:I-519, 1994 [abstract].
45. Evans AE, Poirier O, Kee F, et al: Polymorphisms of the angiotensin-converting-enzyme gene in subjects who die from coronary heart disease. Q J Med 87(4):211–214, 1994.
46. Keating M: Risk, genotype and cardiovascular disease. Circulation 86:688–690, 1992.
47. Zhou X, Daubert JP, Wolf PD, et al: Epicardial mapping of ventricular defibrillation with monophasic and biphasic shocks. Circ Res 72:145–160, 1993.
48. Mirowski M, Reid PR, Mower MM, et al: Clinical performance of the implantable cardioverter-defibrillator. PACE 7:1345, 1984.

49. Mower MM, Reid PR, Watkins L Jr, et al: Automatic implantable cardioverter defibrillator structural characteristics. PACE 7:1331–1337, 1984.
50. Bach S: Engineering aspects of implantable defibrillators. In Saksena S, Goldschlager NF (eds): Electrical Therapy for Cardiac Arrhythmias. Philadelphia, W.B. Saunders, 1990.
51. Winkle RA, Mead H, Ruder MA, et al: Long term outcome with the automatic implantable cardioverter defibrillator. J Am Coll Cardiol 13:1353, 1989.
52. Mitchell JD, Lee R, Garan H, et al: Experience with an implantable tiered therapy device incorporating antitachycardia pacing and cardioverter/defibrillator therapy. J Thorac Cardiovasc Surg 453:105, 1993.
53. Bardy GH, Marchlinski FE, Sharma AD, et al: Multicenter comparison of truncated biphasic shocks and standard damped sine wave monophasic shocks for transthoracic ventricular defibrillation. Circulation 94:2507–2514, 1996.
54. Yamanouchi Y, Brewer JE, Mowrey KA, et al: Sawtooth first phase biphasic defibrillation waveform: A comparison with standard waveform in clinical devices. J Cardiovasc Electrophysiol 8:517–528, 1997.
55. Bardy GH, Gliner BE, Kudenchuk PJ, et al: Truncated biphasic pulses for transthoracic defibrillation. Circulation 91:1768–1774, 1995.
56. Dillon SM, Mehra R: Prolongation of ventricular refractoriness by defibrillation shocks may be due to additional depolarization of the action potential. J Cardiovasc Electrophysiol 3:442–456, 1992.
57. Moubarak JB, Karasik PE, Fletcher RD, et al: High dispersion of ventricular repolarization after an implantable defibrillator shock predicts induction of ventricular fibrillation as well as unsuccessful defibrillation. J Am Coll Cardiol 35:422–427, 2000.
58. Olson WH: Tachyarrhythmia sensing and detection. In Singer I (ed): Implantable Cardioverter-Defibrillator. Armonk, NY, Futura, 1994, pp 71–107.
59. Stiel IG, et al: Improved out of hospital cardiac arrest survival through the inexpensive optimization of an exiting defibrillation program: OPALS study phase II. JAMA 281:1175–1181, 1999.
60. AVID Investigators: A comparison of anti-arrhythmic drug therapy with implantable defibrillators in patients resuscitated from near fatal ventricular arrhythmias. N Engl J Med 337:1576–1583, 1997.
61. Moss AJ, Hall WJ, Cannom DS, et al: Improved survival with an implanted defibrillator in patients with coronary disease at high risk for ventricular arrhythmia. N Engl J Med 335:1933–1940, 1996.
62. Nichol G, Hallstrom AP, Ornato JP, et al: Potential cost-effectiveness of public access defibrillation in the United States. Circulation 97:1315–1320, 1998.
63. Becker L, Eisenberg M, Fahrenbruch C, et al: Public locations of cardiac arrest: Implications for public access defibrillation. Circulation 21:2106–2109, 1998.
64. Kleinman NS, White HD, Ohman EM, et al, for the GUSTO-I Investigators: Global utilization of streptokinase and tissue plasminogen activator for occluded coronary arteries: Mortality within 24 hours of thrombolysis for myocardial infarction. Circulation 90:2658–2665, 1994.
65. Campbell RW, Murray A, Julian DG: Ventricular arrhythmias in first 12 hours of acute myocardial infarction: Natural history study. Br Heart J 146:351–357, 1981.
66. O'Doherty M, Taylor DI, Quinn E, et al: Five hundred patients with myocardial infarction monitored within one hour of symptoms. BMJ 286:1405–1408, 1983.
67. El Sharif N, Myerburg RJ, Sherlag BJ, et al: Electrocardiographic antecedents of primary ventricular fibrillation: Value of the R-on-T phenomenon in myocardial infarction. Br Heart J 38:415–422, 1976.
68. Nichol G, Detsky AS, Stiell IG, et al: Effectiveness of emergency medical services for victims of out of hospital cardiac arrest: A meta-analysis. Ann Emerg Med 27:700–710, 1996.
69. Eisenberg MS, Horwood BT, Cummins RO, et al: Cardiac arrest and resuscitation: A tale of 29 cities. Ann Emerg Med 19:179–186, 1990.
70. Guidelines 2000 for Cardiopulmonary Resuscitation and Emergency Cardiovascular Care: An International Consensus on Science. Part 7: The era of reperfusion. Acute coronary syndromes (acute myocardial infarction). Circulation 102(Suppl I):I-172–I-203, 2000.
71. Kereiakes DJ, Gibler WB, Martin LH, et al: Relative importance of emergency medical system transport and the prehospital electrocardiogram on reducing hospital time delay to therapy for acute myocardial infarction: A preliminary report from the Cincinnati Heart Project. Am Heart J 123:835–840, 1992.
72. Karagounis L, Ipsen SK, Jessop MR, et al: Impact of field transmitted electrocardiography on time to in-hospital thrombolytic therapy in acute myocardial infarction. Am J Cardiol 66:786–791, 1990.

73. Weaver W, Cerqueira M, Hallstrom A, et al: Pre-hospital initiated vs. hospital-initiated thrombolytic therapy: The Myocardial Triage and Intervention Trial (MITI). JAMA 270:1203–1210, 1993.
74. Canto JG, Rogers WJ, Bowlby LJ, et al: National Registry of Myocardial Infarction 2 Investigators: The pre-hospital electrocardiogram in acute myocardial infarction: Is its full potential being realized? J Am Coll Cardiol 29:498–505, 1997.
75. Cummins RO, Eisenberg MS, Litwin PE, et al: Automatic external defibrillators used by emergency medical technicians: A controlled clinical trial. JAMA 257:1605–1610, 1987.
76. Kerber RE, Becker LB, Bourland JD, et al: Automatic external defibrillators for public access defibrillation: Recommendations for specifying and reporting arrhythmia analysis algorithm performance, incorporating new waveforms, and enhancing safety. Circulation 95:1677–1682, 1997.
77. Nichol G, Hallstrom AP, Kerber R, et al: American Heart Association report on the second public access defibrillation conference. Circulation 97:1309–1314, 1998.
78. Koster RW, Dunning J: Intramuscular lidocaine for prevention of lethal arrhythmias in the prehospitalization phase of acute myocardial infarction. N Engl J Med 313:1105, 1985.
79. Josephson ME: Treatment of ventricular arrhythmias after myocardial infarction. Circulation 74:653, 1986.
80. Mehra R, Zeiler RH, Gough WB, et al: Reentrant ventricular arrhythmias in the later myocardial infarction period. IX: Electrophysiologic-anatomic correlation of reentrant circuits. Circulation 67:11, 1983.
81. May GS, Furberg CD, Eberlein KA, et al: Secondary prevention after myocardial infarction. A review of short-term acute phase trials. Prog Cardiovasc Dis 25:335, 1983.
82. Lie KI, Wellens HJ, Van Capelli FJ: Lidocaine in the prevention of primary ventricular fibrillation: A double-blind randomized study of 212 consecutive patients. N Engl J Med 291:1324, 1974.
83. DeSilva RE, Hennekens CH, Lown B, et al: Lidocaine prophylaxis in acute myocardial infarction: An evaluation of methodology. Lancet 1:855, 1981.
84. Alexander JH, Granger CB, Sadowski ZP, et al: Prophylactic lidocaine use in acute myocardial infarction: Incidence and outcomes from two international trials. Am Heart J 137:799–805, 1999.
85. Sadowski ZP, Alexander JH, Skrabucha B, et al: Multicenter randomized trial and a systematic overview of lidocaine in acute myocardial infarction. Am Heart J 137:792–798, 1999.
86. Kessler KM, Kayden DS, Estes DM, et al: Procainamide pharmaco-kinetics in patients with acute myocardial infarction or congestive heart failure. J Am Coll Cardiol 7:1131, 1986.
87. Akiyama T, Pawitan Y, Greenberg H, et al: Increased risk of death and cardiac arrest from encainide and flecainide in patients after non-Q wave myocardial infarction in the cardiac arrhythmia suppression trial. Am J Cardiol 68:1551–1555, 1991.
88. Anderson JL, Platia EV, Hallstrom A, et al: Interaction of baseline characteristics with the hazard of encainide, flecainide and moricizine therapy in patients with myocardial infarction. Circulation 90:2843–2852, 1994.
89. Yusuf S, Sleight P, Rossi P, et al: Reduction of infarct size, arrhythmias and chest pain by early intravenous beta blockade in suspected myocardial infarction. Circulation 67:12, 1983.
90. Hjalmarson A, Herlitz J, Holmberg S, et al: The Goteborg metoprolol trial. Effects on mortality and morbidity in acute myocardial infarction. Circulation 67:26, 1983.
91. Hjalmarson A: Effects of beta blockade on sudden cardiac death during acute myocardial infarction and the post infarction period. Am J Cardiol 80(9B):35J–39J, 1997.
92. Herlitz J, Elmfeldt D, Hjalmarson, et al: Effect of metoprolol on indirect signs of the size and severity of acute myocardial infarction. Am J Cardiol 51:1282–1288, 1983.
93. ISIS-1 (International Study of Infarction Survival) Collaborative Group: Randomized trial of intravenous atenolol among 16,027 cases of suspected acute myocardial infarction. ISIS–1. Lancet 2:57, 1986.
94. ISIS–2. Collaborative Group: Randomized trial of intravenous streptokinase, oral aspirin, both, or neither among 17,187 cases of suspected acute myocardial infarction. ISIS-2. Lancet 2:349, 1988.
95. Gheorghiade M, Schultz L, Tilley B, et al: Effects of propranolol in non Q-wave acute myocardial infarction in the Beta Blocker Heart Attack Trial. Am J Cardiol 66:129–133, 1990.
96. Buxton AE, Lee KL, Fisher JD, et al: A randomized study of the prevention of sudden death in patients with coronary artery disease. N Engl J Med 341:1882–1890, 1999.
97. Waldo AL, Camm AJ, deRuyter H, et al, for the SWORD Investigators: Effect of d-sotalol on mortality in patients with left ventricular dysfunction after recent and remote myocardial infarction. Lancet 348:7–12, 1996.
98. Julian DG, Camm AJ, Frangin G, et al: Randomised trial of effect of amiodarone on mortality in patients with left ventricular dysfunction after recent myocardial infarction: EMIAT. European Myocardial Infarct Amiodarone Trial Investigators. Lancet 349:667–674, 1997.

99. CASCADE Investigators: Randomized antiarrhythmic drug therapy in survivors of cardiac arrest (the CASCADE Study). Am J Cardiol 72:280–287, 1993.
100. CASCADE Investigators: Cardiac Arrest in Seattle: Conventional versus Amiodarone Drug Evaluation (The CASCADE Study). Am J Cardiol 67: 578–584, 1991.
101. Dolack GL, for the CASCADE Investigators: Clinical predictors of implantable cardioverter-defibrillator shocks (results of the CASCADE Trial). Am J Cardiol 73: 237–241, 1994.
102. Gruppo Italiano per lo Studio della Streptochinasi nell'Infarcto Miocardico (GISSI): Effectiveness of intravenous thrombolytic treatment in acute myocardial infarction. Lancet 1:397, 1986.
103. TIMI Study Group: Comparison on invasive and conservative strategies following tissue plasminogen activator in acute myocardial infarction: Results of the thrombolysis in myocardial infarction (TIMI-II) trial. N Engl J Med 320:618, 1989.
104. Roberts R, Rogers RW, Mueller HS, et al: Immediate versus deferred use of beta blockade following thrombolytic therapy in patients with acute myocardial infarction: Results of the thrombolysis in myocardial infarction (TIMI-IIB) Study. Circulation 83:422, 1991.
105. Ellis SG, O'Neill WW, Bates ER, et al: Coronary angioplasty as primary therapy for acute myocardial infarction 6 to 48 hours after symptom onset: report of an initial experience. J Am Coll Cardiol 13:1122, 1989.
106. O'Neill WW, Timmis GC, Bourdillon PD, et al: A prospective randomized clinical trial of intracoronary streptokinase versus coronary angioplasty for acute myocardial infarction. N Engl J Med 314:812, 1986.
107. Ellis SG, Topol EJ, Gallison L, et al: Predictors of success for coronary angioplasty performed for acute myocardial infarction. J Am Coll Cardiol 12:1407, 1988.
108. Verna E, Repetto S, Boscarini M, et al: Emergency coronary angioplasty in patients with severe left ventricular function or cardiogenic shock after acute myocardial infarction. Eur Heart J 10:958, 1989.
109. Bigger JT, for the Coronary Artery Bypass Graft (CABG) Patch Trial Investigators: Prophylactic use of implanted cardiac defibrillators in patients at high risk for ventricular arrhythmias after coronary artery bypass graft surgery. N Engl J Med 337: 1569–1575, 1997.

The Use of Angiotensin-converting Enzyme Inhibitors and Angiotensin Receptor Blockers in the Acute Coronary Syndrome

VENKATESH K. RAMAN, MD

DONALD F. LEON, MD

It has been over 50 years since Hill and colleagues initially demonstrated the interaction between the heart and the renin-angiotensin system (RAS).[1] In the ensuing half-century, our understanding has evolved of both the role of the humoral and so-called tissue RAS in normal and pathophysiologic cardiovascular states and the use of pharmacologic agents (i.e., angiotensin-converting enzyme [ACE] inhibitors and angiotensin receptor blockers [ARBs]) in the treatment of various cardiovascular disorders. This chapter first reviews the current understanding of the RAS and other relevant pathways, including the kinin/kallikrein system, and then examines the clinical literature about the use of ACE inhibitors and ARBs for the acute coronary syndrome (ACS).

The RAS was long viewed as a classical endocrine system, with a dedicated gland secreting substances that traveled through the bloodstream to exert effects at a target organ. In this framework (Fig. 1), angiotensinogen was cleaved by renin to form angiotensin I, which was further metabolized to angiotensin II (Ang II), the end-product octapeptide of the RAS. Ang II, an extremely potent vasoconstrictor, was believed to influence the cardiovascular system via its hemodynamic effects on systemic preload and afterload, in addition to influencing electrolyte balance and volume homeostasis. The emergence in the 1970s and 1980s of experimental evidence documenting the presence of RAS peptides in other tissues, including the heart, and clinical evidence revealing the efficacy of ACE inhibitors in treating hypertensive cardiac hypertrophy and chronic heart failure, despite a dissociation of clinical effectiveness from systemic RAS activity, led to the hypothesis of the existence of separate, "local" tissue RAS.[2,3]

Mounting evidence indicates that Ang II from tissue RAS, particularly in the coronary vasculature and myocardium, plays a central role in the pathogenesis

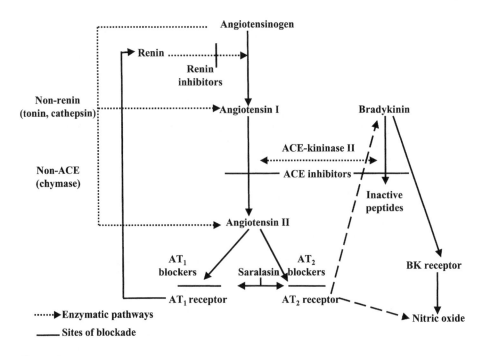

Figure 1. Angiotensin-converting enzyme (ACE) inhibitors block the conversion of angtiotensin I to angiotensin II, a vasoconstrictor. They also block the breakdown of bradykinin to inactive peptides, thus increasing tissue concentrations of bradykinin. Some pathway steps have yet to be characterized, but the final vascular effects include increased nitric oxide production, reduced oxidative stress, and improved endothelial function. (Adapted from Burnier M, Brunner HR: Angiotensin II receptor antagonists. Lancet 355:637–645, 2000.)

of atherosclerosis and ischemic events, primarily by disrupting endothelial function. The normal endothelium is critical to vascular health, and dysfunction of this system is believed to be among the earliest events in the development of atherosclerotic disease. The most important effector of the endothelium is nitric oxide, which exerts a host of vasoprotective effects. It acts as a potent vasorelaxant, inhibits platelet aggregation, and inhibits adhesion of monocytes to the endothelium, an important event in atherogenesis. Most of the known cardiovascular risk factors increase oxidative stress, which effectively reduces nitric oxide production. In this setting, Ang II negatively alters the balance of vascular function by several mechanisms. Ang II is a powerful oxidative stress agent, leading to impairment of endothelial function and setting the stage for atherosclerosis. In addition to powerful vasoconstrictive effects on vascular smooth muscle cells (VSMCs), Ang II also promotes growth and proliferation through activation of growth factors and proto-oncogenes. The balance of hemostasis also can be altered by Ang II via stimulation of plasminogen activator inhibitor-1, which inhibits production of tissue plasminogen activator.[4]

Perhaps more important to acute coronary processes is the kinin/kallikrein system, a companion pathway of the RAS. Bradykinin is a potent stimulus leading to production of nitric oxide and other endothelium-derived vasodilators. ACE is responsible for the metabolism of this compound. By decreasing production of Ang II and breakdown of bradykinin, ACE inhibitors exert significant vasorelaxant, antimitogenic, antithrombotic, and anti-inflammatory effects. ACE inhibitors vary greatly in their ability to bind plasma and tissue ACE. Clinical evidence supports the beneficial effects of such tissue "avid" ACE inhibitors on flow-mediated vasodilatation in coronary and brachial arterial beds.[5,6] It remains to be seen whether this indicator of improved endothelial function translates into better clinical outcomes.

The newer sartanes, or ARBs, also modulate the RAS. These drugs selectively target the Ang II type I (AT-1) receptor, which mediates most of the growth-promoting and proinflammatory effects of Ang II. During chronic ACE inhibition, plasma Ang II levels tend to return to baseline, probably because of Ang II generation by non-ACE pathways, such as chymase. Therefore, ARBs may provide a more complete inhibition of the RAS. Furthermore, this blockade of the AT-1 receptor may allow unopposed stimulation of the Ang II type 2 (AT-2) receptor. Although the physiologic role of AT-2 remains to be fully delineated, it appears to suppress cell growth processes.

With the complementary advances in molecular biology and clinical medicine, our understanding of the RAS and kinin/kallikrein systems continues to evolve. These complex, interrelated systems subserve a number of functions, many of which we have yet to appreciate fully. Within this framework, we can focus on the clinical use of ACE inhibitors and ARBs in the treatment of the acute coronary syndrome.

Unstable Angina

To date, no large, randomized trials have evaluated the use of ACE inhibitors as therapy for patients presenting acutely with unstable angina. The vast majority of clinical data about ACE inhibitors and acute coronary syndromes focuses on acute myocardial infarction (AMI). These trials, to be discussed in the following section, show an unequivocal benefit for the early use of ACE inhibitors in AMI, particularly in high-risk patients, including those with anterior wall involvement and those with left ventricular systolic dysfunction. Because our current understanding of the pathogenesis of the ACS places unstable angina on one end of this spectrum, it stands to reason that ACE inhibitors may be beneficial in unstable angina as well as in AMI.

The most relevant clinical data comes from heart failure and post-MI trials as well as from a more recent primary prevention trial. In the former group is a combined analysis of the treatment and prevention arms of the Study of Left Ventricular Dysfunction (SoLVD) trial,[7] in which 6797 patients with either symptomatic or asymptomatic left ventricular dysfunction were randomly assigned to either enalapril or placebo in two concurrent double-blind trials with a mean follow-up of 40 months. Each trial reported a significant reduction in the number of hospitalizations for unstable angina (RRR = 20%, p < 0.001) as well as in the number of myocardial infarctions (RRR = 23%, p < 0.001) in the combined groups receiving ACE inhibitors compared with placebo. In the Survival and Ventricular Enlargement (SAVE) trial[8] (discussed in greater detail below), post-MI patients with asymptomatic left ventricular systolic dysfunction who were treated with captopril enjoyed a 25% reduction in risk for recurrent myocardial infarction compared with their counterparts receiving placebo (p = 0.015).

Recently published results from the Heart Outcomes Prevention Evaluation Study (HOPE) also provide insight into the role of ACE inhibitors in prevention of coronary events among patients with atherosclerosis.[9] Over 9000 high-risk patients (i.e., patients with known atherosclerotic disease or patients with diabetes and at least one other cardiovascular risk factor but without known heart failure or left ventricular dysfunction) were randomized to either ramipril or placebo for a mean of 5 years. Despite only modest reductions in blood pressure (3 mmHg systolic, 1 mmHg diastolic), the group receiving ramipril had a significant reduction in the combined endpoint of cardiovascular death, MI, or stroke (RR = 0.78, p < 0.001) and in the risk of myocardial infarction (RR = 0.80, p < 0.001). There was no significant difference, however, in the risk of hospitalization for unstable angina (RR = 0.98, p=0.68). The magnitude of the benefits of ACE inhibitors beyond that expected from small changes in hemodynamics indicates the presence of more fundamental mechanisms in modifying the disease process at the level of the vasculature and myocardium. Two additional large trials, EUROPA and PEACE (expected to conclude in 2002 and 2003, respectively) also are designed to address the role of ACE inhibitors in the prevention of ischemic events in patients with established coronary artery disease (CAD). Although the trials to date support the broad use of ACE inhibitors in patients with CAD, there is clearly a need for large-scale, randomized trials to evaluate the use of ACE inhibitors in the treatment of unstable angina. In summary, no clinical data justify the use of ACE inhibitors in the acute phase of unstable angina. However, based on the HOPE trial and others discussed above, it is reasonable, if not fully evidence-based, to use ACE inhibitors in the long-term management of patients with unstable angina.

Myocardial Infarction: Early Initiation, Short-term Use

The ACE-Inhibitor MI Collaborative Group[10] divides trials of ACE inhibitor therapy for AMI into two categories: (1) broad inclusion, early initiation, and short-term treatment and (2) selective inclusion and long-term treatment. The former group includes the CONSENSUS II, GISSI-3, ISIS-4, and CCS-1 studies as well as several smaller trials. In CONSENSUS II, which was the first large trial to assess the short-term effects of ACE inhibition initiated within 24 hours of onset of symptoms of AMI,[11] 6090 patients were randomized to either placebo or enalapril for 6 months. In the group assigned to ACE inhibitor therapy, the first dose was administered as an intravenous infusion, and subsequent doses were given orally. The trial was stopped early, however, because of the high probability that the null hypothesis would apply (i.e., that enalapril was not superior to placebo) and because of concerns for possible adverse effects from hypotensive reactions in elderly patients receiving enalapril. There was no significant difference in the primary endpoint—all-cause mortality at 6 months—between the placebo and enalapril groups (10.2% vs 11.0%, p = 0.26). Analysis of prespecified subgroups, including age ≥ 70 years, female gender, previous MI, and concomitant diabetes or hypertension, also failed to show a benefit for ACE inhibitor treatment.

The results of CONSENSUS II were unexpected, given the promising results of animal studies as well as clinical trials in patients with left ventricular dysfunction. The GISSI-3 study sought to clarify the role of early ACE inhibitor therapy for AMI.[12] Over 19,000 patients were enrolled in the study, which was a multicenter, open trial of 2×2 factorial design to assess the effect of placebo, lisinopril, nitrates, or lisinopril plus nitrates on the primary endpoints of all-cause mortality and the combined endpoint of all-cause mortality plus severe ventricular dysfunction at 6 weeks. Patients with AMI admitted within 24 hours of onset of symptoms were randomized to one of four treatment groups. Those assigned to the ACE inhibitor groups received the drug in oral form and continued treatment for 6 weeks. Patients receiving lisinopril had an 11% lower risk of death compared with controls (6.3% vs. 7.1%, OR = 0.88). Of interest, the survival curves diverged within the first days and continued to separate for the duration of follow-up. As in the CONSENSUS II study, a significant excess of hypotensive episodes was reported in the lisinopril groups, but it was not accompanied by an increase in clinical events.

The promising results of GISSI-3 were confirmed and supported by the much larger and blinded ISIS-4 trial.[13] This study utilized a $2 \times 2 \times 2$ factorial design to assess the efficacy of placebo, captopril, nitrates, and magnesium in nearly 60,000 patients in the acute phase of MI. ACE inhibitors were initiated shortly after randomization, within 24 hours after onset of symptoms, and oral captopril was continued for 1 month. The primary endpoint was all-cause mortality at 5 weeks. The mortality risk was lower in patients assigned to ACE inhibitors complared with placebo (7.19% vs. 7.69%, RRR = 7%). This result corresponds to 5 lives saved per thousand patients treated for 1 month. The benefit of early treatment with captopril was maintained at 1-year follow-up.

The Chinese Cardiac Study (CCS-1) was the last of the large-scale trials to assess the safety and efficacy of early ACE inhibitor therapy for AMI.[14] Over 13,000 patients presenting up to 36 hours from onset of suspected AMI were randomized to captopril or placebo for 1 month. The primary endpoint was mortality at 4 weeks. The nonsignificant reduction in 4-week mortality (9.05% vs. 9.59%, p = 0.3), translated into a comparable reduction of 5 deaths per thousand patients treated.

Recently, the ACE-Inhibitor Myocardial Infarction Collaborative Group published a systematic overview of data from these four large trials, including nearly 100,000 patients.[15] Their analyses revealed a modest but consistent 7% reduction in 30-day mortality. Although the proportional reduction was consistent across a number of subgroups, patients at higher risk for death, such as those with anterior wall involvement, pulmonary edema, or diabetes, enjoyed a greater absolute reduction in mortality. This overview also provided additional insight into the timing of lives saved, revealing that most of the survival benefit conferred by ACE inhibitors occurs within the first week after randomization. Based on this analysis, there are two reasonable strategies for the early, short-term use of ACE inhibitors in AMI. The first involves the early initiation of ACE inhibitor therapy in all patients presenting with AMI without contraindications to treatment (e.g., hypotension, renal failure). A second, more selective approach commits to ACE inhibitors only patients at high risk, such as those with anterior wall involvement, tachycardia, or pulmonary edema. This approach maximizes the number of lives saved while avoiding the risk of hypotensive events or renal failure in the broader population. Long-term management of such patients, however, certainly should entail the use of ACE inhibitors, as supported by the HOPE trial.

Acute Myocardial Infarction:
Long-term Left Ventricular Dysfunction

By the late 1980s and early 1990s, the evidence supporting benefits of ACE inhibitors in patients with left ventricular dysfunction and heart failure was compelling.[16,17] Several studies specifically addressed the use of ACE inhibitors in the population of patients with recent MI and moderate left ventricular systolic dysfunction. This area was of particular concern, given the higher risk of future fatal and nonfatal cardiovascular events in patients who have suffered an MI. Mortality in the post-MI group is a function of several parameters, most importantly left ventricular ejection fraction (LVEF). Small clinical trials[18,19] showing the ability of ACE inhhibitors to prevent post-MI left ventricular dilatation provided the foundation for the larger, long-term SAVE, AIRE and TRACE studies.

The Survival and Ventricular Enlargement Trial (SAVE) was a randomized, double-blind, placebo-controlled study involving patients admitted for AMI with LVEF of 0.40 or less, as assessed by radionuclide ventriculography.[8] Within 3–16 days after an AMI, 2231 of patients without overt heart failure or persistent ischemia were randomized to treatment with either captopril or placebo and followed for an average of 42 months. All-cause mortality was significantly reduced in the captopril group compared with the placebo group (RRR = 19%, p = 0.019). Furthermore, there were significant reductions in cardiovascular mortality (RRR = 21%, p = 0.014), incidence of recurrent MI (RRR = 25%, p = 0.015), and development of severe heart failure (RRR = 37%, p < 0.001).

In the Acute Infarction Ramipril Efficacy Study (AIRE), 2006 patients presenting with AMI complicated by clinical signs of congestive heart failure were randomized between days 3 and 10 to treatment with either ramipril or placebo and followed for an average of 15 months.[20] The group treated with the ACE inhibitor showed a substantial reduction in all-cause mortality compared with those receiving placebo (RRR = 27%, p = 0.002). Unlike the SAVE trial, in which mortality benefits were not observed for 1 year, the AIRE Study revealed mortality benefits by 30 days, with mortality curves continuing to separate for the duration of the trial. There was a trend toward lower reinfarction rates, which did not reach statistical significance, in the ramipril-treated group. This finding may have resulted from the shorter duration of follow-up and, consequently, fewer events in AIRE compared with SAVE.

Of the patients enrolled in the AIRE Study, the 603 recruited from United Kingdom centers continued to be followed for an average of 59 months as part of the AIRE Extension (AIREX) Study,[21] which was undertaken to address duration of benefit and treatment. Patients in the ACE inhibitor group were treated with ramipril for an average of 12 months during the AIRE Study. After cessation of the study, medical management was left entirely to treating physicians; thus, the number of patients subsequently receiving ACE inhibitors was not known. At the end of the additional 3-year follow-up period, analyses revealed persistent mortality benefits in the ACE inhibitor group (RRR = 36%, p = 0.002). The survival curves separated early during AIRE and continued to diverge up to 2 years, running parallel thereafter. These results translate into 114 lives saved at 5 years per 1000 patients treated with ramipril for one year.

The findings of SAVE and AIRE were supported and confirmed by the Trandolapril Cardiac Evaluation (TRACE) Study,[22] in which 2606 patients with

AMI and echocardiographic evidence of left ventricular systolic dysfunction (LVEF < 0.35) (with or without clinical congestive heart failure) were randomized on days 3 through 7 to either trandolapril or placebo for an average of 26 months. As in the trials discussed above, all-cause mortality was reduced significantly in the group treated with trandolapril (RRR = 22%, p = 0.001). The mortality curves separated within the first month and continued to diverge throughout the duration of follow-up. There was also a significant decrease in progression to severe heart failure (RRR = 29%, p = 0.003) as well as a nonsignificant trend toward a reduction in risk of recurrent MI (RRR = 14%, p = 0.29). Of importance, benefits of treatment with trandolapril were observed whether or not clinical heart failure was present. These three trials support unequivocally the long-term use of ACE inhibitors in post-MI patients with left ventricular systolic dysfunction. Combing these results with the broad inclusion trials discussed above, in which patients at greatest risk derived the greatest absolute benefits, it is clear that ACE inhibitors should be initiated early and continued indefinitely in high-risk patients.

Sudden Cardiac Death

Although individual trials have shown a reduction in all-cause and cardiovascular mortality in post-MI patients, they have been too small to reveal any reduction in sudden cardiac death (SCD). To this end, Domanski et al.[23] performed a meta-analysis of 15 trials of ACE inhibitors in over 15,000 post-MI patients. Of the more than 2300 deaths that occurred in these studies, nearly 40% were attributed to SCD. Comparison of the ACE inhibitor- and placebo-treated groups revealed a significant reduction in SCD risk in the group receiving the ACE inhibitor (OR = 0.80, 95% CI = 0.70–0.92). More recent data from the HOPE trial[9] confirmed this beneficial effect. More than 50% of the study population had a history of MI. The group receiving ramipril showed a significant decrease in the risk of cardiac arrest compared with the placebo-treated group (RRR = 38%, p = 0.02). The mechanisms postulated to explain this effect include favorable effects on remodelling and ventricular loading, sympatholysis, potassium-sparing effects (especially in patients treated with diuretics), and, perhaps most importantly, reduction in recurrent ischemic events (given the high incidence of intracoronary thrombus at autopsy in patients dying of SCD). These data support the view that ACE inhibitor therapy may offer secondary prevention benefits with regard to risk of SCD.

Role of Angiotensin Receptor Blockers

Although the efficacy of ARBs in causing regression of left ventricular hypertrophy is becoming clearer, their role in treating heart failure and atherosclerosis is far from established. The generation of Ang II by non-ACE pathways and the postulated beneficial vascular effects of AT-2 receptor stimulation provide the rationale for the interest in ARBs. Promising results from small trials in patients with clinical heart failure await confirmation in larger studies. The Evaluation of Losartan in the Elderly Heart Failure Trial (ELITE), designed primarily to assess the renal safety of losartan in elderly patients with New York Heart Association (NYHA) class II–IV heart failure, randomized 722 ACE inhibitor-naive patients to 48 weeks of treatment with either losartan or captopril.[24] Patients treated with losartan showed a significant reduction in all-cause mortality (RRR = 46%, p = 0.035) and SCD (RRR = 64%) compared with captopril-treated patients. The enthusiasm for these preliminary results was tempered by the presentation of ELITE-II results at the American Heart Association meeting in November 1999.[25] This trial of 3150 older patients with heart failure, randomized to either losartan or captopril with all-cause mortality as the primary endpoint, failed to show superiority of the ARB in reducing mortality, SCD, or other cardiovascular endpoints. Larger studies of ARBs in heart failure are underway to define their role in lieu of or in addition to beta blockers. The Valsartan Heart Failure Trial (Val-HeFT) will compare valsartan plus an ACE inhibitor to placebo plus an ACE inhibitor (in addition to standard heart failure therapy), to determine whether a more complete blockade of the RAS will lead to an improvement in clinical outcomes. This trial of 5000 patients will utilize primary outcome measures of death, worsening heart failure, or a morbid event. The Candesartan Cilexetil in Heart Failure: Reduction in Mortality and Morbidity (CHARM) study, which began in 1999, also will assess combinations of ACE inhibitor and ARB therapy in several heart failure populations. These trials should provide significant insight into a role for the sartanes in heart failure treatment.

As in heart failure, the role for ARBs in acute coronary syndromes remains to be defined. Two large-scale trials are under way to provide answers to this important clinical issue. The Optimal Therapy in Myocardial Infarction with the Ang II Antagonist Losartan (OPTIMAAL) study will evaluate 5000 patients manifesting evidence of heart failure within 10 days of AMI. Patients will be randomized to treatment with either captopril or losartan. This trial, expected to be completed during the first half of 2000, is powered to detect a 20% difference between the two treatments. The other major high-risk, post-MI study is the Valsartan in Myocardial Infarction Trial (VALIANT), which began enrolling patients in 1999 and is expected to reach completion by 2003. In VALIANT, 14,500 patients with AMI, identified as high-risk by evidence of heart failure and/or objective documentation of at least moderate left ventricular dysfunction, will be randomized to one of three arms. In addition to receiving standard therapies, patients will be treated with captopril alone, captopril plus low-dose valsartan, or captopril plus high-dose valsartan. The trial will run until 2700 deaths have occurred in order to detect a 15% difference between treatments. All-cause mortality is the primary endpoint. The results of OPTIMAAL and VALIANT are eagerly awaited to help define the ideal mode of inhibition of the RAS in acute coronary syndromes.

Conclusion

The RAS and kallikrein/kinin systems play an integral part both in normal cardiovascular physiology and in the development and progression of pathologic states. The most convincing proof is the myriad of clinical benefits afforded by the use of ACE inhibitors and by the promise of more effective RAS blockade with ARBs in the management of patients with acute coronary syndromes. Although no evidence supports the use of ACE inhibitors in the acute phase of unstable angina, the HOPE trial and many smaller trials reveal that the broader population of all patients with coronary artery disease may benefit from the long-term use of these drugs. Patients presenting with AMI should receive

ACE inhibitors within 36 hours or once hemodynamic stability is achieved, because the greatest reduction in mortality occurs within the first week after presentation. The clinical literature unequivocally supports the use of long-term ACE inhibitor treatment in high-risk post-MI patients with left ventricular dysfunction, regardless of the presence of heart failure. The role of ACE inhibitor therapy for arrhythmias in patients with acute coronary syndromes appears to be one of prevention. ACE inhibitors are not pharmacologically equivalent. Those with greater potency for inhibiting tissue ACE appear to improve endothelial function. Although the endothelium is central to the pathogenesis of atherosclerotic disease, it remains to be seen whether this surrogate marker is indicative of augmented clinical benefits. Finally, there is not yet an established role for ARBs in the treatment of the acute coronary syndromes; however, several trials currently under way should provide useful insight into this and other issues.

References

1. Hill WHP, Andrus EC: The cardiac factor in the "pressor" effects of renin and antiotonin. J Exp Med 74:91–103, 1941.
2. Dzau VJ: Circulating versus local renin-angiotensin system in cardiovascular homeostasis. Circulation 77(Suppl I):I-4–I-13, 1989.
3. Jin M, Wilhelm MJ, Lang RE, et al: The endogenous tissue renin-angiotensin systems: From molecular biology to therapy. Am J Med 84(Suppl 3A):28–36, 1987.
4. Dzau VJ: Mechanism of protective effects of ACE inhibition on coronary artery disease. Eur Heart J 19(Suppl J):J2–J6, 1998.
5. Mancini GBJ, Henry GC, Macaya C, et al: Angiotensin-converting enzyme inhibition with quinapril improves endothelial vasomotor dysfunction in patients with coronary artery disease: The TREND (Trial on Reversing Endothelial Dysfunction) Study. Circulation 94:258–265, 1996.
6. Anderson TJ, Elstein E, Haber H, Charbonneau F: Comparative study of ACE-inhibition, angiotensin II antagonism, and calcium channel blockade on flow-mediated vasodilation in patients with coronary disease (BANFF study). J Am Coll Cardiol 35:60–66, 2000.
7. Yusuf S, Pepine CJ, Garces C, et al: Effect of enalapril on myocardial infarction and unstable angina in patients with low ejection fractions. Lancet 340:1173–1178, 1992.
8. Pfeffer MA, Braunwald E, Moye LA, et al, on behalf of the SAVE investigators: Effect of captopril on mortality and morbidity in patients with left ventricular dysfunction after myocardial infarction: Results of the Survival and Ventricular Enlargement Trial. N Engl J Med 327:669–677, 1992.
9. Heart Outcomes Prevention Evaluation Study Investigators: Effects of an angiotensin-converting-enzyme inhibitor, ramipril, on cardiovascular events in high-risk patients. N Engl J Med 342:145–153, 2000.
10. Pfeffer MA: ACE inhibitors in acute myocardial infarction: Patient selection and timing. Circulation 97:2192–2194, 1998.
11. Swedberg K, Held P, Kjekshus J, et al, on behalf of the CONSENSUS II Study Group: Effects of the early administration of enalapril on mortality in patients with acute myocardial infarction: Results of the Cooperative New Scandinavian Enalapril Survival Study II (CONSENSUS II). N Engl J Med 327:678–684, 1992.
12. GISSI Investigators: GISSI-3: Effects of lisinopril and transdermal glyceryl trinitrate singly and together on 6-week mortality and ventricular function after acute myocardial infarction. Lancet 343:1115–1122, 1994.
13. ISIS-4 Collaborative Group. ISIS-4: A randomized factorial trial assessing early oral captopril, oral mononitrate, and intravenous magnesium sulphate in 58,050 patients with suspected acute myocardial infarction. Lancet 345:669–685, 1995.
14. Chinese Cardiac Study Collaborative Group: Oral captopril versus placebo among 13,634 patients with suspected acute myocardial infarction: Interim report from the Chinese Cardiac Study (CCS-1). Lancet 345:686–687, 1995.
15. ACE Inhibitor Myocardial Infarction Collaborative Group: Indications for ACE inhibitors in the early treatment of acute myocardial infarction: Systematic overview of individual data from 100,000 patients in randomized trials. Circulation 97:2202–2212, 1998.
16. SOLVD Investigators: Effect of enalapril on survival in patients with reduced ejection fractions and congestive heart failure. N Engl J Med 325:293–302, 1991.

17. CONSENSUS trial study group: Effects of enalapril on mortality in severe congestive heart failure: Results of the Cooperative North Scandinavian Enalapril Survival Study (CONSENSUS). N Engl J Med 316:1529–1535, 1987.
18. Pfeffer MA, Lamas GA, Vaughan DE, et al: Effect of captopril on progressive ventricular dilatation after anterior myocardial infarction. N Engl J Med 319:80–86, 1988.
19. Sharpe N, Murphy J, Smith H, Hannan S: Treatment of patients with symptomless left ventricular dysfunction after myocardial infarction. Lancet 1:255–259, 1988.
20. Acute Infarction Ramipril Efficacy (AIRE) study investigators: Effect of ramipril on mortality and morbidity of survivors of acute myocardial infarction with clinical evidence of heart failure. Lancet 342:821–828, 1993.
21. Hall AS, Murray GD, Ball SG, on behalf of the AIREX study investigators: Follow-up study of patients randomly allocated ramipril or placebo for heart failure after acute myocardial infarction: AIRE Extension (AIREX) Study. Lancet 349:1493–1497, 1997.
22. Kober L, Torp-Pedersen C, Carlsen JE, et al, for the Trancolapril Cardiac Evaluation (TRACE) study group: A clinical trial of the angiotensin-converting-enzyme inhibitor trandolapril in patients with left ventricular dysfunction after myocardial infarction. N Engl J Med 333:1670–1676, 1995.
23. Domanski MJ, Exner DV, Borkowf CB, et al: Effect of angiotensin converting enzyme inhibition on sudden cardiac death in patients following acute myocardial infarction. J Am Coll Cardiol 33:598–604, 1999.
24. Pitt B, Segal R, Martinez FA, Meurers G, et al, on behalf of the ELITE study investigators: Randomised trial of losartan versus captopril in patients over 65 with heart failure (Evaluation of Losartan in the Elderly Study, ELITE). Lancet 349:747–752, 1997.
25. ELITE-II results: presented at the 72nd Scientific Sessions of the American Heart Association, Atlanta, November 7–10, 1999.

Other Pharmacologic Agents for Acute Coronary Syndromes

HENRY DEMOTS, MD

This chapter discusses several pharmacologic and metabolic approaches that are not routinely considered in the management of acute coronary syndromes but may have a role in the future, including anti-inflammatory drugs, the combination of glucose, insulin, and potassium (GIK), and lipid-lowering therapy, especially with an HMG CoA reductase inhibitor (statin). Except for statin drugs, none is mentioned in the practice guidelines recently published by the American College of Cardiology and American Heart Association (ACC/AHA)[1] for management of unstable angina and non–ST-segment elevation myocardial infarction. Nonetheless, these agents have been studied extensively throughout the years.

Anti-inflammatory Agents

The most commonly used anti-inflammatory drug is aspirin, but its use in acute coronary syndromes is predicated on its well-documented antiplatelet activity. Acetylcholine induces the production of vasoconstrictor prostaglandins, and aspirin has been shown to improve the endothelial dysfunction associated with atherosclerosis. Therefore, part of its benefit may relate to factors other than antiplatelet activity.[2] A reduction of acetylcholine-induced vasoconstriction has been demonstrated in patients with heart failure.[3] It is difficult, if not impossible, to separate completely the endothelial effects from the antiplatelet effects in clinical trials, but it is likely that the antiplatelet effects are dominant. At present nonsteroidal anti-inflammatory drugs (NSAIDs) are widely used for a variety of conditions other than coronary artery disease, and their major importance at present relates to their effects when used coincidentally for other conditions.

Although they are not specifically indicated for coronary artery disease, a beneficial effect of anti-inflammatory drugs for patients with coronary artery disease has been postulated throughout the past few decades. Work in the experimental laboratory suggests a role for NSAIDs in acute coronary syndromes.[4] The inflammatory process that attends acute coronary syndromes is known to affect ventricular function in the nonischemic area. This process is attenuated in the experimental setting by anti-inflammatory agents, which may be useful in the management of patients. However, there are continuing concerns about interference with the inflammatory process within the infarcted area because it may be essential to scar formation. Ventricular rupture has been reported in association with use of anti-inflammatory drugs.[5] Most notably, controlled trials using corticosteroids to limit infarct size in the 1970s were terminated early because of an increase in the incidence of myocardial rupture.[6]

Because the outcome for patients depends on a balance between potential positive and negative effects, there is little motivation for a large clinical trial. The use of anti-inflammatory agents cannot be recommended as a specific therapy for acute coronary syndromes. This conclusion leaves open the question of their continued use in patients with acute coronary syndromes and if there are other indications for anti-inflammatory drugs. When NSAIDs are prescribed for arthritis or other inflammatory conditions, it is appropriate to continue the medication because the evidence for their role in myocardial rupture or impaired scar formation is anecdotal and theoretical; it is not based on carefully designed trials.

NSAIDs often are used in the setting of acute coronary syndromes with infarct-related pericarditis. Although no controlled trials have examined these indications, it is widely believed that NSAIDs are useful in reducing the duration and severity of symptoms related to pericarditis. The reports of myocardial rupture raise concerns but do not establish that the incidence is increased by NSAIDs. Careful use of NSAIDs remains an option for pericarditis in acute coronary syndromes, but the preferred agent is aspirin because of its proven benefits in acute coronary syndromes.

Lipid-lowering Therapy

The usefulness of lipid-lowering therapy can be considered in the primary prevention of acute coronary syndromes, the prevention of recurrences of acute coronary syndromes, and the management of the syndrome itself. Although the value of lipid-lowering therapy has been well established in the chronic management of coronary artery disease, physicians do not consider it as readily in patients with acute coronary syndrome. However, if one views the acute coronary syndrome as a dramatic chapter in the continuum of coronary artery disease, lipid management assumes a role in the care of patients with unstable angina or myocardial infarction because it changes their risk profile. The value of lipid-lowering therapy is a function of the patient's future risk.

Primary Prevention of Acute Coronary Syndromes

The West of Scotland Coronary Prevention Study Group (WOSCOPS) used pravastatin, 40 mg/day, to decrease total cholesterol by 20% and low-density lipoprotein (LDL) cholesterol by 26% in patients with a baseline total cholesterol of 272 mg/dl and an LDL cholesterol of 192 mg/dl. The incidence of death or nonfatal myocardial infarction was reduced by 31%.[7]

The Air Force/Texas Coronary Atherosclerosis Prevention Study (AFCAPS/ TexCAPS)[8] examined patients with a lower initial cholesterol. The baseline total cholesterol was 221 mg/dl, and the LDL cholesterol was 150 mg/dl. In this patient population, which included both men and women, the risk of a first major coronary event was decreased by 37%. The trial was terminated prematurely because of the benefit noted in the treatment group. LDL cholesterol was reduced to 115 mg/dl, lending support to more aggressive lipid-lowering therapy.

The two trials establish that reduction in lipids enhances survival and reduces the incidence of acute coronary syndromes in patients without a previous myocardial infarction. A number of trials are currently under way to determine which populations benefit most based on risk profiles. The extent to which clinical trials can determine this issue will always be somewhat limited because coronary artery disease is caused by many risk factors that interact in complex ways.

Secondary Prevention of Acute Coronary Syndromes

Several trials have shown decreased mortality and a decreased incidence of acute coronary syndromes in patients with abnormal lipid profiles, established coronary artery disease, and an acute coronary event. Initial trials included patients with significantly elevated levels of total and LDL cholesterol and high risk status proven by an acute nonfatal event. The Scandinavian Simvastatin Survival Study (4S) studied 4444 patients with hyperlipidemia and acute myocardial infarction. A reduction in total mortality rate was achieved by giving 10–40 mg of simvastatin. Total cholesterol levels were reduced by 25% and LDL cholesterol levels by 35% in the treatment group. The primary endpoint was total mortality, which fell by 30% (p = 0.0003). Similar decreases were found in the combined endpoint of coronary death and myocardial infarction and resuscitated cardiac arrest.

The results of the 4S trial were supported by the work of the Cholesterol and Recurrent Events (CARE) trial,[9] in which 4159 patients with average total cholesterol levels of 209 mg/dl and average LDL cholesterol levels of 139 mg/dl, (considerably lower than in the 4S trial) were randomized to pravastatin or placebo. Pravastatin decreased total cholesterol by 20% and LDL cholesterol by 28%. The reduction in total mortality rate was 22% in this group of patients, who were at lower risk than the 4S study cohort. Similar reductions were found in combined endpoints of fatal coronary artery disease and myocardial infarction (24%) and need for revascularization (27%).

A third secondary prevention trial, the Long Term Intervention with Pravastatin in Ischemic Disease (LIPID),[10] extended the results found in the previous trials by including patients with total cholesterol levels of 218 mg/dl and an average LDL cholesterol of 150 mg/dL. The study included patients who presented without infarction but with unstable angina. Reductions in deaths from coronary artery disease and total mortality were 24% and 22%, respectively. These values reached statistical significance despite a relatively low mortality rate of 1.4% per year in the placebo group. The mean duration of follow-up was 6.1 years.

The Veterans Administration HDL Intervention Trial (HIT) assessed the usefulness of increasing HDL cholesterol in patients with established coronary artery disease and normal LDL cholesterol levels.[11] Gemfibrozil was the chosen agent because it is known to raise HDL cholesterol with modest effects on LDL cholesterol and therefore provided an opportunity to examine the hypothesis that increases in HDL would reduce mortality and morbidity due to coronary artery disease. Treatment with gemfibrozil raised HDL from 32 mg/dl to 34 mg/dl (7%), had no significant effect on LDL cholesterol, and produced a 23% reduction in death or nonfatal myocardial infarction. Confounding the interpretation of the results was a 31% reduction in serum triglycerides (166 vs 115 mg/dl). The study supports the importance of HDL cholesterol as a consideration in deciding whom to treat, a point established in the AFCAPS/TexCAPS study as well, and supports the value of treatment in patients with relatively low LDL cholesterol values, established coronary artery disease, and low HDL levels.

The above studies establish with certainty the efficacy of statin therapy in patients with elevated cholesterol and form the basis for the recommendation by the ACC/AHA expert panel for the treatment at discharge of patients presenting with an acute coronary syndrome. Mortality data from these trials support initiating drug therapy if LDL levels are > 130 mg/dl in patients with coronary artery disease. The expert panel of the National Cholesterol Education Panel[12] designated an LDL level below 100 mg/dl as optimal in patients with known coronary artery disease. Drug therapy is recommended for patients with levels above 130 mg/dl. Many physicians strive to reduce LDL below 100 mg/dl based on trials that use endpoints other than mortality. Clinical trials that explore the impact of more aggressive therapy on mortality rates are currently under way.

The usefulness of statins in the short-term management of acute coronary syndromes has not been examined in randomized or controlled studies. Physicians have not considered their use because lipid management is viewed as a long-term management issue, because the ability to rapidly lower cholesterol values with drugs is limited, and because the measurement of lipid values in the setting of acute illness may not be representative of chronic values.[13]

The major mechanism by which the statins decrease mortality is thought to be lowering of lipid levels. A meta-analysis of major trials concluded that lowering of lipid levels may account for all or nearly all of the reported benefit. However, the trials identified above did not recruit and measure endpoints during the period of coronary insufficiency. Randomization was not allowed prior to 3 months.

Possible mechanisms by which statin may benefit patients with an acute coronary syndrome include an effect on endothelial function,[14–16] changes in platelet function, and anti-inflammatory effects.[17] However, even if these physiologic effects are demonstrated, they may be mediated by changes in lipid concentrations rather than by some other effect of the drug.

Endothelial function has been used as a surrogate for clinical progression of atherosclerosis and the likelihood of acute clinical events. Rapid changes in endothelial function can be demonstrated in patients with high levels of cholesterol who are treated with LDL-apheresis.[18] Theoretically, this approach may be of value in the management of patients with an acute coronary syndrome. The large clinical trials performed to date have specifically excluded patients who presented with an acute coronary syndrome. The addition of LDL-apheresis to other therapies in the setting of an acute coronary syndrome is uncertain and difficult to assess. The high cost is a barrier to testing and implementation in the near future. However, the acute changes observed in endothelial function support the value of testing the use of lipid-lowering therapy in the acute setting.

Pravastatin administered to patients presenting with acute coronary syndromes improved endothelial function at 6 weeks.[19] During this time LDL cholesterol was reduced by 23%. Flow-mediated brachial artery dilation increased by 42%. Because of the correlation between peripheral arterial endothelial function and coronary arterial function, lipid-lowering therapy may be of value in the acute setting. The time course of improvement that can be achieved with pharmacologic therapy is uncertain. Another trial, currently in progress, randomizes patients in the acute setting and may shed light on the value of beginning therapy in the acute setting.[20]

Because it has been established that statin therapy provides benefit by reducing the incidence of recurrent events, it may be prudent to begin statin therapy as a matter of course in all patients who present with an acute coronary syndrome unless it is known that lipid values were low prior to the event. Statin therapy begins a downward course of lipid levels that may be of value in preventing a recurrent event in the months immediately after the acute episode or enhance the likelihood of success with procedures, such as coronary bypass surgery or angioplasty, that may be performed electively. It also ensures that lipid management becomes part of the patient's regimen. Statin therapy can be discontinued or the dosage reduced if subsequent determinations of serum lipid levels indicate that they are not necessary. In one small study, the prescription of a statin drug to patients with an acute coronary syndrome was predictive of mortality across all LDL levels.[21] Routine prescribing of a statin may be the most effective way of ensuring effective management of lipid abnormalities; the number of patients who fail to meet goals for lipid levels remains unacceptably high. Although this approach favors the treatment of all patients who may potentially benefit, the trials performed to date show little difference in survival curves during the first 2 years. Most of the benefit appears from year 3 onward. The value of beginning statin therapy at the time of an acute coronary event may not be evident until a substantial period has elapsed.

The extent to which lipid levels should be lowered is also a matter of ongoing study. The Care Trial[22] demonstrated reductions in mortality of 35% in patients with LDL cholesterol levels of 150–175 mg/dl, a 26% reduction with LDL levels of 125–150 mg/dl, and a 3% reduction with levels < 125 mg/dl. The investigators postulated that decreasing LDL cholesterol below 125 mg/dl offers little or no benefit. In the AVERT study, however, lowering LDL cholesterol to 77 mg/dl vs. 115 mg/dl showed a reduction in the time to next ischemic event in patients with stable coronary artery disease.[23] Ongoing trials will shed more light on the value of this aggressive approach to lipid management.

Glucose-Insulin-Potassium

The combination of glucose, insulin, and potassium (GIK) has been studied intermittently for nearly 40 years but has failed to establish a role in the care of patients with the acute coronary syndromes. Numerous prospective randomized studies have been conducted, but the number of patients included in each trial has been relatively small.

The mechanism of efficacy is not precisely understood. Several possible mechanisms have been postulated. The demonstration that acute myocardial infarction results in a low-flow rather than a zero-flow region of infarction lends credence to the postulated value of GIK because they must enter the infarcted region to produce benefit.[24] Circulating free fatty acids decrease myocardial performance, induce membrane damage, and produce arrhythmias. Free fatty acid levels decrease in response to an infusion of GIK. Some evidence indicates that glycolysis may be enhanced by GIK, although the importance of this finding remains uncertain. It is possible that GIK only slows the development of necrosis and buys time for other interventions. When it was first proposed in 1962, few of the currently available interventions were in use. Thus it is important to study GIK therapy with attention to concurrent treatments such as successful reperfusion. In addition, the dosage required to suppress free fatty acid levels remains uncertain.

A recent meta-analysis included 15 trials examining the role of GIK.[25] The 15 trials that met the criteria for inclusion in the analysis randomized nearly 2000 patients. GIK reduced the mortality rate of acute myocardial infarction from 21% to 16.1% (28%). Despite promising results, GIK has been abandoned because of lack of confidence in the results of the individual trials and possibly because of lack of commercial interest in developing the approach. Each of the 15 trials was relatively small. The mortality rates are the same as those found in the era before reperfusion and beta blockers, the other therapies currently used on a routine basis.

These data provided the impetus for a pilot trial recently reported by Diaz[26] and coworkers in Latin America. Patients were given "usual" medical management and then randomized to high-dose GIK, low-dose GIK, or placebo. The high-dose group received 25% glucose, 50 units of insulin, and 80 mmol of potassium chloride (KCl). The low-dose group received 10% glucose, 20 units of insulin, and 40 mmol of KCl given as an infusion for 24 hours after presentation. The reduction in mortality with GIK (from 11.5% to 6.7%) approached statistical significance. In patients in whom reperfusion was attempted, the difference was a statistically significant decrease from 15.2% to 5.2%. The higher dose of GIK was modestly more effective than the low dose. Complications of therapy (mainly phlebitis) were low.

This pilot trial served as the impetus for a large trial that will enroll 10,000 patients. Despite its impressive difference in survival rates, the pilot trial is limited by the small number of patients and the high mortality rates in the placebo groups. However, if the effectiveness of GIK therapy is validated, it may be a valuable adjunct to current treatments. Possible uses include management during the time required to establish reperfusion either with percutaneous angioplasty or coronary artery bypass surgery. GIK may be useful to emergency medical technicians during transport of patients and to surgeons during operations for acute ischemic conditions. Eventually, studies in each of the clinical circumstances may be required because of the complexity of the various interactions. This complexity includes the importance of reperfusion, the importance of diabetes, and the optimal dose of GIK.

References

1. Committee on the Management of Patients with Unstable Angina: ACC/AHA guidelines for the management of patients with unstable angina and non–ST-segment elevation myocardial infarction J Am College Cardiol 36:970–1056, 2000.
2. Husain S, Andrews NP, Mulcahy D, et al: Aspirin improves endothelial dysfunction in atherosclerosis. Circulation 97:716–720, 1998.
3. Katz SD, Schwarz M, Yuen J, LeJemtel TH: Impaired acetylcholine-mediated vasodilation in patients with congestive heart failure: Role of endothelium-derived vasodilating and vasoconstricting factors. Circulation 88:55–61, 1993.
4. Sulpice T, Boucher F, deLeiris J: Limiting lipid peroxidation in the non-ischemic zone of infarcted rat hearts by indomethacin improves left ventricular function without affecting myocardial healing and remodeling. Am Heart J 131:681–688, 1996.
5. Silverman HS, Pfeiffer MP: Relation between use of anti-inflammatory agents and left ventricular free wall rupture during acute myocardial infarction. Am J Cardiol 59:363–364, 1987.
6. Barzilai D, Plavnick J, Hazani A, et al: Use of hydrocortisone in the treatment of acute myocardial infarction. Summary of a clinical trial in 446 patients. Chest 61:488–491, 1972.

7. West of Scotland Coronary Prevention Study Group: Influence of pravastatin and plasma lipids on clinical events in the West of Scotland Coronary Prevention Study (WOSCOPS). Circulation 97:1440–1445, 1998.

8. Downs JR, Clearfield M, Weis S, et al: Primary prevention of acute coronary events with lovostatin in men and women with average cholesterol levels: Results of AFCAPS/TexCAPS. Air Force/Texas Coronary Atherosclerosis Prevention Study. JAMA 279:1615–1622, 1998.

9. Scandinavian Simvastatin Survival Group: Randomized trial of cholesterol lowering in 4444 patients with coronary heart disease: The Scandinavian Simvastatin Survival Study (4S). Lancet 344:1383–1389, 1994.

10. Long-term Intervention with Pravastatin in Ischaemic Disease (LIPID) Study Group: Prevention of cardiovascular events and death with pravastatin in patients with coronary heart disease and a broad range of initial cholesterol levels. N Engl J Med 339:1349–1357, 1998.

11. Rubins HB, Robins SJ, Collins D, et al, for the Veterans Affairs High-Density Lipoprotein Cholesterol Intervention Trial Study Group: Gemfibrozil for the secondary prevention of coronary heart disease in men with low levels of high-density lipoprotein cholesterol. N Engl J Med 341:410–418, 1999.

12. National Cholesterol Education Program: Second Report of the Expert Panel on Detection, Evaluation, and Treatment of High Blood Cholesterol in Adults (Adult Treatment Panel II). Washington D.C., Department of Health and Human Services, 1993 [NIH Publ. No. 93-3096].

13. Gore JM, Goldberg RJ, Matsumoto AS, et al: Validity of serum total cholesterol level obtained within 24 hours of acute myocardial infarction. Am J Cardiol 54:722–725, 1984.

14. O'Driscoll GO, Green D, Taylor RR: Simvastatin, an HMG-coenzyme A reductase inhibitor, improves endothelial function within one month. Circulation 95:1126–1131, 1997.

15. Anderson TJ, Meredith IT, Yeaung AC, et al: The effect of cholesterol lowering and antioxidant therapy on the coronary endothelium in patients with coronary artery disease. N Engl J Med 332:488–493, 1995.

16. Treasure CB, Klein JL, Weintraub WS, et al: Beneficial effects of cholesterol-lowering therapy on the coronary endothelium in patients with coronary artery disease. N Engl J Med 332:481–487, 1995.

17. Ridker PM, Rifai N, Pfeffer MA, et al: Inflammation, pravastatin, and the risk of coronary events after myocardial infarction in patients with average cholesterol levels. Cholesterol and Recurrent Events (CARE) Investigators. Circulation 98:839–844, 1998.

18. Tamai O, Matsuoka H, Itabe H, et al: LDL apheresis improves endothelium-dependent vasodilation in hypercholesterolemic humans. Circulation 95:76–82, 1997.

19. Dupuis J, Tardif JC, Cernacek P, Theroux P: Cholesterol reduction rapidly improves endothelial function after acute coronary syndromes. The RECIFE (Reduction of Cholesterol in Ischemia and Function of the Endothelium) trial. Circulation 99:3227–3233, 1999.

20. Schwartz GG, Oliver MF, Ezekowitz MD, et al: Rationale and design of the Myocardial Ischemia Reduction with Aggressive Cholesterol Lowering (MIRACL) study that evaluates atorvastatin in unstable angina pectoris and in non-Q wave myocardial infarction. Am J Cardiol 81:578–581, 1998.

21. Muhlestein JB: Post-hospitalization management of high-risk coronary patients. Am J Cardiol 85:13B–20B, 2000.

22. Sacks FM, Pfeffer MA, Moye LA, et al: The effects of pravastatin on coronary events after myocardial infarction in patients with average cholesterol levels. N Engl J Med 335:1001–1009, 1996.

23. Pitt B, Waters D, Brown WV, et al: Aggressive lipid-lowering therapy compared with angioplasty in stable coronary artery disease. N Engl J Med 341:70–76, 1999.

24. Milavetz JJ, Giebel DW, Christian TF, et al: Time to therapy and salvage in myocardial infarction. J Am Coll Cardiol 31:1246–1251, 1998.

25. Fath-Ordoubadi F, Beatt KJ: Glucose-insulin-potassium therapy for treatment of acute myocardial infarction: An overview of randomized placebo-controlled trials. Circulation 96:1152–1156, 1997.

26. Diaz R, Paolasso EC, Peigas LS, et al, on behalf of the ECLA (Estudios Cardiologicos Latinoamerica) Collaborative Group: Metabolic modulation of acute myocardial infarction: The ECLA glucose-insulin-potassium pilot trial. Circulation 98:2227–2234, 1998.

Role of Coronary Angiography in the Evaluation of Patients with Acute Coronary Syndromes

GREGORY J. DEHMER, MD

Selective coronary angiography was first performed in 1957 by Mason Sones, and the angiogram is still considered the gold standard for the evaluation of coronary artery anatomy and pathology.[1] Coronary angiography and newer invasive imaging techniques, such as intravascular ultrasound and angioscopy, have provided considerable insight into the pathophysiology of the acute coronary syndromes. Clinical data from coronary angiography have had a profound effect on the diagnosis and management of ischemic heart disease, and cardiologists have increasingly relied on coronary angiography to guide patient management despite the array of available noninvasive tests. In part, reliance on coronary angiography has been driven by changing therapies for the various acute coronary syndromes—in particular, balloon angioplasty and other percutaneous revascularization techniques. Especially for Q-wave myocardial infarction, treatment over the past 20 years has shifted from a passive approach emphasizing supportive care and management of complications to an active therapeutic approach. Currently it is uncommon to perform coronary angiography during or after myocardial infarction solely for diagnostic purposes. Rather, most procedures are performed to evaluate the patient for a percutaneous or surgical revascularization procedure. Therefore, the appropriateness of performing coronary angiography during or after presentation with an acute coronary syndrome is directly linked to the efficacy of the revascularization procedure as assessed by clinical outcome.

Angiographic Findings in the Acute Coronary Syndromes

As discussed in earlier chapters about the pathophysiology of acute coronary syndromes, we now understand that there is a continuum from the unstable atherosclerotic plaque that frequently is the anatomic basis for the clinical syndrome of unstable angina to the occluded coronary artery initially found in a high percentage of patients presenting with Q-wave myocardial infarction. Many of the initial observations that led to current understanding of the pathophysiology of acute coronary syndromes were derived from coronary angiography.

Coronary Angiography in Unstable Angina

The angiographic findings in unstable angina vary with the population studied and depend on the clinical history and mode of presentation. Of all patients presenting with unstable angina, three-vessel disease is found in approximately 40%, two-vessel disease in about 20%, left main coronary artery disease in 10–20%, single-vessel disease in about 10%, and no critical obstruction in the remaining 10–15%.[2-4] Patients with unstable angina that develops within the context of long-standing stable angina often have multivessel disease, whereas patients who present with a first episode of unstable angina often have disease only in a single coronary artery.[4-7] Approximately one-half of all patients with unstable angina present with this syndrome as the initial manifestation of coronary artery disease. In such patients, the distribution of coronary artery disease is different compared with patients who undergo coronary angiography for chronic stable angina.[3] Patients with a first episode of unstable angina have a higher incidence of single-vessel disease (43% vs. 27%) and a lower incidence of three-vessel disease (23% vs. 35%) and left main disease (5% vs. 10%) compared with patients who have chronic stable angina at the time of coronary angiography.[3,8]

Among the patients initially thought to have unstable angina, 10–15% have no angiographic evidence of coronary atherosclerosis or minimal obstructive disease. In some of these patients, the initial clinical diagnosis may have been incorrect, and their pain syndrome may have some other cause. In the remainder, however, coronary spasm, spontaneous lysis of a coronary thrombus, abnormalities of the microvascular circulation, or a lesion not well-visualized by the angiogram may be responsible.[9] In the TIMI-IIIa trial, patients with ischemic pain at rest underwent coronary angiography within 12 hours of presentation. No luminal diameter stenosis of ≥ 60% was found in 14% of the patients; one-half had no visually detectable coronary stenosis; and the remaining had a noncritical coronary narrowing without morphologic features suggesting an unstable or active coronary plaque. Delayed angiographic filling of the distal artery was present in approximately one-third of the patients without angiographic evidence of a flow-limiting stenosis, suggesting the possibility of coronary microvascular dysfunction.[9] However, because angiography outlines only the arterial lumen, important atherosclerosis that can be detected only by alternative imaging techniques (e.g., intravascular ultrasound) may be present within the arterial wall.[10]

In addition to defining the distribution of disease in patients with unstable angina, coronary angiography has identified certain characteristic morphologic features of the presumed culprit lesion. Correlative studies comparing angiographic and pathologic findings show that an eccentric stenosis with a narrow neck, overhanging edge, or scalloped border corresponds to lesions with plaque rupture or hemorrhage and superimposed partially occlusive or recanalized thrombus.[11-15] In the seminal studies of Ambrose et al., this so called type II eccentric lesion was found in 71% of the presumed culprit arteries in patients with unstable angina compared with only 16% of the arteries from patients with stable angina.[12] In contrast, lesions with concentric, symmetrical narrowing or asymmetrical narrowing with smooth borders and a broad neck are more common in patients with stable angina. In addition, the role of coronary thrombus formation in the pathogenesis of acute coronary syndromes is now well characterized. The angiographic detection of thrombus varies from 6–57% in various series.[16-20] This wide variation in the reporting of coronary thrombus by angiography is related, in part, to the population studied and the definition of thrombus, but the most important factor is the time interval between the last angina attack and the angiographic study. Angiographically evident thrombi are particularly common in patients studied within hours of an episode of angina at rest[16–18, 20–22] (Fig. 1).

More recent observations with angioscopy indicate that coronary mural thrombus is present in nearly all patients with rest angina, even when not detected by angiography.[23] Angioscopy has demonstrated that patients with unstable angina frequently have grayish-white (platelet) thrombi, whereas reddish (fibrin) thrombi are more commonly observed in patients with acute myocardial infarction.[24] Furthermore, occlusive thrombi occur frequently in patients with acute myocardial infarction, but are quite uncommon in patients with unstable angina. Intravascular ultrasound imaging also complements and expands the information derived from angiography. In addition to identifying thrombus more accurately than angiography,[25–27] intravascular ultrasound imaging provides a clinical tool to characterize the underlying morphology of the lesion in

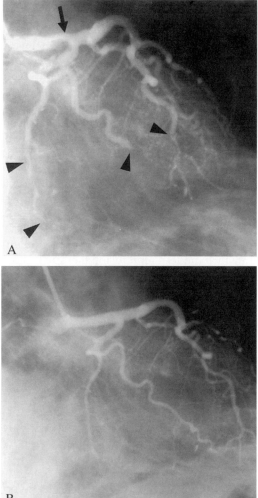

Figure 1. Angiographic demonstration of coronary thrombus with distal embolization. *A,* Right anterior oblique coronary angiogram from a 57-year-old woman who presented with an acute coronary syndrome and ST-segment changes in the anterior and lateral electrocardiographic leads. This angiogram was obtained approximately 8 hours after presentation after the patient had been treated with heparin and a glycoprotein IIb/IIIa inhibitor. An ill-defined narrowing of the left main coronary artery *(arrow)* is present with angiographic evidence of distal embolization into the left anterior descending artery, an obtuse marginal artery, and the distal portion of the circumflex artery *(arrowheads)*. *B,* Coronary angiogram in a similar projection from the same patient after 1 week of therapy with aspirin, ticlopidine, heparin, and a 72-hour infusion of a glycoprotein IIb/IIIa inhibitor. The presumed thrombus in the left main coronary artery has resolved, as has the angiographic evidence of distal embolization.

patients with acute coronary syndromes. Patients with unstable angina have an increased frequency of soft plaque (65% vs. 31%) in the presumed culprit lesion and a lower frequency of plaque calcification (26% vs. 57%) compared with patients with stable angina.[28] In another study of patients with unstable angina, more plaque burden and a higher incidence of plaque thrombus and rupture were found in lesions with adaptive or positive remodeling (compensatory arterial enlargement) than in lesions with constrictive or negative remodeling.[29] The findings of a greater frequency of soft plaque and positive arterial remodeling in unstable angina compared with hard plaque and negative remodeling in stable angina are entirely consistent with the current understanding of the pathophysiology of acute coronary syndromes.[11,30] The former process involves plaque fissuring or ulceration, and often thrombus formation occurs in lesions with only mild luminal narrowing but considerable plaque burden within the arterial wall. Rupture-prone atherosclerotic lesions tend to be relatively soft and cholesterol-rich, with a thin fibrous cap overlying a lipid core. Several studies have indicated this finding as the pathogenic mechanism in most patients presenting with unstable angina or myocardial infarction.[23,31,32] A lipid-rich plaque with associated fresh thrombus is likely to appear soft or echolucent by intracoronary ultrasound. In contrast, stable angina is a slowly progressive process over years, producing advanced fibroatheromatous lesions that may develop focal calcification over time. This appears to be the predominant mechanism of plaque formation in patients presenting with stable angina.

Several studies have shown a correlation between angiographic plaque morphology and clinical status or prognosis. Cardiac events (death, myocardial infarction, and the need for urgent revascularization) are more frequent in patients with coronary thrombus (73%), complex coronary morphology (55%), or multivessel disease (58%) than in patients without these angiographic features (17%, 31%, and 7%, respectively).[33,34] Similarly, intracoronary thrombi were present in 75% of patients requiring urgent coronary arteriography for persistent angina at a later time after admission.[20]

Coronary Angiography in Myocardial Infarction

Coronary angiography has provided many of the pivotal clinical observations on which modern reprefusion therapy is based. The classic angiographic study of DeWood et al. in 1980 not only demonstrated that thrombotic coronary occlusion is the cause of transmural myocardial infarction but also showed the evolution of this process over the next 24 hours.[35] Coronary angiography performed within 4 hours of symptom onset showed coronary occlusion in 87% of patients compared with 65% when angiography was performed 12–24 hours after symptom onset. Subsequent studies during the era of intracoronary streptokinase infusion confirmed this observation with an incidence of coronary occlusion as high as 91% within the first 6 hours.[36–39] Most likely due to spontaneous lysis of the thrombus, the rate of occlusion diminishes during the first month after infarction to 67% between 6 and 24 hours, 53% at 2 weeks, 45% at 4 weeks, 47% at 6–8 weeks, 50% at 6 months, and 46% from 7–12 months after the event[35,40–43] (Fig. 2).

Coronary angiograms in patients who have recently suffered an acute myocardial infarction have been compared with their prior studies, thus providing insight into the coronary artery pathology preceding the infarction. Although severe stenoses certainly may lead to myocardial infarction, in 50–66% of patients, the artery that subsequently occluded had less than 50% stenosis on the

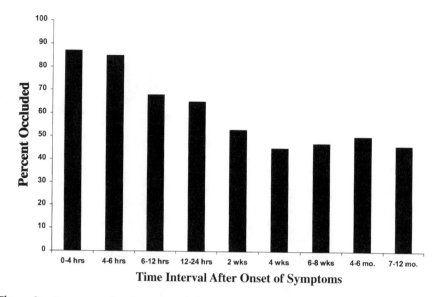

Figure 2. Frequency of total coronary occlusion after the onset of symptoms in acute Q-wave myocardial infarction. The incidence of total occlusion decreases from nearly 90% during the first hours after infarction to approximately 50% by 2 weeks. Thereafter, the incidence of total occlusion remains relatively constant. (Adapted from DeWood MA, Spores J, Notske R, et al: Prevalence of total coronary occlusion during the early hours of transmural myocardial infarction. N Engl J Med 303:897–902, 1980, and deFeyter PJ, van den Brand M, Serruys PW, et al: Early angiography after myocardial infarction: What have we learned? Am Heart J 109:194–199, 1985.)

initial angiogram, and 78–97% of the initial stenoses were less than 70%.[13,44,45] In another study, the risk of myocardial infarction within the next 3 years was related to several angiographic and clinical variables, including percent luminal diameter narrowing and "roughness" of the stenotic surface.[46] Although severity of stenosis was a significant factor, the greatest increase in relative risk for myocardial infarction was found in patients with surface roughness.

In contrast, patients undergoing coronary angiography shortly after suffering a non–Q-wave myocardial infarction have different angiographic findings. In a separate study, DeWood and colleagues examined coronary angiograms from 341 patients suffering a non–Q-wave myocardial infarction within the preceding week.[47] Compared with the high incidence of early coronary occlusion in patients with Q-wave myocardial infarction, the incidence in the entire group with non–Q-wave myocardial infarction was only 32%. Furthermore rather than decreasing over time, the incidence of coronary occlusion increased with passing hours. Patients studied within the first 24 hours had a 26% incidence of total occlusion compared with 42% in patients studied more than 72 hours after their event. The incidence of total occlusion in several other studies ranged from 45% to 79% when coronary angiography was performed relatively late in the clinical course, well after the diagnosis of non–Q-wave myocardial infarction was established.[15,48–51]

In a more contemporary study, Keen et al. performed coronary angiography after the onset of symptoms and before the diagnosis of non–Q-wave infarction was confirmed.[52] Whereas complete occlusion of the presumed culprit artery was present in 91% of patients with Q-wave myocardial infarction, occlusion was present in only 39% of those with non–Q-wave infarction (Fig. 3). Collateral

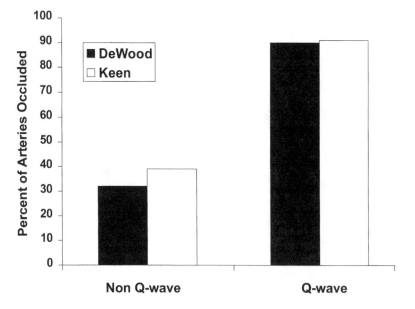

Figure 3.   Frequency of total coronary occlusion within 6 hours after the onset of symptoms in non–Q-wave compared with Q-wave myocardial infarction. The incidence of total occlusion in non–Q-wave myocardial infarction in these two studies was 32% and 39%, whereas the incidence of total occlusion in Q-wave infarction was 90% and 91%. (Adapted from DeWood MA, Spores J, Notske R, et al: Prevalence of total coronary occlusion during the early hours of transmural myocardial infarction. N Engl J Med 303:897–902, 1980; DeWood MA, Stifer WF, Simpson CS, et al: Coronary arteriographic findings soon after non-Q-wave myocardial infarction. N Engl J Med 315:417–423, 1986; and Keen WD, Savage MP, Fischman DL, et al: Comparison of coronary angiographic findings during the first 6 hours of non–Q-wave and Q-wave myocardial infarction. Am J Cardiol 74:324–328, 1994.)

vessels to the infarct-related artery also were found more frequently in patients with non–Q-wave infarction (45% vs. 19%), as was residual perfusion of the infarct related artery (79% vs. 26%) by either anterograde or collateral flow. The angiographic findings in patients with non–Q-wave infarction are congruent with the known clinical course of the disease. Compared with Q-wave infarction, non–Q-wave infarction is associated with lower elevations of the cardiac enzymes, greater preservation of left ventricular function, and an in-hospital mortality rate roughly one-half that of patients with Q-wave myocardial infarction.[49,53–55] Despite their more favorable early outcome, patients with non–Q-wave myocardial infarction have a higher incidence of recurrent myocardial ischemia and infarction and, consequently, a long-term mortality rate that is similar to that of Q-wave myocardial infarction.[55–58] Although the infarct-related artery is usually patent in patients with non–Q-wave infarction, it typically has a complex morphology.[13–15] Therefore, the residual noninfarcted myocardium remains in jeopardy and probably accounts for the higher rate of postinfarction angina and reinfarction in patients with non–Q-wave myocardial infarction.

Coronary Angiography in Survivors of Sudden Cardiac Death

In some circumstances, sudden cardiac death may be a manifestation of an acute coronary syndrome, usually acute myocardial infarction. Ischemic heart disease and its consequences account for at least 80% of sudden cardiac deaths in Western cultures.[59–61] Although sudden cardiac death is the first clinical manifestation of coronary heart disease in approximately 25% of patients with ischemic heart disease, a previous myocardial infarction is identified by some means in up to 75% of patients who die suddenly.[62,63] Although coronary artery disease is the most common underlying pathology in patients with sudden cardiac death, approximately 5% of survivors have no evidence of structural heart disease, and other cardiac etiolgies exist.[64] Therefore, coronary angiography has an important role in the reevaluation of survivors.

The frequency of acute coronary occlusion in survivors of out-of-hospital cardiac arrest ranges from 36% in clinical studies in which coronary angiography was performed late after the event to 95% in series based on autopsies.[61,65] Using current techniques to intervene and treat acute coronary occlusion, Spaulding and colleagues performed immediate coronary angiography in 84 consecutive survivors of out-of-hospital cardiac arrest.[66] The purpose of their study was to determine whether successful coronary intervention affected survival. Clinically significant coronary artery disease was found in 71% of the study group, 8% had insignificant coronary artery disease (< 50% stenosis), and 20% had no coronary disease evident by angiography. Of those with coronary artery disease, two-thirds had a coronary artery occlusion that was judged to be of recent onset. Coronary occlusion prevented characterization of the lesion's morphology, but so-called type II irregular stenoses were found in 90% of the patent coronary vessels. Of note, successful coronary angioplasty was a significant independent predictor of survival in this study.

Lo et al. evaluated stenotic morphology in survivors of cardiac arrest without myocardial infarction.[67,68] Type II irregular stenoses were more prevalent in patients without a demonstrable anatomic or electrophysiologic substrate for reentrant ventricular tachycardia, indirectly implicating ruptured plaque in the pathogeneses of cardiac arrest.

Nonatherosclerotic Causes of Myocardial Infarction and Sudden Cardiac Death

Numerous pathologic processes other than atherosclerosis can affect the coronary arteries and result in myocardial infarction and sudden cardiac death (Table 1). Coronary angiography is an essential diagnostic tool in the evaluation of many of these abnormalities. For example, emboli, most frequently lodging in the distribution of the left anterior descending coronary artery, may result in a coronary occlusion and myocardial infarction.[69,70] The numerous causes of coronary embolism include infective endocarditis, nonbacterial thrombotic endocarditis, mural thrombi, prosthetic valves, and neoplasms. Various inflammatory processes can be responsible for coronary artery abnormalities, some of which mimic atherosclerotic disease, predispose to true atherosclerosis, and cause coronary artery occlusion.[71–75] Therapeutic levels of mediastinal radiation can cause thickening and hyalinization of coronary artery walls, leading to myocardial infarction.[76] Acute myocardial infarction also may result from certain metabolic diseases, such as amyloidosis, Hurler syndrome, and pseudoxanthoma elasticum.[77–79] Cocaine abuse may cause acute myocardial infarction by increasing myocardial oxygen demands or causing coronary artery spasm or coronary thrombosis.[80–84] Finally, in about 6% of all patients suffering an acute myocardial infarction, coronary atherosclerosis is not found by coronary angiography or at autopsy.[35,41,85] In patients under 35

Table 1.   Myocardial Infarction and Sudden Cardiac Death Without Coronary Atherosclerosis

Myocardial infarction
Coronary artery diseases other than atherosclerosis
  Arteritis
    Luetic, granulomatous (Takayasu disease), polyarteritis nodosa, mucocutaneous lymph node
    (Kawasaki) syndrome, disseminated lupus erythematosus, rheumatoid arthritis, ankylosing
    spondylitis
  Trauma to coronary arteries
    Laceration, thrombosis, iatrogenic
  Coronary mural thickening from metabolic or intimal proliferative diseases
    Mucopolysaccharidoses (Hurler disease), Fabry disease, amyloidosis, juvenile intimal sclerosis
    (idiopathic arterial calcification of infancy), pseudoxanthoma elasticum, coronary fibrosis after
    radiation therapy
  Luminal narrowing by other mechanisms
    Dissection of the aorta, spontaneous dissection of a coronary artery, coronary artery spasm
    (Prinzmetal angina or nitrate withdrawal)
Emboli to coronary arteries
  Infective endocarditis, mural thrombus from left atrium, left ventricle or pulmonary veins,
  prosthetic valve emboli, nonbacterial thrombotic endocarditis, mitral valve prolapse, cardiac
  myxoma, paradoxical emboli, papillary fibroelastoma of aortic valve, iatrogenic associated with
  cardiopulmonary bypass or invasive cardiac procedures
Congenital anomalies of the coronary arteries
  Anomalous origin of the left coronary artery from the pulmonary artery, left coronary artery from
  right or noncoronary sinus of Valsalva, coronary arteriovenous or arteriocameral fistulas, coronary
  artery aneurysms
Myocardial oxygen supply-demand disproportion
  Aortic stenosis, aortic insufficiency, carbon monoxide poisoning, thyrotoxicosis, prolonged
  hypotension
Hematologic disorders
  Polycythemia vera, thrombocytosis, disseminated intravascular coagulation, hypercoagulability
  syndromes, thrombocytopenic purpura

Sudden death
Diseases of the coronary arteries
  Congenital anomalies, coronary artery spasm, coronary embolism, spontaneous coronary
  dissection, coronary trauma, arteritis
Myocardial diseases
  Valvular heart disease, cardiomyopathy (dilated, hypertrophic), arrhythmogenic right ventricular
  dysplasia, congenital heart disease, infiltrative diseases of the myocardium (tumor, amyloidosis,
  hemochromatosis), myocarditis
Electrophysiologic disorders
  Long QT syndromes, idiopathic ventricular tachycardia, preexcitation syndromes, conduction
  system disorders

Adapted from Cheitlin MD, McAllister HA, de Castro CM: Myocardial infarction without atherosclerosis. JAMA 231:951–959, 1975, and DiMarco JP, Haines DE: Sudden cardiac death. Curr Probl
Cardiol 15:183–232, 1990.

years of age, this percentage is even greater. Possible causes include coronary
artery spasm, transient thrombosis overlying minimal coronary atherosclerosis
not apparent by angiography, coronary emboli, and various rare conditions
listed in Table 1. In this situation, coronary angiography provides important
prognostic information. The long-term outlook for such patients is considerably better than for those with underlying coronary artery disease.[86]

Certain congenital abnormalities of the coronary arteries are of particular interest because they may present as an episode of sudden cardiac death.
Coronary angiography is required for a definitive diagnosis of these anomalies.[87–89] One of the congenital lesions most relevant to the adult population is

anomalous origin of the left coronary artery from the right (anterior) or non-coronary sinus of Valsalva.[90-92] When the left main coronary artery arises from the anterior sinus, it runs leftward, passing between the aorta and pulmonary artery. The exact mechanism by which this coronary anomaly may produce sudden death is not definitively known. However, in this anatomic position, the left ostium has a slitlike lumen because of its origin at an acute angle. It is postulated that increased physical activity with consequent aortic and pulmonary artery distention may induce a flaplike closure of the stretched anomalous artery, resulting in sudden, fatal ischemia. The mirror image of this condition is anomalous origin of the right coronary artery from the left sinus of Valsalva, with the artery coursing between the aorta and pulmonary trunk.[93,94] The anatomic and pathophysiologic situation at the right coronary ostium is analogous to that of the translocated left coronary artery. Origin of the right coronary artery from the aortic wall behind the left sinus results in an acute rightward take-off of the right coronary artery. Exercise may cause obstruction of this artery because the acute angle increases further as a result of increased stroke volume and aortic dilation. Although this lesion appears to be associated with an increased risk of sudden death, this risk is lower than with an anomalous left coronary artery from the right sinus of Valsalva. Other rare coronary anomalies also may cause sudden death, such as severe hypoplasia of the right coronary artery. Several developmental anomalies (coronary artery fistula, coronary-cameral fistulas, and myocardial bridging) also have been associated with myocardial ischemia and infarction.[95-98] Coronary angiography is the essential diagnostic technique for all of these conditions.

Coronary Angiography for the Evaluation and Management of Acute Coronary Syndromes

In considering the role of coronary angiography in the management of patients with acute coronary syndromes, the distinction among these clinical entities is sometimes imprecise, especially when patients first present for evaluation (Fig. 4). Although a Q-wave acute myocardial infarction ultimately develops in the majority of patients with ST-segment elevation, in a minority of cases ST elevation resolves without developing Q waves. Such patients have only enzyme evidence of infarction, and a few do not even develop enzyme evidence. Alternatively, of the patients who present without ST-segment elevation and are ultimately diagnosed with either unstable angina or a non–Q-wave myocardial infarction, a few with elevated enzymes develop pathologic Q-waves on the electrocardiogram. This overlap is further emphasized by the fact that several major clinical trials combine patients with unstable angina and non–Q-wave myocardial infarction into a single cohort in which a specific therapy or management strategy is compared. These trials, which provide the background for our current management strategies in patients with unstable angina and non–Q-wave myocardial infarction, are reviewed below.

Thrombolysis in Myocardial Infarction IIIb Trial

The Thrombolysis in Myocardial Infarction (TIMI IIIb) study is a randomized trial of thrombolytic therapy with tissue plasminogen activator vs. placebo in 1473 patients with unstable angina or non–Q-wave myocardial infarction.[99] Patients were randomized to undergo either early coronary angiography and revascularization within 18–48 hours after randomization or a conservative

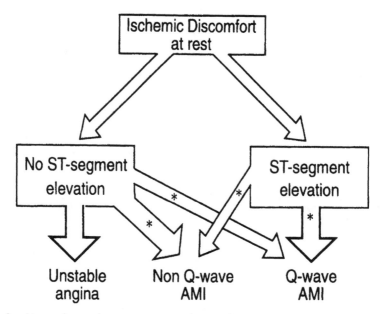

Figure 4. Nomenclature of acute coronary syndromes. The spectrum of clinical conditions ranging from unstable angina to non–Q-wave and Q-wave acute myocardial infarction is referred to as the acute coronary syndromes. Patients with ischemic pain may present with or without ST-segment elevation on the electrocardiogram. The majority *(large arrow)* of patients with ST-segment elevation eventually develop a Q-wave myocardial infarction, whereas a minority *(small arrow)* develop a non–Q-wave myocardial infarction. Of the patients who present without ST-segment elevation, the majority *(large arrows)* have either unstable angina or non–Q-wave infarction based on the presence or absence of an enzyme marker of infarction. A minority of such patients may actually develop a Q-wave acute MI. * Positive serum cardiac enzyme marker of infarction. (From Antman EM, Braunwald E: Acute myocardial infarction. In Braunwald E (ed): Heart Disease: A Textbook of Cardiovascular Medicine, 5th ed. Philadelphia, W.B. Saunders, 1996, with permission.)

strategy with angiography performed only in the presence of demonstrable ischemia. All patients were treated with beta blockers, calcium channel blockers, nitrates, heparin, and aspirin. Thrombolytic therapy was not beneficial and possibly even detrimental in this patient population. The incidence of fatal and nonfatal myocardial infarction after randomization was higher (7.4% vs. 4.9%) in the thrombolytic-treated patients, who also experienced more intracranial hemorrhages. The study showed no significant difference in the composite endpoint of death, myocardial infarction, or failed symptom-limited exercise tolerance test at 6 weeks between patients in the early invasive group (16.2%) and patients in the conservative management group (18.1%). Considerable crossover occurred: 64% of patients in the conservative group had coronary angiography within 42 days of initial presentation. Although there was no difference in the major composite endpoint, patients in the invasive group had a slightly shorter (0.7 days) length of stay, a lower need for second hospitalization within 6 weeks (7.8% vs. 14.1%), and a reduction in the use of antianginal medications.

After 1 year of follow-up, the incidence of death and nonfatal myocardial infarction was similar in patients receiving invasive and conservative management (10.8% and 12.2%, respectively).[100] Revascularization procedures by 1 year were slightly more frequent in the invasive group (64%) compared with the conservative group (58%). This finding was related entirely to a small difference in angioplasty rates (39% vs. 32%); the rates of bypass grafting by 1 year were identical (30%) in the two groups. Fewer patients in the early invasive strategy group required late repeat hospitalization (26% vs. 33%). No formal economic analyses were performed as part of TIMI IIIb. Therefore, it is not known whether the cost of routine coronary angiography and intervention was offset by the reduced need for further hospitalization and antianginal medications, but the impact of these small differences with attendant costs probably is small. Limitations of the TIMI-IIIb trial include a relatively late time to revascularization (mean = 36 hours after presentation) and a preponderance of patients with unstable angina, for whom the risk of death is known to be less than for patients with non–Q-wave myocardial infarction.

Veterans Affairs Non–Q-wave Infarction Strategies In-Hospital Trial

The Veterans Affairs Non–Q-wave Infarction Strategies In-Hospital (VAN-QWISH) Trial focused only on patients with non–Q-wave myocardial infarction.[101] Within 24–72 hours of experiencing a non–Q-wave myocardial infarction, 920 patients (97% male) were randomized to an early invasive strategy with coronary angiography and revascularization, if appropriate, vs. a conservative strategy with noninvasive testing and invasive management only for spontaneous or inducible ischemia. The primary endpoint was a composite of death and nonfatal myocardial infarction, and the average follow-up was 23 months. Coronary angiography was performed less often in the conservative arm of VANQWISH (29% at 30 days) compared with the conservative arm of TIMI IIIb (64% at 42 days), whereas the use of coronary angiography was similar to that of TIMI IIIb (> 95%) in the invasive arm. Revascularization procedures were performed in 44% of patients in the invasive arm compared with 33% in the conservative arm. Although the overall mortality rate did not differ between the two study groups during the duration of follow-up (12–44 months), the rates of death and nonfatal myocardial infarction were higher at hospital discharge, after 30 days, and during the first year in the invasive group.

The results of the VANQWISH trial have been criticized because the difference in mortality rate between the two strategies was related primarily to the considerably higher mortality rate for coronary bypass surgery in the invasive arm (11.6%) compared with the conservative arm (3.4%). Cardiac catheterization procedures in the invasive strategy group were performed electively after admission, with a mean time from randomization to revascularization of 8 days. This interval may be too long for the salvage of threatened myocardium and may have contributed to the lack of beneficial effect for revascularization in the invasive strategy group. Multivessel disease was routinely managed with bypass surgery rather than percutaneous methods, which consisted primarily of balloon angioplasty and, in rare cases, directional atherectomy. Moreover, this study predated the common use of coronary artery stents and glycoprotein IIb/IIIa inhibitors, both of which are known to improve short- and long-term outcomes.

These differences were emphasized by Gersh, who reanalyzed the TIMI IIIb data focusing only on patients with non–Q-wave myocardial infarction.[102] Patients with non–Q-wave myocardial infarction in TIMI IIIb then were compared with patients in the VANQWISH trial. Although one must be cautious in interpreting such a post-hoc subset analysis, the findings are nevertheless of interest. Conservatively treated patients in both trials experienced similar outcomes at 1 year. The mortality rate was 6.3% in TIMI IIIb patients compared

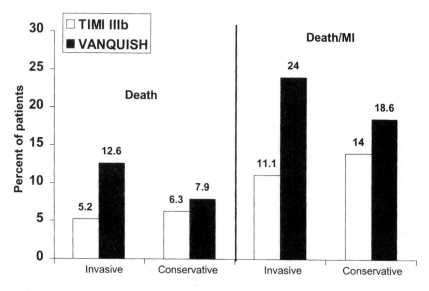

Figure 5. Comparisons of 1-year outcomes of patients with non–Q-wave myocardial infarction (MI) in the TIMI IIIb and VANQWISH trials. (From Gersh BJ, O'Rourke RA: Is coronary revascularization the optimum strategy for patients with non–Q-wave myocardial infarction? A point-counterpoint. Clin Cardiol 21(Suppl II): II-18–II-22, 1998, with permission.)

with 7.9% in VANQWISH patients, whereas the composite endpoint of death or nonfatal myocardial infarction was 14% in TIMI IIIb patients and 18.6% in VANQWISH patients (Fig. 5). Outcomes in the invasive arm of TIMI IIIb were comparable to the conservative arm in VANQWISH (death = 5.2%, death or myocardial infarction = 11%). The highest rate of death or death and nonfatal myocardial infarction occurred in the invasive arm of the VANQWISH trial (12.6% and 24%, respectively). Despite concerns about outcomes in the invasive arm of the VANQWISH trial, these data argue against the necessity of an aggressive approach with early angiography and revascularization for all patients with non–Q-wave myocardial infarction and suggest that a conservative strategy with medical therapy, noninvasive testing, and ischemia-driven invasive therapy is both safe and appropriate.

Fragmin and Fast Revascularization during Instability in Coronary Artery Disease Study

The Fragmin and Fast Revascularization during InStability in Coronary Artery Disease (FRISC II) trial is a prospective, randomized, multicenter trial with parallel treatment groups.[103] A factorial design was used to compare an invasive vs. noninvasive management strategy with prolonged vs. acute-phase therapy with low-molecular-weight heparin (dalteparin). As soon as possible after admission, patients were allocated to one of four treatment strategies: long-term dalteparin and noninvasive strategy; long-term placebo and noninvasive strategy; long-term dalteparin and invasive strategy; and long-term placebo and invasive strategy. The invasive strategy consisted of coronary angiography and revascularization, if appropriate, within 7 days and was compared with a conservative treatment consisting of coronary angiography and revascularization only in patients with refractory or recurrent symptoms despite maximal medical treatment or severe ischemia with symptom-limited exercise before discharge. Before randomization, patients received open-label dalteparin or unfractionated heparin. The study cohort consisted of 2457 patients presenting with either non–Q-wave myocardial infarction or unstable angina; approximately one-half of patients had enzyme evidence of myocardial necrosis. The median age of the study population was 66 years, and 70% were men. The primary endpoint was a composite of death or nonfatal myocardial infarction. In the invasive treatment group, coronary angiography was performed within the first 7 days in 96% and revascularization within the first 10 days in 71% of the patients. In the conservative arm, coronary angiography was performed within the first 7 days in 10% and revascularization within the first 10 days in 9% of the patients. The large difference in revascularization rates between the invasive and conservative groups in FRISC-II are in sharp contrast to those seen in the TIMI IIIb trial (61% vs. 49% at 42 days) and the VANQWISH trial (44% vs. 33% after about 1 year) and may reflect the more contemporary medical therapy, including low-molecular-weight heparin, used in the FRISC-II trial.

The main finding of the FRISC-II study was a significant 22% relative and 2.7% absolute decrease in the composite endpoint of death and myocardial infarction in the invasive treatment group after 6 months (9.4% in the invasive arm vs. 12.1% in the conservative arm). The study also found a significant decrease in myocardial infarction alone (7.8 vs. 10.1%) and a trend toward lower mortality rate (1.9% vs. 2.9%, p = 0.1) in the invasive treatment group. During the first 2 weeks, however, a higher event rate was associated with the procedures in the invasive treatment group, which thereafter had a lower event rate (Fig. 6). The use of abciximab was encouraged during percutaneous interventions, and 60–70% of patients treated in this fashion received a coronary artery stent. Other benefits noted in the invasive treatment group included a 50% relative decrease in symptoms and corresponding difference in Canadian

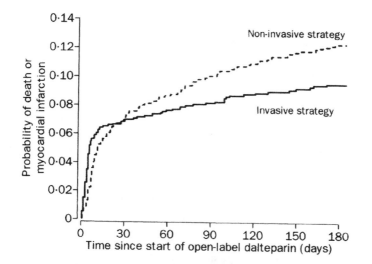

Figure 6. Probability of death or myocardial infarction in invasive and non-invasive groups from the FRISC-II trial. (From Fragmin and Fast Revascularization during InStability in Coronary artery disease (FRISC-II) Investigators: Invasive compared with non-invasive treatment in unstable coronary-artery disease: FRISC-II prospective randomised multicentre study. Lancet 354:708–715, 1999, with permission.)

Cardiovascular Society angina score and a 50% reduction in the need for readmission. Thus, the FRISC-II study clearly shows the benefit of an early invasive strategy following medical treatment with dalteparin, aspirin, and contemporary antianginal medications. The advantages of early invasive treatment were most marked in patients of higher age, male patients, and patients with angina of longer duration, chest pain at rest, or ST-segment depression.

The findings of FRISC II clearly differ from those of previous trials comparing invasive with noninvasive management strategies in patients with acute coronary syndromes. Earlier trials indicated either no difference or an excess in adverse outcomes with an early invasive approach to management.[99-101] This disparity in results may be explained by differences in antianginal and antithrombotic medications, proportion and timing of invasive procedures in each patient group, improvements in technology and equipment during the treatment periods, and the low mortality rate of coronary artery bypass surgery in FRISC II. The timing of the invasive procedures in the FRISC-II study deserves further emphasis because up to 7 days elapsed before early intervention procedures were performed. In both the TIMI IIIb and VANQWISH trials, patients in the invasive treatment arms received coronary angiography followed by revascularization much sooner—at 18–48 hours in TIMI IIIb and within 24–72 hours in VANQWISH. This observation implies that a longer period for plaque stabilization with current antithrombotic therapies may be beneficial. No other study comparing invasive vs. conservative management strategies in acute coronary syndromes has used medical therapy of this intensity, which included not only antithrombotic drugs but also lipid-lowering drugs, angiotensin-converting enzyme inhibitors, and antidiabetic treatments.

Medicine vs. Angiography in Thrombolytic Exclusion Trial

The Medicine vs. Angiography in Thrombolytic Exclusion (MATE) Trial was a small prospective, multicenter, randomized trial to determine whether early-triage coronary angiography with revascularization, if indicated, favorably affected clinical outcome in patients with suspected myocardial infarction who were ineligible for thrombolysis.[104] Patients were considered ineligible for thrombolysis because of a lack of diagnostic electrocardiographic changes, symptoms lasting longer than 6 hours, or increased bleeding or stroke risk. Patients were randomized to early coronary angiography, with therapy based on the results of angiography, or medical therapy consisting of intravenous unfractionated heparin, nitroglycerin, beta blockers and analgesics. In the invasive treatment arm (n = 111), triage angiography was performed at a mean of 16 hours from symptom onset, and 98% of patients underwent invasive study within the first 24 hours of presentation. In the medical therapy group (n = 90), 60% of patients underwent a nonprotocol coronary angiogram. One-half of these were related to an ischemic event, and the remainder were done because of physician or patient preference. Acute myocardial infarction was confirmed by elevated cardiac enzymes in about one-half of each treatment group, and approximately 25% of patients receiving angiography in each group had either noncritical or no angiographic evidence of coronary artery disease. The composite endpoint of all recurrent ischemic events or death occurred in 13% of patients in the triage angiography group compared with 34% in the medical group. These findings indicate a 45% risk reduction with triage angiography. Patients in the triage angiography group had a shorter time to definitive revascularization during the index hospitalization, but this finding did not equate to a significant difference in hospital costs. Finally, long-term follow-up at a median of 21 months showed no differences in the endpoints of late revascularization, recurrent myocardial infarction, or all-cause mortality. Thus, despite more frequent early revascularization after triage angiography, there was no long-term benefit in cardiac outcomes compared with medical therapy and revascularization prompted by recurrent ischemia.

Myocardial Infarction Triage and Intervention Registry

Although not a randomized trial, the Myocardial Infarction Triage and Intervention (MITI) Registry contains detailed data about a cohort of 12,331 consecutive patients with acute myocardial infarction admitted to 19 Seattle area hospitals. From this database, a cohort of 1635 consecutive patients who presented with non–Q-wave myocardial infarction were identified. In a retrospective fashion, the benefits of very early routine cardiac catheterization and revascularization (within 6 hours) vs. a conservative strategy were compared.[105] Two hospitals favored the early invasive approach (n = 308), and the remainder favored the conservative approach to management (n = 1327). Of patients admitted to the invasive hospitals, 59% underwent cardiac catheterization within the first 6 hours after admission. In contrast, 52% of patients admitted to the other hospitals underwent cardiac catheterization during admission, but only 8% within the first 6 hours. Univariate analyses showed that both 30-day and 4-year mortality rates were significantly lower in patients treated at hospitals using the early invasive strategy. In a multivariate analysis, only the 4-year mortality rate was lower in patients treated at hospitals using the early invasive strategy (20% vs. 37%). Based on these data, the authors concluded that an early invasive strategy in patients with non–ST-segment elevation myocardial infarction is associated with a lower long-term mortality rate.

Although the objective of the comparisons was to determine differences in short- and long-term outcomes after early invasive or conservative strategies, the actual comparisons were between treatments in hospitals that favor an early invasive approach and hospitals that favor a more conservative approach to the management of non–Q-wave myocardial infarction. In addition, in any observational study such as the MITI Registry, potentially confounding variables may contribute to the differences in outcome. For example, several potentially important differences in the baseline characteristics of patients admitted to hospitals favoring the conservative approach are associated with a worse short- and long-term outcome after myocardial infarction. Examples include lower socioeconomic status and more comorbidities, such as greater age; higher rates of prior congestive heart failure, angina, or myocardial infarction; new congestive heart failure; diabetes; and current smoking. After adjustment for these factors, the 30-day mortality rate was no longer different between hospitals using the different management strategies, suggesting that the better short-term outcome observed in hospitals favoring the invasive approach may be related more to differences in baseline characteristics than to the early invasive approach.

Recommendations for Coronary Angiography in Patients with Unstable Angina

The rational use of coronary angiography in the management of patients with unstable angina should be based on two factors: (1) the likelihood of underlying coronary artery disease and (2) the short- and long-term risk of death or nonfatal myocardial infarction. This approach is based on the Unstable Angina Clinical Practice Guideline of the Agency for Health Care Research and Policy and the Practice Guidelines for Coronary Angiography of the American College of Cardiology and American Heart Association (ACC/AHA).[106,107] In general, coronary angiography is indicated in unstable angina when a subsequent revascularization procedure is likely to alter the natural history of the syndrome or when important symptoms continue despite aggressive therapy. Table 2 summarizes the clinical features associated with a high, intermediate, or low risk of death or nonfatal myocardial infarction in patients with unstable angina. Patients at high or intermediate risk for adverse outcome who do not respond after an hour of intensive medical therapy or who have recurrent symptoms after initial stabilization should undergo emergent (immediately or within 6 hours) coronary angiography. Fortunately, the incidence of truly refractory angina in the current therapeutic era is low. In one study of patients with > 20 minutes of angina at rest and reversible electrocardiographic changes, 52% were believed to be medically refractory by the referring practitioners.[108] However, with a more aggressive medical regimen including intravenous heparin, aspirin, nitrates, calcium channel blockers, and beta blockers, 83% were rendered pain-free. The incidence of truly medically refractory unstable angina with this five-drug regimen was 8.8%, and coronary angiography showed an increased occurrence of left main or three-vessel disease in such patients.

Table 2.   Clinical Indicators of High, Intermediate and Low Risk
in Patients with Unstable Angina

High Risk	Intermediate Risk	Low Risk
At least 1 of following features must be present:	No high-risk features but must have any of following:	No high- or intermediate-risk features but may have any of following :
Prolonged ongoing (>20 min) chest pain	Prolonged (> 20 min) angina at rest, now resolved, with moderate or high likelihood of coronary artery disease.	Increased frequency, severity or duration of angina
Pulmonary edema, most likely related to ischemia	Angina at rest (> 20 min) relieved with rest or sublingual nitroglycerin	Angina provoked by lower threshold
Angina at rest with dynamic ST changes ≥ 1 mm	Nocturnal angina	New-onset angina within 2 weeks to 2 months before presentation
Angina with new or worsening mitral regurgitation murmur	Angina with dynamic T-wave changes	Normal or unchanged electrocardiogram
Angina with S3 gallop or new or worsening rales	New-onset CCSC III or IV angina in past 2 weeks with moderate or high likelihood of coronary artery disease	
Angina with hypotension	Pathologic Q-waves or resting ST-segment depression ≤ 1 mm in multiple lead groups (anterior, inferior or lateral)	
	Age > 65 years	

CCSC = Canadian Cardiovascular Society classification.
Adapted from Gersh BJ, O'Rourke RA: Is coronary revascularization the optimum strategy for patients with non–Q-wave myocardial infarction? A point-counterpoint. Clin Cardiol 21(Suppl II): II-18–II-22, 1998.

Although no data are available, the likelihood of medically refractory angina is probably even lower with the use of low-molecular-weight heparin and glycoprotein IIb/IIIa inhibitors.

For patients whose clinical instability resolves after initial medical treatment, existing guidelines offer options for either an early invasive or early conservative management strategy.[106,107] Patients managed with an early invasive strategy undergo coronary angiography within 48 hours of presentation, if they have no contraindications to the procedure. In contrast, the intent of the early conservative strategy is to avoid "rushing" into early angiography for all patients. Some patients managed conservatively may be found to have some other cause for their symptoms at presentation and never require coronary angiography. As shown in the MATE trial, approximately 15% of patients undergoing early-triage angiography have no angiographic evidence of coronary artery disease, and another 10% have noncritical disease.[104] However, many patients in this category ultimately have appropriate indications for angiography. Although their symptoms may respond favorably to medical therapy, patients with high-risk or multiple intermediate-risk clinical indicators (see Table 2) should be strongly considered for angiography before hospital discharge. In addition to the indicators in Table 2, patients with a history of previous revascularization, congestive heart failure, left ventricular ejection fraction < 0.50, malignant ventricular arrhythmias, or a functional study indicating high risk should be strongly considered for coronary angiography.

In summary, outcome data from the major randomized trials that included patients with unstable angina (TIMI IIIb, FRISC II, and MATE) suggest that an early invasive strategy with coronary angiography and revascularization, if necessary, is useful and effective. However, data from the most recent of these trials (FRISC II) implies that it may be advantageous to have patience and to embark on invasive studies only after a period of contemporary medical management, including aspirin, standard or low-molecular-weight heparin, and a glycoprotein IIb/IIIa inhibitor.

For patients judged to be at low-risk for adverse outcomes (see Table 2), current guidelines recommend outpatient management.[106,107] The evaluation of such patients should begin promptly. For patients able to perform adequate dynamic exercise, the evaluation should include exercise stress testing with electrocardiographic monitoring or echocardiographic or myocardial perfusion imaging. In patients not able to exercise adequately, pharmacologic stress testing coupled with some type of imaging study of the heart should be used. Evaluation of left ventricular function is also important. Noninvasive test indicators associated with an increased risk of adverse outcome in patients with known or suspected coronary artery disease are shown in Table 3. Patients who initially are believed to be at low risk for adverse outcomes but have one or more of these high-risk indicators should be referred for coronary angiography unless they have contraindications to the procedure.

Recommendations for Coronary Angiography in Patients with Non–Q-wave Myocardial Infarction

Before the era of thrombolytic therapy, short-term mortality in patients with non–Q-wave myocardial infarction was more favorable, averaging about 10% compared with about 20% for Q-wave myocardial infarction.[109] Despite this initial

Table 3. Noninvasive Test Indicators of Increased Risk for Adverse Outcome
in Patients with Coronary Artery Disease

Resting left ventricular dysfunction (LVEF < 35%)
High-risk treadmill score (score ≤ 11)[†]
Severe exercise left ventricular dysfunction (exercise LVEF < 35%)
Stress-induced large perfusion defect (especially if involving the anterior wall)
Stress-induced multiple moderate perfusion defects
Large, fixed perfusion defect with LV dilatation or increased lung uptake (thallium-201)
Stress-induced moderate perfusion defect with LV dilatation or increased lung uptake (thallium-201)
Echocardiographic wall motion abnormality (involving > 2 segments) developing at low doses of dobutamine (≤ 10 mg/kg per minute) or at low heart rate (< 120 beats/min)
Stress echocardiographic evidence of extensive ischemia

LVEF = left ventricular ejection fraction
[†] Treadmill score is calculated using a standard Bruce protocol test as duration of exercise in minutes
 – (5 × maximal ST-segment deviation during or after exercise in mm) – (4 × treadmill angina index).
 The numerical treadmill angina index is 0 for no angina, 1 for nonlimiting angina, and 2 for exercise-
 limiting angina.
Adapted from Mark DB, Shaw L, Harrell FE, et al: Prognostic value of a treadmill exercise score in
outpatients with suspected coronary artery disease. N Engl J Med 325:894–853, 1991.

difference, long-term mortality in patients with non–Q-wave infarction was equal or slightly greater than that of Q-wave myocardial infarction, and the incidence of reinfarction was about 3-fold higher (15.7% vs. 5.7%). Angina also recurs more frequently after non–Q-wave than after Q-wave infarction, affecting 35–50% of patients.[109] Perhaps because of the improvements in early mortality rates due to thrombolytic therapy in patients with Q-wave myocardial infarction, clinicians have focused more attention recently on improving outcomes in patients with non–Q-wave myocardial infarction. Many clinicians have adopted an aggressive approach, including coronary angiography in all such patients. Advocates of this approach argue that it allows a definitive anatomic diagnosis, improves assessment of prognosis, and facilitates formation of a therapeutic plan early during hospitalization.[110] In contrast, a more conservative approach is to perform coronary angiography and revascularization only in patients who have a high risk of adverse outcomes, spontaneous episodes of ischemia, or inducible ischemia during provocative testing.

As noted earlier, four randomized trials have evaluated the merits of an early invasive strategy vs. a conservative approach in patients with non–Q-wave myocardial infarction. Of these, only the most recent, FRISC-II, showed a reduction in the incidence of death or myocardial infarction during follow-up in patients managed with the early invasive strategy. Similar findings were observed in a small retrospective study limited to patients with anterior wall non–Q-wave myocardial infarction. Early angiography with revascularization by balloon angioplasty or bypass surgery resulted in a decrease in recurrent myocardial infarction (7.2% vs. 29%) and improved survival rates after 3 years.[111] However, several issues should be considered when data from these randomized studies are used to make clinical decisions about the management of patients with non–Q-wave myocardial infarction:

1. Newer treatment strategies and medical therapies have emerged since some of these trials were completed. Although patients in all of the trials received aspirin and heparin, only the FRISC-II trial used low-molecular-weight

heparin. Low-molecular-weight heparins have several advantages over unfractionated heparin, including a more predictable anticoagulant effect and resistance to inhibition by activated platelets (see Chapter 6 for a complete discussion of low-molecular-weight heparins). In addition, the dosage of antianginal drugs may not have been optimal by current standards, and the aggressive use of lipid-lowering drugs was not emphasized in all trials. These aspects of medical therapy are currently recommended in daily practice but were not used in these protocol-driven clinical trials.

2. Revascularization procedures in some of the early trials were different from those currently believed to provide better outcomes. For example, in the VANQWISH trial, the majority of percutaneous revascularization procedures were balloon angioplasties, and a few patients had directional arthrectomies. In contrast, 60–70% of patients in the FRISC-II trial received a coronary artery stent. Likewise, in the VANQWISH trial, the number of patients receiving an internal mammary graft was not cited, and the 30-day mortality rate was high, totalling 7.7% in the entire study cohort and 11.6% in the invasive treatment group. In the FRISC-II trial, 95% of patients undergoing bypass surgery received an internal mammary artery graft, and the 30-day mortality rate in the invasive treatment group was only 2.1%. In addition, most of these studies were conducted before the introduction of glycoprotein IIb/IIIa receptor blockers, which have also been shown to improve outcomes in patients with acute coronary syndromes (see Chapter 4).

3. Patients with non–Q-wave myocardial infarction are not a homogeneous population. Coronary pathology varies from single-vessel disease, involving a small vascular territory, to multivessel disease with important stenoses in all vessels. In addition, ventricular function is important prognostically, and most patients included in the major trials had normal or minimal left ventricular dysfunction. In the FRISC-II trial, for example, less than 15% of patients had a left ventricular ejection fraction < 45%. Other variables, such as extent and type of electrocardiographic change and troponin-I release, also have prognostic implications and should be considered.[112]

4. Variations in coronary artery pathology are important. Clinical decisions are based not only on the number of arteries involved but also on the percent stenosis, presence or absence of serial stenoses in the same vessel, location of the stenosis within the vessel (proximal vs. distal), length and morphology of the stenosis, presence of thrombus, TIMI flow grade, and presence or absence of collateral vessels. Certain types of coronary disease patterns may have been excluded by investigator bias in some of the randomized trials. For example, it is unlikely that patients with high-grade proximal stenoses of the left anterior descending artery were uniformly included because of concerns about long-term outcome.[113–115]

Clinical judgment must be used to make decisions about management in patients with non–Q-wave myocardial infarction. A synopsis of current data suggests that emergency coronary angiography is necessary only in a minority of patients, such as those with ongoing chest pain unresponsive to medical therapy or hemodynamic instability. Based solely on the results of the FRISC-II trial, a management strategy of early coronary angiography and revascularization appears to be justified, but after several days of comprehensive medical therapy. In reality, conservative and invasive management should be considered as complementary rather than competing strategies. Early angiography after non–Q-wave myocardial infarction identifies patients who are good candidates for either percutaneous or surgical revascularization. A substantial number of patients with non–Q-wave myocardial infarction are at increased risk for adverse outcomes and are most likely to benefit from early revascularization by an appropriate technique. Until more data are available, individualized therapy based on clinical, noninvasive, or invasive risk stratification seems to be the most effective management.

Recommendations for Coronary Angiography in Patients with Q-wave Myocardial Infarction

Beginning with the advent of thrombolytic therapy, the treatment of Q-wave myocardial infarction shifted from a more passive approach emphasizing supportive care and management of complications to a more active interventional approach. Coronary angiography is rarely performed during or after myocardial infarction solely for diagnostic purposes. Most procedures are performed to evaluate the patient for a revascularization procedure; thus, the appropriateness of coronary angiography is linked directly to the appropriateness and efficacy of the revascularization procedure as assessed by improved outcome. Using the format adopted by the ACC/AHA Guidelines,[107] the use of coronary angiography can be considered in three distinct time periods after infarction. These time periods, however, are somewhat arbitrary and have indistinct boundaries because the diagnosis of myocardial infarction may not be established immediately, patients do not always present at an identical starting point in the event, and patients may evolve through the infarction at different rates. Included in the group with ST-segment elevation are patients with typical ischemic chest pain and a new (or presumed new) bundle-branch block that obscures the electrocardiographic diagnosis of myocardial infarction because clinical outcomes are similar, especially after thrombolysis.

The first time period encompasses the use of coronary angiography during the initial diagnosis and management of patients in the emergency department. Coronary angiography usually is coupled with the intent to perform percutaneous coronary revascularization as an alternative to thrombolytic therapy. Other possible indications for the urgent use of coronary angiography during initial management include the following: (1) for some reason, the diagnosis of acute myocardial infarction is obscure, or (2) other miscellaneous causes of coronary occlusion, such as aortic dissection, are possible.

The second time period includes the use of coronary angiography during hospital management of the patient with myocardial infarction. Performance of coronary angiography usually is driven by a complication of infarction, such as spontaneous recurrent ischemia, heart failure related to ventricular septal defect, papillary muscle dysfunction, or malignant arrhythmias persisting beyond the first 24 hours after infarction.

The final time period during which coronary angiography may be necessary after myocardial infarction is during risk stratification before hospital discharge. In reality, risk stratification does not occur exclusively in the 24–48 hours before discharge. The process occurs throughout the physician's entire encounter with the patient as information is accumulated about the extent and consequences of the infarction.

Coronary Angiography During the Initial Management Phase

There are two main situations in which coronary angiography may be used during the initial management of patients with acute ST-segment elevation myocardial infarction. First, coronary angiography is a requisite part of the strategy to determine whether the patient is a candidate for mechanical reperfusion. Second, coronary angiography may be necessary in patients who have just received thrombolytic therapy, especially if therapy failure is suspected. Whether mechanical or thrombolytic therapy is chosen, rapid triage decisions are mandatory because benefit to the patient is linked directly to the time required to reestablish normal distal blood flow.[116] Both fibrinolytic agents and percutaneous coronary intervention in the treatment of acute coronary syndromes are the subject of individual chapters. On rare occasions, the clinical picture and electrocardiographic findings may be so confusing that coronary angiography is necessary to clarify the diagnosis of acute myocardial infarction.

Coronary Angiography Coupled with Mechanical Reperfusion

Because coronary angiography is an obligatory part of any percutaneous intervention, mechanical reperfusion in fact involves coronary angiography followed by triage to the most appropriate means of reperfusion.[117] Advocates of mechanical reperfusion highlight several possible advantages of initial triage angiography to direct an appropriate revascularization strategy:

1. Although mechanical reperfusion is used for revascularization after coronary angiography in approximately 90% of patients studied, about 5% have severe three-vessel or left main coronary disease or anatomic features that are unfavorable for mechanical revascularization. In such patients, bypass surgery may be more appropriate.[118]

2. Immediate coronary angiography identifies an additional 5% of patients in whom the infarct-related artery has spontaneously opened, leaving a noncritical residual narrowing and normal flow beyond the culprit stenosis. In such patients, conservative management may be used, and perhaps the risks of thrombolytic therapy can be avoided.

3. In unusual circumstances, thrombolytic therapy is inappropriate or unnecessary. For example, in rare cases myocardial infarction is caused by aortic dissection, or in an occasional patient with suspected myocardial infarction and bundle-branch block, immediate angiography shows the absence of coronary occlusion.

4. Immediate angiography during the initial evaluation of patients with myocardial infarction may be valuable for identifying not only high-risk but also low-risk patients. Results from the Primary Angioplasty in Myocardial Infarction-2 (PAMI-2) trial show that a combination of clinical and invasive variables can stratify patients treated successfully by mechanical reperfusion into high- and low-risk subgroups.[119] In PAMI-2, low-risk patients were not hospitalized in an intensive care unit, received no further noninvasive testing, and were discharged on the third day after infarction. Compared with traditional care, this approach resulted in a shorter length of stay, lower hospital costs, and no difference in mortality or nonfatal complications after 6 months. Mortality in patients judged to be high risk was approximately 10 times greater (3.8%) than in low-risk patients (0.4%), and high-risk patients had a higher incidence of in-hospital reinfarction and recurrent ischemic events (for a more complete discussion of percutaneous coronary interventions for acute coronary syndromes, see Chapter 17).

Coronary Angiography after Thrombolytic Therapy

There are two circumstances in which coronary angiography coupled with the intention to perform mechanical reperfusion may be considered after thrombolytic therapy has been given. The first involves the routine use of invasive evaluation and therapy immediately after thrombolytic therapy. Current thrombolytic regimens may fail to open the infarct-related artery by 90 minutes in up to 25% of patients, and reocclusion despite successful initial reperfusion occurs in an additional 12%.[116,120,121] Even when thrombolysis was successful, significant stenosis remained in the infarct-related artery in the majority of patients.[122,123] Because of these issues, three randomized, prospective trials tested the hypothesis that outcome can be improved with coronary angiography followed by balloon angioplasty of a residual stenosis immediately after thrombolytic therapy.[122–124] The Thrombolysis in Acute Myocardial Infarction (TAMI) study,[122] the European Cooperative Study Group trial,[123] and the TIMI IIA study[124] were remarkably concordant in their conclusions that immediate coronary angiography followed by balloon angioplasty neither preserves myocardium nor reduces the incidence of reinfarction or death compared with a more conservative approach in which angiographic evaluation and intervention are reserved for patients with spontaneous or inducible ischemia after infarction. Patients treated with immediate balloon angioplasty within hours of thrombolytic therapy had a higher complication rate at 24 hours and a higher mortality rate at 1 year.[123,125,126] Therefore, the routine performance of coronary angiography followed by balloon angioplasty in all patients immediately after thrombolytic therapy is not indicated.

The second circumstance exists when there is a serious concern that thrombolysis has failed. Recanalization of the infarct-related artery by so-called "rescue" angioplasty has been suggested to establish patency of the affected artery, salvage any remaining viable myocardium, and improve survival. Unfortunately, there is no definitive way to identify patients in whom thrombolytic therapy has failed. This decision is based on the judgment of the clinician. Such patients often have continuing severe chest pain and worsening of clinical and hemodynamic status. Clinical markers of reperfusion, such as relief of chest pain or reperfusion arrhythmias, do not accurately predict the success or failure of thrombolysis.[127] If ST-segment elevation resolves quickly and completely, there is a high likelihood that coronary flow has been restored.[128] However, this marker is fairly insensitive; failure of the ST-segment elevation to resolve cannot be used as an indicator of thrombolytic failure. In the GUSTO-1 study, patency at 90 minutes was correlated with resolution of ST-segment elevation. Compared with patients who received streptokinase, more patients who received tissue plasminogen activator had patent arteries at 90 minutes. ST-segment elevation, however, did not resolve more quickly.[129] No other reliable markers of reperfusion have been thoroughly validated, but newer markers and techniques under study include blood levels of cardiac troponin T, continuous multiple ST-segment monitoring, myocardial contrast echocardiography, magnetic resonance imaging, and nuclear scintigraphy.[130,131]

Randomized studies of coronary angiography coupled with rescue angioplasty are difficult to conduct because many clinicians believe that patients with failed fibrinolysis should undergo angioplasty. In an observational study from one center, 257 patients with acute myocardial infarction underwent angiography 90 minutes after fibrinolytic therapy. Rescue angioplasty was performed in patients with TIMI grade 0 or 1 flow. Rescue and direct angioplasty provided effective early reperfusion to patients in whom thrombolysis failed.[132] In the TAMI-5 study, patients who underwent angiography and angioplasty, if indicated, 90 minutes after starting fibrinolysis had improved regional wall motion in the infarct zone and fewer adverse events compared with patients who underwent angiography 5–10 days later (55% vs 67%, respectively).[133] Three fairly small randomized trials of rescue angioplasty vs. conservative treatment have been published.[134–136] The largest included only 151 patients who had their first anterior infarction and were demonstrated to have an occluded artery within 8 hours of presentation.[135] Patients were allocated to balloon angioplasty to open the occluded artery or conservative therapy consisting of aspirin, heparin, and coronary vasodilators. Although there was no difference in resting ejection fraction 30 days after myocardial infarction, exercise ejection fraction was higher and a composite endpoint of death or severe heart failure was lower in patients treated with rescue angioplasty (6% vs. 17%).

The outcome after rescue angioplasty also was evaluated in the Global Utilization of Streptokinase and Tissue Plasminogen Activator for Occluded Coronary Arteries (GUSTO-I) angiographic substudy.[137] Clinical and angiographic outcomes in 198 patients treated with rescue angioplasty were compared with outcomes of 266 patients managed conservatively after failed thrombolysis and 1,058 patients with successful thrombolysis. The latter two groups were documented by angiography. Although the assignment of thrombolytic therapy was randomized, patients selected for rescue angioplasty tended to be those with clinical predictors of a poor outcome. Rescue angioplasty successfully opened 88.4% of the closed arteries; 68% achieved TIMI grade 3 flow. Despite this favorable angiographic result, left ventricular function and 30-day mortality rates were not different compared with the group who had a closed infarct-related artery and were managed conservatively. Mortality associated with a failed rescue angioplasty attempt was quite high (30.4%), but most patients who died were in cardiogenic shock before the procedure. These data are similar to the experience of the TIMI study, in which rescue angioplasty was successful in 82% of patients, but there was no difference in mortality rate at 21 days (12% for rescue angioplasty vs. 7% for medical therapy) and the mortality rate for failed rescue angioplasty attempt was 33%.[138]

Although the exact role for rescue angioplasty is not known, it is reasonable to consider urgent coronary angiography and possible rescue angioplasty if fibrinolysis appears to have failed by 120 minutes after the start of therapy, especially if the patient has a moderate or large myocardial infarction, as assessed by the electrocardiographic pattern or clinical behavior, and cardiac catheterization facilities are immediately available. Certainly patients with cardiogenic shock or marginal hemodynamic status unresponsive to appropriate treatment should be considered for urgent angiography and possible rescue angioplasty.

Coronary Angiography During the Hospital Management Phase

Coronary angiography can become necessary at several times during the initial hospital management phase of acute myocardial infarction. These situations usually are related to complications of the infarction, such as congestive heart failure, hemodynamic instability, recurrent ischemia, or arrhythmias, and may occur in any type of infarction, regardless of initial treatment. The occurrence of spontaneous myocardial ischemia or ischemia with minimal activity during the early hospital convalescence after infarction is an important indicator of increased risk. Both short- and long-term mortality rates are higher among patients with recurrent ischemia.[139–143] Across the entire spectrum of left ventricular function and severity of coronary disease, survival is related to the frequency, severity, and magnitude of myocardial ischemia.[144] Because revascularization procedures relieve myocardial ischemia, coronary angiography is indicated in patients who are potential candidates for revascularization under the assumption that mortality will be decreased. In patients who develop spontaneous or inducible ischemia after infarction, support for the use of coronary angiography with subsequent revascularization comes from the DANish trial in Acute Myocardial Infarction (DANAMI).[145] One thousand and eight patients with acute Q-wave myocardial infarction who had ischemia after thrombolytic therapy were randomized to coronary angiography and revascularization or medical management. Although there was no long-term difference in mortality rates, patients in the invasive group had a lower incidence of subsequent myocardial infarction and fewer subsequent admissions for unstable angina than patients in the conservative group.

Several mechanical complications of acute MI may require prompt evaluation, which includes coronary angiography. These complications may occur with any infarction but are more likely in patients who develop Q-waves. Examples include mitral regurgitation, acute ventricular septal defect, and subacute rupture of the left ventricular free wall.[146–151] Coronary angiography is indicated before surgical repair as well as for the rare patient who requires early resection of a left ventricular aneurysm because of refractory congestive heart failure, uncontrollable arrhythmias, or systemic embolization despite anticoagulation.

The development of congestive heart failure is an important event during hospital management of acute myocardial infarction. Prognosis after acute myocardial infarction is highly dependent on residual left ventricular function, as determined by left ventricular ejection fraction.[152] In the prethrombolytic era, the 1-year mortality rate was < 5% for patients with an ejection fraction > 0.40 but declined sharply when the ejection fraction was < 0.40 and approached 50% in patients with an ejection fraction < 0.20.[153] More recent trials generally show lower mortality rates, but the mortality rate still increases inversely with decreasing ejection fraction.[154,155] The importance of left ventricular function and coronary anatomy was apparent in a database study of 1214 medically treated patients with coronary artery disease.[156] The incidence of new cardiac events, both fatal and nonfatal, increased with the number of stenotic vessels and decreasing left ventricular function. In patients with multivessel disease, the likelihood that a subsequent event would be fatal was markedly increased by depressed left ventricular function. For example, only 23% of patients with normal left ventricular function suffered a new event during the 5-year follow-up, whereas 64% of patients with impaired left ventricular function had a new event. In patients with well-preserved left ventricular function, 44% of the new events were fatal compared with 86% in patients with impaired left ventricular function. Although not specifically proven in a large randomized study, it seems reasonable to recommend coronary angiography in patients with depressed left ventricular function after a recent myocardial infarction.

Frequently, coronary angiography is performed in patients who have received a thrombolytic agent even when the clinical evidence suggests that reperfusion has been successful. The management strategy of routine coronary angiography followed by balloon angioplasty at various times after successful thrombolytic therapy has been examined in several prospective, randomized trials. As noted above, in the TIMI IIa trial, TAMI trial, and European Cooperative Study Group trial,[122–124] the use of coronary angiography and balloon angioplasty within 2 hours after thrombolytic therapy was shown to have no benefit and to be potentially harmful in such patients. Subsequent studies examined a similar strategy, but the invasive procedure was performed at a later time after the onset of infarction and thrombolytic therapy. It was hoped that this strategy would be safer because of a stable hemostatic environment at the site of the lesion and less chance of bleeding complications at the catheter insertion sites. In the TIMI IIb trial,[157] patients were randomized within 18–48 hours of thrombolysis with tissue plasminogen activator to coronary angiography and balloon angioplasty, if appropriate, or conservative management. After 6 weeks, the investigators found no difference in mortality, nonfatal recurrent myocardial infarction, or left ventricular ejection fraction between the groups, and follow-up reports showed no difference in survival, anginal class, or frequency of bypass surgery after 1 and 3 years.[158,159] In the Should We Intervene Following Thrombolysis (SWIFT) Study, 800 patients who received thrombolytic therapy were randomized to coronary angiography and balloon angioplasty within 2–7 days or conservative management with invasive treatment only for spontaneous or exercise-induced ischemia.[160] Again, no difference was found in left ventricular function, incidence of recurrent myocardial infarction, in-hospital survival, or 1-year survival between the two treatment groups.

Other smaller trials have examined the routine use of coronary angiography coupled with balloon angioplasty at even longer intervals after thrombolysis, which allow further clot maturation and stabilization with remodeling of the infarct-related stenosis, possibly improving outcomes. Coronary angiography with angioplasty of suitable lesions, including occluded arteries, was performed > 72 hours after treatment with tissue plasminogen activator and compared with conservative management and revascularization only for recurrent ischemia in a randomized study of 201 patients.[161] After 10 months, no difference was found in left ventricular function, recurrent infarction, or death between the groups. In another study, 87 asymptomatic patients were randomized to coronary angiography and angioplasty or conservative management 4–14 days after thrombolytic therapy.[162] Patients with postinfarction angina or exercise-induced ischemia were excluded. No difference was found in mortality rates between the two groups, but patients treated with angioplasty had less angina after 1 year of follow-up. However, neither of these trials was of sufficient power to detect small differences among the groups. Based on these trials, the automatic use of coronary angiography and balloon angioplasty in all patients within days after thrombolytic therapy is not justified.

Coronary Angiography During the Risk Stratification Phase

Coronary angiography is an integral part of the risk stratification process. The purpose of risk stratification is to predict prognosis and the need for further therapies that may improve prognosis.[163] Risk stratification occurs throughout the entire encounter with the patient and is not limited to procedures performed in the days before discharge. For example, rales, tachycardia, or hypotension in the early hours after infarction are important predictors of increased risk because

Table 4. Factors Associated with an Adverse Prognosis after Acute Myocardial Infarction

Age > 70 yr

Congestive heart failure or LVEF <0.40

Extent of coronary artery disease

Large infarct size, anterior infarction, or non–Q-wave myocardial infarction

New bundle-branch block of any type, Mobitz 2 or transient third-degree heart block

Recurrent angina, reinfarction, or infarct extension

Frequent VPBs, ventricular tachycardia, or ventricular fibrillation occurring after acute phase or inducible monomorphic ventricular tachycardia during electrophysiologic testing

Supraventricular arrhythmias except sinus bradycardia

Abnormal signal-averaged electrocardiogram

Provokable ischemia during exercise testing or inability to exercise

Diabetes, hypertension

Female sex

LVEF = left ventricular ejection fraction, VPB = ventricular premature beat.
Modified from Hessen SE, Brest AN: Risk profiling the patient after acute myocardial infarction. In Pepine CJ (ed): Acute Myocardial Infarction. Philadelphia, F.A. Davis,1989, p 284.

they most likely indicate depressed left ventricular performance, which, in turn, is highly predictive of survival.[164,165] Numerous factors have been related to prognosis after acute myocardial infarction (Table 4).[163–168] Approximately one-half of deaths in the first year after infarction occur within the first 3 weeks and 75% within the first 3 months.[169] Therefore, it is important to identify patients at increased risk relatively early if they are to be considered for coronary angiography and possible revascularization.

Cardiac catheterization and coronary arteriography can identify many of the major determinants of mortality after myocardial infarction, such as left ventricular ejection fraction and multivessel coronary artery disease.[167,170–174] Because of the higher incidence of cardiac events and mortality early within the first year after infarction, many experts support a management strategy that includes coronary angiography in all survivors, even though it involves a small risk and is expensive.[110,169] Alternatively, considerable data suggest that evaluation by noninvasive methods, such as standard exercise testing, echocardiography, radionuclide ventriculography, thallium scintigraphy, or imaging techniques coupled with dynamic or pharmacologic stress, can identify most high-risk patients who may benefit from revascularization.[163,164,170,171,175–180] Various strategies for the use of coronary angiography after myocardial infarction have been proposed,[110,152,163,179,181] but prospective trials are limited. Ross et al. used outcome data in 1848 patients with acute myocardial infarction to formulate a strategy of conservative management in patients with a 1-year mortality < 3% and coronary angiography in patients with an average 1-year mortality of 16%.[182] Patients over 75 years of age were excluded, and the decision scheme was tested prospectively in an additional 780 patients. The indications for coronary angiography used in this model are as follows:

1. Severe resting ischemia at any time beyond the first 24 hours after infarction (1-year mortality rate = 18%);

2. Hospital survivors with a history of previous infarction and clinical or radiographic signs of left ventricular failure in the hospital (1-year mortality rate = 25%);

3. An ischemic exercise response or poor workload (1-year mortality rate = 11%); and

4. A resting left ventricular ejection fraction of 20–44% (1-year mortality rate = 12%).

Following this decision scheme, approximately 55% of patients who survived to the fifth day after infarction had an indication for coronary angiography, which was avoided in low-risk patients and performed only in high-risk patients. This utilization rate for coronary angiography is higher than the 33% rate in the TIMI II trial[157] but considerably lower than the actual utilization rate of coronary angiography after myocardial infarction determined from survey data. Data from the National Registry of Myocardial Infarction from 1990 through 1993 and the GUSTO trial show that approximately 72% of patients treated by American participants undergo coronary angiography during their initial hospitalization after myocardial infarction.[183,184] Table 5 summarizes recent guidelines for the use of coronary angiography after myocardial infarction.

Clinical Practice Patterns for the Use of Coronary Angiography in Acute Coronary Syndromes

In 1993, cardiac catheterization was the second most frequently performed in-hospital operative procedure in the U.S. and the most frequently performed procedure in patients older than 65 years of age.[185] Medicare data show continued growth in the number of cardiac catheterization procedures from 575,000

Table 5. Recommendations for Coronary Angiography After Q-wave Myocardial Infarction

Initial acute management phase
 Preceding a mechanical reperfusion technique as an alternative to thrombolytic therapy
 Cardiogenic shock or persistent hemodynamic instability unresponsive to medical therapy in patients < 75 years of age—provided revascularization can occur within 18 hours of the onset of shock
 Preceding a mechanical reperfusion technique in patients who are not candidates for thrombolytic therapy
 Evolving large or anterior myocardial infarction after thrombolytic therapy when it is believed that reperfusion has not occurred and the patient is a candidate for rescue angioplasty

Hospital management phase
 Spontaneous myocardial ischemia or myocardial ischemia provoked by minimal exertion during recovery from infarction
 Before definitive therapy of a mechanical complication of infarction such as acute mitral regurgitation, ventricular septal defect, pseudoaneurysm or left ventricular aneurysm
 When the cause of the infarction is suspected to be by a mechanism other than thrombotic occlusion of an atherosclerotic plaque
 Survivors of acute myocardial infarction with a LVEF ≤ 0.40, congestive heart failure, prior revascularization or malignant ventricular arrhythmias
 Clinical heart failure during the acute episode, but subsequent demonstration of preserved left ventricular function (LVEF > 0.40)

Risk stratification phase
 Ischemia at low levels of exercise with electrocardiographic changes (≥ 1 mm ST-segment depression or other predictors of adverse outcome) and/or important imaging abnormalities
 Clinically significant congestive heart failure during the hospital course
 Inability to perform exercise test with LVEF ≤ 0.45

LVEF = left ventricular ejection fraction.
Adapted from Scanlon PJ, Faxon DP, Audet AM, et al: ACC/AHA guidelines for coronary angiography: A report of the American College of Cardiology/American Heart Association Task Force on Practice Guidelines (Committee on Coronary Angiography) J Am Coll Cardiol 33:1756–1824, 1999.

in 1991 to 793,000 in 1995, an increase of 38% over 4 years.[187] In 1994, approximately 10% of cardiac catheterizations were performed in patients with a diagnosis-related group (DRG) diagnosis of acute myocardial infarction.[107,187] Although this population is only a small percentage of patients undergoing coronary angiography, it has been well characterized. From 1987 to 1990, the proportion of Medicare patients with acute myocardial infarction who underwent cardiac catheterization increased from 24% to 33%.[188] The likelihood of undergoing cardiac catheterization is approximately three-fold higher in patients with an acute myocardial infarction who are admitted to hospitals with cardiac catheterization laboratories than in patients admitted to hospitals without such facilities.[189,190]

Substantial regional differences in the use of coronary angiography after myocardial infarction also are found within the United States.[185] In the Global Utilization of Streptokinase and Tissue Plasminogen Activator for Occluded Coronary Arteries (GUSTO)-1 study, the proportion of patients undergoing coronary angiography varied from a low of 52% in New England to 81% in the South.[191] Despite these regional differences, there was no apparent relationship between procedure rates and certain patient outcomes. In another study of only Medicare patients with acute myocardial infarction, the utilization of cardiac catheterization varied from 45% in Texas to 30% in New York.[192] Paradoxically, the use of cardiac catheterization in Texas was higher for all clinical subgroups except patients at greatest risk for reinfarction, specifically patients with non–Q-wave infarction or postinfarction angina. Despite the increased use of coronary angiography in Texas, patients in New York had fewer symptoms and a lower adjusted mortality rate after 2 years.

A difference in the use of coronary angiography after myocardial infarction also has been observed among different countries.[183,193] Coronary angiography is used more frequently after myocardial infarction in the United States than in Canada with no apparent difference in mortality or reinfarction rates between the two countries. Similar conclusions were formed in a recent study comparing elderly patients with myocardial infarction in the U.S. and Canada.[194] In contrast, data from 6851 patients enrolled in a large health maintenance organization show the opposite pattern.[195] The rates of angiography were inversely related to the risk of cardiac mortality and subsequent cardiac events over 1–4 years of follow-up. This association was strongest among patients for whom published criteria indicated that angiography was necessary.

Similar registry data comparing rates of cardiac catheterization with outcome in patients with unstable angina and non–Q-wave myocardial infarction were reported in the Organization to Assess Strategies for Ischaemic Syndromes (OASIS) Registry.[196] Approximately 8000 consecutive patients with unstable angina or myocardial infarction without ST-segment elevation were prospectively recruited from 95 hospitals in 6 countries with clinical follow-up for 6 months. Overall, 48% underwent coronary angiography and 33% underwent a revascularization procedure. Hospitals with vs. hospitals without invasive facilities had higher rates of cardiac catheterization (60% vs. 30%) and revascularization (approximately 40% vs. 20%) during follow-up. However, there was no difference in cardiovascular mortality among hospitals or among countries, and there was a slightly lower mortality rate at 6 months in hospitals without catheterization facilities (10.6% vs. 12.5%).

Variation in use of coronary angiography without an obvious difference in outcome raises questions about the appropriateness of angiography, particularly for patients with myocardial infarction.[197,198] In the Myocardial Infarction Triage and Intervention (MITI) Project, the appropriateness of angiography was evaluated in patients with acute myocardial infarction.[187] Except for recurrent angina, clinical risk factors that predict higher mortality rates were associated with a lower rather than a higher use of angiography, suggesting that many patients who needed angiography did not receive it. Although these data do not determine with certainty whether angiographic procedures are overused in patients at low risk of mortality or underused in patients at greater risk of mortality, they suggest that the current balance between patient risk and procedure utilization may not be the most efficient use of this expensive resource.[187] In contrast to data showing that the performance of coronary angiography may be inappropriate in some patients,[199–204] one study focused on how frequently patients fail to undergo angiography despite firm indications for its use.[205] A "necessary" indication for coronary angiography was defined as a highly positive stress test. Among patients with a necessary indication, only 47% underwent angiography within 3 months of the stress test and 61% within 12 months. After adjustment for demographics and clinical presentation, patients cared for by a cardiologist were more likely to undergo necessary angiography than patients cared for by nonspecialists (74% vs. 44% by 1 year). These data raise concern that widely accepted and effective diagnostic tests and therapies are not used in substantial numbers of patients. They also confirm findings from other studies that specialists in cardiovascular disease are more likely to provide appropriate or "necessary" procedures than generalists.[206,207]

Conclusion

There is no question that coronary angiography has provided a substantial amount of anatomic and pathophysiologic information that has improved understanding of the acute coronary syndromes. Although some data suggest that the test may be overused, the information unique to coronary angiography is indispensable in daily clinical management. Thus, coronary angiography probably will remain a highly valuable clinical test for years to come.

References

1. Sones FM, Shirley EK: Cine coronary angiography. Mod Concept Cardiovasc Dis 31:735–738, 1962.
2. Gersh BJ, Braunwald E, Rutherford JD: Chronic coronary artery disease. In Braunwald E (ed): Heart Disease—A Textbook of Cardiovascular Medicine, 5th ed. Philadelphia, W.B. Saunders, 1997, pp 1289–1365.
3. Plotnick GD, Greene HL, Carliner NH, et al: Clinical indicators of left main coronary artery disease in unstable angina. Ann Intern Med 91:149–153, 1991.
4. Victor MF, Likoff MJ, Mintz GS, et al: Unstable angina pectoris of new onset: A prospective clinical and arteriographic study of 75 patients. Am J Cardiol 47:228–232, 1981.
5. Bugiardini R, Pozzati A, Borghi A, et al: Angiographic morphology in unstable angina and its relation to transient myocardial ischemia and hospital outcome. Am J Cardiol 67:460–464, 1991.
6. Allison HW, Russell RO, Mantel JA, et al: Coronary anatomy and arteriography in patients with unstable angina pectoris. Am J Cardiol 41:204–209, 1978.
7. Chaitman BR, Bourassa MG, Davis K, et al: Angiographic prevalence of high-risk coronary artery disease in patient subsets (CASS). Circulation 64:360–367, 1981.
8. Roberts KB, Califf RM, Harrell FE, et al: The prognosis for patients with new-onset angina who have undergone cardiac catheterization. Circulation 68:970–978, 1983.
9. Diver DJ, Bier JD, Ferreira PE, et al: Clinical and arteriographic characterization of patient with unstable angina without critical coronary arterial narrowing (from the TIMI-IIIA trial). Am J Cardiol 74:531–537, 1994.

10. Topol EJ, Nissen SE: Our preoccupation with coronary luminology: The dissociation between clinical and angiographic findings in ischemic heart disease. Circulation 92:2333–2342, 1995.
11. Fuster V, Stein B, Ambrose JA, et al: Atherosclerotic plaque rupture and thrombosis: Evolving concepts. Circulation 82(Suppl II):II-47–II-59, 1990.
12. Ambrose JA, Winters SL, Stern A, et al: Angiographic morphology and the pathogenesis of unstable angina. J Am Coll Cardiol 5:609–616, 1985.
13. Ambrose JA, Winters SL, Arora RR, et al: Coronary angiographic morphology in myocardial infarction: A link between the pathogenesis of unstable angina and myocardial infarction. J Am Coll Cardiol 6:1233–1238, 1985.
14. Wilson RF, Holida MD, White CW: Quantitative angiographic morphology of coronary stenoses leading to myocardial infarction or unstable angina. Circulation 73:286–293, 1986.
15. Ambrose JA, Hjemdahl-Monsen CE: Arteriographic anatomy and mechanisms of myocardial ischemia in unstable angina. J Am Coll Cardiol 9:1397–1402, 1987.
16. Vetrovec GW, Cowley MJ, Overton H, et al: Intracoronary thrombus in syndromes of unstable myocardial ischemia. Am Heart J 102:1202–1208, 1981.
17. Bresnahan DR Davis JL, Holmes DR, et al: Angiographic occurrence and clinical correlates of intraluminal coronary artery thrombus: Role of unstable angina. J Am Coll Cardiol 6:285–289, 1985.
18. Capone G, Wolf NM, Meyer B, et al: Frequency of intracoronary filling defects by angiography in angina pectoris at rest. Am J Cardiol 56:403–406, 1985.
19. Cowley MJ, DiSciascio G, Rehr RB, et al: Angiographic observations and clinical relevance of coronary thrombus in unstable angina pectoris. Am J Cardiol 63:108E–113E, 1989.
20. Freeman MR, Williams AE, Chisholm RJ, et al: Intracoronary thrombus and complex morphology in unstable angina: Relation to timing of angiography and in-hospital cardiac events. Circulation 80:17–23, 1989.
21. Gotoh K, Minamino T, Katoh O, et al: The role of intracoronary thrombus in unstable angina: Angiographic assessment and thrombolytic therapy during ongoing anginal attacks. Circulation 77:526–534, 1988.
22. Rehr R, DiSciascio G, Vetrovec G, et al: Angiographic morphology of coronary artery stenoses in prolonged rest angina: Evidence of intracoronary thrombosis. J Am Coll Cardiol 14:1429–1437, 1989.
23. Sherman CT, Litvack F, Grundfest W, et al: Coronary angioscopy in patients with unstable angina pectoris. N Engl J Med 315:913–919, 1986.
24. Mizuno K, Satomura K, Miyamoto A, et al: Angioscopic evaluation of coronary-artery thrombi in acute coronary syndromes. N Engl J Med 326:287–291, 1992.
25. Chemarin MJ, Pieraggi MT, Elbaz M, et al: Identification of coronary thrombus after myocardial infarction by intracoronary ultrasound compared with histology of tissue sampled by atherectomy. Am J Cardiol 77:344–349, 1996.
26. Lee DY, Eigler N, Fishbein MC, et al: Identification of intracoronary thrombus and demonstration of thrombectomy by intravascular ultrasound imaging. Am J Cardiol 73:522–523, 1994.
27. Pandian NG, Kries A, Brockway B: Detection of intraarterial thrombus by intravascular high frequency two-dimensional ultrasound imaging in vitro and in vivo studies. Am J Cardiol 65:1280–1283, 1990.
28. Rasheed Q, Nair R, Hodgson J McB: Correlation of intracoronary ultrasound plaque characteristics in atherosclerotic coronary artery disease patients with clinical variables. Am J Cardiol 73:753–758, 1994.
29. Gyongyosi M, Yang P, Hassan A, et al: Arterial remodeling of native human coronary arteries in patients with unstable angina pectoris: A prospective intravascular ultrasound study. Heart 82:68–74, 1999.
30. Davies MJ: A macro and micro view of coronary vascular insult in ischemic heart disease. Circulation 82 (Suppl II): II-38–II-46, 1990.
31. Davies MJ, Thomas AC: Plaque fissuring—the cause of acute myocardial infarction, sudden ischemic death and crescendo angina. Br Heart J 53:363–373, 1985.
32. Moise A, Théroux P, Taeymans Y, et al: Unstable angina and progression of coronary atherosclerosis. N Engl J Med 309:685–689, 1983.
33. Ahmed WH, Bittl JA, Braunwald E: Relation between clinical presentation and angiographic findings in unstable angina pectoris, and comparison with that in stable angina. Am J Cardiol 72:544–550, 1993.
34. Kaski JC, Chester MR, Chen L, et al: Rapid angiographic progression of coronary artery disease in patients with angina pectoris. Circulation 92:2058–2065, 1995.
35. DeWood MA, Spores J, Notske R, et al: Prevalence of total coronary occlusion during the early hours of transmural myocardial infarction. N Engl J Med 303:897–902, 1980.
36. Ganz W, Buchbinder M, Marcus H, et al: Intracoronary thrombolysis in evolving myocardial infarction. Am Heart J 101:4–13, 1981.

37. DeFeyter PJ, van Eenige MJ, de Jong PJ, et al: Experience with intracoronary streptokinase in 36 patients with acute evolving myocardial infarction. Eur Heart J 3:441–448, 1982.

38. Cowley MJ, Hastillo A, Vetrovec GW, et al: Effects of intracoronary streprokinase in acute myocardial infarction. Am Heart J 102:1149–1158, 1981.

39. Timmis GC, Gangadharan V, Hauser AM, et al: Intracoronary streptokinase in clinical practice. Am Heart J 104:925–938, 1982.

40. Bertrand ME, Lefebvre JM, Laisne CL, et al: Coronary arteriography in acute transmural myocardial infarction. Am Heart J 97:61–69, 1979.

41. Betriu A, Castañer A, Sanz GA, et al: Angiographic findings 1 month after myocardial infarction. A prospective study of 259 survivors. Circulation 65:1099–1105, 1982.

42. DeFeyter PJ, van Eenige MJ, van der Wall EE, et al: Effects of spontaneous and streptokinase-induced recanalization on left ventricular function after myocardial infarction. Circulation 67:1039–1044, 1983.

43. Pichard AD, Ziff C, Rentrop P, et al: Angiographic study of infarct-related coronary in the chronic stage of acute myocardial infarction. Am Heart J 106:687–692, 1983.

44. Nobuyoshi M, Tanaka M, Nosaka H, et al: Progression of coronary atherosclerosis: Is coronary spasm related to progression? J Am Coll Cardiol 18:904–910, 1991.

45. Little WC, Constantinescu M, Applegate RJ, et al: Can coronary angiography predict the site of a subsequent myocardial infarction in patients with mild-to-moderate disease? Circulation 78:1157–1166, 1988.

46. Ellis S, Alderman EL, Cain K, et al: Morphology of left anterior descending coronary territory lesions as a predictor of anterior myocardial infarction: A CASS registry study. J Am Coll Cardiol 13:1481–1491, 1989.

47. DeWood MA, Stifer WF, Simpson CS, et al: Coronary arteriographic findings soon after non-Q-wave myocardial infarction. N Engl J Med 315:417–423, 1986.

48. Fuster V, Frye RL, Connolly DC:. Arteriographic pattern early after the onset of the coronary syndromes. Br Heart J 37:1250–1255, 1975.

49. Huey BL, Gheorghiade , Crampton RS, et al: Acute non–Q-wave myocardial infarction associated with early ST segment elevation: Evidence for spontaneous coronary reperfusion and implications for thrombolytic trials. J Am Coll Cardiol 9:18–25, 1987.

50. Timmis AD, Griffin B, Crick JCP, et al: The effects of early coronary patency on the evolution of myocardial infarction: A prospective arteriographic study. Br Heart J 58:345–351, 1987.

51. Fox JP, Beattie JM, Salih MS, et al: Non–Q-wave infarction: Exercise test, characteristics, coronary anatomy and prognosis. Br Heart J 63:151–153, 1990.

52. Keen WD, Savage MP, Fischman DL, et al: Comparison of coronary angiographic findings during the first 6 hours of non–Q-wave and Q-wave myocardial infarction. Am J Cardiol 74:324–328, 1994.

53. Madigan NP, Rutherford BD, Frye RL: The clinical course, early prognosis and coronary anatomy of subendocardial infarction. Am J Med 60:634–641, 1976.

54. Ogawa H, Hiramori K, Haze K, et al: Comparison of clinical features of non–Q-wave and Q-wave myocardial infarction. Am Heart J 111:513–518, 1986.

55. Krone RJ, Friedman E, Thanavaro S, et al: Long-term prognosis after first Q-wave (transmural) or non–Q-wave (nontransmural) myocardial infarction: Analysis of 593 patients. Am J Cardiol 52:234–239, 1983.

56. Cannon D, Levy W, Cohen L: The short- and long-term prognosis of patients with transmural and nontransmural infarction. Am J Med 61:452–458, 1976.

57. Hutter AM, DeSanctis RW, Flynn T, et al: Nontransmural myocardial infarction: A comparison of hospital and late clinical course of patients with that of matched patients with transmural anterior and transmural inferior myocardial infarction. Am J Cardiol 48:595–602, 1981.

58. Hollander G, Ozick H, Greengart A, et al: High mortality and early reinfarction with first non-transmural myocardial infarction. Am Heart J 108:1412–1416, 1984.

59. Liberthson RR, Nagel EL, Hirschman JC, et al: Prehospital ventricular fibrillation: Prognosis and follow-up course. N Engl J Med 291:317–321, 1974.

60. Baum RS, Alvarez H, Cobb LA: Survival after resuscitation from out-of-hospital ventricular fibrillation. Circulation 50:1231–1235, 1974.

61. Myerburg RJ, Conde CA, Sung RJ, et al: Clinical, electrophysiologic, and hemodynamic profile of patients resuscitated from prehospital cardiac arrest. Am J Med 68:568–576, 1980.

62. Kuller LH. Sudden death: Definition and epidemiologic considerations. Prog Cardiovasc Dis 23:1–12, 1980.

63. Myerburg RJ, Kessler KM, Castellanos A: Sudden cardiac death: Epidemiology, transient risk, and intervention assessment. Ann Intern Med 119:1187–1197, 1993.

64. Consensus Statement of the Joint Steering Committees of the Unexplained Cardiac Arrest Registry of Europe and of the Idiopathic Ventricular Fibrillation Registry of the United States: Survivors of out-of-hospital cardiac arrest with apparently normal heart: Need for definition and standardized clinical evaluation. Circulation 95:265–272, 1997.
65. Davies MJ, Thomas A: Thrombosis and acute coronary-artery lesions in sudden cardiac ischemic death. N Engl J Med 310:1137–1140, 1984.
66. Spaulding CM, Joly L-M, Rosenberg A, et al: Immediate coronary angiography in survivors of out-of-hospital cardiac arrest. N Engl J Med 336:1629–1633, 1997.
67. Lo YS, Cutler JE, Blake K, et al: Angiographic coronary morphology in survivors of cardiac arrest. Am Heart J 115:781–785, 1988.
68. Lo YS, Cutler JE, Wright A, et al: Long-segment coronary ulcerations in survivors of sudden cardiac death. Am Heart J 116:1444–1447, 1988.
69. Roberts WC: Coronary embolism: A review of causes, consequences and diagnostic considerations. Cardiovasc Med 3:699–710, 1978.
70. Prizel KR, Hutchins GM, Bulkley BH: Coronary artery embolism and myocardial infarction. Ann Intern Med 88:155–161, 1978.
71. Parillo JE, Fauci AS: Necrotizing vasculitis, coronary angiitis and the cardiologist. Am Heart J 99:547–554, 1980.
72. Heibel RH, O'Toole JD, Curtiss EI, et al: Coronary arteritis in systemic lupus erythematosus Chest 69:700–703, 1976.
73. Fukushige J, Nihill MR, McNamara DG: Spectrum of cardiovascular lesions in mucocutaneous lymph node syndrome: Analysis of 8 cases. Am J Cardiol 45:98–107, 1980.
74. Pick RA, Glover MU, Vieweg WVR: Myocardial infarction in a young woman with isolated coronary arteritis. Chest 82:378–380, 1982.
75. Lie JT, Failoni DD, Davis DCJ: Temporal arteritis with giant cell aortitis, coronary arteritis, and myocardial infarction. Arch Pathol Lab Med 110:857–860, 1986.
76. Joensuu H: Myocardial infarction after heart irradiation in young patients with Hodgkin's disease. Chest 95:388–390, 1989.
77. Brosius FC, Roberts WC: Coronary artery disease in the Hurler syndrome. Am J Cardiol 47:649–653, 1981.
78. Smith RR, Hutchins GM: Ischemic heart disease secondary to amyloidosis of intramyocardial arteries. Am J Cardiol 44:413–417, 1979.
79. Huang S, Kumar G, Steele HD, et al: Cardiac involvement in pseudoxanthoma elasticum: Report of a case. Am Heart J 74:680–686, 1967.
80. Hollander JE, Hoffman RS, Burstein JL, et al: Cocaine-associated myocardial infarction: Mortality and complications. Arch Intern Med 155:1081–1086, 1995.
81. Minor RL, Scott BD, Brown DD, et al: Cocaine-induced myocardial infarction in patients with normal coronary arteries. Ann Int Med 115:797–806,1991.
82. Smith HWB, Liberman HA, Brody SL, et al: Acute myocardial infarction temporararily related to cocaine use. Clinical, angiographic, and pathophysiologic observations. Ann Intern Med 107:13–18, 1987.
83. Stenberg RG, Winniford MD, Hillis LD, et al: Simultaneous acute thrombosis of two major coronary arteries following intravenous cocaine use. Arch Pathol Lab Med 113:521–524, 1989.
84. Isner JM, Estes NAM, Thompson PD, et al: Acute cardiac events temporally related to cocaine abuse. N Engl J Med 315:1438–1443, 1986.
85. Alpert JS: Myocardial infarction with angiographically normal coronary arteries. Arch Intern Med 154:265–269, 1994.
86. Pecora MJ, Roubin GS, Cobbs BW, et al: Presentation and late outcome of myocardial infarction in the absence of angiographically significant coronary artery disease. Am J Cardiol 62:363–367, 1988.
87. Yamanaka O, Hobbs RE: Coronary artery anomalies in 126,595 patients undergoing coronary angiography. Cath Cardiovasc Diagn 21:28–40, 1990.
88. Roberts WC: Major anomalies of coronary arterial origin seen in adulthood. Am Heart J 111:941–963, 1986.
89. Basso C, Maron BJ, Corrado D, et al: Clinical profile of congenital coronary artery anomalies with origin from the wrong aortic sinus leading to sudden death in young competitive athletes. J Am Coll Cardiol 35:1493–1501, 2000.
90. Cheitlin MD, De Castro CM, McAllister HA: Sudden death as a complication of anomalous left coronary artery origin from the anterior sinus of Valsalva: A not-so-minor congenital anomaly. Circulation 50:780–787, 1974.
91. Maron BJ, Epstein SE, Roberts WC: Causes of sudden death in competitive athletes. J Am Coll Cardiol 7:204–214, 1986.

92. Ishikawa T, Brandt PWT: Anomalous origin of the left main coronary artery from the right anterior aortic sinus: Angiographic definition of anomalous course. Am J Cardiol 55:770–776, 1985.

93. Roberts WC, Siegel RJ, Zipes D: Origin of the right coronary artery from the left sinus of Valsalva and its functional consequences: Analysis of 10 necropsy cases. Am J Cardiol 49:863–868, 1982.

94. Kragel AH, Roberts WC: Anomalous origin of either the right or left main coronary artery from the aorta with subsequent coursing between aorta and pulmonary trunk: Analysis of 32 necropsy cases. Am J Cardiol 62:771–777, 1988.

95. Blake HA, Manion WC, Mattingly TW, et al: Coronary artery anomalies Circulation 30:927, 1964.

96. Wolf A, Rockson SG: Myocardial ischemia and infarction due to multiple coronary-cameral fistulae: Two case reports and review of the literature. Cath Cardiovasc Diagn 43:179–183, 1998.

97. Sapin P, Frantz E, Jain A, et al: Coronary artery fistula: An abnormality affecting all age groups. Medicine 69:101–113, 1990.

98. Bestetti RB, Costa RS, Zucolotto S, et al: Fatal outcome associated with autopsy proven myocardial bridging of the left anterior descending coronary artery. Eur Heart J 10:573–576, 1989.

99. TIMI IIIb Investigators: Effects of tissue plasminogen activator and a comparison of early invasive and conservative strategies in unstable angina and non-Q-wave myocardial infarction: Results of the TIMI IIIb Trial. Circulation 89:1545–1556, 1994.

100. Anderson HV, Cannon CP, Stone PH, et al: One-year results of the Thrombolysis in Myocardial Infarction (TIMI) IIIb clinical trial: A randomized comparison of tissue-type plasminogen activator versus placebo and early invasive versus conservative strategies in unstable angina and non-Q-wave myocardial infarction. J Am Coll Cardiol 26:1643–1650, 1995.

101. Boden WE, O'Rourke RA, Crawford MH, et al: Outcomes in patients with acute non-Q-wave myocardial infarction randomly assigned to an invasive as compared with conservative management strategy. Veterans Affairs Non-Q-wave Infarction Strategies In-Hospital (VAN-QWISH) Trial Investigators. N Engl J Med 338:1785–1792, 1998.

102. Gersh BJ, O'Rourke RA: Is coronary revascularization the optimum strategy for patients with non-Q-wave myocardial infarction? A point-counterpoint. Clin Cardiol 21(Suppl II): II-18–II-22, 1998.

103. Fragmin and Fast Revascularization during InStability in Coronary artery disease (FRISC-II) Investigators: Invasive compared with non-invasive treatment in unstable coronary-artery disease: FRISC II prospective randomised multicentre study. Lancet 354:708–715, 1999.

104. McCullough PA, O'Neill WW, Graham M, et al: A prospective randomized trial of triage angiography in acute coronary syndromes ineligible for thrombolytic therapy: Results of the Medicine Versus Angiography in Thrombolytic Exclusion (MATE) Trial. J Am Coll Cardiol 32:596–605, 1998.

105. Scull GS, Martin JS, Weaver D, et al. Early angiography versus conservative treatment in patients with non-ST elevation acute myocardial infarction. J Am Coll Cardiol 35:895–902, 2000.

106. Braunwald E, Mark DB, Jones RH, et al: Clinical Practice Guideline Number 10: Unstable Angina: Diagnosis and Management, 86th ed. Rockville MD, U.S. Dept of Health and Human Services, Agency for Health Care Policy and Research, AHCPR publication 94-0602, 1994.

107. Scanlon PJ, Faxon DP, Audet AM, et al: ACC/AHA guidelines for coronary angiography: A report of the American College of Cardiology/American Heart Association Task Force on Practice Guidelines (Committee on Coronary Angiography) J Am Coll Cardiol 33:1756–1824, 1999.

108. Grambow DW, Topol EJ: Effect of maximal medical therapy on refractoriness of unstable angina pectoris. Am J Cardiol 70:577–581, 1992.

109. Gibson RS: Non-Q-wave myocardial infarction: Diagnosis, prognosis, and management. Curr Probl Cardiol 13:9–72, 1988

110. Kulick DL, Rahimtoola SH: Risk stratification in survivors of acute myocardial infarction: Routine cardiac catheterization and angiography is a reasonable approach in most patients. Am Heart J 121:641–656, 1991.

111. Lotan CS, Jonas M, Rozenman Y, et al: Comparison of early invasive and conservative treatments in patients with anterior wall non-Q-wave acute myocardial infarction. Am J Cardiol 76:330–336, 1995.

112. Conti CR: Optimal therapeutic management of non-Q-wave myocardial infarction. Clin Cardiol 23:1–3, 2000.

113. Samaha JK, Connor MJ, Tribble R, et al: Natural history of left anterior descending coronary artery obstruction: Significance of location of stenoses in medically treated patients. Clin Cardiol 8:415–422, 1985.

114. Brooks N, Cattell M, Jennings K, et al: Isolated disease of the left anterior descending coronary artery: Angiographic and clinical study in 218 patients. Br Heart J 47:71–77, 1982.
115. Califf RM, Tomabechi Y, Lee KL, et al: Outcome in one-vessel coronary artery disease. Circulation 67:283–290, 1983.
116. Simes RJ, Topol EJ, Holmes DR Jr, et al: Link between the angiographic substudy and mortality outcomes in a large randomized trial of myocardial reperfusion: Importance of early and complete infarct artery reperfusion. GUSTO-I Investigators. Circulation 91:1923–1928, 1995.
117. O'Neill WW: The evolution of primary PTCA therapy of acute myocardial infarction: A personal perspective. J Invasive Cardiol 7:2F–11F, 1995.
118. Grines CL, Browne KF, Marco J, et al: A comparison of immediate angioplasty with thrombolytic therapy for acute myocardial infarction: The Primary Angioplasty in Myocardial Infarction Study Group. N Engl J Med 328:673–679, 1993.
119. Grines CL, Marsalese D, Brodie B, et al: Safety and cost-effectiveness of early discharge after primary angioplasty in low-risk patients with acute myocardial infarction: PAMI-II Investigators. Primary Angioplasty in Myocardial Infarction. J Am Coll Cardiol 31:967–972, 1998.
120. Neuhaus KL, von Essen R, Tebbe U, et al: Improved thrombolysis in acute myocardial infarction with front-loaded administration of alteplase: Results of the rt-PA-APSAC patency study (TAPS). J Am Coll Cardiol 19:885–891, 1992.
121. Ohman EM, Califf RM, Topol EJ, et al: Consequences of reocclusion after successful reperfusion therapy in acute myocardial infarction: TAMI study group. Circulation 82:781–791, 1990.
122. Topol EJ, Califf RM, George BS, et al: A randomized trial of immediate versus delayed elective angioplasty after intravenous tissue plasminogen activator in acute myocardial infarction. N Engl J Med 317:581–588, 1988.
123. Simoons ML, Arnold AE, Betriu A, et al: Thrombolysis with tissue plasminogen activator in acute myocardial infarction: No additional benefit from immediate coronary angioplasty. Lancet 1:197–203, 1988.
124. TIMI Research Group: Immediate vs. delayed catheterization and angioplasty following thrombolytic therapy for acute myocardial infarction: TIMI II A results. JAMA 260:2849–2858, 1988.
125. Arnold AE, Simoons ML, Van de Werf F, et al: Recombinant tissue-type plasminogen activator and immediate angioplasty in acute myocardial infarction: One-year follow-up. The European Cooperative Study Group. Circulation 86:111–120, 1992.
126. Rogers WJ, Baim DS, Gore JM, et al: Comparison of immediate invasive, delayed invasive, and conservative strategies after tissue type plasminogen activator: Results of the Thrombolysis in Myocardial Infarction (TIMI) Phase II-A trial. Circulation 81:1457–1476, 1990.
127. Califf RM, O'Neill W, Stack RS, et al: Failure of simple clinical measurements to predict perfusion status after intravenous thrombolysis. Ann Intern Med 108:658–662, 1998.
128. De Lemos JA, Antman EM, Gibson CM, et al: Abciximab improves both epicardial flow and myocardial reperfusion in ST-elevation myocardial infarction: Observations from the TIMI 14 Trial. Circulation 101:239–242, 2000.
129. Langer A, Krucoff MW, Klootwijk P, et al: Noninvasive assessment of speed and stability of infarct-related artery reperfusion: Results of the GUSTO ST segment monitoring study. J Am Coll Cardiol 25:1552–1557, 1995.
130. Abe S, Arima S, Yamashita T, et al: Early assessment of reperfusion therapy using cardiac troponin T. J Am Coll Cardiol 23:1382–1389, 1994.
131. Andrews J, Straznicky IT, French JK, et al: ST-segment recovery adds to the assessment of TIMI 2 and 3 flow in predicting infarct wall motion after thrombolytic therapy. Circulation 101:2138–2143, 2000.
132. Juliard JM, Himbert D, Golmard JL, et al: Can we provide reperfusion therapy to all unselected patients admitted with acute myocardial infarction? J Am Coll Cardiol 30:157–164, 1997.
133. Califf RM, Topol EJ, Stack RS, et al: Evaluation of combination thrombolytic therapy and timing of cardiac catheterization in acute myocardial infarction: Results of the thrombolysis and angioplasty in myocardial infarction–Phase 5 randomized trial. Circulation 83:1543–1556, 1991.
134. Belenkie I, Traboulsi M, Hall CA, et al: Rescue angioplasty during myocardial infarction has a beneficial effect on mortality: A tenable hypothesis. Can J Cardiol 8:357–362, 1992.
135. Ellis SG, da Silva ER, Heyndrix G, et al: Randomized comparison of rescue angioplasty with conservative management of patients with early failure of thrombolysis for acute anterior myocardial infarction Circulation 90:2280–2240, 1994.
136. Vermeer F, Ophuis AJ, Berg EJ, et al: Prospective randomized comparison between thrombolysis, rescue PTCA, and primary PTCA in patients with extensive myocardial infarction admitted to a hospital without PTCA facilities: A safety and feasibility study. Heart 82:426–431, 1999.

137. Ross AM, Lundergan CF, Rohrbeck SC, et al: Rescue angioplasty after failed thrombolysis: Technical and clinical outcomes in a large thrombolysis trial. J Am Coll Cardiol 31:1511–1517, 1998.

138. McKendall GR, Forman S, Sopko G, et al: Value of rescue percutaneous transluminal coronary angioplasty following unsuccessful thrombolytic therapy in patients with acute myocardial infarction: Thrombolysis in Myocardial Infarction Investigators. Am J Cardiol 76:1108–1111, 1995.

139. Epstein SE, Palmeri ST, Patterson RE: Current concepts: Evaluation of patients after acute myocardial infarction: Indications for cardiac catheterization and surgical intervention. N Engl J Med 307:1487–1492, 1982.

140. Benhorin J, Andrews ML, Carleen ED, et al: Occurrence, characteristics and prognostic significance of early postacute myocardial infarction angina pectoris. Am J Cardiol 62:679–685, 1988.

141. Bosch X, Theroux P, Waters DD, et al: Early postinfarction ischemia: Clinical, angiographic, and prognostic significance. Circulation 75:988–995, 1987.

142. Gibson RS, Young PM, Boden WE, et al: Prognostic significance and beneficial effect of diltiazem on the incidence of early recurrent ischemia after non-Q-wave myocardial infarction: Results from the Multicenter Diltiazem Reinfarction Study. Am J Cardiol 60:203–209, 1987.

143. Gibson RS, Beller GA, Gheorghiade M, et al: The prevalence and clinical significance of residual myocardial ischemia 2 weeks after uncomplicated non–Q-wave infarction: A prospective natural history study. Circulation 73:1186–1198, 1986.

144. Rahimtoola SH: A perspective on the three large multicenter randomized clinical trials of coronary bypass surgery for chronic stable angina. Circulation 72:V-123–V-135, 1985.

145. Madsen JK, Grande P, Sannamaki K, et al: Danish multicenter randomized study of invasive versus conservative treatment in patients with inducible ischemia after thrombolysis in acute myocardial infarction (DANAMI): DANish trial in Acute Myocardial Infarction. Circulation 96:748–755, 1997.

146. Clements SD Jr, Story WE, Hurst JW, et al: Ruptured papillary muscle, a complication of myocardial infarction: Clinical presentation, diagnosis, and treatment. Clin Cardiol 8:93–103, 1985.

147. Edwards BS, Edwards WD, Edwards JE: Ventricular septal rupture complicating acute myocardial infarction: Identification of simple and complex types in 53 autopsied hearts. Am J Cardiol 54:1201–1205, 1984.

148. Scanlon PJ, Montoya A, Johnson SA, et al: Urgent surgery for ventricular septal rupture complicating acute myocardial infarction. Circulation 72:II-185–II-190, 1985.

149. Muehrcke DD, Daggett WM Jr, Buckley MJ, et al: Postinfarct ventricular septal defect repair: Effect of coronary artery bypass grafting. Ann Thorac Surg 54:876–882, 1992.

150. Rasmussen S, Leth A, Kjoller E, et al: Cardiac rupture in acute myocardial infarction: A review of 72 consecutive cases. Acta Med Scand 205:11–16, 1979.

151. Pohjola-Sintonen S, Muller JE, Stone PH, et al: Ventricular septal and free wall rupture complicating acute myocardial infarction: Experience in the Multicenter Investigation of Limitation of Infarct Size. Am Heart J 117:809–818, 1989.

152. Lavie CJ, Gersh BJ: Acute myocardial infarction: Initial manifestations, management, and prognosis. Mayo Clin Proc 65:531–548, 1990.

153. Risk stratification and survival after myocardial infarction. N Engl J Med 309:331–336, 1983.

154. Zaret BL, Wackers FJ, Terrin ML, et al: Value of radionuclide rest and exercise left ventricular ejection fraction in assessing survival of patients after thrombolytic therapy for acute myocardial infarction: Results of Thrombolysis in Myocardial Infarction (TIMI) phase II study. The TIMI Study Group. J Am Coll Cardiol 26:73–79, 1995.

155. Rouleau JL, Talajic M, Sussex B, et al: Myocardial infarction patients in the 1990s: their risk factors, stratification and survival in Canada: The Canadian Assessment of Myocardial Infarction (CAMI) Study. J Am Coll Cardiol 27:1119–1127, 1996.

156. Harris PJ, Lee KL, Harrell FE Jr, et al: Outcome in medically treated coronary artery disease: Ischemic events: Nonfatal infarction and death. Circulation 62:718–726, 1980.

157. TIMI Study Group: Comparison of invasive and conservative strategies after treatment with intravenous tissue plasminogen activator in acute myocardial infarction: Results of the Thrombolysis in Myocardial Infarction (TIMI) phase II trial. N Engl J Med 320:618–627, 1989.

158. Williams DO, Braunwald E, Knattererud G, et al: One-year results of the Thrombolysis in Myocardial Infarction investigation (TIMI) Phase II Trial. Circulation 85:533–542, 1992.

159. Terrin ML, Williams DO, Kleiman NS, et al: Two- and three-year results of the Thrombolysis in Myocardial Infarction (TIMI) phase II clinical trial. J Am Coll Cardiol 22:1763–1772, 1993.

160. SWIFT trial of delayed elective intervention vs. conservative treatment after thrombolysis with anistreplase in acute myocardial infarction: SWIFT (Should We Intervene Following Thrombolysis?) Trial Study Group. BMJ 302:555–560, 1991.

161. Barbash Gl, Roth A, Hod H, et al: Randomized controlled trial of late in-hospital angiography and angioplasty versus conservative management after treatment with recombinant tissue-type plasminogen activator in acute myocardial infarction. Am J Cardiol 66:538–545, 1990.

162. Ellis SG, Mooney MR, George BS, et al: Randomized trial of late elective angioplasty versus conservative management for patients with residual stenoses after thrombolytic treatment of myocardial infarction: Treatment of Post-Thrombolytic Stenoses (TOPS) Study Group. Circulation 86:1400–1406, 1992.

163. Krone RJ: The role of risk stratification in the early management of myocardial infarction. Ann Int Med 116:223–237, 1992.

164. Hillis LD, Forman S, Braunwald E: Risk stratification before thrombolytic therapy in patients with acute myocardial infarction: The Thrombolysis in Myocardial Infarction (TIMI) Phase II Co-investigators. J Am Coll Cardiol 16:313–315, 1990.

165. Nicod P, Gilpin E, Dittrich H, et al: Influence on prognosis and morbidity of left ventricular ejection fraction with and without signs of left ventricular failure after acute myocardial infarction. Am J Cardiol 61:1165–1171, 1988.

166. Greenberg H, McMaster P, Dwyer EM Jr: Left ventricular dysfunction after acute myocardial infarction: Results of a prospective multicenter study. J Am Coll Cardiol 4:867–874, 1984.

167. Taylor GJ, Humphties JO, Mellits ED, et al: Predictors of clinical course, coronary anatomy and left ventricular function after recovery from acute myocardial infarction. Circulation 62:960–970, 1980.

168. Madsen EB, Hougaard P, Gilpin E: Dynamic evaluation of prognosis from time-dependent variables in acute myocardial infarction. Am J Cardiol 51:1579–1583, 1983.

169. Gilpin EA, Koziol JA, Madsen EB, et al: Periods of differing mortality distribution during the first year after acute myocardial infarction. Am J Cardiol 52:240–244, 1983.

170. Dittus RS, Roberts SD, Adolph RJ: Cost-effectiveness analysis of patient management alternatives after uncomplicated myocardial infarction: A model. J Am Coll Cardiol 10:869–878, 1987.

171. Sanz G, Castaner A, Betriu A, et al: Determinants of prognosis in survivors of myocardial infarction: A prospective clinical angiographic study. N Engl J Med 306:1065–1070, 1982.

172. Roubin GS, Harris PJ, Bernstein L, et al: Coronary anatomy and prognosis after myocardial infarction in patients 60 years of age and younger. Circulation 67:743–749, 1983.

173. Schulman SP, Achuff SC, Griffith LS, et al: Prognostic cardiac catheterization variables in survivors of acute myocardial infarction: A five year prospective study. J Am Coll Cardiol 11:1164–1172, 1988.

174. Arnold AE, Simoons ML, Detry JM, et al: Prediction of mortality following hospital discharge after thrombolysis for acute myocardial infarction: Is there a need for coronary angiography? European Cooperative Study Group. Eur Heart J 14:306–315, 1993.

175. Rapaport E, Remedios P: The high risk patient after recovery from myocardial infarction: Recognition and management. J Am Coll Cardiol 1:391–400, 1983.

176. DeBusk RF, Blomqvist CG, Kouchoukos NT, et al: Identification and treatment of low-risk patients after acute myocardial infarction and coronary-artery bypass graft surgery. N Engl J Med 314:161–166, 1986.

177. DeBusk RF: Specialized testing after recent acute myocardial infarction. Ann Intern Med 110:470–481, 1989.

178. Moss AJ, Benhotin J: Prognosis and management after a first myocardial infarction. N Engl J Med 322:743–753, 1990.

179. Rogers WJ: Contemporary management of acute myocardial infarction. Am J Med 99:195–206, 1995.

180. Shaw LJ, Petersen ED, Kesler K, et al: A meta-analysis of predischarge risk stratification after acute myocardial infarction with stress electrocardiographic myocardial perfusion and ventricular function imaging. Am J Cardiol 78:1327–1337, 1996.

181. Topol EJ, Holmes DR, Rogers WJ: Coronary angiography after thrombolytic therapy for acute myocardial infarction. Ann Intern Med 114:877–885, 1991.

182. Ross J Jr, Gilpin EA, Madsen EB, et al: A decision scheme for coronary angiography after acute myocardial infarction. Circulation 79:292–303, 1989.

183. Mark DB, Naylor CD, Hlatky MA, et al: Use of medical resources and quality of life after acute myocardial infarction in Canada and the United States. N Engl J Med 331:1130–1135, 1994.

184. Rogers WJ, Bowlby LJ, Chandra NC, et al: Treatment of myocardial infarction in the United States (1990 to 1993): Observations from the National Registry of Myocardial Infarction. Circulation 90:2103–2114, 1994.

185. Graves EJ: National hospital discharge survey: Annual summary, 1993. Vital Health Stat 13:1–63, 1995.

186. Medicare claims data. Provided by the Physician Payment Review Commission, 1996.

187. Spertus JA, Weiss NS, Every NR, et al: The influence of clinical risk factors on the use of angiography and revascularization after acute myocardial infarction: Myocardial Infarction Triage and Intervention project Investigators. Arch Int Med 155:2309–2316, 1995.
188. Pashos CL, Newhouse JP, McNeil BJ: Temporal changes in the care and outcomes of elderly patients with acute myocardial infarction, 1987 through 1990. JAMA 270:1232–1236, 1993.
189. Every NR, Larson EB, Litwin PE, et al: The association between on-site cardiac catheterization facilities and the use of coronary angiography after acute myocardial infarction: Myocardial Infarction Triage and Intervention Project Investigators. N Engl J Med 329:546–551, 1993.
190. Blustein J: High-technology cardiac procedures: The impact of service availability on service use in New York State. JAMA 270:344–349, 1993.
191. Pilote L, Califf RM, Sapp S, et al: Regional variation across the United States in the management of acute myocardial infarction: GUSTO-1 Investigators. Global Utilization of Streptokinase and Tissue Plasminogen Activator for Occluded Coronary Arteries. N Engl J Med 333:565–572, 1995.
192. Guadagnoli E, Hauptman PJ, Ayanian JZ, et al: Variation in the use of cardiac procedures after acute myocardial infarction. N Engl J Med 333:573–578, 1995.
193. Rouleau JL, Moye LA, Pfeifer MA, et al: A comparison of management patterns after acute myocardial infarction in Canada and the United States: The SAVE investigators. N Engl J Med 328:779–784, 1993.
194. Tu JV, Pashos CL, Naylor CD, et al: Use of cardiac procedures and outcomes in elderly patients with myocardial infarction in the United States and Canada. N Engl J Med 336:1500–1505, 1997.
195. Selby JV, Fireman BH, Lundstrom RJ, et al: Variation among hospitals in coronary-angiography practices and outcomes after myocardial infarction in a large health maintenance organization. N Engl J Med 335:1888–1896, 1996.
196. Yusef S, Flather M, Poguee J, et al: Variations between countries in invasive procedures and outcome in patients with suspected unstable angina or myocardial infarction without initial ST elevation. Lancet 352:507–514, 1998.
197. Leape LL, Park RE, Solomon DH, et al: Does inappropriate use explain small-area variations in the use of health care services? JAMA 263:669–672, 1990.
198. Wennberg JE: The paradox of appropriate care. JAMA 258:2568–2569, 1987.
199. Bernstein SJ, Hilbome LH, Leape LL, et al: The appropriateness of use of coronary angiography in New York State. JAMA 269:766–769, 1993.
200. Hampton GD Jr, Cary D, Hampton JR: Methods of establishing criteria for purchasing coronary angiography in the investigation of chest pain. J Public Health Med 16:399–405, 1994.
201. McGlynn EA, Naylor CD, Anderson GM, et al: Comparison of the appropriateness of coronary angiography and coronary artery bypass graft surgery between Canada and New York State. JAMA 272:934–940, 1994.
202. Bengston A, Herlitz J, Karlsson T, et al: The appropriateness of performing coronary angiography and coronary artery revascularization in a Swedish population. JAMA 271:1260–1265, 1994.
203. Bernstein SJ, Hilborne LH, Leape LL, et al: The appropriateness of use of cardiovascular procedures in women and men. Arch Intern Med 154:2759–2765, 1994.
204. Ayanian JZ, Landrum MB, Normand SL, et al: Rating the appropriateness of coronary angiography—do practicing physicians agree with an expert panel and with each other? N Engl J Med 338:1896–1904, 1998.
205. Borowsky SJ, Kravitz RL, Laouri M, et al: Effect of physician specialty on use of necessary coronary angiography. J Am Coll Cardiol 26:1484–1491, 1995.
206. Jollis JG, DeLong ER, Peterson ED, et al: Outcome of acute myocardial infarction according to the specialty of the admitting physician. N Engl J Med 335:1880–1887, 1996.
207. Nash IS, Hash DB, Fuster V: Do cardiologists do it better? J Am Coll Cardiol 29:475–478, 1997.

The Essential Role of Percutaneous Coronary Interventions in the Management of Acute Coronary Syndromes

GARY E. LANE, MD
DAVID R. HOLMES, JR., MD

Andreas Gruentzig's pioneering effort in the mid 1970s established balloon angioplasty as an important treatment option for patients with coronary artery disease. Its extraordinary success has led to enthusiastic growth and continual evolution of the technique. The application of angioplasty has expanded from the initial anatomic indications (single, discrete, concentric proximal stenoses) in stable patients with preserved left ventricular function to include complex lesions in unstable clinical situations. Creative technologic advances have been introduced, tested, and incorporated into the interventional cardiology practice. This spirited progress has occurred largely as a result of observational study, although recent important developments (e.g., stents, glycoprotein IIb/IIIa receptor antagonists) have not been introduced on a widespread basis until after the completion of randomized trials.

The acute coronary syndrome is comprised of three clinical entities; ST-elevation or Q-wave myocardial infarction, unstable angina, and non–ST-elevation or non–Q-wave myocardial infarction. Coronary revascularization by transluminal intervention maintains an integral role in the management of patients with acute coronary syndromes, yet many points of controversy remain.

Unstable Angina and Non–ST-elevation Infarction

At presentation there is little to distinguish the two non–ST-elevation entities. Although most patients share plaque disruption and thrombus formation as an initiating pathogenic event, the prognosis is influenced by multiple variables, including extent of anatomic coronary artery disease, collateral function, vasospasm, degree of left ventricular dysfunction, and associated conditions that may intensify ischemia. In comparison with Q-wave infarction, in which vessel patency and degree of myocardial damage determine prognosis, the outcome of the non–ST-elevation syndromes is affected principally by the severity of plaque injury and associated thrombus accumulation. The complex "type II eccentric" lesions of Ambrose are predictive of an unstable clinical hospital course and are more likely to progress (primarily to complete occlusion) in the months after hospitalization, even when the patient is stabilized on medical therapy.[1–3] The similarity in plaque morphology and thrombus characteristics of the "white," predominantly platelet thrombus in these syndromes mitigates the necessity for clear differentiation between unstable angina and non-Q-wave infarction.[4]

Balloon angioplasty expands the arterial lumen by barotrauma inducing disruption of the atherosclerotic plaque, dissection of the intima from the media, and expansion of medial and adventitial elements.[5,6] These mechanical effects may cause extensive damage to the arterial wall with concomitant platelet deposition and activation of a myriad of coagulation factors, resulting in thrombus formation.

Complex lesion morphology has been shown to increase the likelihood of acute complications after balloon angioplasty.[7] The common presence of thrombus or a thrombotic local environment associated with plaque rupture in acute coronary syndromes also enhances the risk of coronary angioplasty. Several studies have documented the amplified risk of abrupt closure during angioplasty in patients with angiographically or angioscopically identified intracoronary thrombus.[8–13] Although modern advances (particularly glycoprotein IIb/IIIa antagonists) in interventional cardiology have blunted the impact of intracoronary thrombus, it remains a risk factor for in-hospital complications.[9,14,15] Thrombus also appears to promote the occurrence of restenosis primarily by accentuating the risk of subsequent total occlusion.[16]

Unstable Angina

Early reports suggested that coronary angioplasty was an effective treatment method for patients with unstable angina.[17,18] However, the initial report from the Percutaneous Transluminal Coronary Angioplasty (PTCA) Registry of the National Heart, Lung, and Blood Institute (NHLBI) delineated a significantly increased risk of complications (especially myocardial infarction and emergency bypass surgery) compared with patients with stable angina.[19] Although the procedural success of angioplasty is comparable in patients with stable or unstable angina, historically the major complication rate has been consistently higher in patients with unstable angina.[20,21] In concert with the risk of intracoronary thrombus, the increment in complications is due principally to an increased risk of abrupt closure, which translates to an increased incidence of coronary bypass surgery, myocardial infarction, and death.[10,22]

Examination of the overall success and complication rates of several reported series of patients undergoing balloon angioplasty for unstable angina (1984–1996) reveals improving but nonuniform success rates from several centers[17,19,21,23–35,40] (Table 1). In the 1985–1986 NHLBI PTCA Registry there was no overall difference in procedural success between patients with stable or unstable angina. Major complications remained higher in the group with unstable angina, but cumulative 5-year mortality rates, myocardial infarction rates, and repeat revascularization were not significantly different.[20,36] A more contemporary report from the NHLBI Dynamic Registry (1997–1998) reveals that despite

Table 1. Short-term Outcomes with Angioplasty for Unstable Angina

Author	Publication Year	n	Success (%)	Hospital Complications		
				CABG	*MI*	*Death*
Williams[17]	1981	17	76	6.0	—	0.0
Faxon[19]	1983	447	63	29.0	9.6	0.9
Meyer[23]	1983	50	74	2.0	0.0	0.0
Quigley[24]	1986	857	81	12.0	12.0	4.0
Timis[25]	1987	56	70	12.5	7.1	5.4
Steffenino[26]	1987	327	90	2.6	5.0	0.0
Sharma[27]	1988	40	88	12.0	7.5	0.0
Plokker[28]	1988	469	88	3.0	4.9	1.0
Perry[29]	1988	105	87	4.0	9.0	2.0
Kamp[21]	1989	334	87	10.0	9.0	0.6
Halon[30]	1989	90	93	0.0	0.0	1.1
Myler[31]	1990	807	84	5.1	3.6	0.2
Rupprecht[32]	1990	202	83	7.9	6.5	7.9
Stammen[33]	1992	631	91	4.7	3.6	0.3
Bentivoglio[36]	1994	952	79	4.4	3.3	1.3
Morrison[34]	1995	207	95	1.0	4.0	5.0
TIMI IIIB[35]	1996	278	97	1.4	4.3	0.5
Rozenman[40]	1996	872	92	0.3	1.1	1.1

CABG = coronary artery bypass graft, MI = myocardial infarction.

more complex patient and lesion characteristics associated with unstable angina, procedural success and in-hospital outcome are similar to patients with stable angina.[37] The dramatic progress in transluminal revascularization technique for patients with unstable angina is illustrated by the results from the Mayo Medical Center since 1979 (Table 2).[38] The improved acute procedural success led to a reduction in adverse events at 1-year follow-up.

Table 2. Outcomes of Percutaneous Intervention for Unstable Angina at Mayo Medical Center

	1979–1989	1990–1993	1994–1998	p value
Number of patients	2209	2212	3211	
Mean age	62.1	64.8	64.6	
Clinical success (%)	76.5	87.0	94.1	< 0.00001
Hospital mortality (%)	3.0	2.4	1.8	0.009
Q-wave MI (%)	1.8	1.0	0.7	0.001
CABG < 24 hr (%)	4.9	1.8	0.7	< 0.00001
1-year follow-up				
Death (%)	3.1	4.2	2.8	0.004
Q-wave MI (%)	0.7	0.9	0.3	0.0001
CABG (%)	10.7	9.5	7.0	0.0001

MI = myocardial infarction, CABG = coronary artery bypass graft.
From Singh M, Holmes DR, Garratt KN, et al: Changing outcomes of percutaneous intervention in patients with unstable angina. J Am Coll Cardiol 33:31A, 1999, with permission.

It has been reported that coronary angioplasty for unstable angina performed within 1–2 weeks after the onset of symptoms is associated with lower success rates and higher complication rates.[31,39,40] It also has been suggested that complication rates are increased in patients with medically refractory unstable angina.[41] However, Antonucci et al. reported the results (n = 263) of early angioplasty (within 4 hours) for patients with medically refractory unstable angina compared with delayed (> 72 hours) angioplasty of stabilized patients.[42] The success rate for the primary lesion in the refractory (93%) and stabilized (94%) groups was equivalent. The combined adverse hospital event rate was statistically similar (18.6% refractory vs. 12.5% stabilized, p = 0.25) with a significantly shorter hospitalization in the refractory group (3.6 days vs. 6.1 days, p < 0.0001). The composite adverse event rate at 6-month follow-up was also statistically comparable (27% refractory vs. 39% stabilized). Considering data accrued from several trials (including EPIC, CAPTURE, IMPACT, and RESTORE), "passivation" of the plaque with the use of glycoprotein IIb/IIIa antagonists can diminish the hazard of early coronary interventions.[43–46]

Angioplasty of the Culprit Vessel

Most patients with unstable angina have multivessel disease.[47] Angioplasty of the ischemia-generating artery (identified by lesion appearance or localization of the ischemic region) has been advocated as an effective therapeutic option.[48,49] Although incomplete revascularization may lead to recurrent ischemia in the future, this strategy often stabilizes the patient's condition, allowing medical therapy or a more elective strategy for further revascularization.[50] A large trial comparing multivessel angioplasty with coronary artery bypass surgery in patients with unstable angina has not been undertaken. In the BARI (Balloon Angioplasty Revascularization Investigation) trial, however, most patients (64%) were classified as having unstable angina.[51] The angioplasty strategy did not significantly decrease 5-year survival rates compared with surgical treatment except in patients with diabetes. Additional revascularization procedures were significantly more frequent in the patients assigned to the angioplasty strategy (54% vs. 8%, p < 0.001).

Restenosis and Unstable Angina

Unstable angina has been recognized as a risk factor for restenosis after coronary angioplasty.[52–55] Halon et al. identified intracoronary thrombus, multiple lesion irregularities, and decreased flow as risk factors for restenosis in unstable angina.[30] Other studies have confirmed that thrombus demonstrated by angiography or angioscopy is a predictor for restenosis.[16,56] In theory, platelet thrombus may be an integral antecedent of the restenosis process. The mechanism of restenosis in unstable angina appears to be related principally to plaque proliferation, in contrast to the more frequent vessel contracture noted in patients with stable angina.[57] In the EPIC trial a sustained reduction in target vessel revascularization was seen in patients receiving abciximab.[58] However this benefit was not evident in the CAPTURE, EPILOG, RESTORE, or IMPACT trials.[44,46,59,60]

Non–Q-wave Myocardial Infarction

Categorization of acute coronary syndromes as non–Q-wave infarction typically implies an intermediate risk between unstable angina and acute ST-elevation or Q-wave infarction. This distinction is complicated by multiple functional and anatomic variables, resulting in an uncertain prognosis on presentation. The hospital mortality rate appears to be lower for non–Q-wave infarction than for Q-wave infarction. More jeopardized myocardium is present after non–Q-wave than after Q-wave infarction, and the long-term cumulative mortality rate is similar for both conditions.[61,62] Patients with non–Q-wave infarction have an increased risk of reinfarction and death compared with patients with unstable angina.[63]

The boundaries defining infarction and unstable angina have become more obscure with the development of sensitive biochemical markers of myocardial injury. Elevations of myocardial-bound creatine kinase (CK-MB) can occur without pathologic evidence of myocardial necrosis.[64] Recently troponin I and troponin T have been shown to be powerful predictors of myocardial infarction and death in patients with acute coronary syndromes.[6–68] Meta-analysis of 12 studies assessing the importance of elevated troponin levels derived risk ratios of 2.7 (troponin I) and 4.2 (troponin T) for subsequent infarction and death.[69] Approximately 30% of patients with elevated troponin levels show no evidence of necrosis by CK-MB determination.[70] Isolated troponin elevation may represent focal necrosis due to microembolization, and troponin elevation may be a surrogate for an active complex thrombotic coronary lesion.[67,71] Patients with elevated troponin levels have more severe coronary artery disease, and revascularization therapy may equalize their risk with that of patients with normal levels.[72,73] However, elevation of troponin levels predicts angiographic lesion characteristics associated with a higher risk during angioplasty.[74] The excessive risk of intervention in patients with elevated troponin levels is mollified considerably by treatment with abciximab.[75]

The diverse pathogenesis of non–Q-wave myocardial infarction is exemplified by early coronary angiographic findings. Keen et al. found evidence of thrombus in 43% and total occlusion in 39% in 28 patients examined within 6 hours of symptom onset.[76] Collateral vessels to the occluded artery were noted in 45%. The appearance of collateral vessels to the region of the infarct artery is visualized more commonly after non–Q-wave than after Q-wave infarction. In contrast, total occlusion is seen in about 10% of patients with unstable angina.[77] Multivessel disease is noted in most patients with non–Q-wave infarction.[62,78] Compared with ST–elevation infarction, patients with non–ST-elevation infarction included in the recent NHLBI dynamic registry are more likely to have prior coronary artery bypass grafting (CABG; 2.5% vs. 16.4%, p < 0.001), prior infarction (17% vs. 29.4%, p < 0.01), history of congestive heart failure (5.9% vs. 14.9%, p < 0.001) and multivessel disease (51.3% vs. 55.8%, p <0.01).[79]

The range of pathology encountered by the interventional cardiologist may account for variations in success and complication rates of reported series[35,80–85] (Table 3). These studies defined non–Q-wave infarction by elevation of creatine kinase levels. In the TIMI IIIB trial, comparable success rates were attained with angioplasty for unstable angina (96.9%) and non–Q-wave infarction (94.8%) (p = 0.33) despite more severe lesions with lower grades of antegrade flow in the latter patient classification.[35] Of interest, periprocedural myocardial infarction was more common in patients with unstable angina than in patients with non–Q-wave infarction (4.3% vs. 0%, p = 0.007). This finding may relate to difficulties with detection and/or conditions of prior myocardial injury. Studies comparing late outcome reveal similar event rates after angioplasty of patients with non–Q-wave infarction or Q-wave infarction.[81,85] Future classification schemes for patients with acute coronary syndromes incorporating accurate coronary anatomic and ventricular functional status may help to clarify the disparities noted in prognosis and response to therapy.[86]

Table 3.   Short-term Outcomes with Angioplasty for Non–Q-wave Infarction

Author	Publication Year	Patients	Success (%)	Hospital Complications		
				CABG (%)	MI(%)	Death (%)
Safian[83]	1987	68	87	1.4	1.4	0
Holt[82]	1988	38	89	8	—	2.6
Suryapranata[84]	1988	114	88	6	4.4	0
Alfonso[80]	1990	33	91	0	0	0
Welty[85]	1995	231	90	4.3	4	1
Brueren[81]	1997	175	97	0	7.4	0
TIMI IIIB[35]	1996	165	95	1.4	0	0.5

CABG = coronary artery bypass graft, MI = myocardial infarction.

Adjuvant Antithrombotic Therapy

Aspirin reduces the complication of abrupt closure when administered prior to balloon angioplasty. In a randomized trial (n = 376) by Schwartz and colleagues, the combination of aspirin and dipyridamole vs. placebo resulted in significant reduction (1.6% vs. 6.9%, p = 0.011) in periprocedural Q-wave infarction.[55] A retrospective analysis of angiograms revealed a reduction in angiographically apparent thrombus in aspirin-treated patients.[87]

The thienopyridine drugs are necessary adjuncts to stent implantation.[88] The STARS (Stent Anticoagulation And Restenosis Study) trial demonstrated a significant reduction in clinical events reflecting stent thrombosis with the combination of aspirin and ticlopidine (aspirin alone, 3.6%; aspirin and warfarin, 2.7%; aspirin and ticlopidine, 0.5%; p = 0.001).[89] Clopidogrel has recently assumed preeminence as the thienopyridine of choice for prevention of stent thrombosis because of its improved side-effect profile (especially reduced bone marrow suppression).[90]

The infusion of intravenous heparin for 3–6 days prior to balloon angioplasty reduced the incidence of abrupt closure in patients with unstable angina in three observational studies.[91–93] Likewise, prolonged heparin therapy prior to angioplasty has been reported to enhance procedural success in patients with intracoronary thrombus.[94,95]

Direct thrombin inhibitors have been studied in acute ischemic syndromes as a substitute for heparin therapy during angioplasty. In the HELVETICA trial of patients with unstable angina undergoing angioplasty, administration of hirudin compared with heparin was associated with a significant reduction in early adverse events (relative risk = 0.61, 95% confidence interval = 0.41–0.90, p = 0.023).[96] However, the benefit was not apparent at 6 months. In a similar trial hirulog therapy resulted in a reduction of myocardial infarction and abrupt closure in a subset of patients with postinfarction angina, although again no difference was apparent compared with the heparin group at 6 months.[97]

Early observations suggested a role for intracoronary thrombolytic agents as adjuncts to angioplasty in acute coronary syndromes. However, controlled trials have confirmed deleterious effects, possibly due to intramural hemorrhage or prothrombotic effects.[98–100] The TIMI-IIIB trial found no advantage for tissue plasminogen activator (tPA) treatment of non–ST-elevation acute coronary syndromes.[101] Myocardial infarction occurred more frequently in patients treated with tPa. The Thrombolysis and Angioplasty in Unstable Angina

(TAUSA) trial revealed an increase in acute closure (10.2% vs. 4.3%, p < 0.02) and hospital events (ischemia, infarction, or bypass surgery; 12.9% vs. 6.3%, p < 0.02) for patients treated with intracoronary urokinase during angioplasty.[102]

Recent efforts to halt thrombotic complications of angioplasty have focused on the integrin glycoprotein (GP) IIb/IIIa receptor on the platelet surface, which binds fibrinogen.[103] In the EPIC trial of patients undergoing high-risk angioplasty, the subset with unstable angina accrued an enhanced benefit with abciximab treatment.[43] There was a 62% reduction in the primary endpoint of death, myocardial infarction, and urgent repeat revascularization (4.8% vs. 12.8%, p = 0.012). Patients with or without angiographic evidence of intracoronary thrombus received similar benefits in the EPIC trial. The CAPTURE (C7E3 AntiPlatelet Therapy in Unstable REfractory angina) trial examined pretreatment with abciximab for 18–24 hours before intervention and 1 hour afterward.[46] The primary combined endpoint of death, myocardial infarction, and urgent target vessel revascularization was reduced from 15.9% to 11.3% (p = 0.012) with abciximab therapy. A trend toward benefit also was seen in the IMPACT and RESTORE trials of the GP IIb/IIIa antagonists eptifibatide and tirofiban, respectively.[44,45] Results from the EPILOG trial emphasized the importance of modifying the heparin dosage to reduce hemorrhagic complications.[59]

Overall, GP IIb/IIIa receptor antagonists reduce the risk of periprocedural ischemic complications by 50–60% in patients undergoing angioplasty with acute ischemic syndromes. These agents have become integral adjuncts during coronary interventional procedures.

Atherectomy Devices

Several mechanical innovations have been used in patients with acute coronary syndromes, including devices specifically designed for thrombus removal.

Directional coronary atherectomy (DCA) was the first interventional device tested in a randomized, controlled trial. Use of this device has declined steadily. In the National Cardiovascular Network database, the proportion of interventional procedures using DCA fell from 12% to 1%.[104] It was hoped that the excision and containment mechanism of DCA would allow removal of unstable plaque and associated thrombus. Both favorable and unfavorable results have been reported for DCA in the presence of thrombus.[105,106]

The CAVEAT (Coronary Angioplasty Versus Excisional Atherectomy Trial) trial, which compared DCA with balloon angioplasty for focal de novo lesions in native coronary arteries, failed to show a benefit for DCA.[107] Patients treated with DCA had an increased incidence of non–Q-wave infarction and a higher 1-year mortality rate (2.2% vs. 0.6%, p = 0.035).[108] It was proposed that the excessive risk seen with DCA in the CAVEAT trial was possibly due to the significant proportion of patients with unstable angina (65%). Later "optimal" atherectomy techniques (uniform use of a 7-French device with adjunctive balloon angioplasty) were tested in the BOAT (Balloon vs. Optimal Atherectomy Trial) trial.[109] Although angiographic restenosis was reduced in the DCA group (31.4% vs. 39.8%, p = 0.016), the reduction in late clinical events failed to reach statistical significance compared with balloon angioplasty and stent back-up (stents in 9.3%). Recently a small randomized trial (n = 122) demonstrated that more aggressive DCA with intravascular ultrasound guidance may rival the outcomes achieved with stents.[110] Further investigation of these methods and a reduction of device profiles may increase the use of DCA.

The aspiration mechanism of the transluminal extraction catheter (TEC) appears to be ideally suited for treatment of thrombotic lesions. This device has been used primarily in diseased vein grafts. In one observational report, only a modest acute gain in lumen diameter was achieved for patients who underwent TEC for complex lesions in native coronary arteries. Adjunctive balloon angioplasty was necessary in most cases, with a restenosis rate of 61%.[111] A small (n = 250) randomized trial, TOPIT (TEC Or PTCA In Thrombus) in native vessels noted similar efficacy compared with balloon angioplasty and no statistical difference in the occurrence of adverse in-hospital events.[112] TEC remains a niche technique because of its complexity and because it has no clear advantage over balloon angioplasty.

The presence of intracoronary thrombus has been considered a contraindication for the use of the rotational atherectomy device. Rotational atherectomy may micropulverize thrombus, leading to embolization and enhancement of the thrombotic process within an unstable lesion.[113] Excimer laser angioplasty has no clear advantage over balloon angioplasty.[114] The results of laser-assisted angioplasty have been reported to be compromised in the presence of intracoronary thrombus.[115]

The Possis AngioJet catheter uses the Venturi-Bernoulli principle to remove thrombus by rheolytic fragmentation and suction. Thrombus burden was successfully reduced in 91 lesions (57% vein grafts) with an overall clinical success of 87% in the VeGAS I pilot study.[116] In the VeGAS II trial (n = 352), the AngioJet device was compared with prolonged urokinase infusion for thrombotic lesions. Procedural success was higher with use of the AngioJet catheter (88% vs. 72%, p < 0.01). A reduction in in-hospital and 1-year major adverse cardiac events also was demonstrated for the patients treated with the device.[117]

Coronary ultrasound thrombolysis is a developing modality that may have a role in safely reducing the thrombus burden of patients with acute coronary syndromes.[118]

Stents

The promise of coronary stents has been realized. The ascendency of stent technology is clearly illustrated in the temporal trends of interventional device use (Fig. 1) from the National Cardiovascular Network Database.[104] The proportion of cases using stents rose 12-fold from 5.4% in 1994 to 69% in 1997.

Several studies have demonstrated the efficacy of stents as a treatment for abrupt or threatened closure after balloon angioplasty.[119–123] Stents are effective intraluminal scaffolds for intracoronary dissections and efficiently prevent elastic recoil. Complications of balloon coronary angioplasty are reduced when bailout stenting is available.[124]

Controlled randomized investigations of stent implantation compared with balloon angioplasty have been conducted in patients with predominantly stable symptoms and focal lesions. Results demonstrated improved event-free survival, primarily because of a lower restenosis rate and reduction of repeat revascularization procedures.[125,126]

Early experience suggested that stent implantation should be avoided in the presence of intracoronary thrombus.[127,128] Nath et al. identified unstable angina as an independent predictor of early stent thrombosis.[129]

Expansion of stent practice coincided with advances in technique, including adoption of high-pressure deployment and demonstration of the advantage of

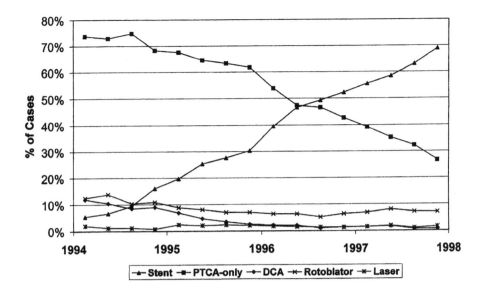

Figure 1. Overall temporal trends in interventional device selection from January 1994 to December 1997 at National Cardiac Network sites. (From Petersen ED, Lansky AJ, Anstrom KJ, et al: Evolving trends in interventional device use and outcomes: Results from the National Cardiovascular Network Database. Am Heart J 139:198–207, 2000, with permission.)

postimplantation antiplatelet therapy over anticoagulation regimens that include warfarin.[88,130,131] These innovations largely surmounted the onerous drawbacks of coronary stenting, including intense anticoagulation with associated complications, prolonged hospitalization, and significant risk of subacute stent thrombosis.

Initial experience with intracoronary stent implantation during acute myocardial infarction documented the feasibility of applying stent technology to patients with acute coronary syndromes.[132–134] Alfonso et al. reported favorable results with stent implantation in 86 patients with angiographic evidence of intracoronary thrombus (75% with unstable angina, 22% with acute myocardial infarction).[135] Angiographic success was seen in 96%; only 1% developed stent thrombosis. Restenosis occurred in 33% of 50 patients undergoing late angiographic follow-up.

The transformation of interventional practice to routine application of stent technology has extended beyond the evidence obtained from randomized trials. The STRESS/BENESTENT "equivalent" lesion constitutes only a small proportion of stenoses currently treated with stents.[136] Many interventional operators believe that the impressive acute gain achieved by stenting may overcome restenotic processes.[137] Some also believe that stents should be used prophylactically for lesions with an increased risk of closure.[138] This tactic is supported by data from the Hirulog Angioplasty Substudy, which determined that "uncomplicated abrupt closure" (supported by stents in 44%) was a strong independent predictor of major adverse cardiac events at 6 months.[139] Furthermore, the risk of subacute stent thrombosis and major adverse cardiac events is enhanced when stents are implanted for abrupt closure.[140,141] The prediction of abrupt closure with balloon angioplasty remains an imprecise task.

Controversy continues over the value of a provisional approach to use of stents after balloon angioplasty. For instance, the OCBAS (Optimal Coronary Balloon Angioplasty versus Stent) trial (n = 115) examined routine vs. provisional stenting after unsatisfactory balloon angioplasty (14% crossover to stents in provisional group).[142] Although a greater acute gain was noted with routine stenting (1.6 vs. 1.0 mm, p < 0.03), 6-month restenosis and target vessel revascularization rates were similar. This provisional stenting approach for patients with acute coronary syndromes has not been examined in a randomized manner. However, Marzocchi et al. retrospectively analyzed the outcome of 135 patients with unstable angina who underwent stent implantation and compared 50 patients who achieved a "stent-like" result with balloon angioplasty.[143] Postprocedural lumen diameter was greater with the stent procedure (2.74 vs. 2.27 mm, p = 0.025), and at 1-year follow-up, the stent group demonstrated a higher event-free survival rate (77.9% vs. 64.6%, p = 0.009), primarily because of less angina and revascularization.

Randomized data related to the use of stents for patients with non–ST-elevation acute coronary syndromes are scarce. Several series (Table 4) have reported excellent procedural success rates for stent implantation.[144–150] In some of these studies, the risk of subacute stent thrombosis remained significant, especially compared with patients with stable angina.[145,149] However, modern stent deployment technique was not uniformly applied in these series, and patients did not receive adjunctive therapy with IIb/IIIa receptor antagonists. Complications such as stent thrombosis were related to stent procedure for bailout, small vessel caliber, longer stent length, and anticoagulant therapy.[145,148] Marzzocchi and colleagues confirmed the necessity of antiplatelet therapy in patients with unstable angina, reporting a stent thrombosis rate of 1.5% compared with 11.4% with an anticoagulation regimen (p = 0.002).[148] Therapy with abciximab appears to augment the advantages of stenting. In the EPISTENT (Evaluation of Platelet IIb/IIIa Inhibitor for Stenting) trial, in which 36% of patients had unstable angina, the primary composite endpoint of death, myocardial infarction, or urgent revascularization was reduced in patients treated with stents plus abciximab (5.3%) compared with stent plus placebo (10.8%) or balloon angioplasty plus abciximab (7.8%) (p < 0.001).[151]

Overall, the preponderance of data supports relatively indiscriminant use of stent technology for transluminal revascularization. Data from the National Cardiovascular Network database noted a significant reduction in complications, such as in-hospital death or in-hospital repeat revascularization, for patients receiving stents compared with patients receiving balloon angioplasty alone (p < 0.01).[104] Although stents are now a firmly entrenched revascularization modality, further innovation and investigation are needed to deal with the limitations in small-vessel disease, diffuse or lengthy lesions, bifurcations, and the vexing problem of in-stent restenosis.

Aortocoronary Vein Graft Disease

Patients undergoing intervention for acute coronary syndromes after previous coronary bypass surgery deserve special consideration. Vein graft lesions are often extensive, bulky, and friable, and thrombus is a frequent component.[152] The presence of angiographically evident thrombus clearly increases the risk of distal embolization and complications during intervention.[153] Despite these risks, balloon angioplasty can be performed successfully in ~90%

Table 4. Stent Deployment for Unstable Angina

Author	Publication Year	n	Procedure Success (%)	Death	MI	CABG	Stent Thrombosis	Deployment Pressure (atm)	Antithrombotic Therapy	
									A/C	A/P
Malosky[149]	1994	48	96	0	4.2	2.1	4.2	NA	100	—
Shimada[150]	1998	91	96	0	0	0	0	≥12	NA	NA
Chauhan[144]	1998	110	100	0	4.5	0.9	3.6	15.8	4	96
Madan[147]	1998	156	99	0.6	1.9	1.9	1.9	12–20	56	63
DeBenedictis[146]	1998	311	96	0.9	1.9	0.9	0.3	NA	NA	NA
Marzocchi[148]	1999	266	98	0.4	4.6	2.9	4.1	13.4	25	75
Clarkson[145]	1999	103	96	NA	NA	NA	10.6	Nominal—12	—	100

MI = myocardial infarction, CABG = coronary artery bypass graft, A/C = anticoagulant therapy with warfarin, A/P = antiplatelet therapy, NA = data not available.

of patients, but the incidence of recurrence is high (> 50%) in proximal or body vein graft stenoses.[154]

Recently it was demonstrated that stent implantation for focal vein graft lesions results in superior efficacy (angiographic success without major hospital complication) compared with balloon angioplasty (92% vs. 69%, p < 0.01).[155] Although angiographic evidence of thrombus was an exclusion criteria in this trial, 80% of patients were classified as exhibiting unstable angina. The number of adverse clinical events at 6 months also was reduced in stent-treated patients.

Despite the encouraging results with stents, vein grafts with extensive lesions and a large thrombus burden continue to be problematic.[156] Results reported with DCA and TEC devices have been disappointing.[157,158] Newer devices, such as the POSSIS AngioJet rheolytic catheter and ultrasound thrombolysis, may hold promise.[116–118] Distal protection devices may enhance procedural safety.[159] Nevertheless, many challenges remain in the treatment of degenerated vein grafts.

Invasive or Conservative Management Strategy

Vigorous debate continues about the optimal management strategy for patients with unstable angina or non–ST-elevation myocardial infarction.[160,161] Advocates of a routine invasive approach cite the value of anatomic definition and expediency of revascularization to abate the early risk of recurrent ischemia.[63] Alternatively, the conservative recurrent ischemia-driven approach to revascularization avoids potentially unnecessary invasive procedures.

These strategies have been compared in three published randomized trials.[78,101,162] Examination of the distinct variations among these trials is instructive for integrating the data into practice (Table 5). For instance, the ultimate revascularization rate in the conservative arm may dampen the discernible advantages of an early invasive strategy.

The TIMI-IIIB trial found no difference in the incidence of death or myocardial infarction with either strategy at 6 weeks or 1 year.[101,163] Repeat hospitalization was decreased by the invasive approach (26% vs. 33% at 1 year, p < 0.05). Patients over age 65 years experienced a reduction of death or myocardial infarction at 6 weeks (7.9% vs. 14.8%, p = 0.02) and 1 year (12.5% vs. 19.5%, p = 0.03).

The invasive strategy of the VANQWISH (Veterans Affairs Non–Q-wave Infarction Stategies in Hospital) trial was associated with higher rates of death and nonfatal infarction during hospitalization and at 1 year, but the mortality curves converged at 23 months.[78] Of note, the surgical mortality rate in the invasive group was 11.6% compared with 3.4% in the conservative group. No patients undergoing angioplasty in the invasive group died. The intervention rate was 44% with the invasive approach and 33% in the conservative group.

The more recent FRISC II (FRagmin and fast Revascularisation during InStability in Coronary artery disease) trial used more contemporary interventional techniques (stents in 61%, abciximab in 10%) and reported a greater disparity in revascularization rates for the early invasive and conservative groups (71% vs. 9% at 10 days; 77% vs. 37% at 6 months) compared with the other two trials.[162] There was a reduction in the composite endpoint of death or myocardial infarction for the invasive strategy (9.4% vs. 12.1%, p = 0.031) at 6 months, with a distinct advantage in higher-risk patients (elderly patients, men, patients with rest pain or ST depression). Moreover, there was a consistent benefit for the invasive approach, regardless of troponin level at admission.[164]

Table 5. Randomized Trials of Early Invasive vs. Conservative Management of Non–ST-elevation Acute Coronary Syndromes

	TIMI IIIB[101,163]			VANQWISH[78]			FRISC II[162]		
	Invasive	Conservative	p value	Invasive	Conservative	p value	Invasive	Conservative	p value
Patients	740	744		462	458		1222	1235	
Age (years)	59	59		62	61		66	65	
Follow-up (months)	12	12		23	23		6	6	
Time to catheterization (days)	0.75–2	–		2	14		4	17	
% Catheterization	99	73		96	48		98	47	
% PCI	39	32*		21	12		43	18	
% CABG	25	23*		23	21		35	19	
CABG mortality rate	NA	NA		11.6	3.4		1.2	0.4	
% PCI with stents	0	0		NA	NA		61	70	
% Non-Q-wave MI	34	30		100	100		57†	58†	
Results									
Death (%)	4.1	4.4	0.79				1.9	2.9	0.1
MI (%)	8.3	9.3	0.51				7.8	10.1	0.045
Combined (%)	10.8	12.1	0.42	29.9	26.9	0.35	9.4	12.1	0.031

PCI = percutaneous coronary intervention, CABG = coronary atery bypass graft, MI = myocardial infarction.
* At 1 year.
† By troponin T > 0.1 µg/L.

Although an invasive approach appears to be validated by the results of the FRISC-II trial, the changing paradigm of interventional practice must be balanced against advances in medical therapy for acute coronary syndromes, such as low-molecular-weight heparin and glycoprotein IIb/IIIa receptor antagonists. Additional data from the RITA III trial and the TACTICS-TIMI-18 trial will enhance the understanding of management strategy for patients with non–ST-elevation acute coronary syndromes.

Acute ST-elevation Myocardial Infarction

In the care of patients with cardiac disease, the development of reperfusion therapy for acute myocardial infarction certainly qualifies as one of the twentieth century's most important medical achievements. Randomized trials involving many thousands of patients have led to a continual succession of meaningful advances, but currently there is a basic dichotomy of practice regarding the primary method of reperfusion: angioplasty or thrombolysis.

Rescue Angioplasty

Few data from randomized trials address the value of salvage or rescue angioplasty for patients who fail to reperfuse after thrombolytic therapy. However, several series have reported reperfusion success in > 80% of patients.[165–167] The high mortality rates (25–39%) among patients who fail an attempted rescue angioplasty have led some to call for caution in considering this strategy.[165,168,169]

The CORAMI (Cohort of Rescue Angioplasty in Myocardial Infarction) study group reported success, defined as TIMI flow grade 3 (Table 6), in 90% of patients (n = 72) with a hospital mortality rate of 4%.[167] In the GUSTO-I Angiographic Substudy,[169] rescue angioplasty was attempted at the operator's discretion in 198 of 464 (43%) patients with occluded infarct arteries studied at 90 or 180 minutes Patients undergoing rescue angioplasty had more impaired left ventricular function at onset than patients managed conservatively. In patients successfully reperfused with angioplasty (88%), left ventricular function and 30-day mortality rates were similar to those in patients with closed infarct arteries managed conservatively but less favorable than in patients with initially successful thrombolysis. This finding is consistent with the time-dependent

Table 6. TIMI Flow Grade Classification Scheme

Flow Grade	Definition
Grade 0	No perfusion. No antegrade flow beyond the point of occlusion.
Grade 1	Penetration without perfusion. Contrast material passes beyond the area of obstruction but fails to opacify the entire coronary bed distal to the obstruction for the duration of the cineangiographic filming sequence.
Grade 2	Partial perfusion. Contrast material passes across the obstruction and opacifies the coronary bed distal to the obstruction. However, the rate of entry of contrast material into the vessel distal to the obstruction or its rate of clearance from the distal bed (or both) is preceptiby slower than its flow into or clearance from comparable areas not perfused by the previously occluded vessel.
Grade 3	Complete perfusion. Antegrade flow into the bed distal to the obstruction occurs as promptly as antegrade flow into the bed proximal to the obstruction, and clearance of contrast material from the involved bed is as rapid as clearance from an uninvolved bed in the same vessel or the opposite artery.

relation of reperfusion to survival, as verified by the GUSTO-I trial.[170] In a corresponding manner patients undergoing successful rescue angioplasty (88%) in the TIMI-4 trial also attained a superior TIMI-3 flow grade (87% vs. 65%, p = 0.002) compared to successful thrombolysis but with slightly worse outcomes for the rescue angioplasty group.[171]

The only randomized trial is RESCUE (Randomized Evaluation of Salvage angioplasty with Combined Utilization of Endpoints), which compared salvage angioplasty with conservative management in 151 patients with anterior wall infarctions. Successful angioplasty (92% of cases) resulted in a nonsignificant decline in mortality and a significant reduction in the combined incidence of death and congestive heart failure[172] (Fig. 2).

Recent advances in the technique of infarct artery angioplasty (stents and glycoprotein IIb/IIIa antagonists) can improve reperfusion success and the clinical benefits of salvage intervention.[173] Nevertheless, the difficulty of noninvasively assessing the status of the infarct artery during the early stages of thrombolytic therapy remains an important limitation for this approach.[174]

Immediate Postthrombolysis Adjunctive Balloon Coronary Angioplasty

A significant residual stenosis (≥ 70% diameter stenosis) is commonly identified after thrombolytic-induced reperfusion of the infarct artery during acute myocardial infarction.[175,176] Concern for the consequences of residual stenosis, limiting myocardial salvage and enhancing the risk for reocclusion, led to routine application of balloon angioplasty soon after thrombolysis. This strategy was tested by three trials that compared routine immediate angioplasty after thrombolysis to thrombolysis followed by deferred angioplasty (TAMI I, TIMI IIA) or conservative therapy (ECSG) (Table 7).[177–179] These three trials reported

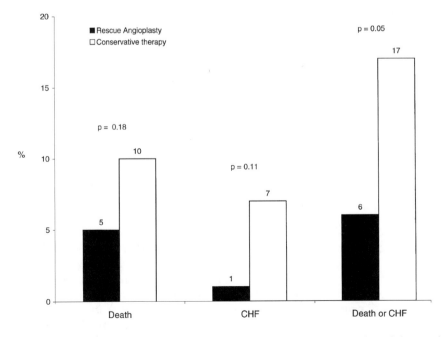

Figure 2. The 30-day adverse clinical outcomes (death and severe congestive heart failure) in the RESCUE trial.

Table 7. Trials of Immediate vs. Delayed Coronary Angioplasty after Thrombolytic Therapy

	Time of PTCA	n	Predischarge LVEF	Emergency CABG (%)	Hospital Mortality Rate (%)
TAMI-I[178]					
Immediate	< 15 hr	99	0.53	7	4
Delayed	7–10 days	98	0.56	2	1
TIMI-IIA[177]					
Immediate	< 2 hr	195	0.50	1	7
Delayed	18–48 hr	194	0.49	1	6
ESCG[179]					
Immediate	< 3 hr	183	0.51	2	7
Conservative	—	184	0.51	0	3

PTCA = percutaneous transluminal coronary angioplasty, LVEF = left ventricular ejection fraction, CABG = coronary artery bypass graft.

similar results despite differences in study design and somewhat limited statistical power. There was no difference in the primary endpoint (predischarge ejection fraction), and a trend toward higher mortality rates was seen in the immediate angioplasty group of each trial. Pooled comparison of the data reveals a significantly higher mortality rate for immediate angioplasty compared with the deferred approach (6.5% vs. 3.4%, $p = 0.04$).[180] The hazard of immediate angioplasty has been presumed to be caused by extensive intramural hemorrhage and/or platelet activation induced by thrombolytic agents.[98–100] Despite advances in transluminal revascularization, routine angioplasty within 24 hours of thrombolysis remains a class III (not useful or effective and may be harmful) recommendation in the August 1999 update to the American College of Cardiology/American Heart Association (ACC/AHA) guidelines for management of acute myocardial infarction.[181]

Delayed Postthrombolysis Adjunctive Balloon Coronary Angioplasty

The DANAMI (DANish trial in Acute Myocardial Infarction) trial documented the necessity for revascularization of patients who exhibit postinfarction angina or inducible ischemia.[182] Patients exhibiting postinfarction ischemia (n = 1008) were randomized to a deferred invasive strategy with revascularization (60% PTCA and 29% CABG) or medical treatment with revascularization (1.6% at 2 months) reserved for refractory angina. The revascularization approach led to a significant reduction in the combined endpoint of mortality, reinfarction, and admission for unstable angina at 2.4 years of follow-up (Fig. 3).

In the United States patients commonly undergo routine deferred coronary angiography and angioplasty after thrombolysis, often without a preceding stress test.[183] This practice prevails despite several trials that have failed to demonstrate a benefit in survival, left ventricular function, or reinfarction. Two large randomized trials compared routine deferred angioplasty (18–48 hours in TIMI IIB, 2–7 days in SWIFT [Should We Intervene Following Thrombolysis]) with revascularization limited to patients with recurrent ischemia.[184,185] (Table 8). No benefit was identified with routine angioplasty for the major endpoints. However, in TIMI-IIB the invasive approach was associated with a lower mortality rate for patients with previous infarction (10.3% vs. 17.0%, $p = 0.030$). Other smaller studies also failed to demonstrate a significant benefit despite an increment in the interval from thrombolysis to routine angioplasty of > 4 days.[186,187]

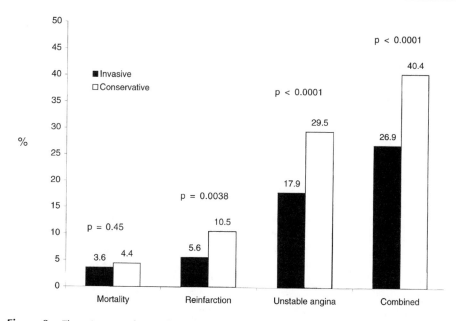

Figure 3. The primary endpoints for patients randomized to conservative or invasive treatment of postinfarction ischemia in the DANish trial in Acute Myocardial Infarction (DANAMI).

Many investigators have concerns about the validity of a negative stress test in excluding a value for revascularization to persistently viable myocardium beyond a severe residual stenosis, particularly after large infarctions. A bias also remains to pursue angiography for accurate risk stratification. Nevertheless, routine coronary angiography and subsequent angioplasty after thrombolytic therapy also remain a class III recommendation according to ACC/AHA guidelines.

Primary Reperfusion in Acute Myocardial Infarction by Coronary Angioplasty

The initial studies of reperfusion therapy in acute myocardial infarction involved the use of intracoronary thrombolysis along with nitroglycerin and a mechanical approach via guidewire recanalization.[188] Intracoronary thrombolysis proved to be an effective (~75% success rate) but somewhat impractical method of reperfusion.[189] Extensive investigation validated the benefits of intravenous thrombolytic therapy.[190] The continuing investigative effort to enhance the success of thrombolysis has clarified the limitations of reperfusion

Table 8. Trials of Delayed Angioplasty vs. Conservative Therapy after Thrombolysis

	n	%PTCA	Mortality Rate at 1 Year (%)	Reinfarction Rate at 1 Year (%)	Ejection Fraction
TIMI IIB[184]	3262				
Invasive	1636	56	6.9	9.4	50.0
Conservative	1626	13	7.4	9.8	50.4
SWIFT[185]	800				
Invasive	397	43	5.8	15.1	50.7
Conservative	403	3	5	12.9	51.7

PTCA = percutaneous transluminal coronary angioplasty.

effectiveness and risks.[191] The GUSTO-I trial verified the critical link between the early attainment of complete reperfusion (TIMI flow grade 3) and survival, but ≤ 54% of patients receiving accelerated tissue plasminogen activator achieved this standard of success.[170] The gradient of hemorrhagic risk resolved by the therapeutic arms of the GUSTO-I trial invokes a degree of caution in applying thrombolysis to patients with comorbid factors (advanced age, hypertension, prior cerebrovascular accident, lower body weight) that enhance the risk of intracranial hemorrhage.[192] In an attempt to overcome the limitations of thrombolysis and provide a therapeutic alternative to patients with thrombolytic contraindications, primary or direct angioplasty continued to be used in several laboratories

Observational Series

Hartzler and colleagues first reported primary balloon coronary angioplasty of an occluded infarct artery in 1983.[193] Multiple centers have described their experience with direct or primary balloon angioplasty over the past 15 years. These observational studies have been reported from a broad spectrum of community and academic centers with frequent inclusion of patients with contraindications to thrombolysis and in the midst of cardiogenic shock. Eckman and colleagues reviewed 10 series, many with contraindications to thrombolysis (n = 2073), and described a weighted average hospital mortality rate of 8.3%.[194] O'Keefe et al. reported the largest consecutive series of 1000 patients (7.9% with cardiogenic shock), which had a successful infarct artery recanalization rate of 94% and an overall hospital mortality rate of 7.8%.[195] The Primary Angioplasty Registry (n = 271) of thrombolytic-eligible patients from 6 experienced centers reported successful reperfusion (TIMI flow grade 3) in 97% with a hospital mortality rate of 4%.[196] Although selection bias may compromise the significance of many of these studies, the persistent practice of primary angioplasty validated an alternative reperfusion modality.

Randomized, Controlled Trials

An early small (n = 56) randomized trial comparing primary angioplasty and intracoronary streptokinase suggested enhanced salvage by angioplasty as reflected by ejection fraction and infarct regional wall motion.[197] Despite the expansion of reperfusion therapy, concerns about the efficacy and complications of intravenous thrombolysis led to comparative investigations with angioplasty as the primary reperfusion modality.

The PAMI (Primary Angioplasty in Myocardial Infarction) trial found no significant improvement in left ventricular function during rest or exercise at 6-week follow-up for angioplasty vs. tissue plasminogen activator—despite a reperfusion success rate of 97% (94% TIMI flow grade 3) within 60 minutes in the angioplasty group.[198] However, the investigators reported a trend for angioplasty to reduce hospital mortality rate (2.6% vs. 6.5%, p = 0.06) with a significant reduction in reinfarction or death (5.1% vs. 12.0%, p = 0.02) and intracranial hemorrhage (0% vs. 2.0%, p = 0.05). Angioplasty demonstrated a significant reduction in mortality rate (2.0% vs. 10.4%, p = 0.01) in patients classified as "not low risk" (age > 70 years, anterior infarction, or heart rate >100 beats/min).

The Mayo Clinic trial examined myocardial salvage as determined by technitium-99m sestamibi tomographic imaging in 108 patients randomized to primary angioplasty or thrombolysis with tissue plasminogen activator.[199]

Recurrent ischemia occurred in 36% of patients assigned to thrombolysis and 15% assigned to angioplasty. No significant difference in salvage was detected for either approach.

The Netherlands (Zwolle) trial randomly assigned 301 patients to primary angioplasty or intravenous streptokinase.[200] There was a significant reduction in reinfarction with angioplasty (0% vs. 13%, p = 0.003). Predischarge left ventricular ejection fraction was 45% in the streptokinase group and 51% in the angioplasty group (p = 0.004).

The results of these three trials, published simultaneously in *The New England Journal of Medicine*, sparked considerable controversy and debate. Concerns were voiced over methods of thrombolytic therapy and applicability to the broad population of reperfusion-eligible patients with acute myocardial infarction.

The GUSTO-IIb Angioplasty Substudy, the largest comparative trial of primary angioplasty and thrombolysis, was conducted in 57 hospitals.[201] Successful reperfusion was achieved in 93% of angioplasty patients, but TIMI flow grade 3 was documented in only 73% by angiographic core laboratory analysis. The primary composite endpoint (death, nonfatal infarction, and disabling stroke) occurred in 9.6% of the angioplasty group and 13.7% of the tissue plasminogen activator group (odds ratio = 0.67, p = 0.033). No benefit for either treatment was found when prespecified subgroups, classified by age, infarct location, hospital angioplasty experience, randomization time, and high vs. low risk, were analyzed. At 6 months there was no significant difference in the composite endpoint, possibly reflecting late reocclusion or restenosis in the angioplasty group.

A meta-analysis of 10 randomized trials (including those above), conducted by Weaver and colleagues, found a significant reduction in mortality rate (4.4% vs. 6.5%, p = 0.02; 34% risk reduction) for angioplasty over thrombolysis[202] (Figs. 4 and 5). This degree of benefit translates to 21 lives saved per 1000 patients treated. The combination of death and nonfatal reinfarction also was reduced in the angioplasty group (7.2% vs. 11.9%, p < 0.001). Primary angioplasty was associated with a reduction in total stroke (0.7% vs. 2.0%, p = 0.007) and hemorrhagic stroke (0.1% vs. 1.1%, p < 0.001). Table 9 details the characteristics of the 10 trials,[198–201,203–208] which compared different thrombolytic regimens and found a relatively consistent advantage in short-term outcomes for angioplasty at dedicated centers. Yet uncertainty remains, primarily because of the lack of a single statistically powered, randomized trial demonstrating a clear survival advantage.[209,210]

Observational Registries

The promising results of randomized trials at dedicated centers contrasts with reports from community-based registries. The MITI (Myocardial Infarction Triage and Intervention) registry analyzed the outcome of 1050 patients treated with primary angioplasty compared with 2095 patients who underwent thrombolysis at 19 hospitals in the Seattle area from 1988 to 1994.[211] No difference in hospital mortality rates was detected between the two treatment approaches (5.6% for angioplasty and 5.5% for thrombolysis, p = 0.93). Risk-stratification analysis also revealed no advantage for angioplasty. Of note, 26% of patients treated primarily with thrombolysis underwent angioplasty within 24 hours of admission.

The Second National Registry of Myocardial Infarction (NRMI-2) examined 28,000 thrombolytic-eligible patients (excluding those with cardiogenic shock) who underwent reperfusion therapy.[212] The hospital mortality rate was similar

Study	No. (%) PTCA	No. (%) Lytic Therapy	Odds Ratio (95% CI)	P
Streptokinase				
Zijlstra et al[2]	3/152 (2.0)	11/149 (7.4)		
Ribeiro et al[19]	3/50 (6.0)	1/50 (2.0)		
Grinfeld et al[26]	5/54 (9.3)	6/58 (10.3)		
Zijlstra et al[28]	1/45 (2.2)	0/50		
Subtotal	12/301 (4.0)	18/307 (5.9)		.38
t-PA				
DeWood[18]	3/46 (6.5)	2/44 (4.5)		
Grines et al[3]	5/195 (2.6)	13/200 (6.5)		
Gibbons et al[6]	2/47 (4.3)	2/56 (3.6)		
Subtotal	10/288 (3.5)	17/300 (5.7)		.28
Accelerated t-PA				
Ribichini et al[25]	0/41	1/42 (2.4)		
Garcia et al[29]	3/95 (3.2)	10/94 (10.6)		
GUSTO IIb[27]	32/565 (5.7)	40/573 (7.0)		
Subtotal	35/701 (5.0)	51/709 (7.2)		.10
Total	**57/1290 (4.4)**	**86/1316 (6.5)**		.02

0.0   0.5   1.0   1.5   2.0
PTCA Better   Lytic Better

Figure 4.   Mortality rates at the end of the study period in trials comparing primary angioplasty with thrombolytic drug treatment. The rates for each study are grouped by thrombolytic drug regimen. The odds ratios with 95% confidence intervals (CIs) are plotted on the right. Tests for homogenicitiy: streptokinase trials, p = 0.08; tissue plasminogen activator (tPA) trials, p = 0.33; accelerated tPA trials, p = 0.21; thrombolytic regimen, p = 0.96; and overall, p = 0.24. Percentages are pooled results, and odds ratios are calculated by exact methods using all trials. (From Weaver WD, Simes RJ, Betriu A, et al: Comparison of primary coronary angioplasty and intravenous thrombolytic therapy for acute myocardial infarction: a quantitative review. JAMA 278:2093–2098, 1997, with permission.)

(5.2% for angioplasty vs. 5.4% for tissue plasminogen activator). The incidence of reinfarction was also similar (2.5% for angioplasty vs. 2.9% for tissue plasminogen activator). Despite a higher rate of stroke in the thrombolytic group (1.6% vs. 0.7% for angioplasty, p <0.0001), the combined endpoint of death and nonfatal stroke was statistically equivalent (6.2% for tissue plasminogen activator and 5.6% for angioplasty). Other smaller registries (Alabama, Nationwide French Survey) also found no survival advantage for primary angioplasty over thrombolysis.[213,214]

In contrast, pooled data about 9906 patients treated with reperfusion therapy in the German MITRA and MIR registries identified a lower hospital mortality rate in patients treated with primary angioplasty compared with thrombolysis (6.4% vs. 11.3%, p < 0.001).[215] An advantage for primary angioplasty was also evident in subgroups analyzed according to gender, age, and infarct location.

Long-term Outcome

Concern has been raised about a long-term attenuation of the benefit of primary angioplasty over thrombolysis. In the GUSTO-IIb trial, the reduction in the composite adverse outcome endpoint (15.7% for tissue plasminogen activator and 13.3% for angioplasty) at 6 months no longer reached statistical significance.[201] This finding was attributed to late reocclusion or restenosis. However, 2-year

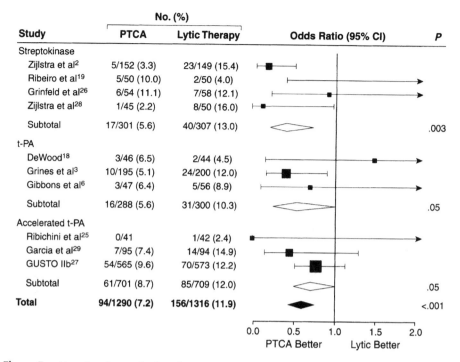

Figure 5.   Mortality plus nonfatal reinfarction rates for each of the studies, with odds ratios and 95% confidence intervals (CIs) for each study, each thrombolytic regimen, and combined trials. Tests for homogenicity: streptokinase trials, p = 0.008; tissue plasminogen activator (tPA) trials, p = 0.35; accelerated tPA trials, p = 0.59; thrombolytic regimen, p = 0.25; and overall, p = 0.04. Percentages are pooled results, and odds ratios are calculated by exact methods using all trials. (From Weaver WD, Simes RJ, Betriu A, et al: Comparison of primary coronary angioplasty and intravenous thrombolytic therapy for acute myocardial infarction: A quantitative review. JAMA 278:2093–2098, 1997, with permission.)

follow-up from the PAMI-I trial demonstrated a reduction in recurrent ischemia (36.4% vs. 48%, p = 0.026) and the combination of death and reinfarction (14.9% vs. 23%, p = .034) for patients treated with angioplasty.[216] Likewise, a sustained advantage for angioplasty over streptokinase reperfusion was noted in a 5-year analysis of patients (n = 395) reported by Zijlstra et al. Reductions were found both in mortality rate (13.4% vs. 23.9%, p = 0.01) and rate of nonfatal reinfarction (6% vs. 22%).[217]

Merits of the Primary Angioplasty Strategy for Reperfusion

Superior Reperfusion Efficacy

The landmark observation linking the early attainment of TIMI flow grade 3 through the infarct artery to myocardial salvage and subsequent survival was clearly demonstrated in the GUSTO-I trial.[170] This relationship between survival and TIMI flow grade 3 also has been verified for patients undergoing angioplasty[218] (Fig 6). The technique of primary angioplasty has been reported to achieve TIMI flow grade 3 in 93–98% of patients when performed at experienced centers.[196,198,219] In contrast, TIMI flow grade 3 is achieved in only 54% of patients undergoing thrombolysis with accelerated tissue plasminogen activator.[170] Therefore, there appears to be a strong theoretical basis for an incremental

Table 9. Randomized Trials Comparing Primary Angioplasty with Thrombolysis

Author	n	Patient Population	Symptom Duration (hr)	Thrombolytic Regimen	Time to Treatment (min)		Primary Follow-up Duration
					PTCA	Thrombolysis	
DeWood[203]	90	<75 yr; ↑ST	<12	Duteplase (4 hr)	126	84	30 days
Grines[198]	395	↑ST	<12	tPA (3 hr)	60	32	Discharge
Zijlstra[200]	294	<75 yr; ↑ST	<6	Streptokinase	68	30	30 days
Gibbons[199]	103	<80 yr; ↑ST	<12	Duteplase (4 hr)	45	20	Discharge
Zijlstra[204]	95	Low risk; ↑ST	<6	Streptokinase	68	30	30 days
Ribeiro[205]	100	<75 yr; ↑ST	<6	Streptokinase	238	179	Discharge
Grinfeld[207]	112	↑ST	<12	Streptokinase	63	18	30 days
Ribichini[206]	83	<80 yr; IWMI	<6	tPA (90 min)	40	43	Discharge
Garcia[208]	189	AWMI	5	tPA (90 min)	84	69	30 days
GUSTO IIB[201]	1138	↑ST, LBBB	<12	tPA (90 min)	114	72	30 days

PTCA = percutaneous transluminal coronary angioplasty, ST = ST segment, tPA = tissue plasminogen activator, IWMI = inferior wall myocardial infarct, AWMI = anterior wall myocardial infarct. (Modified from Weaver WD, Simes RJ, Betriu A, et al: Comparison of primary coronary angioplasty and intravenous thrombolytic therapy for acute myocardial infarction: A quantitative review. JAMA 278:2093–2098, 1997.)

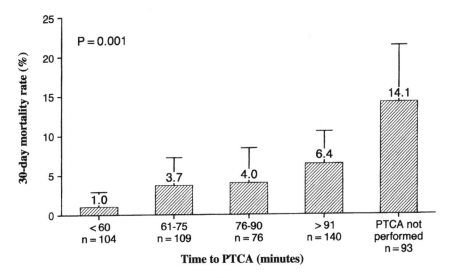

Figure 6.   Relationship between 30-day mortality rates and time from study enrollment to first balloon inflation in the GUSTO-IIB trial. Patients assigned to angioplasty in whom angioplasty was not performed also are shown. (From Berger PB, Ellis SG, Holmes DR Jr, et al: Relationship between delay in performing direct coronary angioplasty and early clinical outcome in patients with acute myocardial infarction: Results from the Global Use of Strategies to Open Occluded Arteries in acute coronary syndromes (GUSTO-IIb) trial. Circulation 100:14–20, 1999, with permission).

improvement in outcome by the enhanced efficacy of primary angioplasty for reperfusion. However, new approaches using the combination of a reduced dose of thrombolytic agent and addition of a glycoprotein IIb/IIIa receptor antagonist have achieved rates of TIMI flow grade 3 at 90 minutes as high as 76% (50 mg alteplase with abciximab bolus, 0.25 mg/kg, plus infusion of 0.125 µg/kg/min).[220] The safety and survival benefit of this approach must be ensured by further trials.

Treatment of Underlying Coronary Artery Stenosis

As mentioned above, significant residual stenosis is commonly identified in coronary arteries after thrombolysis.[175,176] Recurrent ischemia may double the risk of death after infarction.[221] Primary treatment of this stenosis by coronary angioplasty during acute reperfusion appears to result in lower rates of recurrent ischemia and reinfarction.[63,221] In the PAMI-I, Netherlands, and GUSTO-IIb trials, recurrent ischemia was reduced in patients undergoing primary angioplasty compared with thrombolysis. Furthermore, a reduction in reinfarction also was demonstrated in a meta-analysis of the PAMI-I, Netherlands, and Mayo Clinic trials (1.9% vs. 7.6%, p = 0.0008).[222] The less severe stenosis after primary angioplasty also may mitigate adverse left ventricular remodeling after infarction.[223]

Late reocclusion rates (5–20%) compare favorably with those reported with thrombolytic therapy (~30%).[18,224–228] Restenosis after primary angioplasty has been reported in 28–47% of patients.[224–227]

Precise Risk Stratification

Important decision-facilitating data are accumulated at the time of urgent catheterization with planned primary angioplasty. The diagnosis of acute total coronary occlusion is confirmed in patients with equivocal electrocardiographic changes. Approximately 5% of patients undergoing urgent coronary angiography require emergency coronary bypass surgery for critical multivessel or left main coronary artery disease.[229] An additional 5% of patients exhibit spontaneous reperfusion without significant residual stenosis. Mechanical complications such as a ruptured papillary muscle or ventricular septal rupture can be identified during cardiac catheterization.

Patients can be stratified to a low-risk group (age ≤ 70 years, left ventricular ejection fraction $> 45\%$, one- or two-vessel disease, successful angioplasty, no persistent arrhythmias). Because such patients exhibit a low incidence of hospital mortality (0.4%) and reinfarction (0.4%), early hospital discharge is allowed.[219]

Reduced Risk of Intracranial Hemorrhage

Certainly intracranial hemorrhage is the most dreaded complication of thrombolytic therapy for myocardial infarction. This hazard restricts uniform application of reperfusion therapy. The identified risk factors for intracranial hemorrhage are age > 65 years, body weight < 70 kg, hypertension on hospital admission, and treatment with tissue plasminogen activator vs. streptokinase. Their effects are cumulative and must be considered when thrombolytic therapy is used.[192] Primary angioplasty nearly eliminates this risk. Approximately one-third of the reduction in mortality rate by primary angioplasty compared with thrombolysis can be attributed to curtailment of intracranial hemorrhage.[202]

The incidence of death from myocardial rupture also appears to be reduced in patients undergoing reperfusion by angioplasty compared with thrombolysis.[230]

Special Patient Subgroups

Previous Coronary Artery Bypass Graft

Prior coronary bypass surgery is a predictor of thrombolytic failure.[231,232] The large thrombus burden often present within vein grafts during acute infarction may resist the action of lytic agents. No randomized, controlled trials specifically address the reperfusion strategy for patients with previous coronary bypass surgery. In the NRMI-2 registry, 2544 patients with previous bypass surgery were treated with tissue plasminogen activator, and 375 underwent primary angioplasty.[233] There was no significant difference in hospital mortality rates or combined endpoint of death and nonfatal stroke. Primary angioplasty of vein grafts has been associated with a lower procedural success rate (71.4% vs. 86.2%, p = 0.04) and a higher complication rate (30-day CABG: 6.5% vs. 0%, p = 0.04) compared with native vessels in a study of 1073 Mayo Clinic patients.[234] Comparable outcomes were noted in the PAMI-2 trial; TIMI flow grade 3 was achieved in 70.2% of bypass grafts and 94.3% of native arteries (p < 0.001).[235] The mortality rate at 6 months was significantly higher for patients who underwent previous bypass surgery in the PAMI-2 trial (14.3% vs. 4.1%, p = 0.001). Patients with prior CABG are older and have more extensive coronary artery disease, worse ventricular function, and more associated comorbidities.[234,235]

Primary stenting of occluded vein grafts improved procedural success in one retrospective report of 158 patients (TIMI flow grade 3: stents, 96%; PTCA, 72%; p = 0.0001).[236] However, alternate approaches using thrombectomy devices (TEC, rheolytic thrombectomy, ultrasound thrombolysis), distal protection mechanisms, and/or GP IIB/IIIa antagonists may be necessary to optimize results in this cohort.

Thrombolytic-ineligible Patients

True contraindications to the use of thrombolytic agents in patients presenting with acute myocardial infarction are recent major surgery or trauma, recent stroke, previous intracranial hemorrhage, intracranial neoplasm, bleeding diasthesis, recent gastrointestinal or genitourinary hemorrhage, and suspected aortic dissection. In addition, thrombolytic agents are withheld from many patients with comorbid factors (age > 65 years, prior CABG, delayed presentation, prolonged cardiopulmonary resuscitation, hypertension, previous cerebrovascular disease, recent vascular puncture, active peptic ulcer, anticoagulant therapy) because of concerns about the risk-benefit value of treatment. Both groups of patients are at higher risk for death.[237,238]

Nevertheless, angioplasty has been applied to thrombolytic-ineligible patients with a high degree of success.[239] In contrast, the contraindications to primary angioplasty are limited to patients with contraindications to heparin therapy, documented life-threatening contrast allergy, or lack of vascular access.

Cardiogenic Shock

Patency of the infarct artery correlates with improved survival in cardiogenic shock.[240] Thrombolysis is less effective in the setting of cardiogenic shock.[240,241] The hemodynamic derangement during cardiogenic shock reduces perfusion pressure, interfering with delivery of the lytic plasminogen and plasminogen activators to the thrombus.[242] Acidosis in the shock state can impair transformation of plasminogen to plasmin.[243] These limitations are manifest as a persistently high mortality rate for patients in cardiogenic shock reperfused with thrombolytic agents.[244] In the GISSI-I trial, survival was not improved with streptokinase treatment (mortality rate: streptokinase, 69.9%; untreated, 70.1%; p = not significant).[245] Multiple observational series have demonstrated an improvement in hemodynamic status and have suggested an enhanced survival rate for patients in cardiogenic shock treated with angioplasty.[244]

The SHOCK (SHould we emergently revascularize Occluded Coronaries for cardiogenic shocK) trial randomized 302 patients to emergency revascularization (angioplasty, 55%; CABG, 38%) or initial medical stabilization, including use of an intraaortic balloon pump (86% in both groups).[246] The overall mortality rate at 30 days did not differ statistically (47%, revascularization; 56%, medical stabilization; p = 0.11) but was significantly lower in patients ≤ 75 years old treated with emergent revascularization (41% vs. 57%, p = 0.01). Mortality was correlated with infarct artery perfusion grade (39% for TIMI flow grades 2 and 3 vs. 100% for TIMI flow grades 0 and 1).[247] Patients undergoing emergent revascularization also exhibited lower mortality rates at 6 months (50% vs. 63%, p = 0.027).[246] Of note, use of coronary stents in the SHOCK trial was associated with enhanced procedural success, and success was associated with an improved survival rate.[248] Multivessel coronary artery disease is commonly present in patients with cardiogenic shock. Additional studies are needed to refine the revascularization strategy for patients with cardiogenic shock and multivessel disease.[244]

Elderly Patients with Myocardial Infarction

Elderly patients (≥ 65 years) account for 85% of deaths from myocardial infarction.[249] Despite the pivotal influence of reperfusion on outcome in acute myocardial infarction, reperfusion therapy is applied to less than one-half of eligible elderly patients.[250] The major reason is apprehension about the use of thrombolytic agents in the aged population, particularly in regard to the risk of intracranial hemorrhage. Primary angioplasty nearly eliminates this peril and may expand the number of elderly patients who undergo reperfusion.

Various observational series document the efficacy of primary angioplasty in elderly patients.[251] One small (n = 60) randomized trial in patients ≥ 76 years old detected a 30-day survival advantage for primary angioplasty compared with streptokinase thrombolysis (3% vs. 25%, p = 0.02).[252] Pooled analysis of the PAMI, Netherlands, and Mayo Clinic randomized trials revealed a significant reduction in mortality for the elderly subgroup (3.5% vs. 16%, p = 0.02).[222] In the GUSTO-IIB trial, a nonsignificant trend toward lower 30-day mortality rates in the angioplasty arm was noted for patients ≥ 70 years old.[201]

In the NRMI-2 registry, the combined endpoint of death and nonfatal stroke was significantly higher in patients ≥ 75 years who received tissue plasminogen activator (n = 3731) compared with those undergoing primary angioplasty (n = 632) (18.4% vs. 14.6%, p < 0.03).[212] Of 20,683 Medicare beneficiaries (age ≥ 65 years) undergoing reperfusion therapy in the Cooperative Cardiovascular Project (CCP) registry, 30-day (8.7% vs. 11.9%, p = 0.001) and 1-year mortality rates (14.4% vs. 17.6%, p = 0.001) were lower in patients treated with primary angioplasty compared with thrombolysis.[250] This benefit occurred despite a mean time to treatment of 142 minutes (median = 129 min) in the angioplasty group. The advantages of primary angioplasty may be magnified in elderly patients.

Logistic Challenge of Primary Angioplasty

There remains skepticism about the applicability of primary angioplasty for reperfusion in the broad population of patients presenting with acute myocardial infarction. The results of randomized trials from dedicated experienced institutions have not been uniformly reproduced in large community-based registries, as noted above. The discrepancy between treatment intervals—"door-to-balloon time"—in randomized trials (< 60–90 minutes) and community-based studies (100–180 min) is considerable. There appears to be a proportional relationship between the treatment interval and survival with primary angioplasty concordant with evidence from thrombolytic trials[190,218] (see Fig. 6). In some analyses, however, the survival benefit of primary angioplasty over thrombolysis is greater for patients presenting later after the onset of symptoms.[253–255] Increasing the treatment interval for thrombolytic therapy reduces efficacy and enhances the risk of complications such as intracranial hemorrhage and cardiac rupture.[256,257] Although early (< 2 hours) treatment results in the lowest mortality rate, the benefit of later treatment with primary angioplasty may relate to positive remodeling effects, electrical stability, and provision of a conduit for collateral flow without the enhanced risk of complications from thrombolytic agents.[258]

The effectiveness of a widespread primary angioplasty strategy also may be limited by institutional and operator expertise. Several studies have demonstrated a relationship between institutional volume and improved survival rates in large cohorts of patients.[259–261] However, volume alone does not account for discrepant outcomes, and excellent results were seen in the Stent PAMI trial even in inexperienced centers.[262,263]

Less than 20% of hospitals in the United States have cardiac catheterization laboratories, and even fewer are capable of performing coronary artery bypass surgery.[264] Experienced operators have performed primary angioplasty at hospitals without cardiac surgery facilities with a high success rate even in patients with cardiogenic shock.[265,266] Alternatively, the feasibility and safety of urgent transport of patients from a hospital without angioplasty facilities to a center for primary angioplasty have been described in several reports.[267,268] The relative benefits of this strategy compared with on-site thrombolysis remain to be elucidated.[269]

Primary Angioplasty and Glycoprotein IIb/IIIa Receptor Inhibition

Plaque disruption and concomitant thrombus formation underlie the pathophysiology of acute myocardial infarction. Reperfusion therapy (thrombolysis and angioplasty) also activate the coagulation system, creating the risk of recurrent thrombosis.[99,270] Recognition of platelets as a critical component of these thrombotic events led to targeted therapies for acute coronary syndromes and the pharmacologic development of GP IIb/IIIa receptor antagonists.[103,271,272] Multiple trials have documented the benefit of GP IIb/IIIa antagonists in reducing adverse events after transluminal coronary revascularization.[43–46,59,151]

Several trials have evaluated the efficacy of intravenous abciximab as an adjunct to primary angioplasty. In the EPIC trial, 64 patients underwent angioplasty within 12 hours of infarction. At 6 months the composite endpoint of death, myocardial infarction, and target vessel revascularization (TVR) was markedly reduced in the group that received abciximab (4.5% vs. 47.8%, p = 0.002).[273] The RAPPORT (ReoPro in AMI Primary PTCA Organization Randomized Trial) trial blindly randomized 483 patients undergoing primary angioplasty to abciximab or placebo.[274] The composite endpoint of death, reinfarction, or urgent TVR was reduced by intention-to-treat analysis in the abciximab group at 30 days (5.8% vs. 11.1%, p = 0.03) but not at the primary endpoint specified at 6 months (28.2% vs. 28.1%, p = 0.97). Many patients (n = 74) did not receive the study drug or undergo intervention. The composite endpoint at 6 months was reduced in patients who received treatment (10.6% vs. 19.9%, p = 0.004).

Abciximab also has been shown to improve recovery of microvascular perfusion and to enhance contractile function after stenting in acute myocardial infarction.[275] Preliminary results from the ADMIRAL (Abciximab before Direct angioplasty and stenting in Myocardial Infarction Regarding Acute and Long-term results) trial demonstrated a decrease in the primary endpoint (combined incidence of death, recurrent myocardial infarction, and urgent TVR at 30 days) from 20% in the placebo group to 10.7% (p < 0.03) in the abciximab group.[276] In both the RAPPORT and ADMIRAL trials, the gain from abciximab was due primarily to a reduction in urgent TVR. Further insight into the benefits of adjunct treatment with abciximab in patients undergoing primary angioplasty and stenting is forthcoming from the CADILLAC study (see below).

Primary Stenting in Acute Myocardial Infarction

Early studies suggested that the presence of intracoronary thrombus during intervention increased the risk for stent thrombosis.[127,128] The development of high-pressure stent deployment techniques and improved antiplatelet therapy has allowed expansion of the indications for stenting to include patients with acute coronary syndromes.[130,131,135] The impressive angiographic results, improved acute safety profile, and proven decline in restenosis enticed the interventional operator to apply these benefits to patients with acute myocardial infarction.

Stenting initially was used as a bailout procedure after primary angioplasty.[277,278] Suboptimal results after primary angioplasty are predictive of recurrent ischemia or reocclusion.[227,279] Several series documented the feasibility and safety of primary stenting in acute myocardial infarction.[132–134,280]

Randomized trials comparing primary stenting with primary angioplasty have consistently demonstrated a reduction in the composite endpoint of death, nonfatal reinfarction, and repeat TVR[281–286] (Table 10). Both techniques are highly effective at achieving complete reperfusion of the infarct artery; therefore, it is not surprising that the principal benefit of stenting over angioplasty is attributed to a reduction in recurrent ischemia and reocclusion. Most of these trials allowed crossover to stenting in the angioplasty group for suboptimal angiographic results. However the FRESCO (Florence Randomized Elective Stenting in Acute Coronary Occlusios) trial randomized patients after optimal (TIMI flow grade 3, < 30% stenosis) primary angioplasty had been performed.[282]

The PAMI-Stent randomized trial reported a reduction in the 6-month combined endpoint of death, recurrent nonfatal infarction, stroke, and TVR in the stent group (12.6% vs. 20.1%, p < 0.01), related entirely to reduction in TVR (7.7% vs. 17%, p < 0.001).[283] The stent group also demonstrated a significant reduction in recurrent ischemia (9% vs. 28%, p = 0.003) and the incidence of restenosis or reocclusion (17% vs. 43%, p =0.001) (Table 11). Despite the favorable influence of stents on the composite adverse-event endpoint, there is concern about a trend toward increased mortality in the stent group.[287] TIMI flow grade has been noted to decline after stenting. In the PAMI-Stent trial, a nonsignificant trend toward lower rates of TIMI flow grade 3 was seen after routine stenting (89.4% vs. 92.7%, p = 0.10).[283] This finding has been attributed to possible stent deployment-induced embolization, which may contribute to a "no reflow" phenomenon.

The CADILLAC (Controlled Abciximab and Device Investigation to Lower Late Angioplasty Complications) trial compares primary balloon angioplasty with or without abciximab to primary stenting with or without abciximab.[288] Preliminary data (Table 12) reveal the cumulative benefits of abciximab and stenting to reduce recurrent ischemia, with a remarkably low hospital mortality rate. The final clinical results from this trial will provide important information about the relative benefits of adding stents and abciximab to catheter-based reperfusion therapy.

Table 10.   Randomized Trials of Primary Stenting vs. Primary Angioplasty in Acute Myocardial Infarction

	n	PTCA → Stent Crossover (%)	F/U Time (mo)	Composite Endpoint of Death, MI, and TVR		
				Stent (%)	PTCA (%)	p value
Zwolle[281]	227	13	6	5	20	0.0012
FRESCO[282]	150	0	6	9	28	0.003
PASTA[285]	136	10	12	22	49	0.0011
GRAMI[286]	104	25	0.2	4	19	0.03
SENTIM 2[284]	211	26	6	9	28	< 0.01
Stent PAMI[283]	900	15	12	17	25	< 0.01

PTCA = percutaneous transluminal coronary angioplasty, F/U = follow-up, MI = myocardial infarction, TVR = target vessel revascularization.

Table 11. Results of the Stent-PAMI Trial

	Stent	PTCA	p value
Patients	452	448	
Angiographic success (%)	99.3	98.4	0.22
TIMI flow grade 3	89.4	92.7	0.10
Events at 1 month (%)			
Death	3.5	1.8	0.15
Reinfarction	0.4	1.1	0.29
Disabling stroke	0.2	0.2	1.00
TVR	1.3	3.8	0.02
Combined	4.6	5.8	0.46
Events at 1 year (%)			
Death	5.8	3.1	0.07
Reinfarction	2.9	2.7	1.00
Disabling stroke	0.4	0.4	1.00
TVR	10.6	21.0	< 0.0001
Combined	17.0	24.8	< 0.01

PTCA = percutaneous transluminal coronary angioplasty, TVR target vessel revascularization.
Data from Grines CL, Cox DA, Stone GW, et al: Coronary angioplasty with or without stent implantation for acute myocardial infarction. Stent Primary Angioplasty in Myocardial Infarction Study Group. N Engl J Med 341:1949–1956, 1999.

Reperfusion with Alternative Mechanical Devices

Catheter-based reperfusion techniques have emphasized the use of balloon angioplasty and stents. Several other interventional devices, including those designed to remove thrombus directly, have shown promise.

Directional atherectomy has been described as a primary reperfusion modality. Kurisu et al. reported successful reperfusion in 24 patients with a hospital mortality rate of 5.7%.[289] An 86% reperfusion rate was reported in 18 patients with a restenosis rate of 47% on follow-up.[290] There has been no further enthusiasm for use of directional atherectomy as a reperfusion device.

The TEC device has also been used for patients with acute myocardial infarction. Kaplan et al. reported a 94% procedural success rate in 100 patients with acute myocardial infarction and high-risk features, including thrombolysis failure (40%), angiographic thrombus (66%), and saphenous vein graft occlusion (29%).[291] Long-term vessel patency was 90%, but angiographic restenosis occurred in 68% of cases. Experience with this technique has been limited primarily by its large profile and complexity.

Table 12. Hospital Outcomes from the CADILLAC Trial

	PTCA	PTCA + Abciximab	Stent	Stent + Abciximab
Number of patients	488	494	487	492
TIMI flow grade 3 (%)	94.8	95.5	92.1	96.7
Death (%)	1.4	1	1.6	1.6
Reinfarction (%)	0.6	0	0.8	0.2
Disabling stroke (%)	0.4	0	0.6	0
Target vessel revascularization	2.3	0.2	0.8	0.2

PTCA = percutaneous transluminal coronary angioplasty.
Data from Stone GW: CADILLAC (Controlled Abciximab and Device Investigation to Lower Late Angioplasty Complications) Trial. Presented at the American Heart Association 72nd Annual Scientific Meeting, Atlanta, Georgia, 1999.

Intravascular ultrasound thrombolysis also has been used successfully to re-canalize coronary arteries during infarction. Hamm et al. reported successful reperfusion in 13 of 14 patients.[292] This device also induced arterial patency in 94 % (TIMI flow grade 3 in 84%) of 31 patients.[293]

Experience with the Possis AngioJet catheter as a method for reperfusion in acute myocardial infarction is increasing. In 31 patients with acute or recent myocardial infarction, procedural success was achieved in 97% (final TIMI flow grade = 2.84), with adjunctive balloon angioplasty in 30 patients and stenting in 12 patients.[294] Another series of 70 patients underwent rhe-olytic thrombectomy with adjunctive revascularization within 8 hours of acute myocardial infarction. The clinical success rate (defined as angio-graphic success and 30-day freedom from major adverse cardiac events) was reported as 90%.[295]

The Future of Reperfusion Therapy

The impressive survival achieved in recent trials of catheter-based reperfu-sion is a testament to the innovation and investigative effort to improve the care of patients with acute myocardial infarction. Despite this success, the sig-nificant proportion of patients (~50%) who are ineligible for inclusion in these trials suffers a mortality rate that is several-fold greater than that of eligible pa-tients.[296] Continued effort is necessary to reduce the treatment interval, maxi-mize reperfusion efficacy, and minimize complications.

Recently the concept of "facilitated PCI" has emerged to speed and enhance reperfusion. A reduced dose of a short-acting thrombolytic drug, possibly com-bined with a glycoprotein IIb/IIIa antagonist, before the patient's arrival in the catheterization lab may allow improved angioplasty results and enhance my-ocardial salvage. This merging of thrombolytic and catheter-based intervention has been studied in a preliminary fashion in both the PACT (Plasminogen-acti-vator Angioplasty Compatibility Trial) and SPEED (Strategies for Patency Enhancement in the Emergency Department) trials.[297,298] This new strategy awaits confirmation in the GUSTO-IV trial.

Ischemia and Sudden Cardiac Death

Approximately 50% of all cardiac deaths are sudden.[299] The mechanism for sudden death usually is attributed to ventricular arrhythmias.[300] Sudden car-diac death is most commonly a consequence of coronary artery disease, in-cluding the effects of myocardial damage and ischemia. Most patients who experience sudden death are found to have evidence of extensive coronary artery disease. In an autopsy study by Liberthson and colleagues, coronary artery stenosis > 75% was noted in over 90% of patients who died suddenly, with a 60% prevalence of three-vessel disease.[301] Likewise, in an angiographic study by Weaver et al., 94% of 64 patients exhibited stenosis > 70%.[302]

The extent of left ventricular functional impairment in patients with coro-nary artery disease has been clearly identified as a risk factor for symptomatic ventricular arrhythmias and sudden death.[302–305] However, there is less cer-tainty about the role of ischemia. Although some studies have suggested that ischemic symptoms or signs precede cardiac arrest in a significant proportion of patients,[306] no data clearly indicate ischemia alone as predictor for sudden death.[300,307]

Ischemia effects important electophysiologic changes on the myocardium, inducing and enhancing the risk of ventricular arrhythmias. A decrease in the amplitude, duration, and upstroke velocity of the cardiac action potential occurs, along with heterogeneous changes in refractoriness.[308] Polymorphic ventricular tachycardia and ventricular fibrillation typically are seen in the early phases of ischemia.[309] After healing of a myocardial infarction, reentrant mechanisms predominate, leading to monomorphic ventricular tachycardia.

The management of patients who have symptomatic ventricular arrhythmias or survive cardiac arrest involves a multifaceted approach, including consideration of proarrhythmic factors, cardiac catheterization, electrophysiologic testing, pharmacologic treatment, revascularization and increasing use of implantable defibrillators.

The Role of Revascularization

Acute Myocardial Infarction

Patients are at risk for fatal ventricular tachyarrhythmias and occasionally fatal bradyarrhythmias in the earliest phase of acute myocardial infarction. Rapid entry into the medical system ensures restoration of normal rhythm in the prehospital and early hospitalization phases of infarction. Of note, it has been estimated that the incidence of primary ventricular fibrillation during acute myocardial infarction has decreased over time, perhaps reflecting the better overall care of patients with coronary artery disease.[310]

The survival benefits of early reperfusion therapy are emphasized above. Prolonged cardiopulmonary resuscitation for patients who have suffered a cardiac arrest is considered a relative contraindication for thrombolytic therapy. Primary angioplasty allows safer application of reperfusion therapy for such patients. Kahn and colleagues reported the use of primary angioplasty for acute ST-elevation myocardial infarction in 11 patients after out-of-hospital cardiac arrest.[311] The infarct artery was the left anterior descending in 9 patients, and 7 were in cardiogenic shock. Primary angioplasty was successful in 7, and 6 patients survived with neurologic recovery.

Coronary angioplasty also has been reported to affect favorably the outcome of a few patients with acute myocardial infarction and intractable ventricular arrhythmias.[312,313] These patients underwent transluminal revascularization within hours and at 19 days and 10 weeks after the onset of the infarction.

The incidence of sudden cardiac death has declined in the United States since the early 1980s.[314] Although this improvement is likely multifactorial, the time period coincides with the expansion of reperfusion therapy for acute myocardial infarction. In a study of 173 patients, Hohnloser and colleagues identified the presence of an occluded infarct artery as the strongest independent predictor of ventricular arrhthymic complications after acute myocardial infarction.[315] Patients who have received thrombolytic therapy have a lower incidence of inducible sustained ventricular tachycardia. The risk was reduced (8% vs. 88%, p =0.0008) in a study of 32 patients after anterior infarction with aneurysm formation.[316] Likewise, patients receiving thrombolysis in a randomized study had a marked reduction in the incidence of inducible ventricular tachycardia (48% vs. 100%, p = 0.001).[317]

Late potentials detected by signal-averaged electrocardiography are a marker for the electrophysiologic substrate that facilitate ventricular tachycardia.[318] An occluded infarct artery is a strong predictor for the detection of late potentials.[315,319] An open infarct artery may lessen adverse ventricular remodeling and impede development of a substrate for reentry. Of note, reperfusion by angioplasty has been shown to reduce the prevalence of late potentials compared with thrombolytic reperfusion in a study of 109 patients (13.6% vs. 17.4%, p < 0.05).[320] Late (6–15 days) angioplasty also has been shown to eliminate late potentials after myocardial infarction.[321]

Acute Coronary Syndromes and Sudden Death

Previous data have indicated that less than one-third of patients with sudden cardiac death present with an acute myocardial infarction.[304,321,322] However, "active" coronary lesions (plaque rupture, thrombosis) are noted in the majority of patients who suffer sudden cardiac death.[304,323] The plaque disruption, thrombus formation, and microembolization seen in sudden death are comparable to the morphology seen with acute coronary syndromes.[324]

Acute coronary occlusion may play a greater role in the pathogenesis of sudden cardiac death than previous data suggest. In a study of 89 consecutive patients who underwent immediate coronary angiography after presenting with out-of-hospital cardiac arrest, Spaulding et al. documented total occlusion (TIMI flow grades 0 and 1) in 48%.[325] Angioplasty was performed successfully in 28 of 37 patients. Clinical and electrocardiographic findings were poorly predictive of total occlusion. Successful angioplasty was an independent predictor of survival.

Prevention of Sudden Death

The prevalence of sudden cardiac death is reduced by coronary artery bypass surgery. In the Coronary Artery Surgery Study (CASS) registry (n = 13,476) the incidence of sudden death was 1.8% in patients treated surgically compared with 4.6% in patients treated with medical therapy.[326] A similar reduction in cumulative risk (3% vs. 9%) was noted in the European Coronary Surgical Study.[327] Coronary bypass surgery appeared to reduce the risk of subsequent cardiac arrest in a study of 265 survivors of out-of-hospital ventricular fibrillation.[328] Surgical revascularization also appeared to eliminate inducible ventricular fibrillation in 11 survivors of cardiac arrest.[329] In contrast, in the same series inducible ventricular tachycardia persisted after surgery in 80% of 22 patients, possibly reflecting a less important role for ischemia in the pathophysiology of ventricular tachycardia.

Little information is available about the role of transluminal revascularization in the prevention of sudden cardiac death. In a study of 82 postinfarct patients admitted with sustained ventricular tachycardia or ventricular fibrillation, 14 patients had severe (> 90%) stenosis supplying viable myocardium. After treatment (angioplasty in 8, CABG in 3, medical therapy in 3) no recurrence of arrhythmia was reported.[330] However, concern has been raised about the danger of restenosis in such patients.[331]

Small series or case reports have documented the efficacy of coronary angioplasty in the elimination of exercise-induced arrhythmias (ventricular tachycardia/fibrillation and asystole) associated with ischemia.[332,333]

More thorough investigation using modern techniques is necessary to define the preventative and therapeutic roles of transluminal intervention in the management of patients who suffer sudden cardiac death.

Future Promise

Percutaneous coronary interventions have assumed an essential position in the management of patients with acute coronary syndromes. The evidence validating current practice is increasingly substantiated by randomized scientific investigation. The promise of the future will rely on persistent technical innovation and application of the lessons learned from more thorough understanding of the pathobiology responsible for the acute coronary syndromes.

References

1. Ambrose JA, Israel DH: Angiography in unstable angina. Am J Cardiol 68:78B–84B, 1991.
2. Bugiardini R, Pozzati A, Borghi A, et al: Angiographic morphology in unstable angina and its relation to transient myocardial ischemia and hospital outcome. Am J Cardiol 67:460–464, 1991.
3. Chen L, Chester MR, Redwood S, et al: Angiographic stenosis progression and coronary events in patients with 'stabilized' unstable angina. Circulation 91:2319–2324, 1995.
4. Zaacks SM, Liebson PR, Calvin JE, et al: Unstable angina and non–Q-wave myocardial infarction: Does the clinical diagnosis have therapeutic implications? J Am Coll Cardiol 33:107–118, 1999.
5. Waller BF: Pathology of transluminal balloon angioplasty used in the treatment of coronary heart disease. Cardiol Clin 7:749–770, 1989.
6. Steele PM, Chesebro JH, Stanson AW, et al: Balloon angioplasty: Natural history of the pathophysiological response to injury in a pig model. Circ Res 57:105–112, 1985.
7. Mehran R, Ambrose JA, Bongu RM, et al: Angioplasty of complex lesions in ischemic rest angina: Results of the Thrombolysis and Angioplasty in Unstable Angina (TAUSA) trial. J Am Coll Cardiol 26:961–966, 1995.
8. Sugrue DD, Holmes DR, Smith HC, et al: Coronary artery thrombus as a risk factor for acute vessel occlusion during percutaneous transluminal coronary angioplasty: Improving results. Br Heart J 56:62–66, 1986.
9. Ellis SG, Guetta V, Miller D, et al: Relation between lesion characteristics and risk with percutaneous intervention in the stent and glycoprotein IIb/IIIa era: An analysis of results from 10,907 lesions and proposal for new classification scheme. Circulation 100:1971–1976, 1999.
10. Detre KM, Holmes DR Jr, Holubkov R, et al: Incidence and consequences of periprocedural occlusion: The 1985–1986 National Heart, Lung, and Blood Institute Percutaneous Transluminal Coronary Angioplasty Registry. Circulation 82:739–750, 1990.
11. Holmes DR Jr, Simpson JB, Berdan LG, et al: Abrupt closure: The CAVEAT I experience. Coronary Angioplasty Versus Excisional Atherectomy Trial. J Am Coll Cardiol 26:1494–1500, 1995.
12. Waxman S, Sassower MA, Mittleman MA, et al: Angioscopic predictors of early adverse outcome after coronary angioplasty in patients with unstable angina and non–Q-wave myocardial infarction. Circulation 93:2106–2113, 1996.
13. Tenaglia AN, Fortin DF, Califf RM, et al: Predicting the risk of abrupt vessel closure after angioplasty in an individual patient. J Am Coll Cardiol 24:1004–1011, 1994.
14. Khan MM, Ellis SG, Aguirre FV, et al: Does intracoronary thrombus influence the outcome of high risk percutaneous transluminal coronary angioplasty? Clinical and angiographic outcomes in a large multicenter trial. EPIC Investigators. Evaluation of IIb/IIIa Platelet Receptor Antagonist 7E3 in Preventing Ischemic Complications. J Am Coll Cardiol 31:31–36, 1998.
15. Singh M, Ting HH, Araujo NA, et al: Influence of thrombus on the outcome of coronary interventions in the current era. J Am Coll Cardiol 35:90A, 2000.
16. Violaris AG, Melkert R, Herrman JP, Serruys PW: Role of angiographically identifiable thrombus on long-term luminal renarrowing after coronary angioplasty: A quantitative angiographic analysis. Circulation 93:889–897, 1996.
17. Williams DO, Riley RS, Singh AK, et al: Evaluation of the role of coronary angioplasty in patients with unstable angina pectoris. Am Heart J 102:1–9, 1981.
18. Meijer A, Verheugt FW, Werter CJ, et al: Aspirin versus coumadin in the prevention of reocclusion and recurrent ischemia after successful thrombolysis: A prospective placebo-controlled angiographic study. Results of the APRICOT Study. Circulation 87:1524–1530, 1993.
19. Faxon DP, Detre KM, McCabe CH, et al: Role of percutaneous transluminal coronary angioplasty in the treatment of unstable angina: Report from the National Heart, Lung, and Blood Institute Percutaneous Transluminal Coronary Angioplasty and Coronary Artery Surgery Study Registries. Am J Cardiol 53:131C–135C, 1984.

20. Bentivoglio LG, Holubkov R, Kelsey SF, et al: Short- and long-term outcome of percutaneous transluminal coronary angioplasty in unstable versus stable angina pectoris: A report of the 1985-1986 NHLBI PTCA Registry. Cathet Cardiovasc Diagn 23:227–238, 1991.
21. Kamp O, Beatt KJ, De Feyter PJ, et al: Short-, medium-, and long-term follow-up after percutaneous transluminal coronary angioplasty for stable and unstable angina pectoris. Am Heart J 117:991–996, 1989.
22. de Feyter PJ, van den Brand M, Laarman GJ, et al: Acute coronary artery occlusion during and after percutaneous transluminal coronary angioplasty. Frequency, prediction, clinical course, management, and follow-up. Circulation 83:927–936, 1991.
23. Meyer J, Schmitz HJ, Kiesslich T, et al: Percutaneous transluminal coronary angioplasty in patients with stable and unstable angina pectoris: Analysis of early and late results. Am Heart J 106:973–980, 1983.
24. Quigley PJ, Erwin J, Maurer BJ, et al: Percutaneous transluminal coronary angioplasty in unstable angina: Comparison with stable angina. Br Heart J 55:227–230, 1986.
25. Timmis AD, Griffin B, Crick JC, Sowton E: Early percutaneous transluminal coronary angioplasty in the management of unstable angina. Int J Cardiol 14:25–31, 1987.
26. Steffenino G, Meier B, Finci L, Rutishauser W: Follow up results of treatment of unstable angina by coronary angioplasty. Br Heart J 57:416–419, 1987.
27. Sharma B, Wyeth RP, Kolath GS, et al: Percutaneous transluminal coronary angioplasty of one vessel for refractory unstable angina pectoris: Efficacy in single and multivessel disease. Br Heart J 59:280–286, 1988.
28. Thijs Plokker HW, Ernst SM, Bal ET, et al: Percutaneous transluminal coronary angioplasty in patients with unstable angina pectoris refractory to medical therapy: Long-term clinical and angiographic results. Cathet Cardiovasc Diagn 14:15–18, 1988.
29. Perry RA, Seth A, Hunt A, Shiu MF: Coronary angioplasty in unstable angina and stable angina: A comparison of success and complications. Br Heart J 60:367–372, 1988.
30. Halon DA, Merdler A, Shefer A, et al: Identifying patients at high risk for restenosis after percutaneous transluminal coronary angioplasty for unstable angina pectoris. Am J Cardiol 64:289–293, 1989.
31. Myler RK, Shaw RE, Stertzer SH, et al: Unstable angina and coronary angioplasty. Circulation 82:II88–II95, 1990.
32. Rupprecht HJ, Brennecke R, Kottmeyer M, et al: Short- and long-term outcome after PTCA in patients with stable and unstable angina. Eur Heart J 11:964–973, 1990.
33. Stammen F, De Scheerder I, Glazier JJ, et al: Immediate and follow-up results of the conservative coronary angioplasty strategy for unstable angina pectoris. Am J Cardiol 69:1533–1537, 1992.
34. Morrison DA, Sacks J, Grover F, Hammermeister KE: Effectiveness of percutaneous transluminal coronary angioplasty for patients with medically refractory rest angina pectoris and high risk of adverse outcomes with coronary artery bypass grafting. Am J Cardiol 75:237–240, 1995.
35. Williams DO, Braunwald E, Thompson B, et al: Results of percutaneous transluminal coronary angioplasty in unstable angina and non–Q-wave myocardial infarction: Observations from the TIMI IIIB Trial. Circulation 94:2749–2755, 1996.
36. Bentivoglio LG, Detre K, Yeh W, et al: Outcome of percutaneous transluminal coronary angioplasty in subsets of unstable angina pectoris: A report of the 1985–1986 National Heart, Lung, and Blood Institute Percutaneous Transluminal Coronary Angioplasty Registry. J Am Coll Cardiol 24:1195–1206, 1994.
37. Kapoor C, Williams DO, Yeh W, et al: Contemporary coronary intervention for unstable angina: A report from the NHLBI Dynamic Registry. J Am Coll Cardiol 33:35A, 1999.
38. Singh M, Holmes DR, Garratt KN, et al: Changing outcomes of percutaneous intervention in patients with unstable angina. J Am Coll Cardiol 33:31A, 1999.
39. Hartzler GO, Rutherford BD, McConahay DR, et al: "High-risk" percutaneous transluminal coronary angioplasty. Am J Cardiol 61:33G–37G, 1988.
40. Rozenman Y, Gilon D, Zelingher J, et al: Importance of delaying balloon angioplasty in patients with unstable angina pectoris. Clin Cardiol 19:111–114, 1996.
41. Tung C, Sauri D, Fintel D, Gheorghiade M: Management of high-risk subsets in unstable angina. Cardiol Clin 17:415–437, 1999.
42. Antoniucci D, Santoro GM, Bolognese L, et al: Early coronary angioplasty as compared with delayed coronary angioplasty in patients with high-risk unstable angina pectoris. Coron Artery Dis 7:75–80, 1996.
43. EPIC Investigators: Use of a monoclonal antibody directed against the platelet glycoprotein IIb/IIIa receptor in high-risk coronary angioplasty. The EPIC Investigation. N Engl J Med 330:956–961, 1994.

44. IMPACT II Investigators: Randomised placebo-controlled trial of effect of eptifibatide on complications of percutaneous coronary intervention: IMPACT-II. Integrilin to Minimise Platelet Aggregation and Coronary Thrombosis-II. Lancet 349:1422–1428, 1997.

45. RESTORE Investigators: Effects of platelet glycoprotein IIb/IIIa blockade with tirofiban on adverse cardiac events in patients with unstable angina or acute myocardial infarction undergoing coronary angioplasty. The RESTORE Investigators. Randomized Efficacy Study of Tirofiban for Outcomes and REstenosis. Circulation 96:1445–1453, 1997.

46. CAPTURE Investigators: Randomised placebo-controlled trial of abciximab before and during coronary intervention in refractory unstable angina: the CAPTURE Study. Lancet 349:1429–1435, 1997.

47. TIMI IIIA Investigators: Early effects of tissue-type plasminogen activator added to conventional therapy on the culprit coronary lesion in patients presenting with ischemic cardiac pain at rest: Results of the Thrombolysis in Myocardial Ischemia (TIMI IIIA) Trial. Circulation 87:38–52, 1993.

48. Wohlgelernter D, Cleman M, Highman HA, Zaret BL: Percutaneous transluminal coronary angioplasty of the "culprit lesion" for management of unstable angina pectoris in patients with multivessel coronary artery disease. Am J Cardiol 58:460–464, 1986.

49. de Feyter PJ, Serruys PW, Arnold A, et al: Coronary angioplasty of the unstable angina related vessel in patients with multivessel disease. Eur Heart J 7:460–467, 1986.

50. Kussmaul WGd, Krol J, Laskey WK, et al: One-year follow-up results of "culprit" versus multivessel coronary angioplasty trial. Am J Cardiol 71:1431-1433, 1993.

51. Bypass Angioplasty Revascularization Investigation (BARI) Investigators: Comparison of coronary bypass surgery with angioplasty in patients with multivessel disease. N Engl J Med 335:217–225, 1996.

52. Holmes DR Jr, Vlietstra RE, Smith HC, et al: Restenosis after percutaneous transluminal coronary angioplasty (PTCA): A report from the PTCA Registry of the National Heart, Lung, and Blood Institute. Am J Cardiol 53:77C–81C, 1984.

53. Bourassa MG, Lesperance J, Eastwood C, et al: Clinical, physiologic, anatomic and procedural factors predictive of restenosis after percutaneous transluminal coronary angioplasty. J Am Coll Cardiol 18:368–376, 1991.

54. Serruys PW, Luijten HE, Beatt KJ, et al: Incidence of restenosis after successful coronary angioplasty: A time- related phenomenon: A quantitative angiographic study in 342 consecutive patients at 1, 2, 3, and 4 months. Circulation 77:361–371, 1988.

55. Schwartz L, Bourassa MG, Lesperance J, et al: Aspirin and dipyridamole in the prevention of restenosis after percutaneous transluminal coronary angioplasty. N Engl J Med 318:1714–1719, 1988.

56. Bauters C, Lablanche JM, McFadden EP, et al: Relation of coronary angioscopic findings at coronary angioplasty to angiographic restenosis. Circulation 92:2473–2479, 1995.

57. Higuchi Y, Hirayama M, Adachi T, et al: Differing coronary arterial responses to balloon angioplasty between stable and unstable lesions: A combined study of intravascular ultrasound and angioscopy. J Am Coll Cardiol 33:93A, 1999.

58. Topol EJ, Ferguson JJ, Weisman HF, et al: Long-term protection from myocardial ischemic events in a randomized trial of brief integrin beta$_3$ blockade with percutaneous coronary intervention. EPIC Investigator Group. Evaluation of Platelet IIb/IIIa Inhibition for Prevention of Ischemic Complication JAMA 278:479–484, 1997.

59. EPILOG Investigators: Platelet glycoprotein IIb/IIIa receptor blockade and low-dose heparin during percutaneous coronary revascularization. N Engl J Med 336:1689–1696, 1997.

60. Gibson CM, Goel M, Cohen DJ, et al: Six-month angiographic and clinical follow-up of patients prospectively randomized to receive either tirofiban or placebo during angioplasty in the RESTORE trial. Randomized Efficacy Study of Tirofiban for Outcomes and Restenosis. J Am Coll Cardiol 32:28–34, 1998.

61. Mahon NG, Codd MB, McKenna CJ, et al: Characteristics and outcomes in patients with acute myocardial infarction with ST-segment depression on initial electrocardiogram. Am Heart J 139:311–319, 2000.

62. Liebson PR, Klein LW: The non–Q-wave myocardial infarction revisited: 10 years later. Prog Cardiovasc Dis 39:399–444, 1997.

63. Armstrong PW, Fu Y, Chang WC, et al: Acute coronary syndromes in the GUSTO-IIb trial: Prognostic insights and impact of recurrent ischemia. The GUSTO-IIb Investigators. Circulation 98:1860–1868, 1998.

64. Heyndrickx GR, Amano J, Kenna T, et al: Creatine kinase release not associated with myocardial necrosis after short periods of coronary artery occlusion in conscious baboons. J Am Coll Cardiol 6:1299–1303, 1985.

65. Hamm CW, Ravkilde J, Gerhardt W, et al: The prognostic value of serum troponin T in unstable angina. N Engl J Med 327:146–150, 1992.

66. Antman EM, Tanasijevic MJ, Thompson B, et al: Cardiac-specific troponin I levels to predict the risk of mortality in patients with acute coronary syndromes. N Engl J Med 335:1342–1349, 1996.

67. Hamm CW, Goldmann BU, Heeschen C, et al: Emergency room triage of patients with acute chest pain by means of rapid testing for cardiac troponin T or troponin I. N Engl J Med 337:1648–1653, 1997.

68. Ohman EM, Armstrong PW, Christenson RH, et al: Cardiac troponin T levels for risk stratification in acute myocardial ischemia. GUSTO IIA Investigators. N Engl J Med 335:1333–1341, 1996.

69. Olatidoye AG, Wu AH, Feng YJ, Waters D: Prognostic role of troponin T versus troponin I in unstable angina pectoris for cardiac events with meta-analysis comparing published studies. Am J Cardiol 81:1405–1410, 1998.

70. White H: Optimal treatment of patients with acute coronary syndromes and non–ST-elevation myocardial infarction. Am Heart J 139:S105–S114, 1999.

71. Haft JI, Saadeh SA: Cardiac troponins in acute coronary syndromes [letter; comment]. N Engl J Med 336:1257; discussion 1258–1259, 1997.

72. Fuchs S, Kornowski R, Mehran R, et al: Cardiac troponin I levels and clinical outcomes in patients with acute coronary syndromes: The potential role of early percutaneous revascularization. J Am Coll Cardiol 34:1704–1710, 1999.

73. Goldmann BU, Ohman EM, Hamm CW, et al: Is the adverse outcome with positive troponin T neutralized by revascularization? Results from GUSTO-IIa. Circulation 100:I-810, 1999.

74. Benamer H, Steg PG, Benessiano J, et al: Elevated cardiac troponin I predicts a high-risk angiographic anatomy of the culprit lesion in unstable angina. Am Heart J 137:815–820, 1999.

75. Hamm CW, Heeschen C, Goldmann B, et al: Benefit of abciximab in patients with refractory unstable angina in relation to serum troponin T levels. c7E3 Fab Antiplatelet Therapy in Unstable Refractory Angina (CAPTURE) Study Investigators. N Engl J Med 340:1623–1629, 1999.

76. Keen WD, Savage MP, Fischman DL, et al: Comparison of coronary angiographic findings during the first six hours of non–Q-wave and Q-wave myocardial infarction. Am J Cardiol 74:324–328, 1994.

77. Ambrose JA: Plaque disruption and the acute coronary syndromes of unstable angina and myocardial infarction: If the substrate is similar, why is the clinical presentation different? [editorial]. J Am Coll Cardiol 19:1653–1658, 1992.

78. Boden WE, O'Rourke RA, Crawford MH, et al: Outcomes in patients with acute non–Q-wave myocardial infarction randomly assigned to an invasive as compared with a conservative management strategy. Veterans Affairs Non–Q-Wave Infarction Strategies in Hospital (VANQWISH) Trial Investigators. N Engl J Med 338:1785–1792, 1998.

79. Williams DO, Yeh W, Detre KM, etal: Percutaneous coronary intervention for non-ST elevation myocardial infarction: A report from the NHLBI dynamic registry. J Am Coll Cardiol 35:39A, 2000.

80. Alfonso F, Macaya C, Iniguez A, et al: Percutaneous transluminal coronary angioplasty after non-Q-wave acute myocardial infarction. Am J Cardiol 65:835–839, 1990.

81. Brueren BR, Rosseel MP, Bal ET, et al: Are there differences in late outcome after PTCA for angina pectoris after non–Q-wave vs. Q-wave myocardial infarction? Eur Heart J 18:1903–1912, 1997.

82. Holt GW, Gersh BJ, Holmes DR Jr, et al: Results of percutaneous transluminal coronary angioplasty for angina pectoris early after acute myocardial infarction. Am J Cardiol 61:1238–1242, 1988.

83. Safian RD, Snyder LD, Synder BA, et al: Usefulness of percutaneous transluminal coronary angioplasty for unstable angina pectoris after non–Q-wave acute myocardial infarction. Am J Cardiol 59:263–266, 1987.

84. Suryapranata H, Beatt K, de Feyter PJ, et al: Percutaneous transluminal coronary angioplasty for angina pectoris after a non–Q-wave acute myocardial infarction. Am J Cardiol 61:240–243, 1988.

85. Welty FK, Mittleman MA, Lewis SM, et al: Significance of location (anterior versus inferior) and type (Q-wave versus non–Q-wave) of acute myocardial infarction in patients undergoing percutaneous transluminal coronary angioplasty for postinfarction ischemia. Am J Cardiol 76:431–435, 1995.

86. Phibbs B, Marcus F, Marriott HJ, Moss A, Spodick DH: Q-wave versus non–Q-wave myocardial infarction: A meaningless distinction. J Am Coll Cardiol 33:576–582, 1999.

87. Barnathan ES, Schwartz JS, Taylor L, et al: Aspirin and dipyridamole in the prevention of acute coronary thrombosis complicating coronary angioplasty. Circulation 76:125–134, 1987.

88. Schomig A, Neumann FJ, Kastrati A, et al: A randomized comparison of antiplatelet and anticoagulant therapy after the placement of coronary-artery stents. N Engl J Med 334:1084–1089, 1996.

89. Leon MB, Baim DS, Popma JJ, et al: A clinical trial comparing three antithrombotic-drug regimens after coronary-artery stenting. Stent Anticoagulation Restenosis Study Investigators. N Engl J Med. 339:1665–1671, 1998.

90. Berger PB, Bell MR, Rihal CS, et al: Clopidogrel versus ticlopidine after intracoronary stent placement. J Am Coll Cardiol 34:1891–1894, 1999.

91. Laskey MA, Deutsch E, Barnathan E, Laskey WK: Influence of heparin therapy on percutaneous transluminal coronary angioplasty outcome in unstable angina pectoris. Am J Cardiol 65:1425–1429, 1990.

92. Hettleman BD, Aplin RL, Sullivan PR, et al: Three days of heparin pretreatment reduces major complications of coronary angioplasty in patients with unstable angina. J Am Coll Cardiol 15:154A, 1990.

93. Pow TK, Varricchione TR, Jacobs AJ, et al: Does pretreatment with heparin prevent abrupt closure following PTCA? J Am Coll Cardiol 11:238A, 1988.

94. Hartman D, Wolf NM, Schecter JA, et al: Effect of heparin on intracoronary thrombi in unstable ischemic syndromes. J Am Coll Cardiol 7:107A, 1986.

95. Laskey MA, Deutsch E, Hirshfeld JW Jr, et al: Influence of heparin therapy on percutaneous transluminal coronary angioplasty outcome in patients with coronary arterial thrombus. Am J Cardiol 65:179–182, 1990.

96. Serruys PW, Herrman JP, Simon R, et al: A comparison of hirudin with heparin in the prevention of restenosis after coronary angioplasty. Helvetica Investigators. N Engl J Med 333:757–763, 1995.

97. Bittl JA, Strony J, Brinker JA, et al:Treatment with bivalirudin (Hirulog) as compared with heparin during coronary angioplasty for unstable or postinfarction angina. Hirulog Angioplasty Study Investigators. N Engl J Med 333:764–769, 1995.

98. Aronson DL, Chang P, Kessler CM: Platelet-dependent thrombin generation after in vitro fibrinolytic treatment. Circulation 85:1706–1712, 1992.

99. Owen J, Friedman KD, Grossman BA, et al: Thrombolytic therapy with tissue plasminogen activator or streptokinase induces transient thrombin activity. Blood 72:616–620, 1988.

100. Waller BF, Rothbaum DA, Pinkerton CA, et al: Status of the myocardium and infarct-related coronary artery in 19 necropsy patients with acute recanalization using pharmacologic (streptokinase, r-tissue plasminogen activator), mechanical (percutaneous transluminal coronary angioplasty) or combined types of reperfusion therapy. J Am Coll Cardiol 9:785–801, 1987.

101. TIMI IIIB Investigators: Effects of tissue plasminogen activator and a comparison of early invasive and conservative strategies in unstable angina and non–Q-wave myocardial infarction: Results of the TIMI IIIB Trial. Thrombolysis in Myocardial Ischemia. Circulation 89:1545–1556, 1994.

102. Ambrose JA, Almeida OD, Sharma SK, et al: Adjunctive thrombolytic therapy during angioplasty for ischemic rest angina: Results of the TAUSA Trial. TAUSA Investigators. Thrombolysis and Angioplasty in Unstable Angina trial. Circulation 90:69–77, 1994.

103. Lefkovits J, Plow EF, Topol EJ: Platelet glycoprotein IIb/IIIa receptors in cardiovascular medicine. N Engl J Med 332:1553–1559, 1995.

104. Peterson ED, Lansky AJ, Anstrom KJ, et al: Evolving trends in interventional device use and outcomes: Results from the National Cardiovascular Network Database. Am Heart J 139:198–207, 2000.

105. Holmes DR, Ellis SG, Garrat KN: Directional atherectomy for thrombus containing lesions. Circulation 84:II-26, 1991.

106. Emmi R, Movsowitz H, Manginas A, et al: Directional atherectomy in lesions with coexisting thrombus. Circulation 88:I-596, 1993.

107. Topol EJ, Leya F, Pinkerton CA, et al: A comparison of directional atherectomy with coronary angioplasty in patients with coronary artery disease. The CAVEAT Study Group. N Engl J Med 329:221–227, 1993.

108. Elliott JM, Berdan LG, Holmes DR, et al: One-year follow-up in the Coronary Angioplasty Versus Excisional Atherectomy Trial (CAVEAT I). Circulation 91:2158–2166, 1995.

109. Baim DS, Cutlip DE, Sharma SK, et al: Final results of the Balloon vs Optimal Atherectomy Trial (BOAT). Circulation 97:322–331, 1998.

110. Tsuchikane E, Sumitsuji S, Awata N, et al: Final results of the STent versus directional coronary Atherectomy Randomized Trial (START). J Am Coll Cardiol 34:1050–1057, 1999.

111. Safian RD, May MA, Lichtenberg A, et al: Detailed clinical and angiographic analysis of transluminal extraction coronary atherectomy for complex lesions in native coronary arteries. J Am Coll Cardiol 25:848–854, 1995.

112. Schreiber T, Kaplan B, Gregory M, et al: Transluminal extraction atherectomy vs. balloon angioplasty in acute ischemic syndromes (TOPIT): Hospital outcome and 6 month status. J Am Coll Cardiol 29:132A, 1997.

113. Whitlow PL: Rotational atherectomy: When and how. In Ellis SG, Holmes DR (eds): Stategic Approaches in Coronary Intervention, 2nd ed. Philadelphia, Lippincott Williams & Wilkins, 2000, pp 7–22.

114. Reifart N, Vandormael M, Krajcar M, et al: Randomized comparison of angioplasty of complex coronary lesions at a single center. Excimer Laser, Rotational Atherectomy, and Balloon Angioplasty Comparison (ERBAC) Study. Circulation 96:91–98, 1997.

115. Estella P, Ryan TJ Jr, Landzberg JS, Bittl JA: Excimer laser-assisted coronary angioplasty for lesions containing thrombus. J Am Coll Cardiol 21:1550–1556, 1993.

116. Ramee SR, Kuntz RE, Schatz RA, et al: Preliminary experience with the POSSIS coronary AngioJet rheolytic thrombectomy catheter for intracoronary thrombus. J Am Coll Cardiol 27:69A, 1996.

117. Dohad S, Parris TM, Setum C, et al: AngioJet rheolytic thrombectomy: An important tool for percutaneous coronary interventions in high risk patients; VeGAS II trial. J Am Coll Cardiol 35:75A, 2000.

118. Rosenschein U, Gaul G, Erbel R, et al: Percutaneous transluminal therapy of occluded saphenous vein grafts: Can the challenge be met with ultrasound thrombolysis? Circulation 99:26–29, 1999.

119. Antoniucci D, Valenti R, Santoro GM, et al: Bailout coronary stenting without anticoagulation or intravascular ultrasound guidance: Acute and six-month angiographic results in a series of 120 consecutive patients. Cathet Cardiovasc Diagn 41:14–19, 1997.

120. Dean LS, George CJ, Holmes DR Jr, et al: The use of the Gianturco-Roubin intracoronary stent: The New Approaches to Coronary Intervention (NACI) registry experience. Am J Cardiol 80:89K–98K, 1997.

121. George BS, Voorhees WDd, Roubin GS, et al: Multicenter investigation of coronary stenting to treat acute or threatened closure after percutaneous transluminal coronary angioplasty: Clinical and angiographic outcomes. J Am Coll Cardiol 22:135–143, 1993.

122. Nakano Y, Nakagawa Y, Yokoi H, et al: Initial and follow-up results of the ACS multi-link stent: A single center experience. Cathet Cardiovasc Diagn 45:368–374, 1998.

123. Schomig A, Kastrati A, Mudra H, et al: Four-year experience with Palmaz-Schatz stenting in coronary angioplasty complicated by dissection with threatened or present vessel closure. Circulation 90:2716–2724, 1994.

124. Altmann DB, Racz M, Battleman DS, et al: Reduction in angioplasty complications after the introduction of coronary stents: Results from a consecutive series of 2242 patients. Am Heart J 132:503–507, 1996.

125. Fischman DL, Leon MB, Baim DS, et al: A randomized comparison of coronary-stent placement and balloon angioplasty in the treatment of coronary artery disease. Stent Restenosis Study Investigators. N Engl J Med 331:496–501, 1994.

126. Serruys PW, de Jaegere P, Kiemeneij F, et al: A comparison of balloon-expandable-stent implantation with balloon angioplasty in patients with coronary artery disease. Benestent Study Group. N Engl J Med 331:489–499, 1994.

127. Agrawal SK, Ho DS, Liu MW, et al: Predictors of thrombotic complications after placement of the flexible coil stent. Am J Cardiol 73:1216–1219, 1994.

128. Schatz RA, Baim DS, Leon M, et al: Clinical experience with the Palmaz-Schatz coronary stent: Initial results of a multicenter study. Circulation 83:148–161, 1991.

129. Nath FC, Muller DW, Ellis SG, et al: Thrombosis of a flexible coil coronary stent: Frequency, predictors and clinical outcome. J Am Coll Cardiol 21:622–627, 1993.

130. Colombo A, Hall P, Nakamura S, et al: Intracoronary stenting without anticoagulation accomplished with intravascular ultrasound guidance. Circulation 91:1676–1688, 1995.

131. Karrillon GJ, Morice MC, Benveniste E, et al: Intracoronary stent implantation without ultrasound guidance and with replacement of conventional anticoagulation by antiplatelet therapy: 30- day clinical outcome of the French Multicenter Registry. Circulation 94:1519–1527, 1996.

132. Garcia-Cantu E, Spaulding C, Corcos T, et al: Stent implantation in acute myocardial infarction. Am J Cardiol 77:451–454, 1996.

133. Neumann FJ, Walter H, Richardt G, et al: Coronary Palmaz-Schatz stent implantation in acute myocardial infarction. Heart 75:121–126, 1996.

134. Wong PH, Wong CM: Intracoronary stenting in acute myocardial infarction. Cathet Cardiovasc Diagn 33:39–45; discussion 46, 1994.

135. Alfonso F, Rodriguez P, Phillips P, et al: Clinical and angiographic implications of coronary stenting in thrombus-containing lesions. J Am Coll Cardiol 29:725–733, 1997.

136. Sawada Y, Nokasa H, Kimura T, Nobuyoshi M: Intial and six months outcome of Palmaz-Schatz stent implantation: STRESS/BENENTENT equivalent vs. non-equivalent lesions. J Am Coll Cardiol 27:252A, 1996.

137. Kuntz RE, Gibson CM, Nobuyoshi M, Baim DS: Generalized model of restenosis after conventional balloon angioplasty, stenting and directional atherectomy. J Am Coll Cardiol 21:15–25, 1993.
138. Pepine CJ, Holmes DR Jr: Coronary artery stents. American College of Cardiology. J Am Coll Cardiol 28:782–794, 1996.
139. Piana RN, Ahmed WH, Chaitman B, Ganz P, et al: Effect of transient abrupt vessel closure during otherwise successful angioplasty for unstable angina on clinical outcome at six months. Hirulog Angioplasty Study Investigators [see comments]. J Am Coll Cardiol 33:73–78, 1999.
140. Mak KH, Belli G, Ellis SG, Moliterno DJ: Subacute stent thrombosis: Evolving issues and current concepts. J Am Coll Cardiol 27:494–503, 1996.
141. Schuhlen H, Kastrati A, Dirschinger J, et al: Intracoronary stenting and risk for major adverse cardiac events during the first month. Circulation 98:104–111, 1998.
142. Rodriguez AE, Bernardi VH, Ayala FP, et al: Optimal coronary balloon angioplasty vs. stent: Angiographic long term follow-up results of a randomized trial. Circulation 96:I-593, 1997.
143. Marzocchi A, Ortolani P, Piovaccari G, et al: Long-term follow-up of stent implantation versus stent-like angioplasty in unstable angina. Cardiologia 44:261–268, 1999.
144. Chauhan A, Vu E, Ricci DR, et al: Multiple coronary stenting in unstable angina: Early and late clinical outcomes. Cathet Cardiovasc Diagn 43:11–16, 1998.
145. Clarkson PB, Halim M, Ray KK, et al: Coronary artery stenting in unstable angina pectoris: A comparison with stable angina pectoris. Heart 81:393–397, 1999.
146. De Benedictis M, Scrocca I, Borrione M, et al: Coronary stenting in unstable angina: Angiographic and clinical implications. G Ital Cardiol 28:1099–1105, 1998.
147. Madan M, Marquis JF, de May MR, et al: Coronary stenting in unstable angina: Early and late clinical outcomes. Can J Cardiol 14:1109–1114, 1998.
148. Marzocchi A, Ortolani P, Piovaccari G, et al: Coronary stenting for unstable angina: Predictors of 30-day and long-term clinical outcome. Coron Artery Dis 10:81–88, 1999.
149. Malosky SA, Hirshfeld J Jr, Herrmann HC: Comparison of results of intracoronary stenting in patients with unstable vs. stable angina. Cathet Cardiovasc Diagn 31:95–101, 1994.
150. Shimada K, Kawarabayashi T, Komatsu R, et al: Efficacy and safety of early coronary stenting for unstable angina. Cathet Cardiovasc Diagn 43:381–385, 1998.
151. EPISTENT Investigators: Randomised placebo-controlled and balloon-angioplasty-controlled trial to assess safety of coronary stenting with use of platelet glycoprotein- IIb/IIIa blockade. The EPISTENT Investigators. Evaluation of Platelet IIb/IIIa Inhibitor for Stenting. Lancet 352:87–92, 1998.
152. White CJ, Ramee SR, Collins TJ, et al: Percutaneous angioscopy of saphenous vein coronary bypass grafts. J Am Coll Cardiol 21:1181–1185, 1993.
153. Reeves F, Bonan R, Cote G, et al: Long-term angiographic follow-up after angioplasty of venous coronary bypass grafts. Am Heart J 122:620–627, 1991.
154. de Feyter PJ, van Suylen RJ, de Jaegere PP, et al: Balloon angioplasty for the treatment of lesions in saphenous vein bypass grafts. J Am Coll Cardiol 21:1539–1549, 1993.
155. Savage MP, Douglas JS Jr, Fischman DL, et al: Stent placement compared with balloon angioplasty for obstructed coronary bypass grafts. Saphenous Vein De Novo Trial Investigators. N Engl J Med 337:740–747, 1997.
156. Holmes DR Jr, Berger PB: Percutaneous revascularization of occluded vein grafts: Is it still a temptation to be resisted? [editorial; comment]. Circulation 99:8–11, 1999.
157. Holmes DR Jr, Topol EJ, Califf RM, et al: A multicenter, randomized trial of coronary angioplasty versus directional atherectomy for patients with saphenous vein bypass graft lesions. CAVEAT-II Investigators. Circulation 91:1966–1974, 1995.
158. Safian RD, Grines CL, May MA, et al: Clinical and angiographic results of transluminal extraction coronary atherectomy in saphenous vein bypass grafts. Circulation 89:302–312, 1994.
159. Carlino M, De Gregorio J, Di Mario C, et al: Prevention of distal embolization during saphenous vein graft lesion angioplasty: Experience with a new temporary occlusion and aspiration system. Circulation 99:3221–3223, 1999.
160. Lange RA, Hillis LD: Use and overuse of angiography and revascularization for acute coronary syndromes [editorial; comment]. N Engl J Med 338:1838–1839, 1998.
161. Topol EJ: What role for catheter laboratories in unstable angina? [comment]. Lancet 352:500–501, 1998.
162. FRISC II Investigators: Invasive compared with non-invasive treatment in unstable coronary-artery disease: FRISC II prospective randomised multicentre study. FRagmin and Fast Revascularisation during InStability in Coronary artery disease Investigators. Lancet 354:708–715, 1999.

163. Williams DO, Braunwald E, Knatterud G, et al: One-year results of the Thrombolysis in Myocardial Infarction investigation (TIMI) Phase II Trial. Circulation 85:533–542, 1992.

164. Lagerqvist B, Diderholm E, Lindahl B, et al: An early invasive treatment strategy reduces cardiac events regardless of troponin levels in unstable coronary artery (UCAD) with and without troponin-elevation: A FRISC II substudy. Circulation 100:I-497, 1999.

165. Bar FW, Ophnis TJ, Frederiks J, et al: Rescue PTCA following failed thrombolysis and primary PTCA: A retrospective study of angiographic and clinical outcome. J Thromb Thrombol 4:281–288, 1997.

166. Beauchamp GD, Vacek JL, Robuck W: Management comparison for acute myocardial infarction: direct angioplasty versus sequential thrombolysis-angioplasty. Am Heart J 120:237–242, 1990.

167. CORAMI Study Group: Outcome of attempted rescue coronary angioplasty after failed thrombolysis for acute myocardial infarction. The CORAMI Study Group. Cohort of Rescue Angioplasty in Myocardial Infarction. Am J Cardiol 74:172–174, 1994.

168. Abbottsmith CW, Topol EJ, George BS, et al: Fate of patients with acute myocardial infarction with patency of the infarct-related vessel achieved with successful thrombolysis versus rescue angioplasty. J Am Coll Cardiol 16:770–778, 1990.

169. Ross AM, Lundergan CF, Rohrbeck SC, et al: Rescue angioplasty after failed thrombolysis: Technical and clinical outcomes in a large thrombolysis trial. GUSTO-1 Angiographic Investigators. Global Utilization of Streptokinase and Tissue Plasminogen Activator for Occluded Coronary Arteries. J Am Coll Cardiol 31:1511–1517, 1998.

170. GUSTO Angiographic Investigators: The effects of tissue plasminogen activator, streptokinase, or both on coronary artery patency, ventricular function, and survival after acute myocardial infarction. N Engl J Med 329:1615–1622, 1993.

171. Gibson CM, Cannon CP, Greene RM, et al: Rescue angioplasty in the thrombolysis in myocardial infarction (TIMI) 4 trial. Am J Cardiol 80:21–26, 1997.

172. Ellis SG, da Silva ER, Heyndrickx G, et al: Randomized comparison of rescue angioplasty with conservative management of patients with early failure of thrombolysis for acute anterior myocardial infarction. Circulation 90:2280–2284, 1994.

173. Miller JM, Smalling R, Ohman EM, et al: Effectiveness of early coronary angioplasty and abciximab for failed thrombolysis (reteplase or alteplase) during acute myocardial infarction (results from the GUSTO-III trial). Global Use of Strategies To Open occluded coronary arteries. Am J Cardiol 84:779–784, 1999.

174. Califf RM, O'Neil W, Stack RS, et al: Failure of simple clinical measurements to predict perfusion status after intravenous thrombolysis. Ann Intern Med 108:658–662, 1988.

175. Reiner JS, Lundergan CF, van den Brand M, et al: Early angiography cannot predict postthrombolytic coronary reocclusion: Observations from the GUSTO angiographic study. Global Utilization of Streptokinase and t-PA for Occluded Coronary Arteries. J Am Coll Cardiol 24:1439–1444, 1994.

176. Satler LF, Pallas RS, Bond OB, et al: Assessment of residual coronary arterial stenosis after thrombolytic therapy during acute myocardial infarction. Am J Cardiol 59:1231–1233, 1987.

177. TIMI Research Group: Immediate vs delayed catheterization and angioplasty following thrombolytic therapy for acute myocardial infarction. TIMI II A results. The TIMI Research Group. JAMA 260:2849–2858, 1988.

178. Topol EJ, Califf RM, George BS, et al: A randomized trial of immediate versus delayed elective angioplasty after intravenous tissue plasminogen activator in acute myocardial infarction. N Engl J Med 317:581–588, 1987.

179. Simoons ML, Arnold AE, Betriu A, et al: Thrombolysis with tissue plasminogen activator in acute myocardial infarction: No additional benefit from immediate percutaneous coronary angioplasty. Lancet 1:197–203, 1988.

180. O'Neill WW: The evolution of primary PTCA therapy of acute myocardial infarction: A personal perspective. J Invas Cardiol 7:F2–F11, 1995.

181. Ryan TJ, Antman EM, Brooks NH, et al: 1999 update: ACC/AHA Guidelines for the Management of Patients with Acute Myocardial Infarction: Executive Summary and Recommendations: A report of the American College of Cardiology/American Heart Association Task Force on Practice Guidelines (Committee on Management of Acute Myocardial Infarction). Circulation 100:1016–1030, 1999.

182. Madsen JK, Grande P, Saunamaki K, et al: Danish multicenter randomized study of invasive versus conservative treatment in patients with inducible ischemia after thrombolysis in acute myocardial infarction (DANAMI). DANish trial in Acute Myocardial Infarction. Circulation 96:748–755, 1997.

183. Pilote L, Miller DP, Califf RM, et al: Determinants of the use of coronary angiography and revascularization after thrombolysis for acute myocardial infarction. N Engl J Med 335:1198–1205, 1996.

184. TIMI Study Group: Comparison of invasive and conservative strategies after treatment with intravenous tissue plasminogen activator in acute myocardial infarction: Results of the thrombolysis in myocardial infarction (TIMI) phase II trial. N Engl J Med 320:618–627, 1989.
185. SWIFT (Should We Intervene Following Thrombolysis?) Trial Study Group: SWIFT trial of delayed elective intervention v conservative treatment after thrombolysis with anistreplase in acute myocardial infarction. BMJ 302:555–560, 1991.
186. Barbash GI, Roth A, Hod H, et al: Randomized controlled trial of late in-hospital angiography and angioplasty versus conservative management after treatment with recombinant tissue-type plasminogen activator in acute myocardial infarction. Am J Cardiol 66:538–545, 1990.
187. Ellis SG, Mooney MR, George BS, et al: Randomized trial of late elective angioplasty versus conservative management for patients with residual stenoses after thrombolytic treatment of myocardial infarction. Treatment of Post-Thrombolytic Stenoses (TOPS) Study Group. Circulation 86:1400–1406, 1992.
188. Rentrop KP, Blanke H, Karsch KR, et al: Acute myocardial infarction: intracoronary application of nitroglycerin and streptokinase. Clin Cardiol 2:354–363, 1979.
189. Health and Public Policy Committee ACoP: Thrombolysis for evolving myocardial infarction. Ann Intern Med 103:463–469, 1985.
190. Fibrinolytic Therapy Trialists' (FTT) Collaborative Group: Indications for fibrinolytic therapy in suspected acute myocardial infarction: Collaborative overview of early mortality and major morbidity results from all randomised trials of more than 1000 patients. Lancet 343:311–322, 1994.
191. GUSTO Investigators: An international randomized trial comparing four thrombolytic strategies for acute myocardial infarction. N Engl J Med 329:673–682, 1993.
192. Simoons ML, Maggioni AP, Knatterud G, et al: Individual risk assessment for intracranial haemorrhage during thrombolytic therapy. Lancet 342:1523–1528, 1993.
193. Hartzler GO, Rutherford BD, McConahay DR, et al: Percutaneous transluminal coronary angioplasty with and without thrombolytic therapy for treatment of acute myocardial infarction. Am Heart J 106:965–973, 1983.
194. Eckman MH, Wong JB, Salem DN, Pauker SG: Direct angioplasty for acute myocardial infarction: A review of outcomes in clinical subsets. Ann Intern Med 117:667–676, 1992.
195. O'Keefe JH Jr, Bailey WL, Rutherford BD, Hartzler GO: Primary angioplasty for acute myocardial infarction in 1,000 consecutive patients: Results in an unselected population and high-risk subgroups. Am J Cardiol 72:107G–115G, 1993.
196. O'Neill WW, Brodie BR, Ivanhoe R, et al: Primary coronary angioplasty for acute myocardial infarction (the Primary Angioplasty Registry). Am J Cardiol 73:627–634, 1994.
197. O'Neill W, Timmis GC, Bourdillon PD, et al: A prospective randomized clinical trial of intracoronary streptokinase versus coronary angioplasty for acute myocardial infarction. N Engl J Med 314:812–818, 1986.
198. Grines CL, Browne KF, Marco J, et al: A comparison of immediate angioplasty with thrombolytic therapy for acute myocardial infarction. The Primary Angioplasty in Myocardial Infarction Study Group. N Engl J Med 328:673–679, 1993.
199. Gibbons RJ, Holmes DR, Reeder GS, et al: Immediate angioplasty compared with the administration of a thrombolytic agent followed by conservative treatment for myocardial infarction. The Mayo Coronary Care Unit and Catheterization Laboratory Groups. N Engl J Med 328:685–691, 1993.
200. Zijlstra F, de Boer MJ, Hoorntje JC, et al: A comparison of immediate coronary angioplasty with intravenous streptokinase in acute myocardial infarction. N Engl J Med 328:680–684, 1993.
201. GUSTO IIb Angioplasty Substudy Investigators: A clinical trial comparing primary coronary angioplasty with tissue plasminogen activator for acute myocardial infarction. The Global Use of Strategies to Open Occluded Coronary Arteries in Acute Coronary Syndromes (GUSTO IIb) Angioplasty Substudy Investigators. N Engl J Med 336:1621–1628, 1997.
202. Weaver WD, Simes RJ, Betriu A, et al: Comparison of primary coronary angioplasty and intravenous thrombolytic therapy for acute myocardial infarction: A quantitative review. JAMA 278:2093–2098, 1997.
203. DeWood MA: Direct PTCA vs. intravenous t-Pa in acute myocardial infarction: Results from a prospective randomized trial. In The Thrombolysis and Interventional Therapy in Acute Myocardial Infarction Symposium VI. Washington, DC, George Washington University, 1990, pp 28–29.
204. Zijlstra F, Beukema WP, van't Hof AW, et al: Randomized comparison of primary coronary angioplasty with thrombolytic therapy in low risk patients with acute myocardial infarction. J Am Coll Cardiol 29:908–912, 1997.

205. Ribeiro EE, Silva LA, Carneiro R, et al: Randomized trial of direct coronary angioplasty versus intravenous streptokinase in acute myocardial infarction. J Am Coll Cardiol 22:376–380, 1993.

206. Ribichini F, Steffiano G, Dellavalle A, et al: Pimary angioplasty versus thrombolysis in inferior acute myocardial infarction with anterior ST-segment depression: A single center randomized study. J Am Coll Cardiol 27:221A, 1996.

207. Grinfeld L, Berrocal D, Belardi J, et al: Fibinolytics vs. primary angioplasty in acute myocardial infarction (FAP). J Am Coll Cardiol 27:222A, 1996.

208. Garcia E, Elizaga J, Soriano J, et al: Primary angioplasty versus thrombolysis with t-Pa in the anterior myocardial infarction. J Am Coll Cardiol 29:389A, 1997.

209. Yusuf S, Pogue J: Primary angioplasty compared with thrombolytic therapy for acute myocardial infarction [editorial; comment]. JAMA 278:2110–2111, 1997.

210. Ryan TJ, Ryan TJ Jr, Jacobs AK: Primary PTCA versus thrombolytic therapy: An evidence-based summary. Am Heart J 138:96–104, 1999.

211. Every NR, Parsons LS, Hlatky M, et al: A comparison of thrombolytic therapy with primary coronary angioplasty for acute myocardial infarction. Myocardial Infarction Triage and Intervention Investigators. N Engl J Med 335:1253–1260, 1996.

212. Tiefenbrunn AJ, Chandra NC, French WJ, et al: Clinical experience with primary percutaneous transluminal coronary angioplasty compared with alteplase (recombinant tissue-type plasminogen activator) in patients with acute myocardial infarction: A report from the Second National Registry of Myocardial Infarction (NRMI- 2). J Am Coll Cardiol 31:1240–1245, 1998.

213. Rogers WJ, Dean LS, Moore PB, et al: Comparison of primary angioplasty versus thrombolytic therapy for acute myocardial infarction. Alabama Registry of Myocardial Ischemia Investigators. Am J Cardiol 74:111–118, 1994.

214. Danchin N, Vaur L, Genes N, et al: Treatment of acute myocardial infarction by primary coronary angioplasty or intravenous thrombolysis in the "real world": One-year results from a nationwide French survey. Circulation 99:2639–2644, 1999.

215. Zahn R, Schiele R, Gitt AK, et al: Primary angioplasty is superior to intravenous thrombolysis in all subgroups of patients: Results of 9906 patients with acute myocardial infarction. Circulation 99:I-359, 1999.

216. Nunn CM, O'Neill WW, Rothbaum D, et al: Long-term outcome after primary angioplasty: Report from the primary angioplasty in myocardial infarction (PAMI-I) trial. J Am Coll Cardiol 33:640–646, 1999.

217. Zijlstra F, Hoorntje JC, de Boer MJ, et al: Long-term benefit of primary angioplasty as compared with thrombolytic therapy for acute myocardial infarction. N Engl J Med 341:1413–1419, 1999.

218. Berger PB, Ellis SG, Holmes DR Jr, et al: Relationship between delay in performing direct coronary angioplasty and early clinical outcome in patients with acute myocardial infarction: Results from the Global Use of Strategies to Open Occluded Arteries in acute coronary syndromes (GUSTO-IIb) trial. Circulation 100:14–20, 1999.

219. Grines CL, Marsalese DL, Brodie B, et al: Safety and cost-effectiveness of early discharge after primary angioplasty in low risk patients with acute myocardial infarction. PAMI- II Investigators. Primary Angioplasty in Myocardial Infarction. J Am Coll Cardiol 31:967–972, 1998.

220. Antman EM, Giugliano RP, Gibson CM, et al: Abciximab facilitates the rate and extent of thrombolysis: Results of the thrombolysis in myocardial infarction (TIMI) 14 trial. The TIMI 14 Investigators. Circulation 99:2720–2732, 1999.

221. Stone GW, Grines CL, Browne KF, et al: Implications of recurrent ischemia after reperfusion therapy in acute myocardial infarction: A comparison of thrombolytic therapy and primary angioplasty. J Am Coll Cardiol 26:66–72, 1995.

222. O'Neill WW, De Boer MJ, Gibbons RJ, et al: Lessons from the pooled outcome of the PAMI, ZWOLLE, and Mayo Clinic randomized trials of primary angioplasty versus thrombolytic therapy of acute myocardial infarction. J Inv Cardiol 10:4A–10A, 1998.

223. Leung W-H, Lau C-P: Effects of severity of the residual stenosis of the infarct-related coronary artery on left ventricular dilation and function after acute myocardial infarction. J Am Coll Cardiol 20:307–313, 1992.

224. Brodie BR, Grines CL, Ivanhoe R, et al: Six-month clinical and angiographic follow-up after direct angioplasty for acute myocardial infarction. Final results from the Primary Angioplasty Registry. Circulation 90:156–162, 1994.

225. de Boer MJ, Reiber JH, Suryapranata H, et al: Angiographic findings and catheterization laboratory events in patients with primary coronary angioplasty or streptokinase therapy for acute myocardial infarction. Eur Heart J 16:1347–1355, 1995.

226. Miller PF, Brodie BR, Weintraub RA, et al: Emergency coronary angioplasty for acute myocardial infarction. Results from a community hospital. Arch Intern Med 147:1565–1570, 1987.

227. Nakagawa Y, Iwasaki Y, Kimura T, et al: Serial angiographic follow-up after successful direct angioplasty for acute myocardial infarction. Am J Cardiol 78:980–984, 1996.

228. Verheugt FW, Meijer A, Lagrand WK, Van Eenige MJ: Reocclusion: The flip side of coronary thrombolysis. J Am Coll Cardiol 27:766–773, 1996.

229. Grines CL: Aggressive intervention for myocardial infarction: Angioplasty, stents, and intra-aortic balloon pumping. Am J Cardiol 78:29–34, 1996.

230. Brodie BR, Stuckey TD, Hansen CJ, et al: Timing and mechanism of death determined clinically after primary angioplasty for acute myocardial infarction. Am J Cardiol 79:1586–1591, 1997.

231. De Franco AC, Abramowitz B, Krichbaum D, Topol EJ: Substantial (three-fold) benefit of accelerated t-PA over standard thrombolytic therapy in patients with prior bypass surgery and acute MI: Results of the GUSTO Trial. J Am Coll Cardiol 23:345A, 1994.

232. Reiner JS, Lundergan CF, Kopecky SL, et al: Ineffectiveness of thrombolysis for acute MI following vein graft occlusion. Circulation 94:I-570, 1996.

233. Peterson LR, Chandra NC, French WJ, et al: Reperfusion therapy in patients with acute myocardial infarction and prior coronary artery bypass graft surgery (National Registry of Myocardial Infarction-2). Am J Cardiol 84:1287–1291, 1999.

234. Suwaidi JA, Velianou JL, Berger PB, et al: Primary PTCA in patients with acute myocardial infarction and prior coronary artery bypass grafting. J Am Coll Cardiol 35:19A, 2000.

235. Stone GW, Brodie BR, Griffin JJ, et al: Clinical and angiographic outcomes in patients with previous coronary artery bypass graft surgery treated with primary balloon angioplasty for acute myocardial infarction. Second Primary Angioplasty in Myocardial Infarction Trial (PAMI-2) Investigators. J Am Coll Cardiol 35:605–611, 2000.

236. Mattos L, Sousa A, Neto CC, et al: Primary stenting versus balloon PTCA for the treatment of acute vein graft occlusion in myocardial infarction: In-hospital results from the Brazilian Coronary Interventional Registry (CENIC). J Am Coll Cardiol 35:39A, 2000.

237. Stone GW, Grines CL, Browne KF, et al: Outcome of different reperfusion strategies in patients with former contraindications to thrombolytic therapy: A comparison of primary angioplasty and tissue plasminogen activator. Primary Angioplasty in Myocardial Infarction (PAMI) Investigators. Cathet Cardiovasc Diagn 39:333–339, 1996.

238. Cragg DR, Friedman HZ, Bonema JD, et al: Outcome of patients with acute myocardial infarction who are ineligible for thrombolytic therapy. Ann Intern Med 115:173–177, 1991.

239. Himbert D, Juliard JM, Steg PG, et al: Primary coronary angioplasty for acute myocardial infarction with contraindication to thrombolysis. Am J Cardiol 71:377–381, 1993.

240. Bengtson JR, Kaplan AJ, Pieper KS, et al: Prognosis in cardiogenic shock after acute myocardial infarction in the interventional era. J Am Coll Cardiol 20:1482–1489, 1992.

241. Kennedy JW, Gensini GG, Timmis GC, Maynard C: Acute myocardial infarction treated with intracoronary streptokinase: A report of the Society for Cardiac Angiography. Am J Cardiol 55:871–877, 1985.

242. Zidansek A, Blinc A: The influence of transport parameters and enzyme kinetics of the fibrinolytic system on thrombolysis: Mathematical modelling of two idealised cases. Thromb Haemost 65:553–559, 1991.

243. Becker RC: Hemodynamic, mechanical, and metabolic determinants of thrombolytic efficacy: A theoretic framework for assessing the limitations of thrombolysis in patients with cardiogenic shock [editorial]. Am Heart J 125:919–929, 1993.

244. Lane GE, Holmes DR: Aggressive management of cardiogenic shock. In Cannon CP (ed): The Management of Acute Coronary Syndromes. Totowa, NJ, Humana Press, 1999.

245. Gruppo Italiano per lo Studio della Streptochinasi nell'Infarto Miocardico (GISSI): Effectiveness of intravenous thrombolytic treatment in acute myocardial infarction. Lancet 1:397–402, 1986.

246. Hochman JS, Sleeper LA, Webb JG, et al: Early revascularization in acute myocardial infarction complicated by cardiogenic shock. SHOCK Investigators. Should We Emergently Revascularize Occluded Coronaries for Cardiogenic Shock. N Engl J Med 341:625–634, 1999.

247. Sanborn TA, Webb JG, French JK, et al: Final core laboratory angiographic analysis from the randomized SHOCK trial: Relationship of outcome and treatment effect. Circulation 100:I-370, 1999.

248. Webb JG, Sanborn TA, Carere RG, et al: Coronary stenting in the SHOCK trial. Circulation 100:I-87, 1999.

249. Biostatistical Fact Sheet: Older Americans and cardiovascular diseases. American Heart Association, 1998.

250. Berger AK, Schulman KA, Gersh BJ, et al: Primary coronary angioplasty vs thrombolysis for the management of acute myocardial infarction in elderly patients. JAMA 282:341–348, 1999.

251. Lane GE, Holmes J: Primary angioplasty for acute myocardial infarction in the elderly. Coronary Artery Disease. 2000 [in press].
252. de Boer M, Zijilstra F, Liem AL, et al: A randomized comparison of primary angioplasty and thrombolytic therapy in elderly patients with acute myocardial infarction. Circulation 98:I-772, 1998.
253. Zahn R, Schiele R, Hauptmann KE, et al: Longer pre-hospital delays are associated with increasing mortality in patients with acute myocardial infarction treated with intravenous thrombolysis but not in patients treated with primary angioplasty. Circulation 100:I-358, 1999.
254. Weaver WD: Relation of time to treatment on relative effects of primary angioplasty vs. thrombolytic therapy. J Am Coll Cardiol 35:376A, 1999.
255. Cannon CP, Gibson M, Lambrew CT, et al: Relationship of time to treatment and door-to-balloon time to mortality in 27,080 patients with acute myocardial infarction treated with primary angioplasty. Circulation 100:I-360, 1999.
256. Newby LK, Rutsch WR, Califf RM, et al: Time from symptom onset to treatment and outcomes after thrombolytic therapy. GUSTO-1 Investigators. J Am Coll Cardiol 27:1646–1655, 1996.
257. Becker RC, Gore JM, Lambrew C, et al: A composite view of cardiac rupture in the United States National Registry of Myocardial Infarction. J Am Coll Cardiol 27:1321–1326, 1996.
258. Brodie BR, Stuckey TD, Wall TC, et al: Importance of time to reperfusion for 30-day and late survival and recovery of left ventricular function after primary angioplasty for acute myocardial infarction. J Am Coll Cardiol 32:1312–1319, 1998.
259. Cannon CP, Gibson M, Lambrew CT, et al: Higher institutional volume of primary angioplasty is associated with lower mortality in acute myocardial infarction: An analysis of 27,080 patients. Circulation 100:I-809, 1999.
260. Canto JG, Every NR, Magid D, et al: The relationship of primary angioplasty volume and survival among interventional hospitals in the National Registry of Myocardial Infarction. J Am College Cardiol 35:20A, 2000.
261. Grassman ED, Johnson SA, Krone RJ: Predictors of success and major complications for primary percutaneous transluminal coronary angioplasty in acute myocardial infarction: An analysis of the 1990 to 1994 Society for Cardiac Angiography and Interventions registries. J Am Coll Cardiol 30:201–208, 1997.
262. Christian TF, O'Keefe JH, Dewood MA, et al: Intercenter variability in outcome for patients treated with direct coronary angioplasty during acute myocardial infarction. Am Heart J 135:310–317, 1998.
263. Cox DA, Stone GW, Brodie B, et al: Stent PAMI: Are excellent outcomes achieved only by experienced sites? J Am Coll Cardiol 35:363A, 2000.
264. Landau C, Glamann DB, Willard JE, et al: Coronary angioplasty in the patient with acute myocardial infarction. Am J Med 96:536–543, 1994.
265. Wharton TP, McNamara NS, Lew DC, et al: Cardiogenic shock at community hospitals with no surgery on site: Outcomes after primary angioplasty in 101 patients in a multicenter registry. Circulation 98:I-307, 1998.
266. Wharton TP Jr, McNamara NS, Fedele FA, et al: Primary angioplasty for the treatment of acute myocardial infarction: Experience at two community hospitals without cardiac surgery. J Am Coll Cardiol 33:1257–1265, 1999.
267. Vermeer F, Oude Ophuis AJ, vd Berg EJ, et al: Prospective randomised comparison between thrombolysis, rescue PTCA, and primary PTCA in patients with extensive myocardial infarction admitted to a hospital without PTCA facilities: A safety and feasibility study. Heart 82:426–431, 1999.
268. Straumann E, Yoon S, Naegeli B, et al: Hospital transfer for primary coronary angioplasty in high risk patients with acute myocardial infarction. Heart 82:415–419, 1999.
269. Grines CL, Balestrini C, Westerhausen DR, et al: A randomized trial of thrombolysis vs. transfer for primary PTCA in high risk AMI patients: Results of the AIR PAMI trial. J Am Coll Cardiol 35:376A, 2000.
270. Uchida Y, Hasegawa K, Kawamura K, Shibuya I: Angioscopic observation of the coronary luminal changes induced by percutaneous transluminal coronary angioplasty. Am Heart J 117:769–776, 1989.
271. Coller BS: GPIIb/IIIa antagonists: Pathophysiologic and therapeutic insights from studies of c7E3 Fab. Thromb Haemost 78:730–735, 1997.
272. Topol EJ: Toward a new frontier in myocardial reperfusion therapy: Emerging platelet preeminence. Circulation 97:211–218, 1998.
273. Lefkovits J, Ivanhoe RJ, Califf RM, et al: Effects of platelet glycoprotein IIb/IIIa receptor blockade by a chimeric monoclonal antibody (abciximab) on acute and six-month outcomes after percutaneous transluminal coronary angioplasty for acute myocardial infarction. EPIC investigators. Am J Cardiol 77:1045–1051, 1996.

274. Brener SJ, Barr LA, Burchenal JE, et al: Randomized, placebo-controlled trial of platelet glyco-protein IIb/IIIa blockade with primary angioplasty for acute myocardial infarction. ReoPro and Primary PTCA Organization and Randomized Trial (RAPPORT) Investigators. Circulation 98:734–741, 1998.

275. Neumann FJ, Blasini R, Schmitt C, et al: Effect of glycoprotein IIb/IIIa receptor blockade on recovery of coronary flow and left ventricular function after the placement of coronary-artery stents in acute myocardial infarction. Circulation 98:2695–2701, 1998.

276. Montalescot G, Barragan P, Wittenberg O, et al: Abciximab associated with primary angio-plasty and stenting in acute myocardial infarction: The ADMIRAL study, 30-day final results. Circulation 100:I-87, 1999.

277. Cannon AD, Roubin GS, Macander PJ: Intracoronary stenting as an adjunct to angioplasty in acute myocardial infarction. J Invas Cardiol 3:255–258, 1991.

278. Steffenino G, Dellavalle A, Ribichini F, Uslenghi E: Coronary stenting after unsuccessful emer-gency angioplasty in acute myocardial infarction: Results in a series of consecutive patients. Am Heart J 132:1115–1118, 1996.

279. Stone GW, Marsalese D, Brodie BR, et al: A prospective, randomized evaluation of prophylac-tic intraaortic balloon counterpulsation in high risk patients with acute myocardial infarction treated with primary angioplasty. Second Primary Angioplasty in Myocardial Infarction (PAMI-II) Trial Investigators. J Am Coll Cardiol 29:1459–1467, 1997.

280. Stone GW, Brodie BR, Griffin JJ, et al: Prospective, multicenter study of the safety and feasibil-ity of primary stenting in acute myocardial infarction: In-hospital and 30-day results of the PAMI stent pilot trial. Primary Angioplasty in Myocardial Infarction Stent Pilot Trial Investigators. J Am Coll Cardiol 31:23–30, 1998.

281. Suryapranata H, van't Hof AW, Hoorntje JC, et al: Randomized comparison of coronary stent-ing with balloon angioplasty in selected patients with acute myocardial infarction. Circulation 97:2502–2505, 1998.

282. Antoniucci D, Santoro GM, Bolognese L, et al: A clinical trial comparing primary stenting of the infarct-related artery with optimal primary angioplasty for acute myocardial infarction: Results from the Florence Randomized Elective Stenting in Acute Coronary Occlusions (FRESCO) trial. J Am Coll Cardiol 31:1234–1239, 1998.

283. Grines CL, Cox DA, Stone GW, et al: Coronary angioplasty with or without stent implantation for acute myocardial infarction. Stent Primary Angioplasty in Myocardial Infarction Study Group. N Engl J Med 341:1949–1956, 1999.

284. Maillard L, Hamon M, Monassier J, Raynaud P: STENTIM 2: Six months angiographic results. Elective Witkor stent implantation in acute myocardial infarction compared with balloon an-gioplasty. Circulation 98:1–21, 1998.

285. Saito S, Hosokawa G, Tanaka S, Nakamura S: Primary stent implantation is superior to bal-loon angioplasty in acute myocardial infarction: Final results of the primary angioplasty versus stent implantation in acute myocardial infarction (PASTA) trial. PASTA Trial Investigators. Catheter Cardiovasc Interv 48:262–268, 1999.

286. Rodriguez A, Bernardi V, Fernandez M, et al: In-hospital and late results of coronary stents versus conventional balloon angioplasty in acute myocardial infarction (GRAMI trial). Gianturco-Roubin in Acute Myocardial Infarction. Am J Cardiol 81:1286–1291, 1998.

287. Grines CL, Cox DA, Stone GW, et al: Stent PAMI: 12 month results and predictors of mortality. J Am Coll Cardiol 35:402A, 2000.

288. Stone GW: CADILLAC (Controlled Abciximab and Device Investigation to Lower Late Angioplasty Complications) Trial. Presented at the American Heart Association 72nd Annual Scientific Sessions, Atlanta, 1999.

289. Kurisu S, Sato H, Tateishi H, et al: Usefulness of directional coronary atherectomy in patients with acute anterior myocardial infarction. Am J Cardiol 79:1392–1394, 1997.

290. Saito S, Kim K, Hosokawa G, et al: Short- and long-term clinical effects of primary directional coronary atherectomy for acute myocardial infarction [see comments]. Cathet Cardiovasc Diagn 39:157–165, 1996.

291. Kaplan BM, Larkin T, Safian RD, et al: Prospective study of extraction atherectomy in patients with acute myocardial infarction. Am J Cardiol 78:383–388, 1996.

292. Hamm CW, Steffen W, Terres W, et al: Intravascular therapeutic ultrasound thrombolysis in acute myocardial infarctions. Am J Cardiol 80:200–204, 1997.

293. Rosenschein H, Hertz I, Tenebaum-Koren E, et al: Coronary ultrasound thrombolysis in acute myocardial infarction: Results from the acute study. J Am Coll Cardiol 31:192A, 1998.

294. Nakagawa Y, Matsuo S, Kimura T, et al: Thrombectomy with AngioJet catheter in native coro-nary arteries for patients with acute or recent myocardial infarction. Am J Cardiol 83:994–999, 1999.

295. Silva JA, Saucedo JF, Lanoue AS, et al: Rheolytic thrombectomy using the POSSIS angiojet catheter in patients with acute myocardial infarction presenting within 8 hours of symptom onset. Circulation 98:I-147, 1998.

296. Dauerman HL, Pinto DS, Ho KK, et al: Outcome of patients with acute myocardial infarction who are ineligible for primary angioplasty trials. Catheter Cardiovasc Interv 49:237–243, 2000.

297. Ross AM, Coyne KS, Reiner JS, et al: A randomized trial comparing primary angioplasty with a strategy of short-acting thrombolysis and immediate planned rescue angioplasty in acute myocardial infarction: The PACT trial. PACT investigators. Plasminogen-activator Angioplasty Compatibility Trial. J Am Coll Cardiol 34:1954–1962, 1999.

298. Ohman EM, Lincoff AM, Bode C, et al: Enhanced early reperfusion at 60 minutes with low-dose reteplase combined with full-dose abciximab in acute myocardial infarction: Preliminary results from the GUSTO-4 pilot (SPEED) dose-ranging trial. Circulation 98:I-504, 1998.

299. Gillum RF: Sudden coronary death in the United States: 1980–1985. Circulation 79:756–765, 1989.

300. Bayes de Luna A, Coumel P, Leclercq JF: Ambulatory sudden cardiac death: Mechanisms of production of fatal arrhythmia on the basis of data from 157 cases. Am Heart J 117:151–159, 1989.

301. Liberthson RR, Nagel EL, Hirschman JC, et al: Pathophysiologic observations in prehospital ventricular fibrillation and sudden cardiac death. Circulation 49:790–798, 1974.

302. Weaver WD, Lorch GS, Alvarez HA, Cobb LA: Angiographic findigs and prognostic indicators in patients resuscitated from sudden cardiac death. Circulation 54:895–900, 1976.

303. Bigger JT Jr, Fleiss JL, Kleiger R, et al: The relationships among ventricular arrhythmias, left ventricular dysfunction, and mortality in the 2 years after myocardial infarction. Circulation 69:250–258, 1984.

304. Farb A, Tang AL, Burke AP, et al: Sudden coronary death: Frequency of active coronary lesions, inactive coronary lesions, and myocardial infarction. Circulation 92:1701–1709, 1995.

305. Roy D, Waxman HL, Kienzle MG, et al: Clinical characteristics and long-term follow-up in 119 survivors of cardiac arrest: Relation to inducibility at electrophysiologic testing. Am J Cardiol 52:969–974, 1983.

306. Marcus FI, Cobb LA, Edwards JE, et al: Mechanism of death and prevalence of myocardial ischemic symptoms in the terminal event after acute myocardial infarction. Am J Cardiol 61:8–15, 1988.

307. Amsterdam EA: Relation of silent myocardial ischemia to ventricular arrhythmias and sudden death. Am J Cardiol 62:241–271, 1988.

308. Janse MJ, Wit AL: Electrophysiological mechanisms of ventricular arrhythmias resulting from myocardial ischemia and infarction. Physiol Rev 69:1049–1169, 1989.

309. Lazzara R, Scherlag BJ: Generation of arrhythmias in myocardial ischemia and infarction. Am J Cardiol 61:20A–26A, 1988.

310. Antman EM, Berlin JA: Declining incidence of ventricular fibrillation in myocardial infarction: Implications for the prophylactic use of lidocaine. Circulation 86:764–773, 1992.

311. Kahn JK, Glazier S, Swor R, et al: Primary coronary angioplasty for acute myocardial infarction complicated by out-of-hospital cardiac arrest. Am J Cardiol 75:1069–1070, 1995.

312. Bhaskaran A, Seth A, Kumar A, et al: Coronary angioplasty for the control of intractable ventricular arrhythmia. Clin Cardiol 18:480–483, 1995.

313. Fitzpatrick AP, Dawkins K, Conway N: Emergency percutaneous transluminal coronary angioplasty for intractable ventricular arrhythmias associated with acute anterior myocardial infarction. Br Heart J 69:453–454, 1993.

314. Goldberg RJ: Declining out-of-hospital sudden coronary death rates: Additional pieces of the epidemiologic puzzle. Circulation 79:1369–1373, 1989.

315. Hohnloser SH, Franck P, Klingenheben T, et al: Open infarct artery, late potentials, and other prognostic factors in patients after acute myocardial infarction in the thrombolytic era. A prospective trial. Circulation 90:1747–1756, 1994.

316. Sager PT, Perlmutter RA, Rosenfeld LE, et al: Electrophysiologic effects of thrombolytic therapy in patients with a transmural anterior myocardial infarction complicated by left ventricular aneurysm formation. J Am Coll Cardiol 12:19–24, 1988.

317. Kersschot IE, Brugada P, Ramentol M, et al: Effects of early reperfusion in acute myocardial infarction on arrhythmias induced by programmed stimulation: A prospective, randomized study. J Am Coll Cardiol 7:1234–1242, 1986.

318. el-Sherif N: Electrophysiologic basis of ventricular late potentials. Prog Cardiovasc Dis 35:417–427, 1993.

319. Vatterott PJ, Hammill SC, Bailey KR, et al: Late potentials on signal-averaged electrocardiograms and patency of the infarct-related artery in survivors of acute myocardial infarction. J Am Coll Cardiol 17:330–337, 1991.

320. Karam C, Golmard J, Steg PG: Decreased prevalence of late potentials with mechanical versus thrombolysis-induced reperfusion in acute myocardial infarction. J Am Coll Cardiol 27:1343–1348, 1996.

321. Boehrer JD, Glamann DB, Lange RA, et al: Effect of coronary angioplasty on late potentials one to two weeks after acute myocardial infarction. Am J Cardiol 70:1515–1519, 1992.

322. Greene HL: Sudden arrhythmic cardiac death—mechanisms, resuscitation and classification: The Seattle perspective. Am J Cardiol 65:4B–12B, 1990.

323. Davies MJ, Thomas A: Thrombosis and acute coronary-artery lesions in sudden cardiac ischemic death. N Engl J Med 310:1137–1140, 1984.

324. Falk E: Unstable angina with fatal outcome: Dynamic coronary thrombosis leading to infarction and/or sudden death. Autopsy evidence of recurrent mural thrombosis with peripheral embolization culminating in total vascular occlusion. Circulation 71:699–708, 1985.

325. Spaulding CM, Joly LM, Rosenberg A, et al: Immediate coronary angiography in survivors of out-of-hospital cardiac arrest. N Engl J Med 336:1629–1633, 1997.

326. Holmes DR Jr, Davis KB, Mock MB, et al: The effect of medical and surgical treatment on subsequent sudden cardiac death in patients with coronary artery disease: A report from the Coronary Artery Surgery Study. Circulation 73:1254–1263, 1986.

327. Varnauskas E: Survival, myocardial infarction, and employment status in a prospective randomized study of coronary bypass surgery. Circulation 72:V90–V101, 1985.

328. Every NR, Fahrenbruch CE, Hallstrom AP, et al: Influence of coronary bypass surgery on subsequent outcome of patients resuscitated from out of hospital cardiac arrest. J Am Coll Cardiol 19:1435–1439, 1992.

329. Kelly P, Ruskin JN, Vlahakes GJ, et al: Surgical coronary revascularization in survivors of prehospital cardiac arrest: Its effect on inducible ventricular arrhythmias and long-term survival [see comments]. J Am Coll Cardiol 15:267–273, 1990.

330. Wiesfeld AC, Crijns HJ, Hillege HL, et al: The clinical significance of coronary anatomy in post-infarct patients with late sustained ventricular tachycardia or ventricular fibrillation. Eur Heart J 16:818–824, 1995.

331. O'Rourke RA: Role of myocardial revascularization in sudden cardiac death. Circulation 85:I112–117, 1992.

332. Molajo AO, Summers GD, Bennett DH: Effect of percutaneous transluminal coronary angioplasty on arrhythmias complicating angina. Br Heart J 54:375–377, 1985.

333. Hilton TC, Aguirre F, Greenwalt T, et al: Successful treatment of complex ventricular arrhythmias with percutaneous transluminal coronary angioplasty. Am Heart J 122:230–231, 1991.

Surgical Intervention for Acute Coronary Syndromes

J. MICHAEL TUCHEK, DO

BRADFORD BLAKEMAN, MD

Heart disease currently affects 1 in 4 Americans. Atherosclerosis of the coronary arteries and myocardial infarction (MI) remain the most common serious forms of heart disease. When surgeons approach the acute occlusion of an artery in the periphery, reestablishing blood flow by removal of the clot or bypassing a critical stenosis usually results in the restoration of oxygenated blood to the ischemic tissue. If the procedure is done early enough, complete recovery of the ischemic tissue can be expected. This "mechanistic" view is not as applicable when it comes to the surgical management of an acute MI.

Our understanding of the cause of acute MI has a long and controversial history. In 1912, Herrick was the first to describe "coronary thrombosis," which is now commonly called an acute MI.[1] He speculated that coronary thrombosis results in acute MI. Coronary angiography finally resolved the debate as to whether coronary thrombosis was the result or cause of MI. We now know that unstable angina and MIs result from plaque rupture and thrombus formation,[2] involving the acute deposition of platelet thrombi, plaque hemorrhage, arterial spasm, and release of arterial wall metabolites, all of which result in acute myocardial ischemia downstream to the obstruction. Angiographic studies have clearly shown that the degree of the coronary obstruction determines the various clinical syndromes, including angina, MI, infarct-related arrhythmias, and sudden death. However, the extent of the anatomic obstruction does not necessarily correlate with the severity of the clinical symptoms. If blockage does occur, the myocardium must continue to function; otherwise cardiogenic shock or death may occur. Once the patient is in cardiogenic shock, the in-hospital mortality rate can approach 80% with medical treatment.[3] Until the blockage is removed, opened, or bypassed, the heart muscle is clearly in jeopardy.

As a result of the dismal results of medical therapy for acute MI and cardiogenic shock, in the early 1970s surgeons began looking at the results of coronary revascularization in the setting of acute MI. Berg and colleagues from Spokane, Washington published one of the first papers advocating the use of coronary artery bypass grafting (CABG) for the treatment of acute MI. Before the advent of thrombolytic therapy and angioplasty, Berg showed the benefits of surgical intervention by decreasing mortality rates significantly when revascularization was accomplished in < 6 hours. In the 1980s, first intracoronary and then intravenous treatment with thrombolytics was shown to be effective in the setting of acute MI. Shortly thereafter, angioplasty was used successfully in the setting of an acute MI. In the 1990s, the use of intracoronary stents has been shown to be of added benefit.

Cardiac surgeons now have a sophisticated armamentarium to treat coronary artery disease, MI, and their sequelae. As a testament to its success, nearly half a million CABG operations are performed yearly in the United States, making it the most commonly performed surgical procedure.

As we were gaining experience in treating acute MIs surgically, advances in cardioplegia techniques and in the use of the heart/lung machine also were showing promise. "Resting" the heart on the heart/lung machine and providing tailored delivery of cardioplegic solutions to the infarct areas led to better recovery of the injured myocardium—a goal that is not possible using either thrombolytic therapy or interventional techniques.

Postinfarct ventricular aneurysms, ischemic mitral insufficiency, ruptured papillary muscle, and infarct-related ventricular septal defects are among the devastating consequences of acute MI. Although surgical intervention is the only appropriate treatment in most cases, the timing and type of surgical procedure are controversial and are covered in other chapters within this book.

The surgeon's role in the treatment of acute MI has changed over the past 25 years; it is hoped that a review of such changes will be enlightening.

Early Research and Acute Myocardial Infarctions

Canine experiments by Tennant and Wiggens,[4] dating back to 1935, showed that temporary occlusion of a coronary artery resulted in localized myocardial dysfunction and that reperfusion of the affected area frequently resulted in complete recovery of the muscle's function. Not until the 1970s did more sophisticated studies elucidate the functional, cellular, and metabolic deficits associated with acute coronary occlusion.

Because the heart is an obligate aerobic organ, its myocardium requires a continuous supply of oxygenated blood to perform well. Even at rest, maximal oxygen extraction takes place; the heart has no ability to increase oxygen extraction significantly if coronary flow is limited. At normothermia, complete coronary occlusion in a canine model shows no ischemic injury if blood flow is completely restored within 20 minutes. However, if ischemic time is longer than 40 minutes, permanent cellular damage occurs despite complete restoration of coronary blood flow.[5]

Acute MI resulting from coronary occlusion causes significant regional depression of cardiac wall motion, build-up of toxic myocardial metabolites, and depletion of intracellular adenosine triphosphate (ATP).[6] When glucose is used during anaerobic metabolism, lactic acid generation increases and ATP sources are diminished. Cardiac myocyte membrane integrity is then compromised, resulting in calcium diffusion and eventually leading to free radical formation. Myocardial cellular edema takes place during the reperfusion phase and significantly alters the biochemical composition of both intracellular and extracellular spaces. Calcium accumulation soon follows. Increased leukocyte activity can then result in increased free radical formation and cellular injury. Anaerobic glycolysis stops, and the overall result is an irreversible myocardial ischemic contractile state.[3,6,8–10] Some of these effects are reversible with early reperfusion.[11,12]

The subendocardium is the most susceptible portion of the heart to decreased coronary blood flow. Thus, transmural infarcts begin in the subendocardium and extend to the subepicardium in a progressive fashion.[13] One avenue of early investigation into limiting MI size was to decrease myocardial oxygen demand to levels equivalent to the diminished oxygen now available as a result of coronary occlusion. Pharmacologic manipulation to increase collateral flow and thus increase oxygen delivery resulted in the use of vasodilating drugs, such as nitroglycerine, with some success.

Clinical investigators recognized the limitations of acute canine studies. Most animal studies looked at single-vessel disease with otherwise normal coronaries and normal myocardial function as opposed to a typical patient with MI, who has a preexisting atherosclerotic process, multiple stenoses of single or multiple vessels with collateral formation from chronic plaque build-up, varying degrees of myocardial hypertrophy, and varying degrees of coronary reperfusion. Therefore, unlike human infarctions, experimentally induced acute infarctions in the canine model led to rapid and extensive necrosis of the affected canine myocardium. Caution must be used in attempting to extrapolate to humans.

The chronicity of coronary atherosclerosis in humans led to Berg's concept of the acute evolving myocardial infarction.[14] A subacute or chronic MI behaves and is treated differently from an acute evolving MI. Clinicians also began classifying MIs as transmural and nontransmural infarcts. Nontransmural infarcts were thought to be related to significant coronary stenoses, whereas transmural infarcts usually were associated with a totally occluded artery. The evolving nature of the ischemic process was somewhat predictable, depending on the degree of stenosis and surrounding coronary anatomy.[15–18] For example, in a heart with multiple areas of coronary atherosclerosis, the acute decrease or complete loss of coronary flow to one portion of the myocardium may result in an acute loss of collateral blood flow to other areas with diseased coronary arteries. With the acute loss of collateral vessels, the other surrounding stenotic coronary arteries cannot compensate for the deficits and myocardial oxygen needs of the nearby tissues. Further ischemic insults may result from the decreased coronary perfusion pressure secondary, in part, to increases in pulmonary artery wedge pressures during the acute phase of myocardial ischemia. The reversibility of these processes and the functional recovery of the myocardium were shown to be possible in the laboratory setting.[11,12,19]

Early Surgical Therapy for Acute Myocardal Infarction

Generally speaking, emergency surgical revascularization for an acute coronary occlusion attempts to protect the uninvolved nonischemic myocardium, to prevent further damage to the ischemic area, to ameliorate reperfusion injury, and to resuscitate both the normal and damaged myocardium.[20] In this setting, cardiac resuscitation involves restoring the lost energy substrates and stabilization of the cellular homeostatic state, which hopefully translates into better myocardial cellular function.

As data were gathered about the reversibility of myocardial ischemia secondary to coronary atherosclerosis, the first real treatment by coronary revascularization was developed by Favaloro et al.[21] Coronary bypass grafting using reversed saphenous veins was the first effective surgical therapy to treat both chronic and acute occlusions of coronary arteries. Favaloro operated on 11 patients in the setting of acute MI within 4–10 hours of onset of symptoms. Four of the 7 patients studied postoperatively had improved left ventricular function after coronary bypass grafting. Favaloro concluded that treating an acute MI with coronary bypass grafting within 6 hours of onset could reverse the effects of acute MI, limit infarct size, and improve MI postoperatively. Pifarre et al. reported a series of 20 patients undergoing emergency coronary artery bypass, 8 of whom were operated in the acute phase of MI. These patients had single-, double-, and triple-vessel disease and underwent surgery within 4–12 hours after onset of acute infarction. In the acute-phase group, one patient underwent surgery 18 days after the initial infarct because of ongoing angina and recurrent hypotension. One patient underwent surgery in cardiogenic shock. The only patient who died suffered cardiac arrest with ventricular fibrillation before opening of the pericardium. An infarctectomy was performed along with a bypass, but the patient died 6 hours postoperatively. The other 7 survivors were followed for 6–12 months, and most were asymptomatic through the follow-up period. Pifarre concluded that early bypass surgery was generally beneficial even in the most unstable patients with MI.[109] Soon afterward, several programs, including Favaloro's, showed that CABG in patients with acute MI can be done with acceptable mortality rates of 5–6%.[22–24]

A landmark article by Berg et al. in 1975 outlined the Spokane experience in treating acute MI with CABG.[14] From 1971 to 1975 the authors operated on a total of 96 patients in a nonrandomized fashion. Patients who presented to the emergency department with persistent chest pain and ST-segment changes were diagnosed with acute evolving MI. Cardiac enzyme elevations were used to distinguish between acute evolving MI and unstable angina. If angiography showed vessel occlusion with target vessel wall motion abnormalities, the patient was taken to the operating room by the cardiac surgeon who was present at the time of the cardiac catheterization. Also included in this study were patients with acute evolving MI after their established 6-hour period from onset of symptoms who still had angina as well as patients with a stuttering infarct hours or days later. A significant percentage of patients in cardiogenic shock were also included. Some patients were excluded from the study, including those with occlusion of small vessels in which little myocardium was affected. In addition, patients who were pain-free, stable, and late into the infarction were not sent for acute angiography. Patients with infarct-related mitral regurgitation, infarct-related ventricular septal defects, ruptured papillary muscles, and myocardial rupture also were not included.

Once in the operating room, patients underwent rapid-sequence intubation with central venous access and placement of arterial lines. No pulmonary line was used. Each patient was placed on bypass and cooled to 25°; crystalloid antegrade cardioplegia with intermittent cross-clamping was used. The infarcted vessel was grafted first, performing both proximal and distal anastomosis. The cross- clamp was then temporarily removed to allow systemic cold blood to perfuse the affected myocardium through the new bypass graft. Once the remaining coronary bypasses were completed, the patient was weaned from cardiopulmonary bypass. A pulmonary catheter usually was placed before transfer to the intensive care unit. In 1981, when percutaneous placement of an intraaortic balloon pump (IABP) became available, IABPs frequently were placed in the catheterization laboratory prior to surgery for patients with large infarctions or cardiogenic shock. In Berg's report of 96 patients, the in-hospital mortality rate was 5.2%, and the 1-year mortality rate was only 6.3%. The authors noted that the same patient population had a 20% mortality rate if treated medically during the same study years.[14]

In 1983, DeWood et al.[25] updated the Spokane experience to 701 patients who underwent surgery within 24 hours of onset of symptoms. In the nontransmural infarct group (261 patients), 82% had double- or triple-vessel coronary artery disease. The overall hospital mortality rate was 3.1%. With single- and double-vessel disease, the mortality rate was 2.1%. With triple-vessel disease, the mortality rate was 4.2%. Long-term survival rates were > 90% at a mean follow-up of over 4 years. In the transmural infarction group (440 patients), the hospital mortality rate was 5.2%. The mortality rate for anterior infarcts was 5.2% and for inferior infarctions 5.1%. The mortality rates for single-, double-, and triple-vessel disease were 2.3%, 4.4%, and 9%, respectively. In patients who were placed on bypass in < 6 hours from onset of symptoms, the mortality rate was 3.8%. However, in patients placed on bypass after 6 hours, the mortality rate jumped to 8%. Not surprisingly, over one-half of the patients who died after CABG for transmural infarction were in cardiogenic shock preoperatively. If the group of patients who were not in shock was considered independently, the mortality rate was only 2.8%, whereas the mortality rate for patients in cardiogenic shock was 28%. During the same study time, DeWood reviewed similar patients with MI who received medical therapy and IABP placement; the mortality rate was 52%.[26]

Because surgical reperfusion demonstrated such beneficial results in the treatment of acute evolving MI, DeWood et al.[27] compared outcomes in conventional medical therapy groups and surgical groups who were historically matched. A total of 387 patients were studied, 200 of whom received medical therapy and 187 received CABG. The mean follow-up was 11.4 years. The mortality rate of the in-hospital medical group was 11.5%, whereas the mortality rate of the in-hospital surgical group was 5.8%. The mortality rate was 2% for early reperfusion and 10.3% for late reperfusion. In the 10-year follow-up, the early surgical reperfusion group had a mortality rate of 17%, the late surgical reperfusion group had a mortality rate of 34%, and the medical group had a mortality of 41%. In patients with inferior wall MI, the overall surgical mortality rate was 30% vs 32% with medical treatment at late follow-up. For patients undergoing early reperfusion, the mortality rate was only 19% (vs. 32% for patients treated medically). In patients with anterior wall MI, the overall surgical mortality rate was 31% vs. 54% for similar patients treated medically. The early surgical reperfusion group had a much lower long-term mortality rate (33%) compared with patients receiving medical therapy (54%). Over the mean follow-up period of 11.4 years, of the 85 patients who were still alive after conventional medical therapy, 35% eventually underwent CABG.

DeWood et al. also found that surgically treated patients had the same rate of recurrent MIs as the medically treated group (25%). However, the mortality rate due to recurrent infarction was significantly lower in the CABG group (17.5%) compared with the medical group (36.6%). The incidence of sudden death in the early surgical reperfusion group was 3% compared with 12% in the late surgical reperfusion group and 17% in the medical group. When overall ejection fractions after an anterior MI were compared, the early and late surgical reperfusion groups had better anterior wall motion than the medically treated group. After an inferior wall MI, only the early surgical reperfusion group had better inferior wall motion than the medically treated group. Even the New York Heart Association (NYHA) classification was better in the early surgical reperfusion group than in the medically treated group.

In DeWood's study, the surgically treated group had better early mortality rates, better late mortality rates, similar recurrent MI rates but with decreased mortality, decreased incidence of sudden death, better NYHA functional classification, and better overall ejection fractions compared with the medically treated group. These differences were even more pronounced across the board when patients undergoing early reperfusion (< 6 hours) were compared with patients undergoing late reperfusion (> 6 hours).

Another landmark article published in 1983 by Phillips et al.[28] examined the Iowa experience with 339 patients who underwent emergency coronary artery intervention in the face of acute evolving MI. In this nonrandomized study, 112 patients received intracoronary streptokinase, 46 patients received intracoronary streptokinase in addition to percutaneous transluminal coronary angioplasty (PTCA), and 181 patients underwent saphenous vein bypass grafting as the primary reperfusion procedure. This study began in 1975 when emergency bypass surgery was the only interventional therapy for acute evolving MI. From 1979 through the end of their study in 1982, thrombolytics and angioplasty became therapeutic options. Of the 181 patients in the surgical revascularization group, 160 were sent directly to surgery from the catheterization lab. The other 21 patients were crossover patients secondary to failure of streptokinase alone (20 patients) or streptokinase plus PTCA (1 patient). Twenty-six of the 181 patients who received surgical revascularization were in cardiogenic shock preoperatively. Two of these patients were in full cardiac arrest preoperatively. In the bypass group, 79% underwent thrombectomy of the infarct vessel before saphenous vein bypass. There were 12 deaths, 4 early and 8 late, in the surgical group, 2 deaths in the streptokinase-only group, and no deaths in the streptokinase plus PTCA group. All 4 early deaths in the primary CABG group (160 patients) were in cardiogenic shock preoperatively. In fact, all deaths in the three groups occurred in patients with cardiogenic shock before intervention.

Unlike other studies, Phillips et al. found no correlation between the time from onset of symptoms to reperfusion and good or bad outcome. The authors intervened from 1 to 36 hours from onset of symptoms with an average interval of 8 hours. In other words, unlike other studies, they found no magic window for the initiation of treatment and successful outcome.

Based on this study, Phillips et al. recommended streptokinase therapy for single coronary involvement. In patients with significant residual coronary stenosis, PTCA was recommended. If PTCA failed, surgical revascularization was recommended. With significant multivessel disease in the face of an acute evolving MI, they recommended emergency surgical revascularization as the primary therapy.[28] This protocol resulted in a 3.5% mortality rate for patients presenting with acute evolving MI at their institution. All deaths occurred in patients who presented in cardiogenic shock; there were no deaths in the 303 patients who were hemodynamically stable.

Unlike DeWoods, Phillips reported that neither extent of coronary disease nor time from onset of symtoms was a predictor of in-hospital risk. Unfortunately, both studies lacked randomization and were criticized at the time. For example, patients with preexisting left ventricular dysfunction, known multivessel disease, or underlying rhythm problems were not necessarily entered into Phillips' study.

Soon after these experiences were published, DeWood reviewed many other studies reporting similar results from around the world. In a summary of 18 centers involving 1098 patients receiving emergency CABG for acute evolving MI, the overall hospital mortality rate was 4.9%.[29]

Thrombolytics, Percutaneous Transluminal Coronary Angioplasty, and Stents: Impact on Surgical Treatment of Myocardial Infarction

About the same time that Phillips and DeWood were studying the results of surgical revascularization for acute MI, Rentrop outlined the use of intracoronary nitroglycerine and streptokinase for successful reperfusion in patients with acute MI secondary to "coronary thrombosis."[30] This report led to a flurry of studies demonstrating the benefits of intracoronary thrombolytics.

In 1983, the Western Washington randomized multicenter study examined the use of intracoronary streptokinase in 250 patients.[31] Compared with medical therapy, the 30-day mortality rate was significantly lower in the streptokinase-treated group. In the same year, the *New England Journal of Medicine* published two randomized studies showing that patients with acute MI who were treated with streptokinase had a lower mortality rate[32,33] and overall improved myocardial function[33] compared with patients treated medically.

Shortly after the above studies showed the benefits of intracoronary streptokinase, the GISSI trial[34] and the ISIS-2[35] collaborative group study demonstrated the benefits of intravenous thrombolysis. The GISSI trial showed a 47% reduction in mortality if intravenous thrombolytics were given within 1 hour of onset of chest pain, a 23% reduction if treatment began within 3 hours, and no benefit if thrombolytics were given after 6 hours. In the Thrombolysis in Myocardial Infarction (TIMI)-1 trial, the postthrombolytic patency of the infarct artery was related to improved overall long-term survival, even though it had little if any effect on local or global myocardial function.[36,37]

These and other trials of systemic thrombolytics set the stage for the widespread treatment of acute MIs in the emergency departments of most hospitals. This protocol was especially useful in hospitals which did not possess a catheterization lab but were now able to administer thrombolytics within the magic first few hours after the onset of symptoms.

Unfortunately, several studies, including that of Topal et al.,[38] revealed one of the Achilles' heels in thrombolytic therapy: despite clot dissolution, the reocclusion rate within 3 months is approximately 25–30%, partly due to the remaining coronary stenosis.[39] In one study, a cross-sectional area < 0.4 mm^2 correlated with a 54% reocclusion rate.[40] With fibrinolytic therapy for acute MI, only about 50% of the target vessels are patent at 90 minutes after infusion, and the results vary with the fibrinolytic agent used (54% for tissue-type plasminogen activator [tPA] vs. 29% for streptokinase).[41]

In 1978, Gruentzig developed percutaneous coronary angioplasty in patients with stable coronary artery disease. In the 1990s this procedure became the preferred method for treating acute MI, especially in patients who were ineligible for thrombolytic therapy. Emergency angioplasty was shown to be superior to thrombolytic therapy in the treatment of acute MI with a lower incidence of nonfatal reinfarction and death compared with thrombolytics.[42,43]

Because of the success of PTCA in primary treatment of coronary stenosis and acute MI, several studies examined thrombolytic therapy followed by coronary angioplasty in an attempt to address the high incidence of reocclusion at the stenotic site after thrombolytics only. The concept of early angioplasty after the use of thrombolytic therapy has not been found to be broadly beneficial and, in fact, may be harmful.[44-46] For example, coronary reocclusion occurs twice as frequently after rescue angioplasty compared with thrombolytic therapy only.[47] PTCA failures also have a higher mortality rate than thrombolytic failures.[48] For a number of reasons, patients who present with an acute coronary occlusion have become almost exclusively candidates for primary angioplasty without prior thrombolytic therapy,[48,49] even if they present in cardiogenic shock. The mortality rate for primary angioplasty in patients who present in cardiogenic shock is just under 50%—a rate that compares favorably with conventional therapy mortality rates of 70–80%.[50]

The Primary Angioplasty and Myocardial Infarction (PAMI) trial was a multicenter study randomly comparing angioplasty with tPA.[43] Along with similar trials, the PAMI trial found that angioplasty had a high success rate (97%) and a significantly lower in-hospital mortality rate. It also had higher patency rates, lower recurrent angina rates, and lower recurrent infarction rates. Angioplasty in the setting of acute MI has a 2% mortality rate over the course of the first year[51] compared with 5–9% for thrombolytic therapy.

In general, despite opinions to the contrary, the prevailing consensus based on current data justifies primary angioplasty in the setting of acute MI when experienced interventional cardiologists and adequately equipped and staffed cardiac catheterization labs are readily available.

Despite its overwhelming general acceptance, angioplasty in the face of acute MI has several known drawbacks, such as a 30–45% restenosis rate, a 10–20% reintervention rate for the target vessel, total reocclusion rate of 10–20%, reinfarction rates of 3–5%, and coronary artery dissection rate of 20%. In addition, a TIMI flow rate less than grade 3 is found in 20% of infarcted vessels.[42,43,52-55] Coronary artery stents became popular recently to combat some of these shortcomings.

The use of coronary artery stenting for patients with acute MI was initially thought to be relatively contraindicated because of the potential for stent thrombosis with early-generation stents.[56] Later-generation stents, which were less and less thrombogenic, have all but eliminated this problem. The PAMI stent pilot study, which compared 452 patients treated with heparin-coated stents and 448 patients treated with PTCA alone, found that stented arteries had a greater luminal diameter, decreased angiographic restenosis, decreased mortality, decreased recurrent MIs, decreased cerebrovascular accidents, and decreased target vessel revascularization due to angina or ischemia.[57] Thirty-one percent of patients were ineligible for stent placement because of vessel size, excessive residual thrombus, osteal left anterior descending or osteal circumflex lesions, major side branches jeopardized by stent placement, or technical inability to deliver and place the stent appropriately.

Mehta and Bates[58] reviewed all published data about the use of intracoronary stents in patients with acute MI. They concluded that stent implantation is both safe and effective for patients with acute MI. Compared with PTCA alone, procedural success rates are slightly better for the stent patients. Stents had lower reocclusion rates, lower restenosis rates, and less need for target vessel revascularization. Larger luminal diameters also were achieved with stents. Postprocedural mortality, MI, and recurrent ischemia tended to be lower in the stent group. Hansen et al.[59] reported the results of primary stenting in patients with acute MI. They reported a 95% establishment of normal flow in the infarct vessel and acceptably low 6-month morbidity and mortality rates, thus supporting primary stenting as a safe and acceptable strategy with immediate and short-term (6-month) follow-up. Studies by Stone[60] and Antoniucci[61] support these findings.

Interventional vs. Surgical Reperfusion

Since the introduction of interventional reperfusion techniques, including thrombolytics, PTCA, atherectomy, and stents, the treatment of patients with acute MI has changed dramatically. The controversy about the most appropriate method for successful reperfusion of ischemic myocardium has been equally dramatic in some institutions. In the past 20 years, the standard aggressive treatment has changed from emergency CABG to thrombolytics and now to interventional therapies using angioplasty and stent placement. These interventional therapies have all but replaced surgery as the primary treatment for patients with acute MI. Surgical intervention is now used only in salvage situations when interventional therapy has failed, in patients who remain unstable despite interventional attempts, or in patients with other cardiac complications related to acute MI, such as ruptured papillary muscles, ventricular rupture, and ischemic mitral regurgitation. In fact, surgical revascularization after interventional failure is now the most common reason for emergency surgery in patients with uncomplicated acute MI.

In 1983, Phillips et al.[28] reported a 1.3% rate for both early and late mortality in patients with acute MI who were treated primarily with surgical reperfusion. In patients who underwent CABG after failure of interventional reperfusion, the mortality rate was 29%. In patients undergoing emergency CABG for failed PTCA, some recent studies report an operative mortality rate and an incidence of MI of almost 10%.[62,63] This rate has remained stable or increased over the past 10 years despite improved myocardial protection and surgical advances, primarily because patients who present to the hospital with MI have become sicker and older. They have more multivessel disease, poor left ventricular ejection fractions, and high frequency of comorbid problems. Patients who then present for primary angioplasty or surgery after failed angioplasty are proportionately sicker. However, with the advent of intracoronary stents, the incidence of emergency surgical intervention after failed angioplasty is on the decline, so much so that most hospitals require surgical stand-by for only a handful of coronary interventions. With the recent use of stents, the incidence of failed PTCA requiring emergency CABG has fallen to < 3%.[64,65,67] Despite the fact that emergency CABG after stent failure carries a high incidence of Q-wave infarction, patients have a surprisingly good short-term and long-term survival rate (88%).[68]

Based on a large number of small nonrandomized studies, the outcomes of emergent revascularization in patients with cardiogenic shock (especially when ischemic mitral regurgitation, papillary muscle rupture, ventricular septal defect, or rupture/tamponade is involved) are superior when emergency surgical intervention is used rather than interventional revascularization. Among

830 patients in 26 studies who had bypass surgery, the mortality rate was 36% compared with 44% among 1167 patients in 24 studies who had angioplasty.[69,70] Geighteon et al. showed a remarkable hospital and long-term (3-year) survival rate of 88% in patients who presented in cardiogenic shock and were surgically revascularized.[71] Eighty-five percent of these patients were categorized as NYHA class I or II. In the SHOCK Trial Registry, which included patients who were not selected for randomization for the SHOCK Trial, the mortality rate for patients with shock due to left ventricular failure was 28% among 136 CABG treated-patients compared with 46% among 290 PTCA-treated patients.[72]

Only two randomized trials have compared emergency intervention with standard care for postinfarction cardiogenic shock. The Swiss MASH study was terminated early and showed no differences in outcome for patients randomized to angioplasty vs. conventional shock therapy.[73] The SHOCK Trial randomized 152 patients with shock due to left ventricular failure after MI to revascularization and 150 to medical treatment.[69] Eighty-seven percent of the patients assigned to revascularization underwent a revascularization procedure; angioplasty accounted for 64% of the first revascularization attempts and surgery for 36%. Nine patients underwent surgery after attempted angioplasty. Surgically treated patients had more left main disease (40% vs. 14%, p < 0.001) and three-vessel disease (79% vs. 60%, p < 0.0008) than patients treated with angioplasty. The overall mortality rate at 30 days did not differ significantly between the revascularization and medical groups (46.7% and 56.0%, respectively, p = 0.11). At 6 months the mortality rate was lower in the revascularization group than in the medical group (50.3% vs. 63.1%, p = 0.027). Outcome was somewhat better with surgery than with angioplasty but not significantly so; furthermore, the study was not designed to compare surgery with angioplasty.

Preoperative Care

General Surgical Principles

Once a patient enters the emergency room with a diagnosis of acute MI, the emergency physician, cardiologist, and catheterization lab personnel should be mobilized immediately. The patient should be evaluated as quickly as possible with routine blood work, electrocardiography, cardiac enzymes, and physical examination. Thrombolytic therapy may be an option in certain cases. As soon as acute MI is diagnosed, the patient should be taken immediately to the catheterization lab (if available), where a definitive diagnosis can be made. At that point, treatment with PTCA or stent placement may be definitive. If surgery is considered the primary therapy because of anatomic considerations such as infarct-related ventricular septal defect, ventricular rupture, or cardiogenic shock with ischemic mitral regurgitation, resuscitation of the patient in the catheterization lab should begin immediately while the operating room is made ready. Surgery also may be the primary therapy if the patient's anatomy makes PTCA or stent placement difficult or if the patient has severe triple-vessel or left main disease that the cardiologist and cardiac surgeon believe would be best treated with expeditious surgical intervention.

Likewise, if the patient has failed angioplasty or stent therapy and requires surgical therapy, the resuscitative process should begin in the catheterization lab until the operating room is ready. Airway management to maximize oxygenation, manipulation of both preload and afterload along with maintainance of cardiac output using ionotropic therapy, and correction of acid–base deficits or other biochemical abnormalities should begin in the catheterization lab. Placement of an IABP may stabilize hemodynamics until the patient is in the operating room. These procedures should not be done if they delay moving the patient to the operating room; they should be begun and continued only until the patient can be transferred to the operating room.

Once the patient is in the operating room, rapid induction of general anesthesia, along with placement of necessary central venous access lines, should be performed expeditiously. If not already placed in the catheterization lab, an intraaortic balloon can be placed at induction if time permits. Prompt placement on cardiopulmonary bypass is the immediate goal in the operating room. If thrombolytics have been used, antifibrinolytics such as aminocaproic acid or aprotinin should be started before initiation of bypass. Resuscitation can then continue, and reversible cardiogenic shock with some hemodynamic stability can be achieved on the heart-lung machine. Depending on the situation, placement of an IABP before the patient comes off bypass may facilitate weaning.

Role of the Intraaortic Balloon Pump

Percutaneous placement of an IABP became available in the early 1980s. Balloon pumps can easily be placed percutaneously in the catheterization lab, in the operating room before surgery, or even at the bedside, if necessary. Balloon pump complications are not insignificant, especially in patients with severe peripheral vascular disease or small arteries. Thirty-four French and even smaller sheathless balloons are currently available and certainly decrease the complications of percutaneous placement of an IABP in the femoral arteries. Aortic arch balloon pump placement may need to be performed intra-operatively when peripheral vascular disease prohibits percutaneous placement. However, arch placement is associated with high morbidity and mortality rates (58% and 54%, respectively).[7]

The IABP reduces ventricular wall myocardial stress, decreases myocardial oxygen use, improves coronary blood flow, stabilizes overall hemodynamics, and may decrease the need for significant ionotropic support preoperatively. The IABP also may stabilize the patient so that CABG can be performed on an elective rather than an emergent basis.[74–76]

Balloon pump counterpulsation during cardiopulmonary bypass is controversial. Theoretically, pulsatile flow distal to the cross-clamp during the normal nonpulsatile pump run may improve organ function[77,78] and intestinal perfusion.[79] Preoperative, intraoperative, or postoperative use must be evaluated carefully and continually, weighing advantages against possible complications.

Surgery after Thrombolytics and Antiplatelet Therapy

Bleeding disorders are not infrequent after routine cardiopulmonary bypass. Rates of return for bleeding range from 1–5% in the U.S. The need for blood products both intra- and postoperatively ranges from 10–50%. Although these numbers may be decreased with the use of antifibrinolytic agents such as aminocaproic acid or aprotinin, surgery on patients who have received irreversible thrombolytic or antiplatelet therapies requires significantly increased amounts of blood products. Careful, meticulous surgical hemostasis is always mandatory in open heart surgery but cannot be overemphasized in patients who have received these agents.

Failed thrombolytic therapy resulting in emergency CABG in the setting of acute MI or cardiogenic shock carries high morbidity and mortality rates. Skinner et al. reported a 25% mortality rate and a 25% rate of return for bleeding in 24 such patients.[80]

Because of the additional need for blood products and the inherent risks in their use (e.g., excessive blood volume, transmittable diseases), patients who are relatively stable may be better served by delaying the operation for 24–48 hours until the coagulopathic state has reversed.

Right Ventricular Infarcts

Preoperative MI is an independent predictor of mortality after CABG.[81] Acute evolving MIs of the inferior wall secondary to proximal right coronary artery occlusion are among the most challenging problems for coronary revascularization by surgical means. Right heart failure, cardiac arrhythmias, hypotension, and cardiogenic shock are common with right ventricular infarcts.[82–84] Complete revascularization of the right coronary artery and adequate myocardial protection are crucial to surgical intervention for right ventricular infarcts. Patients who present early in the course of right ventricular infarct have a greater chance of successful surgical revascularization than patients who are more than 6–12 hours into the infarct. Factors such as early recognition, early intervention, and collateralization to the right ventricle play a role in the success of surgical intervention. If the patient is well into the infarct (significantly more than 6–12 hours), most surgeons prefer to "ride out the storm" with conservative treatment. Aggressive intervention, anticoagulation, ionotropic support, and IABP (to name a few measures) should be tried if the patient is well into the infarct. Delayed surgery allows the infarcted right ventricle to recover and minimizes the risk of eventual surgical revascularization. Operating on an acute right ventricular infarction is fraught with complications. Cardioplegic protection is paramount. Yet despite adequate protection using retrograde and antegrade cardioplegia, topical cooling, and early grafting of the right coronary artery, irreversible damage to the right ventricle may result in difficulty in weaning the patient from bypass. When a surgeon's hand is forced early in the process because of significant hemodynamic instability, extraordinary measures, including right ventricular assist devices, are not uncommon after surgical revascularization.

Intraoperative Care

The use of an internal mammary artery (IMA) imparts distinct advantages over an all-vein bypass operation. In one study comparing cardiac bypass with and without the use of an IMA, the IMA imparted both early and late survival benefits along with longer graft patency, fewer hospitalizations, fewer MIs, fewer reinterventions (PTCA or reoperation), and a lower mortality rate compared with an all saphenous vein bypass.[85,86]

Although the IMA is always preferable, time constraints and hemodynamic instability may force some surgeons to use all saphenous vein bypass grafts. Others argue that because of the benefits of using the left IMA, the patient should be placed immediately on bypass. While the heart is decompressed and some cooling is performed, the IMA can be taken down. While the conduits are harvested and before the cross-clamp is placed, the surgeon must avoid any distention of the left or right ventricle, which may involve placement of a left ventricular vent through the superior pulmonary vein.

After the cross-clamp is placed, the infarct vessel should be bypassed first to ensure adequate protection of the injured myocardium. Cardioplegia can be given down the graft as soon as the distal anastomosis is completed. Because the right ventricle may not be as well protected as one would like using retrograde and antegrade cardioplegia, early bypass grafting of the right coronary artery may improve right ventricular protection. Performing the bypasses in an efficient fashion minimizing cross-clamp times should be one of the most important goals of the operation.

Reperfusion Strategies

Once the patient is clamped, several protective cardioplegic techniques are available to the surgeon. Understanding the different protocols for cardioplegia gives the surgeon flexibility to match specific protocols with specific types of patients.

Buckberg's reperfusion strategy involves normothermic induction followed by hypothermia, during which bypasses are performed. The final step is normothermic terminal reperfusion.[70,87,88] Another protocol involves continuous normothermic retrograde cardioplegic delivery, which has several myocardial biochemical advantages, including superior regeneration of ATP.

Surgeon's preferences include blood vs. crystalloid cardioplegia, hot vs. cold cardioplegia, warm continuous vs. cold intermittent cardioplegia, and numerous variations between. Although some surgeons believe that continuous warm cardioplegia at near normothermia is cardioprotective, others believe that colder is better and that cooling to 22–25°C may impart better protection. We generally prefer a hypothermic (22–28°) perfusate, cold blood intermittent cardioplegia, and a final "hot shot" of cardioplegia before the cross-clamp is removed. Because continuous cardioplegia makes it difficult to suture distal anastomoses, we prefer intermittent cardioplegia. Completion of the distal anastomosis is followed by cardioplegia down the graft; then the proximal anastomosis is performed, first for the infarcted vessel. This protocol ensures early and frequent cardioplegia to the infarct zone.

Reperfusion strategies and the composition of the reperfusate are complicated subjects. General recommendations have been made by numerous authorities, including decompression of the heart on cardiopulmonary bypass (which significantly decreases myocardial oxygen needs), control of the reperfusion pressure (40–50 mmHg), maintenance of normothermia (which normalizes cellular biochemical reactions), and prolonged reperfusion periods to allow cellular repair while the heart is arrested.

Use of appropriate ionotropic agents should begin at the end of the pump run to prepare the heart for coming off cardiopulmonary bypass. Maintenance of cardiopulmonary bypass for severely injured ventricles allows time for the heart to recover, restoring its own homeostatic state before coming off bypass.

Reperfusion Injury

Ischemic injury to the myocardium can result in the loss of certain homeostatic mechanisms at the cellular level, including the sodium-potassium exchange pump. This energy-requiring pump depletes phosphate stores because of the inability of the myocardium to form enough energy stores via anaerobic glycolytic pathways to maintain normal myocardial cellular function. After flow into a previously ischemic area is reestablished, days may be required to repair structural damage, to replenish lost high-energy phosphate stores, and to restore normal myocardial contractility at the cellular level.

Acutely, once flow is restored, a wave-like reaccumulation of sodium and water produces myocardial edema, which perpetuates the ischemic process and is known as the "no-reflow phenomenon."[5] This phenomenon also increases intracellular calcium levels in the mitochondria and myocardial cytoplasm. This calcium overload results in the so-called "stone heart," which may lead to permanently injured myocardial cells and worsen ischemic injury to the heart. Such reperfusion injury and stone-heart phenomenon were so pervasive at one time that some people argued that surgical intervention was contraindicated in patients with MI.

Both thrombolytics and PTCA/stents restore blood flow to an ischemic area, but they do not control the ultimate reperfusion injury that takes place once the intervention is completed. Advocates of interventional reperfusion techniques argue that there is less delay in treating patients in the catheterization lab (or emergency department if thrombolytics are used), whereas surgeons believe that surgical reperfusion results in less overall myocardial damage and an overall improvement in postoperative myocardial function.

In one study comparing medical and surgical therapy for acute MI, after a few hours of regional ischemia the amount of myocardial necrosis in the medical group was twice that in the surgical group.[89] In addition, overall myocardial function, acutely and chronically, was significantly better after surgical reperfusion.[90]

During PTCA the infarcted muscle is reperfused with "unmodified" whole blood in a normothermic, pressurized, contracting myocardium with normal or increased oxygen needs. Surgical reperfusion of the acutely ischemic myocardium takes place in an arrested, decompressed heart and can be tailored to the patient by altering the timing of reperfusion, temperature, and chemical make-up of the reperfusate. This customized surgical approach may ameliorate the reperfusion injury during treatment of the ischemic myocardium.[3] Thus, resting the heart on the heart-lung machine results in decreased myocardial oxygen needs, and resuscitating the heart with the appropriate reperfusion solutions may limit the amount of ischemic damage and perhaps result in improved survival compared with medically treated/interventional patients.[70]

The benefits of controlled reperfusion were nicely outlined by Allen et al. in 1993.[70] Their multicenter study examined 156 patients who presented with acute MI and underwent emergency CABG using a modified reperfusion protocol. In the surgically reperfused group, despite the fact that left anterior descending occlusion, multivessel disease, and even cardiogenic shock were more common, the mortality rate was 3.9% compared with contemporary angioplasty mortality rates of 9%.[91,92] Twelve patients went to the operating room with cardiopulmonary resuscitation in progress! Furthermore, the time to intervention was almost twice as long in the surgical group (6.3 hours) as in the angioplasty group (3.9 hours). From this study it follows that by the time surgery is required, the patient is many more hours into the acute MI, perhaps making the operation more difficult, the results less rewarding, and comparison between the two more difficult.

Postoperative Care

Once off pump, patients need to remain in a euvolemic state. Although the use of a Swan-Ganz catheter is controversial, it may be helpful in some settings to optimize cardiac output, preload, and afterload with the help of ionotropic support. Correction of acid–base and electrolyte abnormalities is essential in the early postoperative period. Rhythm disturbances must be addressed with antiarrhythmic agents such as lidocaine or amiodarone. Beta blockers are especially useful for prevention of atrial fibrillation and tachyarrhythmias and have been shown to have a beneficial effect on survival after acute MIs.[93] Angiotensin-converting enzyme inhibitors are particularly effective, especially in the setting of postoperative heart failure and poor ventricular function. Antiplatelet therapy, typically aspirin, is almost universally accepted. Low-dose anticoagulation may be indicated in patients with low ejection fractions to prevent mural thrombus formation.

Timing of Surgery

One of the many questions surrounding the surgical treatment of acute MI is the timing of elective CABG. In stable patients who clearly need CABG after acute MI, the question of timing remains controversial. Some studies show a benefit to delaying elective CABG after acute MI, whereas other studies have demonstrated the safety of early CABG.

Survival after acute MI is affected by infarct size and the ability of the surrounding nonischemic myocardium to support cardiac hemodynamics.[20] A large infarct may result in hemodynamic compromise, even cardiogenic shock, which is the leading cause of death in hospitalized patients with acute MI[106] (60–70% mortality rate[107,108]). Advocates of early surgery point to the risk of additional ischemic injury to the infarcted area; extension of the infarction into the surrounding myocardium, which may lead to hemodynamic compromise; increased length of hospital stay; and increased overall hospital costs. Early surgical reperfusion has been shown by VanHaecke et al. to decrease the size of the infarct and thus maintain and improve overall myocardial function.[105] If surgical intervention was begun within 4 hours of onset of symptoms, smaller infarcts and better overall left ventricular myocardial function were noted compared with patients who had emergency surgery after 4 hours from onset of symptoms. The overall improvement in patients with anterior MIs was even more significant with early vs. late revascularization, thus supporting the concept that early surgical reperfusion is even more paramount for anterior wall MIs than for inferior wall MIs. DeWood et al.[25] showed a significantly lower mortality rate (3.8%) for patients with acute MI who underwent surgery within 6 hours as opposed to later than six hours (8% mortality rate). At 5 years, the mortality rate was 8% in patients who underwent surgery within 6 hours and 21% in patients who underwent surgery more than 6 hours after onset of symptoms.

Some surgeons loosely apply the logic gleaned from interventional data to the surgical treatment of patients with stable MI. Early thrombolytic therapy is associated with better outcomes than later thrombolytic therapy. The ISIS-II trial[35] examined the timing of thrombolytic reperfusion and found benefits up to 24 hours from onset of symptoms, although the benefits diminished over time, confirming that earlier is better. Like surgical intervention, both angioplasty and thrombolytics were more successful if used within a few hours of onset of acute MI. Of interest, not unlike the surgical data, both interventional techniques showed a greater benefit to reperfusion of anterior infarctions compared with inferior infarctions. Anterior infarcts seemed to benefit even as long as 12 hours after onset of infarction.

Rodgers et al.[94] found that emergency CABG can be performed successfully well beyond the 4–6-hour window if patients have a stenotic but nonoccluded infarct vessel or if the myocardium is well collateralized. Phillips et al.[28] could not identify the "magic window" in their series. Emergency surgery was performed from 1–36 hours into the course of an infarct whenever there was clinical evidence of ongoing progression of MI. Unfortunately, unlike the DeWood study, the authors did not report the overall morbidity and mortality rates based on timing of the operation. Although early studies showed a relatively high mortality rate associated with operating on patients early after acute MI,[95] like Phillips, more recent studies have shown that the timing of CABG after acute MI is unimportant.[96]

Advocates of delayed surgery argue that allowing the stunned myocardium to recover from the acute MI before CABG is performed can reduce morbidity and mortality rates. Waiting also avoids reperfusion injuries, including hemorrhagic infarction with infarct extension into surrounding viable myocardium and myocardial scar formation. In a retrospective study comparing groups with both nontransmural and transmural acute MIs, Roberts et al. concluded that a waiting period of 3–5 days after a nontransmural acute MI results in an optimal decrease in morbidity and mortality rates, whereas a 5–7-day waiting period after transmural acute MI results in postoperative morbidity and mortality rates similar to those in patients with nonacute MI undergoing elective CABG. Thus, they concluded that a short waiting period is justified.[97] Nunley[98] also studied the interval from acute MI to surgical revascularization. If revascularization was done within the first 48 hours of acute MI, the mortality rate was 7.7% vs. 0% if the revascularization was done after the first 48 hours. Cresell[99] found that surgical revascularization within 2 weeks of acute MI resulted in a mortality rate of 6.5% compared with 2.9% in patients who underwent surgery more than 2 weeks after an acute myocardial event. Waiting has some support, but waiting too long to perform CABG after acute MI may result in ventricular remodeling and perhaps eventual infarct expansion.[100] The infarcted area eventually dilates, and the ventricular wall thins out, resulting in ventricular aneurysm formation and even ventricular rupture.[101]

Others have found no correlation between morbidity or mortality and timing of the surgery. Every et al. studied 1299 patients after surgical revascularization for acute MI.[102] They found no statistical difference in hospital mortality rates in patients undergoing surgery < 24 hours after acute MI vs. patients undergoing surgery > 24 hours after acute MI (8.8% vs. 7%). Other surgeons believe that other risk factors have a greater effect on morbidity and mortality than the actual timing of surgery.[103]

With the advent of off-pump coronary artery bypass (OPCAB), questions have been raised about its role in the surgical armamentarium for acute MI. Unlike standard CABG, OPCAB does not use cardiopulmonary bypass. Like PTCA and thrombolytics, it provides more immediate, albeit uncontrolled, reperfusion of both the infarcted coronary artery and other stenotic arteries. What it lacks in control of reperfusion through various cardioplegic strategies may be outweighed by the theoretical advantages of avoiding the heart-lung machine in certain patients with end-stage chronic obstructive pulmomary disease, renal failure, or recent stroke. Although the role and clinical efficacy of OPCAB are under evaluation in multiple centers around the country for elective CABG, its role in patients with acute MI is less studied. Mohr et al.[104] studied 57 patients, using OPCAB as their primary therapy within the first week of acute MI. More than one-half underwent emergency OPCAB within 48 hours of acute MI, and 12.5% of operations were done because of failed PTCA. Twenty-two percent of patients were in cardiogenic shock preoperatively, and 31% required preoperative IABP. Forty-four percent underwent OPCAB 2–7 days after acute MI. The operative mortality rate was only 1.7%, with an average length of stay of 6.8 days. One- and 5-year actuarial survival rates were 95% and 82%, respectively. Renal failure and preoperative cardiogenic shock were found to be independent predictors of mortality by multivariate analysis. These results clearly show that OPCAB may play an important role in the treatment of certain patients after acute MI.

Other surgical reperfusion strategies, such as Heartport CABG, are used in limited settings by some surgeons. Because many minimally invasive strategies take longer to perform (e.g., longer to get on pump and to harvest a mammary artery through a minithoracotomy incision), their use is infrequent and even less studied. As these technologies evolve, their use may expand. Until that time, few authorities recommend their general use in the treatment of acute MI.

CONCLUSION

The ideal treatment of acute MI remains controversial. Interventional treatments have all but replaced surgery as the primary initial treatment of the acute evolving MI. Surgery has been relegated to patients who fail interventional techniques or have acute mechanical complications of MI. Few recent trials have included surgical therapy as a primary treatment for acute MI; thus little evidence compares the benefits of current surgical therapy and current interventional techniques. CABG is an effective therapy for acute MI with generally low morbidity and mortality rates, even in patients with cardiogenic shock. Unlike interventional techniques, surgery can modify the timing of reperfusion; alter the temperature and type of reperfusate; decrease preload, afterload, and oxygen consumption on the heart/lung machine; and limit reperfusion injury after revascularization. Although the timing of CABG after acute MI remains controversial, its role remains important. It is our hope that future studies will compare modern surgical therapy with current nonsurgical treatment of acute MI.

References

1. Herrick JB: Clinical features of sudden destruction of the coronary arteries. JAMA 59:220–228, 1912.
2. Ahmed WH, Bittel JA, Braunwald E: Relation between clinical presentation and angiographic findings in unstable angina pectoris and comparison with that in stable angina. Am J Cardiol 72:544–550, 1993.
3. Braunwald E, Kloner PA: Myocardial reperfusion: A double-edged sword? J Clin Invest 76:1713–1719, 1985.
4. Tennant R, Wiggens CJ: The effect of coronary occlusion on myocardial contraction. Am J Physiol 112:351, 1935.

5. Jennings RB, Reimer KA: Factors involved in salvaging ischemic myocardium: Effect of reperfusion of arterial blood. Circulation 68(Suppl I):I25–I36, 1983.

6. Schaper J: Effects of anoxia and ischemia on the ultrastructure and metabolism of the myocardium. Ultrastructure of the myocardium after ischemia and reperfusion. Coeur Med Intern 18:617–618, 1979.

7. Mueller DK, Stout M, Blakeman B: Morbidity and mortality of intra-aortic balloon pumps placed through the aortic arch. Chest 114:85–88, 1998.

8. Ferrari R, Ceconi C, Curello S, et al: Intracellular effects of myocardial ischemia and reperfusion: Role of calcium and oxygen. Eur Heart J 7(Suppl A):3–12, 1986.

9. Bodwell W: Ischemia, reperfusion, and reperfusion injury: Role of oxygen free radicals and oxygen free radical scavengers. J Cardiovasc Nurs 4:5–32, 1989.

10. Kingsley PB, Sako EY, Yang MQ, et al: Ischemic contracture begins when anaerobic glycolysis stops: A 31 P-NMR study of isolated rat hearts. Am J Physiol 261:469–478, 1991.

11. Costantini C, Corday E, Lang T, et al: Revascularization after three hours of coronary arterial occlusion: Effects on regional cardiac metabolic function and infarct size. Am J Cardiol 36:368, 1975.

12. Maroko PR, Libby P, Ginks WR, et al: Coronary artery reperfusion: Early effects on local myocardial function and the extent of myocardial necrosis. J Clin Invest 51:2710, 1972.

13. Reimer KA, Lowe JE, Rasmussen MM, et al: The wave front phenomenon of ischemic cell death. I: Myocardial infarct size versus duration of coronary occlusion in dogs. Circulation 56:786–798, 1977.

14. Berg R Jr, Kendall RW, Duvoisin GE, et al: Acute MI: A surgical emergency. J Thorac Cardiovasc Surg 70:432-439, 1975.

15. Shell WE, Covell JW, Lavelle JF, et al: Early estimation of myocardial damage in conscious dogs and patients with evolving acute MI. J Clin Invest 52:2579–2590, 1973.

16. Page, DL, Caulfield, JB, Kastor, JA, et al: Myocardial changes associated with cardiogenic shock. N Engl J Med 285:133–137, 1971.

17. Schuster EH, Bulkley BH: Ischemia at a distance after acute MI: A cause of early post-infarction angina. Circulation 62:509–515, 1980.

18. Corday E, Kaplan L, Meerbaum S, et al: Consequences of coronary arterial occlusion on remote myocardium: Effects of occlusion and reperfusion. Am J Cardiol 36:385–394, 1975.

19. Darsee JR, Kloner RA, Braunwald E: Time course of regional function after coronary occlusions of one to one hundred twenty minutes duration. Am J Physiol 240:399–407, 1981.

20. Beyersdorf F, Acar C, Buckberg GD, et al: Studies on prolonged acute regional ischemia. Early natural history of simulated single and multivessel disease with emphasis on remote myocardium. J Thorac Cardiovasc Surg 98:368–380, 1989.

21. Favaloro RG, Effler DV, Cheanvechai C, et al: Acute coronary insufficiency (impending MI and myocardial ischemia): Surgical treatment by the saphenous vein graft technique. Am J Cardiol 28:598–607, 1971.

22. Cheanvechai C, Effler DB, Loop FD, et al: Emergency myocardial revascularization. Am J Cardiology 32:901–908, 1973.

23. Dawson JT, Hall RJ, Hallman GL, et al: Mortality in patients undergoing coronary artery bypass surgery after MI. Am J Cardiol 33:483, 1974.

24. Keon W, Badard P, Shankar K, et al: Experience with emergency aortocoronary bypass grafts in the presence of acute MI. Circulation 47(Suppl 3):151–155, 1973.

25. DeWood MA, Spores J, Berg R Jr, et al: Acute MI: A decade of experience with surgical reperfusion in 701 patients. Circulation 68(Suppl II):II8–II16, 1983.

26. DeWood MA, Notske RN, Hensley GR, et al: Intra-aortic balloon counterpulsation with and without reperfusion for MI shock. Circulation 61:1105–1112, 1980.

27. DeWood MA, Notske RN, Berg R Jr, et al: Medical and surgical management of early Q-wave MI. Effects of surgical reperfusion on survival: Recurrent MI, sudden death, and functional class at 10 or more year follow-up. J Am Coll Cardiol 14:65–77, 1989.

28. Phillips SJ, Kongtahworn C, Skinner JR, et al: Emergency coronary artery reperfusion: A choice therapy for evolving MI. J Thorac Cardiovasc Surgery 86:679–688, 1983.

29. DeWood MA, Berg R Jr: The role of surgical reperfusion in MI. Cardiol Clin 2:113–122, 1984.

30. Rentrop P, Blanke H, Kostering K, et al: Acute MI: Intracoronary application of nitroglycerine and streptokinase in combination with transluminal recanalization. Clin Cardiol 5:354–363, 1979.

31. Kennedy JW, Ritchie JL, Davis KB, Fritz JK: Western Washington randomized trial of intracoronary streptokinase in acute MI. N Eng J Med 309:1477–1482, 1983.

32. Khaja F, Walton JA, Blymer J, et al: Intracoronary fibrinolytic therapy in acute MI. N Engl J Med 308:1305–1311, 1983.

33. Anderson JL, Marshall HW, Bray BE, et al: A randomized trial of intracoronary streptokinase in the treatment of acute MI. N Engl J Med 308:1312–1318, 1983.

34. Gruppo Italiano per lo Studio della Streptochinasi nell'Infarto Miocardico (GISSI): Effectiveness of intravenous thrombolytic treatment in acute myocardial infarction. Lancet 1:397–402, 1986.
35. ISIS-2 Collaborative Groups: Randomized trial of intravenous streptokinase, oral aspirin, both or neither among 17,187 cases of suspected acute MI. Lancet 2:349–360, 1988.
36. Dalen JE, Gore JM, Braunwald E, et al: Six and 12 month follow-up of the phase I thrombolysis in Myocardial Infarction (TIMI) trial. Am J Cardiol 62:179–185, 1988.
37. TIMI Research Group: Immediate versus delayed catheterization in angioplasty following thrombolytic therapy for acute MI: TIMI-IIA results. JAMA 260:2849–2858, 1988.
38. Topal EL, Morris DC, Smalling RW, et al: A multicenter, randomized, placebo-controlled trial of a new form of intravenous recombinant tissue-type plasminogen-activator (activase) in acute MI. J Am Coll Cardiol 9:1205–1213, 1987.
39. Meijer A, Verheugt FWA, Werter CJ, et al. Aspirin versus Coumadin in the prevention of re-occlusion and recurrent ischemia after successful thrombolysis: a prospective placebo-controlled angiographic study. Circulation 87:1524–1530, 1993.
40. Harrison DG, Ferguson DW, Collins SM, et al: Rethrombosis after reperfusion with streptokinase: Importance of geometry of residual lesions. Circulation 69:991–999, 1984.
41. GUSTO Study Group: The effects of tissue plasminogen activator, streptokinase, or both on coronary artery patency, ventricular function, and survival after acute MI. N Engl J Med 329:615–622, 1993.
42. Zijlstra F, DeBoer MJ, Hoorntje JC, et al: A compromise of immediate coronary angioplasty with intravenous streptokinase in acute MI. N Engl J Med 328:680–684, 1993.
43. Grines CL, Browne KF, Marco J, et al: A comparison of immediate angioplasty with thrombolytic therapy for acute MI. N Engl J Med 328:673–679, 1993.
44. Simoons MF, Arnold AER, Betriu A, et al: Thrombolysis with tissue plasminogen activator in acute MI: No additional benefit from immediate percutaneous coronary angioplasty. Lancet 1:197–203, 1988.
45. Topal EL, Califf RM, George BS, et al: A randomized trial of immediate versus delayed elective angioplasty after intravenous tissue plasminogen activator in acute MI. N Engl J Med 317:581–588, 1987.
46. Lange RA, Hillis LD: Immediate angioplasty for acute MI. N Engl J Med 328:726–728, 1993.
47. Abbottsmith CW, Topol EG, George BS, et al: Fate of patients with acute MI with patency of infarct related vessel achieved with successful thrombolysis versus rescue angioplasty. J Am Coll Cardiol 16:770–778, 1990.
48. Garrahy PJ, Henzlova NJ, Farman S, et al: Has thrombolytic therapy improved survival from cardiogenic shock? Thrombolysis in Myocardial Infarction (TIMI-II) results. Circulation 80(Suppl II):II-623, 1989.
49. GISSI Trial: Effectiveness of intravenous thrombolytic treatment in acute MI. Lancet 1:397–401, 1986.
50. Bate ER, Topol EJ: Limitation of thrombolytic therapy for MI complicated by congestive heart failure and cardiogenic shock. J Am Coll Cardiol 18:1077–1084, 1991.
51. Stack RS, Cliff RM, Hinohara T, et al: Survival and cardiac event rates in the first year after emergency coronary angioplasty for acute MI. J Am Coll Cardiol 11:1141–1149, 1988.
52. Stone GW, Grines CL, Browne KF, et al: Predictors of in-hospital and six month outcome after acute MI in the reperfusion era: The Primary Angioplasty in Myocardial Infarction Trial (PAMI). J Am Coll Cardiol 25:370–377, 1995.
53. Weaver WD, Simes J, Amadeo B, et al: Comparison of primary coronary angioplasty and intravenous thrombolytic therapy for acute MI: A quantitative review. JAMA 278:2093–2098, 1997.
54. Global Use of Strategies to Open Coronary Arteries in Acute Coronary Syndromes (GUSTO IIB). Angioplasty Substudy Investigators: A clinical trial comparing primary coronary angioplasty with tissue plasminogen activator for acute MI. N Engl J Med 336:1621–1628, 1997.
55. Michels KB, Yusuf S: Does PTCA and acute MI affect mortality and reinfarction rates? Circulation 91:476–485, 1995.
56. Nath FC, Muller DW, Ellis SG, et al: Thrombosis of flexible coil coronary stent: Frequency, predictors and clinical outcome. J Am Coll Cardiol 21:622–627, 1993.
57. Grines CL, Cox DA, Garcia E, et al: Stent PAMI: Primary endpoint results of a multicenter randomized trial of heparin coated stenting versus primary PTCA for acute MI. Circulation 98(Suppl I):I22, 1998 [abstract].
58. Mehta RH, Bates ER: Coronary stent implantation in acute MI. Am Heart J 137:603–611, 1999.
59. Hansen PS, Rasmussen HH, Vinen J, et al: A primary stenting strategy as an alternative to fibrinolytic therapy in acute MI: An analysis of results in-hospital and at six weeks and six months. Med J Austr 170:537–540, 1999.

60. Stone GW, Brodie B, Griffin J, et al: Prospective multicenter study of the safety and feasibility of primary stenting in acute MI: In-hospital and 30 day results of the PAMI stent pilot trial. J Am Coll Cardiol 31:23–30, 1998.
61. Antoniucci D, Santoro GM, Bolognese L, et al: A clinical trial comparing primary stenting of the infarct-related artery with optimal primary angioplasty for acute MI: Results from the Florence Randomized Elective Stenting in acute Coronary Occlusions trial (FRESCO). J Am Coll Cardiol 31:1234–1239, 1998.
62. Lazar HL, Jacobs AK, Aldea GS, et al: Factors influencing mortality after emergency coronary artery bypass grafting for failed percutaneous transluminal coronary angioplasty. Ann Thorac Surg 64:1747–1752, 1997.
63. Boylan MJ, Loop FD, Lytle BW, et al: Have PTCA failures requiring emergency coronary bypass changed? Ten year experience with 253 patients. Ann Thorac Surg 59:283–287, 1995.
64. Altmann DB, Racz N, Battlema, DS, et al: Reduction in angioplasty complications after the introduction of coronary stents: Results from a consecutive series of 2242 patients. Am Heart J 132:503–507, 1996.
65. Thompson RC, Holmes DR, Grill DE, et al: Changing outcome of angioplasty in the elderly. J Am Coll Cardiol 27:8–14, 1996.
66. George BS, Voorhees WD, Roubin GS, et al: Multicenter investigation of coronary stenting to treat acute or threatened closure after percutaneous transluminal coronary angioplasty: Clinical and angiographic outcomes. J Am Coll Cardiol 22:135–143, 1993.
67. Schomig A, Kastrati A, Mudra H, et al: Four year experience with Palmaz-Schatz stenting in coronary angioplasty complicated by dissection with threatened or present vessel closure. Circulation 90:2716–2724, 1994.
68. Craver JM, Justicz AG, Weintraub WS, et al: Coronary artery bypass grafting in patients after failure of intra-coronary stenting. Ann Thorac Surg 60:60–66, 1995.
69. Hochman JS, Sleeper LA, Webb JG, et al: Early revascularization in acute myocardial infarction compicated by cardiogenic shock. N Engl J Med 341:625–634, 1999.
70. Allen BS, Buckberg GD, Fontan FM, et al: Superiority of controlled surgical reperfusion versus percutaneous transluminal coronary angioplasty in acute coronary occlusions. J Thorac Cardiovasc Surg 105:864–879, 1993.
71. Michels KB, Yusuf S: Does PTCA and acute MI effect mortality and reinfarction rates? Circulation 91:476–485, 1995.
72. Hochman JS, Buller CD, Sleeper LA, et al: Cardiogenic shock complicating acute myocardial infarction: Etiologies, management and outcome: A report from the SHOCK Trial Registry. J Am Coll Cardiol 36(Suppl A):1063–1070, 2000.
73. Urban P, Stauffer JC, Bleed D, et al: A randomized evaluation of early revascularization to treat shock complicating acute myocardial infarction: The (Swiss) Multicenter Trial of Angioplasty for Shock–(S)MASH. Eur Heart J 20:1030–1038, 1999.
74. Watson JT, Willerson JT, Fixler DE, et al: Temporal changes in collateral coronary blood flow in ischemic myocardium during intra aerative balloon pumping. Circulation 100:47–48, 1973.
75. Bardet J, Masquet C, Kahn JC, et al: Clinical and hemodynamic results of intra aortic balloon counterpulsation and surgery for cardiogenic shock. Am Heart J 93:280–288, 1977.
76. Fuchs RM, Brin KP, Brinker JA, et al: Augmentation of regional myocardial blood flow by intra-aortic balloon counterpulsation in patients with unstable angina. Circulation 68:117–123, 1983.
77. Taylor KM, Bain WH, Davidson KG, et al: Comparative clinical study of pulsatile and nonpulsatile perfusion in 350 consecutive patients. Thorax 37:324–330, 1982.
78. Hickey PR, Buckely MJ, Philbin DM: Pulsatile and nonpulsatile cardiopulmonary bypass: Review of a counterproductive controversy. Ann Thorac Surg 36:720, 1983.
79. Mulay AV, Hansbro SD, Catchpole RW, et al: Should intra-aortic balloon counterpulsation be coninued during cardiopulmonary bypass? J Thor Cardiovasc Surg 114:1128–1129, 1997.
80. Skinner JR, Phillips SJ, Zeff RH, et al: Immediate coronary bypass following failed streptokinase infusion in evolving MI . J Thorac Cardiovasc Surg 87:567–570, 1984.
81. Fremes SE, Goldman BS, Weisel RD, et al: Recent pre-operative MI increases the risk of surgery for unstable angina. J Card Surg 6: 2–12, 1991.
82. Kinch JW, Ryan TJ: Right ventricular infarction. N Engl J Med 330:1211–1217, 1994.
83. Zehender M, Kasper W, Kauder E, et al: Right ventricular infarction as an independent predictor of prognosis after acute inferior MI. N Engl J Med 328:981–988, 1993.
84. Rich JB, Akins CW, Daggett WM: Right ventricular failure following cardiopulmonary bypass: Inadequate myocardial protection or incomplete revascularization? Ann Thorac Surg 45:693–696, 1988.
85. Zeff RH, Kongtahworn C, Iannone LA, et al: Internal mammary artery versus saphenous vein graft to the left anterior descending coronary artery: Prospective randomized study with ten year follow-up. Ann Thorac Surg 45:533–536, 1988.

86. Edwards F, Clark R, Schwartz M: Impact of internal mammary artery conduits on operative mortality and coronary revascularization. Ann Thorac Surg 57:27–32, 1994.

87. Vinten-Johansen J, Buckberg GD, Okamoto F, et al: Studies of controlled reperfusion after ischemia. V: Superiority of surgical versus medical reperfusion after regional ischemia. J Thorac Cardiovasc Surg 92:525–534, 1986.

88. Lazar HL, Buckberg GD, Manganara AM, et al: Myocardial energy replenishment in reversible ischemic damage by substrate enhancement of secondary blood cardioplegia with amino acids during reperfusion. J Thorac Cardiovasc Surg80:350–359, 1980.

89. Quillen J, Kofsk, ER, Buckberg GD, et al: Studies of controlled reperfusion after ischemia. XXII: Deleterious effects of simulated thrombolysis preceding simulated coronary artery bypass grafting with controlled blood cardioplegic reperfusion. J Thorac Cardiovasc Surg 101:455–464, 1991.

90. Cheung EH, Arcidi JM Jr, Dorothy LM, et al: Reperfusion of infarcting myocardium: Benefit of surgical reperfusion in a chronic model. Ann Thoracic Surg 48:331–338, 1989.

91. Miller PF, Brodie BR, Weintraub RA, et al: Emergency coronary angioplasty for acute MI. Results from a community hospital. Arch Intern Med 147:1565–1570, 1987.

92. Sanborn TA, Sleeper LA, Webb JG, et al: Impact of thrombolysis, aortic contrapulsation, and their combination in cardiogenic shock: The SHOCK trial registry. Circulation 98(Suppl I):I-778, 1998 [abstract].

93. Metangi, MF, Neutze, JM, Graham, KJ, et al: Arrythmia prophylaxis after aortocoronary bypass. J Thorac Cardiovasc Surg 89:439–443, 1985.

94. Rodgers WJ, Hood WP, Mantle JA, et al: Return of left ventricular function after reperfusion in patients with MI: Importance of subtotal stenosis or intact collaterals. Circulation 69:338–349, 1984.

95. Dawson JT, Hall RJ, Hallman GL, et al: Mortality in patients undergoing coronary artery bypass surgery after MI. Am J Cardiol 33:483–486, 1974.

96. Lee JH, Murrell HK, Strony J, et al: Risk analysis of coronary bypass surgery after acute MI. Surgery 122: 675–681, 1997.

97. Roberts CS, Schoen FJ, Kloner RA: Effects of coronary reperfusion on myocardial hemorrhage and infarct healing. Am J Cardiol 52:610–614, 1983.

98. Nunley DL, Grunkemeier GL, Teply JF, et al: Coronary bypass operation following acute complicated MI. J Thorac Cardiovasc Surg 85:485–491, 1983.

99. Creswell LL, Moulton MJ, Cox JL, et al: Revascularization after acute MI. Ann Thorac Surg 60:19–26, 1995.

100. Braunwald E: Myocardial reperfusion, limitation of infarct size, reduction of left ventricular dysfunction and improved survival. Should the paradigm be expanded? Circulation 79:441–444, 1999.

101. Alhaddad IA, Kloner RA, Hakim I, et al: Benefits of late coronary artery reperfusion on infarct expansion progressively diminish over time: Relation to viable eyelets of myocytes within the scar. Am Heart J 131:451–457, 1996.

102. Every NR, Maynard C, Cochran RP, et al: Characteristics, management, and outcome of patients with acute MI treated with bypass surgery: MI triage and intervention investigators. Circulation 94(Suppl II):81–86, 1996.

103. Applebaum R, House R, Rademaker A, et al: Coronary artery bypass grafting within 30 days of acute MI. J Thorac Cardiovasc Surg 102: 745–752, 1991.

104. Mohr R, Moshkovitch Y, Shapira I, et al: Coronary artery bypass without cardiopulmonary bypass for patients with acute MI. J Thorac Cardiovasc Surg 118:50–56, 1999.

105. VanHaecke J, Flaming W, Sergeant P, et al: Emergency bypass surgery: Late effects on size of infarction and ventricular function. Circulation 72(Suppl II):179–184, 1985.

106. Goldberg RJ, Gore JM, Alpert J, et al: Cardiogenic shock, acute MI: Incident and mortality from a community-wide perspective, 1975–1988. N Engl J Med 325:1117–1122, 1991.

107. Menon V, Hochman JS, Holmes D, et al: Lack of progress in cardiogenic shock. Lessons from the GUSTO trials. J Am Coll Cardiol 31:1057–1127, 1998.

108. Brodie B, Stuckey T, Weintraub R, et al: Timing and mechanism of death after direct angioplasty for acute MI. J Am Coll Cardiol 25:295a–296a, 1995.

109. Pifarre R, Spinazzola A, Nemickas R, et al: Emergency aortocoronary bypass for acute myocardial infarction. Arch Surg 103: 525–528, 1971.

Anesthetic Considerations for Patients with Acute Myocardial Infarction Undergoing Cardiac Surgery

WILLIAM C. OLIVER, JR., MD

GREGORY A. NUTTALL, MD

MARK H. ERETH, MD

Patients with acute coronary syndromes (ACS) may undergo revascularization within the first month of the episode to reperfuse occluded coronary arteries. Revascularization may improve ventricular function, reduce the risk of recurrent myocardial infarction (MI) or ischemia, and improve survival rates.[1] Revascularization for ACS includes one or some combination of thrombolysis, percutaneous transluminal coronary angioplasty (PTCA), or coronary artery bypass grafting (CABG). CABG has been infrequent since the early 1970s, but with the current approach to acute MI its frequency is increasing (Fig.1). In a large multicenter trial of thrombolytic therapy, 58% of patients were revascularized—27% with CABG and 73% with PTCA.[2] Three indications for CABG with ACS include (1) failed thrombolysis and PTCA, (2) severe three-vessel coronary artery disease (CAD) or left main disease; and (3) postinfarction angina. CABG is performed within 24 hours of MI, but more patients undergo CABG 1–2 weeks after acute MI. CABG is now performed successfully without cardiopulmonary bypass (CPB) in patients with cardiogenic shock.[3]

Because CABG is rarely the initial therapy for reperfusion after MI, patients may present for surgery with severe three-vessel CAD or left main artery disease after emergency angiogram and failed PTCA. They are at increased risk for morbidity and mortality compared with patients who undergo elective CABG.[4] Mortality rates depend on hemodynamics, timing of CABG, and left ventricular (LV) function.[5] Postinfarction angina is a serious risk factor. Because of improvements in anesthesia, surgical technique, and myocardial protection, the mortality rate has dropped to 2–6% for CABG following ACS.[6] Anesthetic management of patients undergoing CABG encompasses a wide range of clinical situations. Each interval—before, after, and during CPB—has

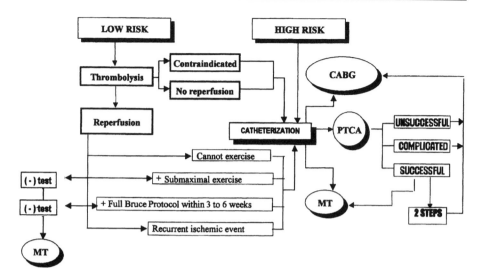

Figure 1.   Present approach to acute myocardial infarction. MT = medical therapy, PTCA = percutaneous transluminal coronary angioplasty, CABG = coronary artery bypass grafting.

specific concerns that influence anesthetic management. This chapter review these anesthetic considerations.

Preoperative Evaluation

Patient characteristics, hemodynamics, operative risk, and timing of surgery vary greatly among patients undergoing CABG with ACS. A comprehensive, preanesthetic evaluation depends to a degree on the urgency of surgery. Contrary to routine preoperative anesthetic evaluation, which focuses mainly on prevention and correction of conditions that may affect the patient intraoperatively, evaluation for urgent surgery focuses on information that will prepare the anesthetist for the most likely intraoperative situations. Time for evaluation often is limited to restrict the interval from onset of MI until CABG to less than 6 hours.

Knowledge of risk factors that predict postoperative morbidity and mortality assists in the preanesthesia evaluation. Surprisingly, risk factors for CABG after ACS are similar to those for elective CABG.[7,8] The most important determinants of risk include cardiogenic shock, preoperative intra-aortic balloon pump (IABP), MI within 21 days, emergency operation, pulmonary disease, and diabetes mellitus (DM). These risk factors are derived from the Society of Thoracic Surgeons database of more than 80,000 CABGs performed during 1980–1990.[8] Other important risk factors in regardto anesthesia include previous sternotomy, gender, small size, advanced age, and poor LV function.[9] DM is particularly important because it is an independent predictor of mortality in patients having CABG.[10] Renal function also should be assessed carefully and monitored if DM is present.

Risk may be estimated quickly with a weighted score derived from an analysis of preoperative risk factors associated with morbidity after CABG[11] (Table 1). The risk factors are creatinine (>1.2 mg/dl), age (> 70 yr), body mass index

Table 1. Short Manual Model with Seven Risk Factors

Variable	Negative	Positive	Weight
Creatinine (μmol/L)	≤ 110*	≥ 111	2
Age (yr)	≤ 69	≥ 70	1
Body mass index	≤ 27	≥ 28	1
Diabetes	No	Yes	2
Emergency operation	No	Yes	2
Abnormal electrocardiogram	No	Yes	1
Lung disease	No	Yes	1

* 110 μmol/L = 1.2 mg/dl.
From Kurki TSO, Kataja M: Preoperative prediction of postoperative morbidity in coronary artery bypass grafting. Ann Thorac Surg 61:1740–1745, 1996, with permission.

(>28), DM, emergency surgery, abnormal electrocardiogram, and severe obstructive pulmonary disease.[11] This method of risk assessment may be more valuable for the anesthesiologist because it represents short-term morbidity in patients having CABG. It is a crude assessment of the patient's anesthesia risk.

Other cardiac-related factors that influence the risk of CABG include previous MI, congestive heart failure, and arrhythmias. Previous MI is a risk factor for postoperative MI.[12] An echocardiogram after diagnosis of ACS helps to identify the newly infarcted myocardium and the condition of the remaining myocardium.[13] Preoperative congestive heart failure is an undisputed risk factor for surgery.[12] The importance of MI and congestive heart failure to anesthesia risk is probably related to depressed LV function as a major risk factor for surgery.[9] Although arrhythmias may influence the prognosis of a patient with congestive heart failure and CAD, the anesthetic significance is still unclear.

Because CABG with ACS is often an emergency, smoking is a serious anesthetic risk factor. Normally, abstinence from smoking for 4–6 weeks is recommended to ensure pulmonary benefit, but cessation of smoking even for 12–24 hours has cardiovascular advantages. The direct effects of coronary vasoconstriction and indirect effects of hypoxemia and carboxyhemoglobin (COHb) formation increase cardiac morbidity.[14] COHb is detrimental because it reduces the available hemoglobin to bind with oxygen. As a result, oxygen content is reduced, and the oxygen dissociation curve shifts to the left so that oxygen also dissociates less readily from hemoglobin. Because of its high oxygen extraction ratio, myocardium is sensitive to minimal amounts of COHb.

Preoperative assessment of the risk of excessive bleeding is important because it influences the morbidity and mortality of cardiac surgery.[15] Patients having CABG after ACS are at high risk for excessive bleeding because of the likelihood of exposure to heparin, thrombolytic agents, aspirin, thienopyridines, and glycoprotein (GP) IIb/IIIa platelet receptor antagonists.[16] Because GPIIb/IIIa platelet receptor antagonists affect platelet activity at the end of the clotting cascade, they increase the risk of excessive bleeding after CPB. Thienopyridines (ticlopidine, clopidogrel) inhibit platelet aggregation for the duration of the platelet's life by blocking ADP receptors. Thrombolysis before CABG also is associated with increased postoperative bleeding (Fig. 2) and transfusion[17] (Table 2). Significantly more packed red blood cells and fresh frozen plasma, and ten times the amount of cryoprecipitate are required in patients who have had thrombolysis before CABG. Even if a thrombolytic infusion is brief in duration,

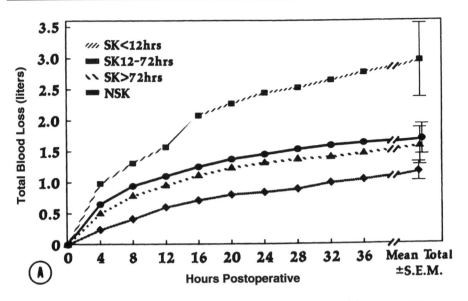

Figure 2. Cumulative postoperative blood loss (mean ± standard error of the mean). NSK = non-streptokinase, SK < 12 = early operation within 12 hrs of streptokinase administration, SK 12–72 = delayed operation between 12 and 72 hr of streptokinase administration, SK > 72 = late operation more than 72 hr after streptokinase administration.

coagulopathy may persist for 24 hours. However, if a thrombolytic infusion is stopped more than 12 hours before CABG, bleeding, transfusion requirements, morbidity, and mortality are significantly less than if the infusion is stopped less than 12 hours before CABG. A delay in the surgery should be considered if thrombolysis for ACS has not been discontinued for 12 hours.

Monitoring

Monitoring before induction of anesthesia depends on hemodynamic stability and surgical urgency. Beyond routine monitoring for general anesthesia, an arte-

Table 2.   Postoperative Coagulation Parameters, Total Blood Loss, and Total Blood Product Use

	NSK	SK < 12	SK 12–72	SK > 72
Total blood loss (ml)*	1174 ± 148	2957 ± 595	1678 ± 244	1585 ± 300
Total blood product use (ml)				
Packed red blood cells	897 ± 158	2756 ± 847[†]	1776 ± 244	558 ± 145
Fresh frozen plasma	856 ± 162	1886 ± 359[‡]	1019 ± 381	704 ± 222
Cryoprecipitate	18 ± 13	194 ± 28	63 ≠ 36	74 ± 25
Platelets	99 ± 47	294 ± 103	253 ± 109	72 ± 50

NSK = no streptokinase, SK < 12 = surgery within 12 hr after streptokinase, SK 12–72 = surgery within 12–72 hr after streptokinase, SK > 72 = surgery after more than 72 hr since streptokinase.
[†] $p < 0.001$
[‡] $p < 0.05$

From Lee KF, Mandell J, Rankin JS, et al: Immediate versus delayed coronary grafting after streptokinase treatment: Postoperative blood loss and clinical results. J Thorac Cardiovasc Surg 95:216–222, 1988, with permission.

rial catheter should be inserted for continuous blood pressure (BP) and arterial blood gas (ABG) determination. Although the radial artery is the cannulation site usually chosen for cardiac surgery, a clinically significant gradient between the central aortic and radial pressure begins to develop early during CPB.[18] This gradient often reaches 35 mmHg and may persist well beyond CPB despite changes in systemic vascular resistance (Fig. 3). A femoral artery catheter for BP monitoring usually approximates central aortic pressure even upon separation from CPB. A radial or femoral indwelling catheter may be inserted under local anesthesia without difficulty or much patient discomfort. Femoral catheters are not associated with increased infection or complications, as previously believed, because of the size of the catheters now used and meticulous site care. Frezza et al.[19] found no difference in the incidence of complications or infection in over 4900 patients who received either femoral or radial artery catheters in the intensive care unit (ICU). A femoral artery catheter was even preferred over a radial artery catheter in patients requiring longer hospitalization.[19]

A pulmonary artery catheter (PAC) may be placed before CABG if the patient is in cardiogenic shock (2–10% of cases).[7] The benefit and timing of PAC insertion in cardiac surgical patients are unclear. In many institutions, a PAC is routine for patients having CABG.[20] PAC was justified on the basis of being a sensitive indicator of myocardial ischemia.[21] It is no longer recognized as such, even if the waveform is abnormal or the pulmonary capillary wedge pressure (PCWP) is elevated. Leung et al.[22] found that less than 10% of all ischemic episodes identified by transesophageal echocardiography (TEE) were preceded by a change in pulmonary artery diastolic pressure. At present, cardiac index (CI) determination alone may justify a PAC until a more reliable and accurate noninvasive monitor is available. Measurement of CI and PCWP may be helpful for patients with early signs of LV deterioration and cardiogenic shock.[13] However, a PAC may mislead the clinician about volume status as well as LV function after CABG. Such errors may be particularly detrimental (Fig. 4). Both false negative and false positives have occurred with assessment of ventricular

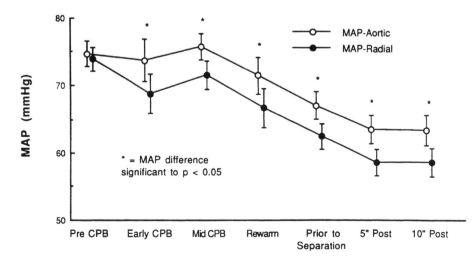

Figure 3. Comparison of the mean aortic and mean radial artery pressures associated with cardiopulmonary bypass (mean ± SEM). SEM = standard error of the mean.

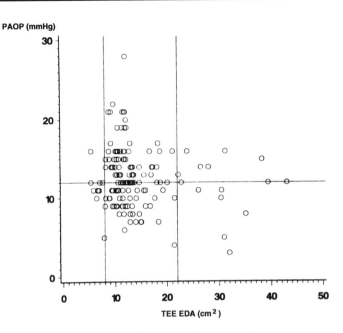

Figure 4.   Measurement of preload by echocardiography and pulmonary artery catheter occlusion pressures (PAOP). Vertical lines identify normal end-diastolic area (EDA). Preload estimated by PAOP is highly influenced by ventricular compliance; for the same pressure, the ventricular dimension can vary considerably (horizontal line). Consequently, a poor correlation (r = 0.541) is found between ventricular EDA and PAOP.

function. Fontes et al.[23] examined ventricular function and management in the ICU after CABG to analyze the accuracy of the PAC in critically ill patients. The PAC in patients with an ejection fraction (EF) below 40% misdiagnosed all nine cases of ventricular dysfunction, even though the CI may have been adequate. The value of the PAC to identify early LV dysfunction is uncertain; however, hemodynamic variables obtained from the PAC may provide benefit beyond only hemodynamic guidance. Reich et al.[10] performed a retrospective analysis of detailed hemodynamic data in 2152 patients having CABG at two hospitals over 2 years. Outcomes were analyzed, and hemodynamic data were obtained from computerized anesthesia records, in which hemodynamic variables were entered every 15 seconds. Indices of poor LV function, including elevated mean pulmonary artery pressures, heart rate after CPB, and diastolic pulmonary artery pressure after CPB, predicted increased mortality and poor outcome. This information may some day allow for improved utilization of health care resources.

To determine the value of a PAC in patients undergoing CABG, Tuman et al.[20] prospectively examined 1094 consecutive patients undergoing elective CABG with either PAC or central venous catheter (CVC). Although type of catheter did not affect mortality or morbidity, patients were not randomized to type of catheter and physicians were not restricted to management with only one type. Seven percent of patients scheduled for CVC required PAC in the opinion of the managing anesthesiologist. It is possible to insert a CVC at the beginning of a case and later replace it with a PAC without increasing morbidity, even in higher-risk patients.[20] Recently, the American Society of Anesthesiologists (ASA) formed a task force to determine practice guidelines for insertion of a PAC.[24]

Patients with ACS and impending CABG satisfy ASA criteria for PAC monitoring based on likelihood of hemodynamic disturbances, severe associated disease,[24] and clinical recommendations.[13]

If a PAC is not present before surgery, the benefit of placing it with local anesthesia and sedation before induction of general anesthesia is questionable, particularly if an IABP is present. Much of the information that is useful for induction of anesthesia is available from cardiac catheterization or preoperative echocardiography. Although there is a relatively low incidence of morbidity with PAC insertion, insertion of a PAC in a conscious patient may cause sympathetic stimulation and myocardial ischemia.[25] Sedation for PAC placement may cause hypercarbia and hypoxia, placing the patient with reduced cardiovascular reserve at greater risk.[25] It may be safer to induce anesthesia and secure the airway before PAC insertion.

Most patients with ACS undergoing CABG have some venous access, but central venous monitoring and access are necessary. Low CI and anticoagulation increase the chance of serious complications, such as puncture or large-bore catheter insertion into the carotid artery with attempted central venous cannulation.[16] The incidence of carotid puncture alone varies between 1% and 10%; arterial cannulation occurs in 0.1–0.5% of cases.[26] Jobes et al.[27] reported that 5 of 43 patients who sustained a punctured carotid artery during central venous cannulation also had large-bore catheter insertion. One patient died from surgical delay and the other from hemorrhage. Surgery was postponed for 2 hours to 13 days in 3 patients.

Several measures can reduce the incidence of carotid puncture and cannulation. An external jugular vein may be used for insertion that avoids the carotid artery, but it has a lower success rate for flotation to the pulmonary artery. Ultrasound is useful to locate and guide cannulation of the internal jugular vein. Its use increases the success rate and reduces carotid artery puncture in comparison with conventional methods of visual and palpable landmarks for central vein cannulation.[28] If an ultrasound device is not available, another technique involves continuous monitoring of the pressure in the cannulation needle (Fig. 5) to detect carotid puncture and reduce large-bore cannulation of the carotid artery[26] (Fig. 6).

Additional monitoring for CABG after ACS may include TEE after induction of anesthesia and intubation. The value of TEE is established for valvular surgery but not for CABG. The earliest indicator of myocardial ischemia is regional wall motion abnormalities (RWMA), but they also may be due to other causes.[22] TEE may be useful to direct and confirm many intraoperative clinical decisions[29] (Table 3). Fluid administration and ischemia therapy are the most common interventions guided by TEE during CABG (Fig. 7). Anesthesiologists estimate global function with TEE more effectively than by attempting discriminate RWMA in a dysfunctional ventricle.

Airway Assessment

If the patient comes to the operating room with a tracheal tube in place, bilateral breath sounds are confirmed and appropriate ventilator settings are established before induction of anesthesia. Some patients may require emergency intubation for pulmonary edema or severe hemodynamic instability. ABGs should be drawn immediately after intubation to determine arterial oxygenation, carbon dioxide, and acid–base status.

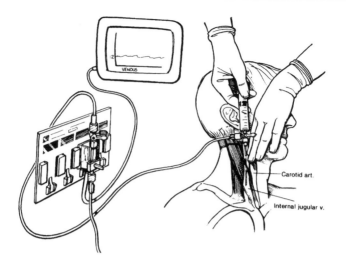

Figure 5.   The apparatus for pressure monitoring the needle used for central venous cannulation. The steel needle does not kink in the vessel like a Teflon catheter. Kinking may lead to an erroneous conclusion about the vessel entered.

The patient who is not intubated should be is evaluated for potential difficulty with ventilation and/or intubation. Difficulties in laryngoscopy may occur in 5–10%[30,31] of patients with general anesthesia, but poor intubating conditions and inability to achieve adequate mask ventilation occur in only 1% and 0.07% of patients, respectively.[30] Anatomic characteristics of the airway are sensitive but not specific for predicting difficult intubation. Visualization of the soft palate alone and short distance from larynx to the mandible identify many patients who may be difficult to intubate, but in nearly 50% of these cases, intubation is easy.[31] Improved risk stratification for difficult intubation may be possible with the preoperative multivariate airway risk index[30] (Table 4). A simplified

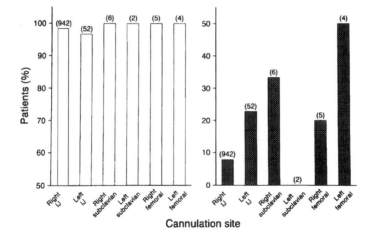

Figure 6.   Success rate *(left)* and incidence of arterial puncture *(right)* associated with central venous cannulation at certain sites. IJ = internal jugular vein; ( ) = number of patients.

Table 3. Comparison of Transesophageal Echocardiography
with Other Intraoperative Monitors*

Type of Interventions	TEE (n)	Arterial Catheter (n)	Pulmonary Artery Catheter (n)	EKG (n)	Other[†]
Fluid bolus	82	44	20	0	131
Vasopressors	4	73	7	1	30
Change in anesthetic depth	1	56	1	0	14
Anti-ischemic therapy	8	4	1	18	7
Vasodilator therapy	1	29	2	2	4
Antiarrhythmic therapy	0	0	0	14	2
Surgical intervention	2	2	0	6	4
Miscellaneous	0	6	0	0	8
Total	98	214	31	41	200

EKG = electrocardiography.
* This table illustrates the number of times that the most influential monitor contributed to each type
of intervention. The interventions were described in Table 1.
† "Other" indicates that the interventions were not based on information from any of the four monitors
examined. More than 50% of these interventions were transfusion of either pump blood or bank
blood for low hematocrit; others include administering volume to increase preload at the time of
separation from bypass.
From Berquist BD, Bellows WH, Leung JM: Transesophageal echocardiography in myocardial
resvascularizations. II: Influence on intraoperative decision making. Anesth Analg 82:1139–1145,
1996, with permission.

airway risk index score of 0 or 1 is rarely associated with difficult intubation.
Availability of a laryngeal mask airway may prevent morbidity and mortality in
patients with a difficult mask ventilation or failed intubation[32] (Fig. 8).

Because CABG after ACS is often an emergency, patients have not fasted
properly and thus have an increased risk of regurgitation with induction of
anesthesia. The risk of aspiration is increased further in patients with DM,

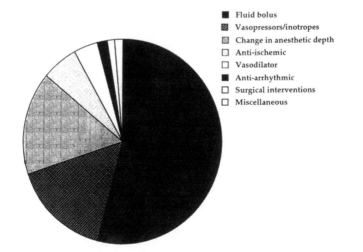

■ Fluid bolus
▨ Vasopressors/inotropes
▨ Change in anesthetic depth
☐ Anti-ischemic
☐ Vasodilator
■ Anti-arrhythmic
☐ Surgical interventions
☐ Miscellaneous

Figure 7. Clinical interventions in which transesophageal echocardiography was deemed to be
"supportive." Fluid bolus administration, vasopressor and inotropic therapy, and changes in anesthetic
depth accounted for most of the interventions.

Table 4.   Multivariate Predictors of Difficult Intubation

Variable	Simplified Airway Risk Index Weighing
Mouth opening	
4 cm	0
< 4 cm	1
Thyromental distance	
> 6.5 cm	0
6.0–6.5 cm	1
> 6.0	2
Mallampati class	
I	0
2	1
3	2
Neck movement	
> 90°	0
80–90°	1
< 80°	2
Ability to prognath	
Yes	0
No	1
Body weight	
< 90 kg	0
90–100 kg	1
> 110 kg	2
History of difficult intubation	
None	0
Questionable	1
Definite	2

From El-Ganzouri AR, McCarthy RJ,Tuman KJ, et al: Preoperative airway assessment: Predictive value of a multivariate risk index. Anesth Analg 82:1197–1204, 1996, with permission.

hiatal hernia, or delays in gastric emptying due to medications. The two most common ways to reduce the risk of aspiration with general anesthesia are rapid-sequence induction with cricoid pressure and "awake" intubation. An "awake" intubation requires upper pharyngeal anesthesia and insertion of the laryngoscope or fiberoptic with little or no sedation. It may result in dangerous tachycardia, hypertension, and arrhythmias. Any level of sedation for either a fiberoptic or laryngoscopic intubation places the patient at risk for aspiration. If the airway appears to be easy to manually ventilate and intubate, a rapid-sequence induction is the most common and expeditious option. Rapid-sequence induction requires cricoid pressure, rapid muscle paralysis (often with succinylcholine), and intravenous administration of anesthetic medications to minimize the time to intubation. Unfortunately, it often is associated with significant hypotension. Patients with marginal hemodynamics may develop profound hemodynamic disturbances. In patients with ACS undergoing CABG, aspiration may be less of a threat than severe hypotension. In a retrospective review of over 150,000 anesthetics, aspiration occurred in only 0.11% of emergency surgical procedures.[33] A reasonable approach to maximize protection for both airway and hemodynamics is a more deliberate induction of anesthesia with routine cardiac medications and maintenance of cricoid pressure. This technique does not provide the same protection against aspiration as rapid-sequence induction with cricoid pressure but may reduce the incidence and severity of hypotension.

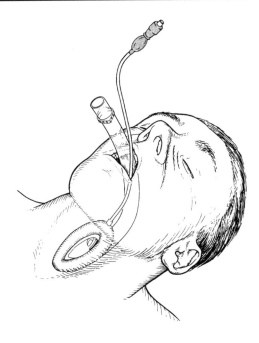

Figure 8. The laryngeal mask airway is inserted blindly into the pharynx. A low-pressure seal is created around the laryngeal inlet to allow positive-pressure ventilation. The laryngeal mask airway does not protect the airway from aspiration. It also may be used as a guide for introduction of a fiberoptic bronchoscope to aid in intubation of a difficult airway.

Induction and Maintenance of Anesthesia

Many authorities consider the period before CPB as the most crucial period of cardiac anesthesia.[34] A poorly managed pre-CPB period may greatly affect outcome.[35] Hemodynamic stability and control of the airway are particularly critical during induction of anesthesia in patients with ACS undergoing CABG.

In general, patients are now older, have more associated diseases, and are more likely to have had CABG, PTCA, or both prior to CABG. Consequently, induction of anesthesia is more likely to cause hemodynamic instability. The diminished response to catecholamines in older patients increases the risk of severe hypotension. If an IABP has not been inserted before induction of anesthesia, it should be considered. IABP before induction of anesthesia significantly improves CI in high-risk patients undergoing CABG.[36] Pre-CPB insertion of IABP reduces the amount of ischemic myocardium before placement of the aortic cross-clamp. If the IABP is present for only 2 hours before CPB, the benefit is similar to placement of IABP 24 hours preoperatively. Waiting to place an IABP after separation from CPB may lead to increased complications, a significantly longer stay in the ICU, and greater duration of mechanical ventilation compared with pre-CPB insertion.[36] In addition, the surgical team should be present and ready to respond, if necessary, with rapid institution of CPB, either by sternotomy or femoral approach, after induction of anesthesia.

A major consideration for induction of anesthesia in patients with ACS is the degree of LV dysfunction. LV dysfunction is one of the major factors determining outcome in patients undergoing CABG.[37] If LV function is relatively good, induction and intubation may produce a significant sympathetic response, resulting in excessive tachycardia, hypertension, and myocardial ischemia. If LV function is poor, hemodynamic status may deteriorate rapidly. The extreme of poor LV function is the occurrence of cardiogenic shock, which is the leading cause of death for patients with ACS and occurs in about 7% of MIs with a mortality rate of 80%.[38] The choice and rate of delivery of medications for induction of anesthesia are critical for patients with impaired myocardium or cardiogenic shock.

The occurrence of ischemia with induction of anesthesia is also a concern. Kleinman et al.[39] studied 22 patients with good LV function undergoing elective CABG. Thallium-201 scans were used to determine the occurrence of ischemia during induction with either thiopental/halothane or the narcotic fentanyl. Although no difference in HR, BP, rate-pressure product, PCWP, CI, or ST changes was found between the two groups, 45% of patients developed evidence of myocardial perfusion defects and ischemia, suggesting a lack of myocardial supply rather than increased demand. This theory is supported by the fact that the intraoperative ischemic pattern during CABG is no worse than the patient's preoperative pattern.[40]

Medications for Induction and Maintenance of Anesthesia

Because some authorities have labeled certain anesthetic techniques as "best," Tuman et al.[41] prospectively studied 1094 primarily "high-risk" patients undergoing CABG. One of five anesthetic regimens was administered: (1) high or (2) moderate doses of fentanyl, (3) sufentanil, (4) diazepam with ketamine, or (5) halothane (0.5–2.5% inspired concentration after thiopental induction). Diazepam with ketamine was supplemented with a volatile secondary anesthetic, such as isoflurane. There was no difference among the five regimens in occurrence of low CI; postoperative MI; serious pulmonary, renal, or neurologic morbidity; or death. There was also no difference in outcome variables among the intravenous anesthetic groups, with or without a volatile agent. The study failed to demonstrate a difference between volatile and narcotic anesthetic techniques. An anesthetic agent associated with a better physiologic profile does not inevitably improve outcome. However, Tuman et al.[41] acknowledge that in certain subsets of patients, anesthetic agents may modulate specific perioperative factors that influence outcome. A thorough knowledge of the actions of anesthetic medications for induction and rigid control of hemodynamics and ischemia is probably more important than the *choice* of anesthetic agents in relationship to the outcome of CABG.[41]

High-dose narcotics were popularized in the late 1970s as the anesthetic of choice for cardiac surgery based on the maintenance of "hemodynamic stability." Lack of histamine release (as seen with morphine) and its pharmacokinetic profile rapidly made fentanyl the drug of choice for narcotic induction and maintenance of anesthesia for cardiac surgery. For induction of anesthesia in patients having CABG with poor LV function (EF < 0.3 and left ventricular end- diastolic pressure > 20 mmHg), fentanyl (30 μg/kg) provided sufficient anesthesia with good hemodynamics.[42] In another study including patients with New York Heart Association (NYHA) class III and IV LV impairment, fentanyl induction (50 μg/kg) decreased systolic BP by only 17%.[43] Fentanyl is not a myocardial depressant but may depress the myocardium if administered with other anesthetic agents.

Other agents that may be used for induction of anesthesia with excellent hemodynamic stability are ketamine (0.1–0.3 mg/kg) and etomidate (0.1–0.3 mg/kg). Although ketamine has been criticized for use in patients undergoing CABG, it strongly attenuates the stress response and maintains BP.[44] Ketamine may increase heart rate and cause delirium, but these effects are blunted or eliminated by the administration of fentanyl and a benzodiazepine.[44] Etomidate and a low-dose narcotic cause minimal myocardial depression. Etomidate is a particularly good choice for diabetic patients because autonomic dysfunction may result in unstable hemodynamics during anesthesia. Propofol, a new agent with a very short half-life, has rarely been used for anesthetic induction during CABG. It may decrease BP by 20–40% during induction in cardiac patients but provides good hemodynamics as a continuous infusion.[45] Patients awaken rapidly after propofol is discontinued, but it has no analgesic properties. Analgesia must be provided while the patient is unconscious. Severe pain in the ICU may precipitate myocardial ischemia.

Another major concern during induction and maintenance of anesthesia is the prevention of myocardial ischemia. Previously, three major goals of anesthetic technique were to minimize perioperative stress, to maintain low myocardial oxygen demand, and to ensure high myocardial oxygen supply. High-dose fentanyl (150 µg/kg) was believed to achieve all three goals. However, some patients developed tachycardia and hypertension as well as intraoperative awareness because a narcotic is not a total anesthetic.[46] Subsequently, other agents were added, such as benzodiazepines and volatile agents (with or without nitrous oxide).

The benefit of a volatile agent for anesthesia is its rapid elimination compared with most other intravenous anesthetics. Volatile agents help to control hypertensive responses as well as reduce the total requirement of narcotics and benzodiazepines.[46] In a double-blind trial comparing a narcotic anesthetic alone with the combination of a narcotic and volatile agent, hemodynamics were best maintained by the combination.[46] Volatile anesthetics are effective as *adjunctive or primary* anesthetic agents for CABG.

Volatile anesthetics depress the contractile state of the normal human myocardium.[47] They need to be administered carefully to patients with ACS and decreased LV function because myocardial depression is dose-dependent. However, Lowenstein et al.[48] reported good hemodynamics even with the addition of a volatile agent if less than 25% of the myocardium is ischemic. Hemodynamic stability is also evident in a dog model of MI followed by volatile anesthesia 7–10 days later. Hemodynamic parameters in dogs were essentially unaffected, including LV dp/dt and left ventricular end-diastolic pressure.[49] Volatile agents are myocardial depressants clinically only at higher concentrations. Two new volatile agents, desflurane and sevoflurane, may result in less myocardial depression than halothane or even isoflurane.

Coronary steal is a concern for patients undergoing CABG with volatile anesthetic agents. Coronary steal (Fig. 9) causing myocardial ischemia is rare because 80–90% of patients with CAD do not have "steal-prone" coronary anatomy.[50] The most commonly used volatile agent, isoflurane, is a coronary vasodilator of distal coronary arterioles.[51] Slogoff and Keats[52] studied isoflurane in a prospective randomized trial as the primary or secondary anesthetic in over 1000 patients undergoing CABG. They found no evidence of an increase in new myocardial ischemia, postoperative MI, or mortality in comparison with other volatile agents or other commonly used anesthetics.

Isoflurane is safe in most patients undergoing CABG. A newer agent, sevoflurane, although similar to isoflurane, has more rapid uptake and shorter duration of action, but its potent direct coronary vasodilation does not induce coronary steal.[53] There is no difference between isoflurane and sevoflurane in incidence of myocardial ischemia in patients with severe CAD.[54] The hemodynamic profile of

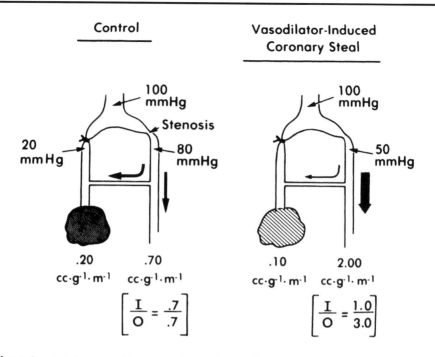

Control

Vasodilator-Induced Coronary Steal

Figure 9.   Arteriolar vasodilator-induced steal. During the control state, the collateral flow to the underperfused area distal to the obstruction is determined by the pressure gradient between the collateral supplying artery (80 mmHg) and the vascular bed distal to the obstruction (20 mmHg). At rest, the proximal stenosis of the supply artery results in an insignificant distal pressure drop (100–80 mmHg). Following distal coronary vasodilation, flow to the normally perfused area increases significantly. The significant change in the gradient from 100 to 50 mmHg is due to vasodilation, which reduces the flow across the collateral vessel and subsequently to the already underperfused area.

sevoflurane is similar to that of isoflurane. A BP decrease of at least 20% from baseline may occur with either agent in patients undergoing CABG. A decrease in BP reduces flow beyond distal coronary obstructions secondary to reduced coronary perfusion pressure.[41] Desflurane, another volatile agent with a short duration of action, is also available. It is not recommended for patients undergoing CABG, particularly those with hemodynamic instability.[55] In comparison with sufentanil, desflurane was associated with more hypotension, tachycardia, and myocardial ischemia before CPB, but there was no difference in adverse cardiac outcomes.[55]

A volatile agent may be administered with or without nitrous oxide during cardiac surgery. The use of nitrous oxide in cardiac surgery has been disparaged on the basis of previous studies of its effect on coronary circulation and myocardial function.[56,57] Direct effects of nitrous oxide on coronary tone, resulting in myocardial ischemia and decreased function, have been disputed.[57] Cahalan et al.[58] administered nitrous oxide with moderate-dose fentanyl to 18 patients with CAD and detected no ischemia. They concluded that nitrous oxide was safe as long as the patient's hemodynamic status was carefully controlled. It appears safe for patients with ACS undergoing CABG.

Muscle relaxants are necessary for cardiac surgery but may cause tachycardia and ischemia.[59] A narcotic-based anesthetic often attenuates the tachycardia. Pancuronium is one of the most commonly used muscle relaxants for cardiac surgery. It is inexpensive and effective, but because it is excreted primarily by the kidneys, it may accumulate, along with its metabolites, in patients with renal impairment. Vecuronium has no hemodynamic effects and is not affected by renal dysfunction.[60] Many of the newer, more expensive muscle relaxants (e.g., cisatracurium, doxacurium, pipecuronium) have little additional benefit compared with pancuronium but are acceptable for neuromuscular blockade during CABG.[60] Cisatracurium is not affected by renal or hepatic dysfunction or associated with histamine release, even at 8 times the normal dose.[61]

As many as 50% of patients with CAD develop ischemia during intubation.[62] Hemodynamic responses associated with intubation in patients with CAD include increases in heart rate, mean arterial pressure (MAP), and PCWP and a decrease in EF.[63] Coronary arteries respond with vasoconstriction due to the sympathetic response generated by intubation. The value of prophylactic nitroglycerin to prevent ischemia is unclear. Hart et al.[64] found a benefit using 1 µg/kg/min—a higher dose than previously reported. It is critical to maintain coronary perfusion pressure if nitroglycerin is used; otherwise its effect may be deleterious.

Considerations Before Cardiopulmonary Bypass

The period after induction of anesthesia until initiation of CPB is unpredictable for patients with ACS undergoing CABG. The incidence of pre-CPB myocardial ischemia varies from 18–45%.[39,40] Pre-CPB ischemia is important because of its apparent relationship with postoperative MI,[66] which may occur in 1–25% of CABGs, depending on the method of detection.[10,66] MI after CABG is associated with mortality rate as high as 34%.[67] Although MI after CABG is associated with various factors, it may be difficult to prevent.[10,66] Post-CABG MI is associated more closely with the technical quality of the coronary grafts and aortic cross-clamp time.[68] Postoperative ischemia is not related to postoperative MI.

Pre-CPB ischemia occurs primarily after sternotomy and aortic cannulation, but hemodynamic changes are not always evident.[66] The classic concept of myocardial oxygen supply and demand is complemented by maintenance of stable hemodynamics. However, ischemia often is not preceded by acute changes in HR, BP, or pulmonary artery diastolic pressure.[40] Knight et al.[40] evaluated 50 patients with severe CAD and 60 patients with previous MI awaiting CABG. Eighteen percent of patients developed intraoperative ischemia. Hemodynamic abnormalities at the onset of ischemia were absent in the preoperative period but present in 42% of intraoperative and 46% of postoperative episodes. Ischemia may occur with a reduction in regional coronary perfusion that reduces myocardial oxygen supply *without* increased demand (Fig.10).[22] Most episodes of intraoperative myocardial ischemia are related to factors beyond simple myocardial oxygen demand, such as thrombosis, platelet function, coronary vasomotion, and anesthetic interaction.[46] Consequently, few ischemic episodes are prevented by careful hemodynamic control, but better detection of ischemia may initiate earlier treatment.[68] Most TEE episodes of RWMA were not associated with any change in hemodynamics.[22] Only 28% of TEE changes were associated with one hemodynamic change (Fig. 11). Electrocardiographic changes were preceded by hemodynamic changes in only about 30% of cases. Lieberman et al.[69] analyzed hemodynamic variables in patients with variable LV function and pre-CPB ischemia. A systolic BP < 90 mmHg was associated with

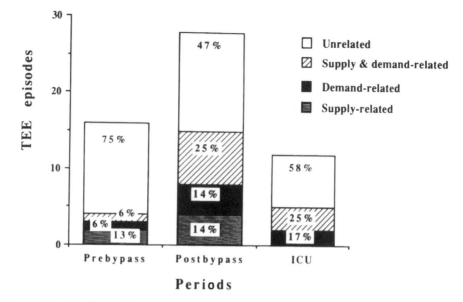

Figure 10.   Distribution of transesophageal echocardiography episodes in the pre-CPB, post-CPB, and ICU periods and their association with hemodynamic indices of supply and demand. CPB = cardiopulmonary bypass, ICU = intensive care unit.

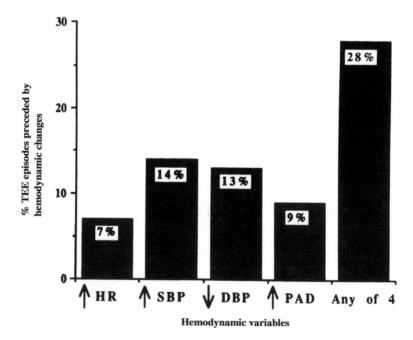

Figure 11.   Episodes of transesophageal echocardiocardiography (TEE) associated with hemodynamic changes. Hemodynamics measured at 5 or 10 minutes before the onset of TEE episodes were used as controls. TEE episodes with hemodynamic changes were preceded by increases > 20% in heart rate, systolic blood pressure, and pulmonary artery diastolic pressure or decreases > 20% in diastolic blood pressure from control values.

ischemia more often than other hemodynamic variables, such as PCWP and heart rate. Severe preoperative LV dysfunction also was more likely to be associated with ischemia. TEE may be more important in patients with impaired ventricular function because it is more sensitive as an ischemia monitoring modality than the electrocardiogram.[70] Although the benefit of intraoperative hemodynamic control and its relationship to outcome have not been firmly established, careful management is still important.

For patients with ACS undergoing CABG, cardiac arrhythmias are not a surprise, particularly with ongoing myocardial ischemia. All types of arrhythmias have been reported with myocardial ischemia. The arrhythmia is related to location of the MI. Ventricular arrhythmias and Mobitz-II heart block are associated with anterior MI. During the initial phase of ACS, the arrhythmia is more likely to have a re-entry mechanism because the myocardium is ischemic, but a previous MI has a necrotic focus that is more likely to generate an ectopic focus. Prophylaxis with antiarrhythmic agents is no longer recommended and may increase mortality in patients with ACS.[71] Procainamide is recommended in patients with malignant ventricular dysrhythmias. It is a myocardial depressant and must be used cautiously in patients with low CI. Hypomagnesemia should be treated with supplemental magnesium because it is associated with an increased incidence of ventricular and atrial dysrhythmias.[72]

Considerations During Cardiopulmonary Bypass

Once the patient is on CPB, hemodynamics are no longer a primary concern. Many patients may have had repeated episodes of myocardial ischemia, and some have developed cardiogenic shock before initiation of CPB. CPB entails a period of ischemia before the heart is revascularized, but also an opportunity to rest the heart and optimize conditions for eventual separation from CPB.

Recent evidence suggests a benefit in maintaining a MAP of 80 mmHg instead of 50 mmHg during CPB. A prospective study evaluated outcome in patients managed at a MAP of 50 mmHg vs. 80 mmHg.[73] Although the mortality rate for each group was the same at 6 months, the incidence of major cardiac and neurologic complications was 12.9% and 4.8% (p = 0.026) in the low and high MAP groups, respectively. Because patients with ACS undergoing CABG often have multisystem disease processes, a higher MAP may be beneficial.

Because of the amount of fluid required in the oxygenator to initiate CPB, hemodilution during CPB is a concern. Patients with more severe medical conditions and cardiac disease may require a greater hemoglobin concentration. An acceptable hemoglobin concentration is based on adequate oxygen delivery to all regions of the body. The myocardium is sensitive to reduced oxygen supply because of its high demand and low reserve of oxygen. During the first minute of hypothermic CPB, aortic cross-clamping, and rewarming, the myocardium is more susceptible to the effects of anemia.[74] Although hypothermia may offer some cellular protection related to reduced metabolic demand for oxygen, even with a $PaO_2 > 350$ mmHg, tissue PO_2 may be only 14 mmHg (Fig. 12). This finding suggests redistribution of blood flow. Once hypothermic CPB has been established, peripheral perfusion generally improves. As a result, blood lactate level will usually decrease. Increases in lactate levels during the rewarming period of CPB may indicate inadequate oxygen delivery (Fig. 13). Mixed venous saturation during CPB helps to assess peripheral perfusion. Hemoglobin should

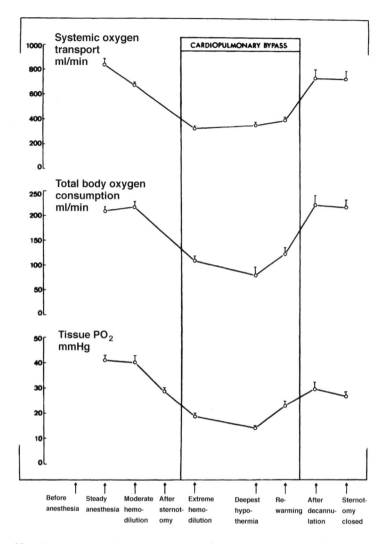

Figure 12. Tissue oxygenation in 12 patients undergoing coronary artery bypass grafting during moderate (mean HCT = 0.33) and extreme hemodilution (mean HCT = 0.16). During extreme hemodilution, the tissue PO_2 fell to a nadir of 14 mmHg. Each value indicates the mean and standard error of the mean of the 12 patients. HCT = hematocrit, PO_2 = partial pressure of oxygen.

be monitored carefully during CPB for maintenance of oxygen delivery. Because of severe anemia and concerns about oxygen delivery during CPB, oxygen demand should be minimized by muscle paralysis and continuous administration of a volatile anesthetic agent. On rewarming, ultrafiltration removes excessive fluid and increases the hemoglobin concentration. If normothermic CPB is used, the hemoglobin concentration should be maintained above 7.5 gm/dl. A higher hemoglobin concentration may be required for various reasons.

In addition to the routine amount of colloid and crystalloid during CPB, patients with ACS undergoing CABG may have been in cardiogenic shock with

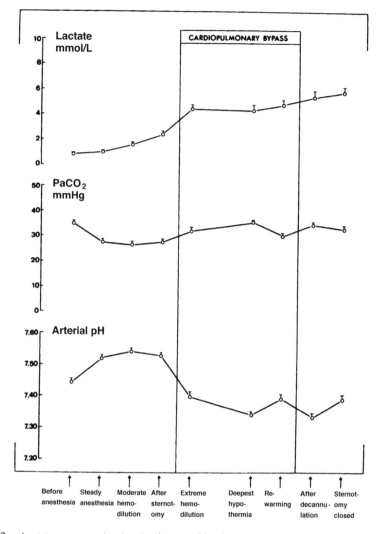

Figure 13. Lactate concentration in mixed venous blood as well as arterial blood carbon dioxide tension ($PaCO_2$) and pH for patients undergoing coronary artery bypass grafting (CABG) with moderate and extreme hemodilution. Twelve patients had CABG with severe (mean HCT + 0.16) or moderate hemodilution (mean HCT + 0.33). Each value represents the mean and standard error of the mean of 12 patients. HCT = hematocrit.

pulmonary edema. The added effect of the whole-body inflammatory response associated with CPB[75] may cause serious respiratory, cardiac, renal, and hemostatic complications. Zero-balanced ultrafiltration minimally reduces inflammatory mediators and improves pulmonary function in low-risk patients undergoing CABG; however, high-risk patients derive greater benefits.[76] Ultrafiltration should be considered for adults undergoing CABG after ACS.

Renal dysfunction after CPB is associated with significant morbidity and mortality.[77] Many patients with ACS have undergone angiography with poor hemodynamics that increase the risk of renal impairment. The mortality rate of patients with renal dysfunction or renal failure was found to be 19% and 63%, respectively, in a prospective, observational multicenter trial of 2222 patients that underwent CABG with or without valvular surgery.[77] Patients with IABP and severe LV dysfunction had a fourfold risk of renal dysfunction compared with patients with other risk factors. Although strategies to prevent or reduce the deleterious effects of renal failure are not proven, mannitol, renal vasodilation, and furosemide may be used individually or together in an attempt to protect the kidneys. Fenoldopam, a selective dopamine type-1 receptor agonist, may prove to be the most effective renal vasodilator. The risk of arrhythmias may also be less for patients with fenoldopam because it lacks alpha and beta receptor activity.

Considerations After Cardiopulmonary Bypass

Permanent left ventricular function determines much of the long-term success of CABG after ACS. However, in the initial hours after separation from CPB, patients have a diminution of myocardial function that is not fully understood[78] but critical to recognize.[79] Both left and right ventricles are moderately depressed, but the depression typically resolves in about 4 hours. Ventricular depression lasting longer often does not resolve. Preoperative EF and dyssynergy may predict the degree of post-CPB left ventricular impairment.[79] Patients with low preoperative EF, prolonged CPB, and prolonged duration of aortic cross-clamp are likely to require hemodynamic support.[78] However, ischemic myocardium does not respond well to inotropes; nitroglycerin, increased perfusion pressure, or further revascularization is needed to improve hemodynamics.

Separation from CPB may be difficult for patients undergoing CABG after ACS. Inotropic agents should not be started immediately after aortic cross-clamp removal because they may further injure a heart that has been subjected to infarction and ischemia from the cross-clamp.[80] The IABP contributes to successful weaning from CPB. After CPB, patients that received an IABP preoperatively had a CI of 3.2 ± 0.7 L/min/m^2 compared with a CI of 1.99 ± 0.54 L/min/m^2 in patients without IABP.[36] The CI remained higher for 72 hours in patients with preoperative rather than post-CPB placement of the IABP. Inotropic support may be needed as well as an IABP, depending on the degree of myocardial impairment and CI. However, inotropes may cause arrhythmias, vasoconstriction (peripheral and coronary), and increased myocardial oxygen consumption in a heart that has been ischemic.

Inotropic support may include epinephrine, dopamine, dobutamine, and the phosphodiesterase inhibitors (amrinone, milrinone). Although dopamine is popular for weaning from CPB, the effect may be selective. Dopamine is more effective for inotropic support after a valve procedure than after CABG. Dobutamine causes moderate vasodilation that may decrease coronary perfusion pressure but has little effect on pulmonary vascular resistance in patients having CABG.[81] Improved CI with dobutamine during CABG is due primarily to increasing heart rate at doses above 8 μg/kg/min. Tachycardia may become severe with dobutamine, despite long-held beliefs that it provides excellent inotropic support without tachycardia.[81] An HR more than 120 beats/min is more of a concern in patients with recent ACS. In contrast to dobutamine, low-dose epinephrine results in a lower HR but increases CI by 14% and BP by 10% in patients with normal left ventricular function.[82] Several studies have indicated that epinephrine in low doses (< 50 ng/kg/min) causes less tachycardia than dopamine or dobutamine at equivalent inotropic doses.[82,83] A study that randomized patients with EF < 0.4 to either epinephrine and placebo or amrinone and epinephrine after CABG found that amrinone is effective compared with epinephrine rescue (as control) in facilitating separation from CPB.[84] This study also demonstrated that amrinone and epinephrine were more effective together than either alone in patients with poor left ventricular function. CI improved from 2.0 to 2.7 L/min/m². Amrinone may reduce the required dose of epinephrine. Milrinone is as effective as amrinone with fewer side effects. Acid–base balance must be maintained to obtain the full effect of any inotropes.

In patients with an impaired ventricle, particularly with myocardial stunning and reduced myocardial compliance, it is important to reduce afterload and myocardial wall tension. Increased afterload reduces ventricular ejection and CI. Vasodilators such as nitroprusside reduce myocardial wall tension and oxygen consumption as well as increase CI.

Optimal oxygen delivery after aortic cross-clamping and CPB is enormously important. Patients with depressed left ventricular function may benefit from higher hemoglobin concentrations.[85] Patients with poor left ventricular function and CAD usually cannot compensate for moderate anemia with an increased CI; therefore, a hemoglobin concentration of at least 9.0 gm/dl is preferred.

Although attention has focused on prevention of ischemia before CPB, the post-CPB period is characterized by increased catecholamines.[40] Post-CPB ischemia may play a role in long-term cardiac morbidity. A continuous infusion of narcotics can reduce the incidence and severity of myocardial ischemia after CPB;[86] however, extubation will be delayed. The average duration of intubation associated with CABG is 2–6 hours after arrival in the ICU. Patients undergoing CABG after ACS are unlikely to be candidates for such early extubation. IABP, significant inotropic support, or massive transfusion requires longer intubation. During intubation, analgesia and sedation should be generous. Fentanyl infusion provides excellent analgesia and reduces sympathetic activation without myocardial depression.

Hemostasis After Cardiopulmonary Bypass

Excessive blood loss after CPB in patients with ACS is common because of the medications and procedures to which many patients are exposed during the course of their illness. Data were collected from 1988 to 1994 in all patients with MI admitted to any of 19 metropolitan-based hospitals.[7] Of approximately 11,000 patients reviewed, 11.6% had CABG, 67% medical therapy, and 21% PTCA. Before CABG, 24% and 14% had thrombolysis or PTCA, respectively. Aspirin, heparin infusion, and newer anticoagulants such as GPIIb/IIIa receptor antagonists (tirofiban, abciximab) and thienopyridines (ticlopidine, clopidogrel) may have been administered to the patient with ACS.[16] As a result, coagulation is impaired before CPB, which increases the chance of excessive bleeding.[13,87]

A blood conservation strategy for patients having CABG after ACS depends on the urgency of surgery. If patients undergo CABG days to weeks after MI, blood conservation options are similar to those for other elective cardiac surgical cases.[88] However, 17% of patients have CABG within 24 hour of ACS, which eliminates certain conservation measures. Blood conservation for such patients may include heparin-coated circuit, antifibrinolytic agent, ultrafiltration, red blood cell salvage, concentration-directed heparin dosing, point-of-care coagulation tests, and algorithm-directed transfusion.

The antifibrinolytic agent of choice for patients undergoing CABG after ACS is not clear. Aprotinin, tranexamic acid (TA), and epsilon-aminocaproic acid (EACA) decrease mediastinal chest tube drainage (MCTD); however, only aprotinin consistently reduces the proportion of patients who require transfusion.[89] Aprotinin reduces MCTD and transfusion requirements in patients at high risk for bleeding who undergo CABG without previous sternotomy.[90] However, if the patient is at low risk for bleeding, aprotinin is not beneficial. Aprotinin, a serine protease inhibitor, also possesses an anti-inflammatory property (secondary to kallikrein inhibition) that is absent in TA and EACA. It may attenuate the whole-body inflammatory response, resulting in clinical benefits beyond hemostasis.

Although an antifibrinolytic agent may be recommended from a transfusion standpoint, the safety of such drugs is a concern, particularly in patients who have shown a predisposition to coronary thrombosis (as with ACS). Cosgrove et al.[91] reported an increased incidence of perioperative Q-wave MI in patients with previous sternotomy for CABG who received aprotinin compared with placebo. Thrombi were detected in 6 of 12 vein grafts in 9 patients who received aprotinin. It was suggested that aprotinin may be more risky for patients with small coronary grafts or low-flow conditions.[91] In contrast, other studies have not found an increased incidence of MIs[92] or graft thrombosis[90] with aprotinin. Table 5 shows the incidence of MI in patients receiving various doses of aprotinin compared with placebo. Only patients who received a priming dose of aprotinin for CPB showed some tendency for MI, as identified by highly sensitive tests.[90] In 1998, results of the International Multicenter Graft Patency Experience Trial, which had a sample large enough to determine any adverse effects of aprotinin, were presented at a meeting of the American Association for Thoracic Surgeons.[93] Of 870 patients, 50% received aprotinin and 50% placebo. Patients receiving aprotinin showed reductions of 43% and 49% in MCTD and red blood cell usage, respectively. Use of non-red blood cell products also was significantly less in the aprotinin group. There was no difference in the number of MIs between aprotinin and placebo patients. Graft patency was 98% in both groups.[93] TA and EACA have not undergone trials in cardiac

Table 5.   Incidence of Myocardial Infarction*

Category	High Dose (n = 165)	Low Dose (n = 169)	Pump Prime-only Dose (n = 166)	Placebo (n = 170)
Definite MI	10 (6%) p = 0.284	11 (7%) p = 0.344	9 (5%) p = 0.443	7 (4%)
Definite or probable MI	14 (8%) p = 0.978	17 (10%) p = 0.870	21 (13%) p = 0.234	16 (9%)
Definite, probable, or possible MI	18 (11%) p = 0.461	22 (13%) p = 0.286	26 (16%) p = 0.045	16 (9%)
No MI	147 (89%) p = 0.461	147 (87%) p = 0.286	140 (84%) p = 0.045	154 (91%)

MI = myocardial infarction.
* Patients valid for safety who answered yes or no to each MI question.
All probability values refer to pairwise comparison of treatment group vs. placebo.
From Lemmer JHJ, Dilling EW, Morton JR, et al: Aprotinin for primary coronary artery bypass grafting: a multicenter trial of three dose regimens. Ann Thorac Surg 62:1659–1668, 1996, with permission.

surgery to assess graft patency or MI; however, meta-analysis of antifibrinolytic agents for cardiac surgery have not shown an increased risk of thrombosis or graft occlusion.[89,94]

In patients undergoing CABG 2–14 days after ACS, it is possible to remove fresh whole blood intraoperatively before heparinization. This blood can be transfused after protamine neutralization to reduce transfusion requirements and MCTD.[95] Newer technical capabilities to increase platelet yield may improve the efficacy of platelet plasmapheresis to reduce transfusion requirements in patients in whom anemia prevents withdrawal of fresh whole blood. These procedures should not be performed unless the patient is hemodynamically stable.

Conclusion

CABG in patients with ACS is more common today. Newer surgical and anesthetic techniques and monitoring capabilities have reduced the mortality and morbidity rates of these high-risk cases. However, they still pose significant anesthetic challenges. The focus should be to institute CPB as safely as possible and to prepare for the hemodynamic and hemostatic challenges after separation from CPB.

References

1. Verheugt FWA: Acute coronary syndromes: Interventions. Lancet 353(Suppl II):16–19, 1999.
2. Pilote L, Miller DP, Califf RM, et al: Determinants of the use of coronary angiography and revascularization after thrombolysis for acute myocardial infarction. N Engl J Med 335:1198–1205, 1996.
3. Mohr R, Moshkovitch Y, Shapira I, et al: Coronary artery bypass without cardiopulmonary bypass for patients with acute myocardial infarction. J Thorac Cardiovasc Surg 118:50–56, 1999.
4. Hochman JS, Sleeper LA, Webb JG, et al: Early revascularization in acute myocardial infarction complicated by cardiogenic shock. N Engl J Med 341:625–634, 1999.
5. Bana A, Yadava OP, Ghadiok R, et al: Myocardial revascularization after acute myocardial infarction. Int J Cardiol 69:209–216, 1999.
6. Pagano D, Townend JN, Bonser RS: What is the role of revascularization in ischemic heart failure? [editorial]. Heart 81:8–9, 1999.
7. Every NR, Maynard C, Cochran RP, et al: Characteristics, management, and outcome of patients with acute myocardial infarction treated with bypass surgery. Circulation 94(Suppl II):II-81–II-86, 1996.
8. Edwards FH, Clark RE, Schwartz M: Coronary artery bypass grafting: The Society of Thoracic Surgeons National database experience. Ann Thorac Surg 57:12–19, 1994.
9. Yau TM, Fedak PWM, Weisel RD, et al: Predictors of operative risk for coronary bypass operations in patients with left ventricular dysfunction. J Thorac Cardiovasc Surg 118:1006–1013, 1999.
10. Reich DL, Bodian CA, Krol M, et al: Intraoperative hemodynamic predictors of mortality, stroke, and myocardial infarction after coronary artery bypass surgery. Anesth Analg 89:814–822, 1999.
11. Kurki TSO, Kataja M: Preoperative prediction of postoperative morbidity in coronary artery bypass grafting. Ann Thorac Surg 61:1740–1745, 1996.
12. Rao TLK, Jacobs KH, El-Etr AA: Reinfarction following anesthesia in patients with myocardial infarction. Anesthesiology 59:499–505, 1983.
13. Favaloro RG: 50th anniversary historical article: Surgical treatment of acute myocardial infarction. JACC 33:1435–1441, 1999.
14. Pearce AC, Jones RM: Smoking and Anesthesia: Preoperative abstinence and perioperative morbidity. Anesthesiology 61:576–584, 1984.
15. Moulton MJ, Creswell LL, Mackey ME, et al: Reexploration for bleeding is a risk factor for adverse outcomes after cardiac operations. J Thorac Cardiovasc Surg 111:1037–1046, 1996.
16. Verheugt FWA: Acute coronary syndromes: Drug treatments. Lancet 353(Suppl II):20–23,1999.
17. Lee KF, Mandell J, Rankin JS, et al: Immediate versus delayed coronary grafting after streptokinase treatment: Postoperative blood loss and clinical results. J Thorac Cardiovasc Surg 95:216–222, 1988.

18. Rich GF, Lubanski RE Jr, McLoughlin TM: Differences between aortic and radial artery pressure associated with cardiopulmonary bypass. Anesthesiology 77:63–66, 1992.
19. Frezza EE, Mezghebe H: Indications and complications of arterial catheter use in surgical or medical intensive care units: Analysis of 4932 patients. Am Surg 64:127–131, 1998.
20. Tuman KJ, McCarthy RJ, Spiess BD, et al: Effect of pulmonary artery catheterization on outcome in patients undergoing coronary artery surgery. Anesthesiology 70:199–206, 1989.
21. Kaplan JA, Wells PH: Early diagnosis of myocardial ischemia using the pulmonary artery catheter. Anesth Analg 60:789–793, 1981.
22. Leung JM, O'Kelly BF, Mangano DT, et al: Relationship of regional wall motion abnormalities to hemodynamic indices of myocardial oxygen supply and demand in patients undergoing CABG surgery. Anesthesiology 73:802–814, 1990.
23. Fontes ML, Bellows W, Ngo L, et al: Assessment of ventricular function in critically ill patients: Limitations of pulmonary artery catheterization. J Cardiothorac Vasc Anesth 13:521–527,1999.
24. Practice guidelines for pulmonary artery catheterization. A report by the American Society for Anesthesiologists task force on pulmonary artery catheterization. Anesthesiology 78:380–394, 1993.
25. Dzelzkalns R, Stanley TH: Placement of the pulmonary arterial catheter before anesthesia for cardiac surgery: A stressful, painful, and unnecessary crutch. J Clin Monit 1:197–200, 1985.
26. Oliver Jr WC, Nuttall GA, Beynen FM, et al: The incidence of artery puncture with central venous cannulation using a modified technique for detection and prevention of arterial cannulation. J Cardiothorac Vasc Anesth 11:851–855, 1997.
27. Jobes DR, Schwartz AJ, Greenhow DE, et al: Safer jugular vein cannulation: Recognition of arterial puncture and preferential use of the external jugular route. Anesthesiology 59:353–355, 1983.
28. Troianos CA, Jobes DR, Ellison N: Ultrasound-guided cannulation of the internal jugular vein. A prospective, randomized study. Anesth Analg 72:823–826, 1991.
29. Bergquist BD, Bellows WH, Leung JM: Transesophageal echocardiograpy in myocardial revascularization. II: Influence on intraoperative decision making. Anesth Analg 82:1139–1145, 1996.
30. El-Ganzouri AR, McCarthy RJ, Tuman KJ, et al: Preoperative airway assessment: Predictive value of a multivariate risk index. Anesth Analg 82:1197–1204, 1996.
31. Lewis M, Keramati S, Benumof JL, et al: What is the best way to determine oropharyngeal classification and mandibular space length to predict difficult laryngoscopy? Anesthesiology 81:69–75, 1994.
32. Pennant JH, White PF: The laryngeal mask airway: Its uses in anesthesiology. Anesthesiology 79:144–163, 1993.
33. Warner MA, Warner ME, Weber JG: Clinical significance of pulmonary aspiration during the perioperative period. Anesthesiology 78:56–62, 1993.
34. Mangano DT: Anesthetics, coronary artery disease, and outcome: Unresolved controversies. Anethesiology 70:175–177, 1989.
35. Slogoff S, Keats AS: Does perioperative myocardial ischemia lead to postoperative myocardial infarction? Anesthesiology 62:107–114, 1985.
36. Christenson JT, Simonet F, Badel P, et al: Optimal timing of preoperative intraaortic balloon pump support in high-risk coronary patients. Ann Thorac Surg 68:934–939, 1999.
37. Tu JV, Sykora K, Naylor CD, et al: Assessing the outcomes of coronary artery bypass graft surgery: How many risk factors are enough? J Am Coll Cardiol 30:1317–1323, 1997.
38. Goldberg RJ, Gore JM, Alpert JS, et al: Cardiogenic shock after acute myocardial infarction. Incidence and mortality from a community-wide perspective, 1975 to 1988. N Engl J Med 325:1117–1122, 1991.
39. Kleinman B, Henkin RE, Glisson SN, et al: Qualitative evaluation of coronary flow during anesthetic induction using thallium-201 perfusion scans. Anesthesiology 64:157–164, 1986.
40. Knight AA, Hollenberg M, London MJ, et al: Perioperative myocardial ischemia: Importance of the preoperative ischemic pattern. Anesthesiology 68:681–688, 1988.
41. Tuman KJ, McCarthy RJ, Spiess BD, et al: Does choice of anesthetic agent significantly affect outcome after coronary artery surgery? Anesthesiology 70:189–198, 1989.
42. Wynands JE, Wong P, Whalley DG, et al: Oxygen-fentanyl anesthesia in patients with poor left ventricular function: Hemodynamics and plasma fentanyl concentrations. Anesth Analg 62:476–482, 1983.
43. Quintin L, Whalley DG, Wynands JE, et al: High dose fentanyl anaesthesia with oxygen for aorto-coronary bypass surgery. Can Anaesth Soc J 28:314–320, 1981.
44. Raza SMA, Masters RW, Zsigmond EK: Haemodynamic stability with midazolam-ketamine-sufentanil analgesia in cardiac surgical patients. Can J Anaesth 36:617–623, 1989.
45. Mora CT, Dudek C, Torjman MC, et al: The effects of anesthetic technique on the hemodynamic response and recovery profile in coronary revascularization patients. Anesth Analg 81:900–910, 1995.

46. Ramsay JG, DeLima LGR, Wynands JE, et al: Pure opioid versus opioid-volatile anesthesia for coronary artery bypass graft surgery: A prospective, randomized double-blind study. Anesth Analg 78:867–875, 1994.

47. Lynch III C: Effects of halothane and isoflurane on isolated human ventricular myocardium. Anesthesiology 68:429–432, 1988.

48. Lowenstein E, Foex P, Francis CM, et al: Regional ischemic ventricular dysfunction in myocardium supplied by a narrowed coronary artery with increasing halothane concentration in the dog. Anesthesiology 55:349–359, 1981.

49. Prys-Roberts C, Roberts JG, Foex P, et al: Interaction of anesthesia, beta-receptor blockade, and blood loss in dogs with induced myocardial infarction. Anesthesiology 45:326–329, 1976.

50. Priebe H-J: Isoflurane and coronary hemodynamics. Anesthesiology 71:960–976, 1989.

51. Sill JC, Bove AA, Nugent M, et al: Effects of isoflurane on coronary arteries and coronary arterioles in the intact dog. Anesthesiology 66:273–279, 1987.

52. Slogoff S, Keats AS: Randomized trial of primary anesthetic agents on outcome of coronary artery bypass operations. Anesthesiology 70:179–188, 1989.

53. Kitahata H, Kawahito S, Nozaki J, et al: Effects of sevoflurane on regional myocardial blood flow distribution: Quantification with myocardial contrast echocardiography. Anesthesiology 90:1436–1445, 1999.

54. Ebert TJ, Kharasch ED, Rooke GA, et al: Myocardial ischemia and adverse cardiac outcomes in cardiac patients undergoing noncardiac surgery with sevoflurane and isoflurane. Anesth Analg 85:993–999, 1997.

55. Helman JD, Leung JM, Bellows WH, et al: The risk of myocardial ischemia in patients receiving desflurane versus sufentanil anesthesia for coronary artery bypass graft surgery. Anesthesiology 77:47–62, 1992.

56. Philbin DM, Foex P, Drummond G, et al: Postsystolic shortening of canine left ventricle supplied by a stenotic coronary artery when nitrous oxide is added in the presence of narcotics. Anesthesiology 62:166–174, 1985.

57. Nathan HJ: Control of hemodynamics prevents worsening of myocardial ischemia when nitrous oxide is administered to isoflurane-anesthetized dogs. Anesthesiology 71:686–694, 1989.

58. Cahalan MK, Prakash O, Rulf ENR, et al: Addition of nitrous oxide to fentanyl anesthesia does not induce myocardial ischemia in patients with ischemic heart disease. Anesthesiology 67:925–929, 1987.

59. Thompson IR and Putnins CL: Adverse effects of pancuronium during high-dose fentanyl anesthesia for coronary artery bypass grafting. Anesthesiology 62:708–713, 1985.

60. Searle NR, Thomson I, Dupont C, et al: A two-center study evaluating the hemodynamic and pharmacodynamic effects of cisatracurium and vecuronium in patients undergoing coronary artery bypass surgery. J Cardiothorac Vasc Anesth 13:20–25, 1999.

61. Lien CA, Belmont MR, Abalos A, et al: The cardiovascular effects and histamine-releasing properties of 51W89 in patients receiving nitrous oxide/opioid/barbiturate anesthesia. Anesthesiology 82:1131–1138, 1995.

62. Thomson IR, Mutch WAC, Culligan JD: Failure of intravenous nitroglycerin to prevent intraoperative myocardial ischemia during fentanyl-pancuronium anesthesia. Anesthesiology 61:385–393, 1984.

63. Giles RW, Berger HJ, Barash PG, et al: Continuous monitoring of left ventricular performance with the computerized nuclear probe during laryngoscopy and intubation before coronary artery bypass surgery. Am J Cardiol 50:735-741, 1982.

64. Hart AP, Camporesi EM, Sell TL, et al: The effect of nitroglycerin on response to tracheal intubation: Assessment by radionuclide angiography. Anesth Analg 68:718–723, 1989.

65. Warltier DC, Pagel PS, Kersten JR: Approaches to the prevention of perioperative myocardial ischemia. Anesthesiology 92:253–259, 2000.

66. Cheng DCH, Chung F, Burns RJ, et al: Postoperative myocardial infarction documented by technetium pyrophosphate scan using single-photon emission computed tomography: Significance of intraoperative myocardial ischemia and hemodynamic control. Anesthesiology 71:818–826, 1989.

67. Eugene J, Ott RA, Piters KM, et al: Operative risk factors associated with unstable angina pectoris. Arch Surg 120:279–282, 1985.

68. Slogoff S and Keats AS: Further observations on perioperative myocardial ischemia. Anesthesiology 65:539–542, 1986.

69. Lieberman RW, Orkin FK, Jobes DR, et al: Hemodynamic predictors of myocardial ischemia during halothane anesthesia for coronary-artery revascularization. Anesthesiology 59:36–41, 1983.

70. Comunale ME, Body SC, Ley C, et al: The concordance of intraoperative left ventricular wall-motion abnormalities and electrocardiographic S-T segment changes. Association with outcome after coronary revascularization. Anesthesiology 88:945–954, 1998.

71. Teo KK, Yusuf S, Furberg CD: Effects of prophylactic antiarrhythmic drug therapy in acute my-ocardial infarction: An overview of results of from randomized controlled trials. JAMA 270:1589–1595, 1993.

72. Teo KK, Yusuf S: Role of magnesium in reducing mortality in acute myocardial infarction: A review of the evidence. Drugs 46:347–359, 1993.

73. Gold JP, Charlson ME, Williams-Russo P, et al: Improvement of outcomes after coronary artery bypass: A randomized trial comparing intraoperative high versus low mean arterial pressure. J Thorac Cardiovasc Surg 110:1302–1314, 1995.

74. Niinikoski J, Laaksonen V, Meretoja O, et al: Oxygen transport to tissue under normovolemic moderate and extreme hemodilution during coronary bypass operation. Ann Thorac Surg 31:134–143, 1981.

75. Kirklin JK, Westaby S, Blackstone EH, et al: Complement and the damaging effects of car-diopulmonary bypass. J Thorac Cardiovasc Surg 86:845–857, 1983.

76. Tassani P, Richter JA, Eising GP, et al: Influence of combined zero-balanced and modified ultra-filtration on the systemic inflammatory response during coronary artery bypass grafting. J Cardiothorac Vasc Anesth 13:285–291, 1999.

77. Mangano CM, Diamondstone LS, Ramsay JG, et al: Renal dysfunction after myocardial revas-cularization: Risk factors, adverse outcomes, and hospital resource utilization. Ann Intern Med 128:194–203, 1998.

78. Royster RL: Myocardial dysfunction following cardiopulmonary bypass: Recovery patterns, predictors of inotropic need, theoretical concepts of inotropic administration. J Cardiothorac Vasc Anesth 7 (4 Suppl 2):19–25, 1993.

79. Mangano DT: Biventricular function after myocardial revascularization in humans: Deterioration and recovery patterns during the first 24 hours. Anesthesiology 62:571–577, 1985.

80. Lazar HL, Buckberg GD, Foglia RP, et al: Detrimental effects of premature use of inotropic drugs to discontinue cardiopulmonary bypass. J Thorac Cardiovasc Surg 82:18–25, 1981.

81. Romson JL, Leung JM, Bellows WH, et al: Effects of dobutamine on hemodynamics and left ventricular performance after cardiopulmonary bypass in cardiac surgical patients. Anesthesiology 91:1318–1328, 1999.

82. Royster RL, Butterworth JF, Prielipp RC, et al: A randomized, blinded, placebo-controlled eval-uation of calcium chloride and epinephrine for inotropic support after emergence from car-diopulmonary bypass. Anesth Analg 74:3–13, 1992.

83. Butterworth JF, Prielipp RC, Royster RL, et al: Dobutamine increases heart rate more than epi-nephrine in patients recovering from aortocoronary bypass surgery. J Cardiothorac Vasc Anes 6:535–541, 1992.

84. Butterworth JFT, Royster RL, Prielipp RC, et al: Amrinone in cardiac surgical patients with left-ventricular dysfunction: A prospective, randomized placebo-controlled trial. Chest 104:1660–1667, 1993.

85. Estafanous FG, Smith CE, Selim WM, et al: Cardiovascular effects of acute normovolemic he-modilution in rats with disopyramide-induced myocardial depression. Basic Res Cardiol 85:227–236, 1990.

86. Mangano DT, Siliciano D, Hollenberg M, et al: Postoperative myocardial ischemia. Therapeutic trials using intensive analgesia following surgery. The Study of Perioperative Ischemia (SPI) Research Group. Anesthesiology 76:342–353, 1992.

87. Despotis GJ, Filos KS, Zoys TN, et al: Factors associated with excessive postoperative blood loss and hemostatic transfusion requirements: A multivariate analysis in cardiac surgical pa-tients. Anesth Analg 82:13–21, 1996.

88. Ereth MH, Oliver WC Jr, Santrach PJ: Perioperative interventions to decrease transfusion of al-logeneic blood products. Mayo Clin Proc 69:575–586, 1994.

89. Fremes SE, Wong BI, Lee E, et al: Metaanalysis of prophylactic drug treatment in the preven-tion of postoperative bleeding. Ann Thorac Surg 58:1580–1588, 1994.

90. Lemmer JHJ, Dilling EW, Morton JR, et al: Aprotinin for primary coronary artery bypass graft-ing: a multicenter trial of three dose regimens. Ann Thorac Surg 62:1659–1668, 1996.

91. Cosgrove DM III, Heric B, Lytle BW, et al: Aprotinin therapy for reoperative myocardial revas-cularization: A placebo-controlled study. Ann Thorac Surg 54:1031–1038, 1992.

92. Levy JH, Pifarre R, Schaff HV, et al: A Multicenter, double-blind, placebo-controlled trial of aprotinin for reducing blood loss and the requirement for donor-blood transfusion in patients undergoing repeat coronary artery bypass grafting. Circulation 92:2236–2244, 1995.

93. Rich JB: The efficacy and safety of aprotinin use in cardiac surgery. Ann Thorac Surg 66:S6–S11, 1998.

94. Munoz JJ, Birkmeyer NJO, Birkmeyer JD, et al: Is epsilon-aminocaproic acid as effective as apro-tinin in reducing bleeding with cardiac surgery? A meta-analysis. Circulation 99:81–89, 1999.

95. Nuttall GA, Oliver Jr WC, Ereth MH, et al: Comparison of blood-conservation strategies in car-diac surgery patients at high risk for bleeding. Anesthesiology 92:674–682, 2000.

Myocardial Protection for Patients with Acute Evolving Myocardial Infarction Undergoing Cardiac Surgery

MARK A. CHANEY, MD

In the United States each year, more than 1.5 million people suffer acute myocardial infarction (AMI). Although prognosis varies considerably, approximately one-half of all deaths associated with AMI occur within 1 hour and are due to ventricular arrhythmias. Of patients who survive acutely, most deaths occur approximately 4 days after infarction and are due to left ventricular failure. Although recent dramatic technologic advances (e.g., intravenous and intracoronary thrombolysis) are responsible for the continually decreasing mortality rate, AMI is fatal in approximately 1 of every 3 patients.[1]

Pathophysiology of Acute Myocardial Infarction

Myocardial infarction is a dynamic process and almost always is associated with coronary atherosclerosis and superimposed coronary thrombosis. The term "acute coronary syndrome" represents a spectrum of increasing severity, which includes unstable angina, non–Q-wave myocardial infarction, and Q-wave myocardial infarction. Intracoronary plaque rupture is considered to be the common pathophysiologic substrate of the acute coronary syndrome.[2]

Myocardial ischemia and/or infarction causes a multitude of hemodynamic abnormalities. Systolic function declines because loss of functioning myocardium leads to decreases in blood pressure, stroke volume, and cardiac output. End-systolic volume increases, left ventricular compliance decreases (impairing diastolic function), and left ventricular end-diastolic volume and pressure increase. Decreases in blood pressure (along with increases in left ventricular end-diastolic pressure) can lead to catastrophic decreases in coronary perfusion pressure. Such hemodynamic abnormalities may be aggravated by complications associated with AMI (e.g., arrhythmias, mitral regurgitation, ventricular septal rupture). Various hemodynamic compensatory mechanisms (e.g., increased left ventricular end-diastolic volume) may or may not prevent the development of congestive heart failure.

Importance of Myocardial Protection

Myocardial protection for patients with acute evolving myocardial infarction is extremely important because infarct size is an important determinant of prognosis. Many investigators have reported associations between infarct size and prognosis, including incidence and severity of congestive heart failure, left ventricular dysfunction, and frequency and severity of ventricular arrhythmias. Because myocardial infarction is a dynamic process that evolves over hours, selected physiologic, pharmacologic, and/or surgical interventions can be initiated to alter favorably the ultimate extent of infarction. Efforts to limit myocardial infarct size generally involve three often overlapping approaches: early reperfusion, optimization of myocardial oxygen supply: demand ratio, and manipulation of myocardial energy dynamics (Table 1). Early reperfusion (via pharmacologic or mechanical routes) remains the primary goal and affects infarct size most profoundly, yet even late reperfusion conveys several benefits that may contribute to mortality reduction. Early reperfusion is attempted most commonly with intravenous or intracoronary thrombolysis, and these techniques are detailed elsewhere in this text. Surgical reperfusion is used only when coronary thrombolysis and/or coronary angioplasty is unsuccesful or under certain limited circumstances.

Role of Myocardial Revascularization

Of all patients experiencing AMI, 10–20% are referred for myocardial revascularization because of persistent angina despite coronary thrombolysis and/or coronary angioplasty, high-risk coronary anatomy discovered during catheterization, or development of complications (e.g., ventricular septal rupture, mitral regurgitation secondary to papillary muscle dysfunction). In essence, coronary artery bypass grafting (CABG) is reserved for patients in whom other procedures (thrombolysis and/or catheter intervention) have failed.[3] Timing of myocardial revascularization is of utmost importance. Myocardial salvage (like all methods attempting to limit infarct size) is most successful when surgery is performed within 4–6 hours of infarction. Myocardial infarction may result in development of intravascular thrombus or coronary spasm followed by extension

Table 1.   Efforts to Limit Myocardial Infarct Size

Early reperfusion
    Coronary thrombolysis
    Coronary angioplasty
    Surgical reperfusion

Optimization of myocardial oxygen supply:demand ratio
    Decrease myocardial oxygen demand
    Increase myocardial oxygen supply

Manipulation of myocardial energy dynamics
    Standard cardioplegia
    Modification of standard cardioplegia
    Additional protective agents

of myocardial necrosis. Once the infarcted area extends, mortality increases substantially. However, it is next to impossible to perform emergent myocardial revascularization within this time frame simply because it takes too long for the usual patient who develops an AMI outside the hospital to progress through clinical evaluation, possible thrombolytic treatment, cardiac catheterization, and operating room preparation (instruments and personnel). Thus, myocardial revascularization is not routinely used in patients who experience AMI. Indeed, myocardial revascularization is contraindicated in patients with uncomplicated transmural infarcts more than 6 hours after onset of symptoms because surgical reperfusion at this time may produce marked hemorrhage into the infarction area. The mortality rate in patients requiring emergency myocardial revascularization within 24–48 hours of AMI is high (15–20%). Long-term mortality is also increased when such surgery is performed in patients with triple-vessel disease, active ongoing myocardial ischemia, and/or cardiogenic shock. Elderly patients are also at higher risk. At autopsy, patients exhibit extensive myocardial necrosis that is often hemorrhagic. Patients undergoing cardiac surgery with acute evolving myocardial infarction are often hemodynamically unstable (for a wide variety of reasons) and have increased morbidity and mortality rates; therefore, all efforts that improve myocardial protection (i.e.. limit infarct size) should be explored.

Myocardial Protection

Before the Operating Room

Many options are available for myocardial protection before the patient enters the operating room. However, heparin, aspirin, and magnesium deserve mention here because of their important role in management of patients with acute evolving myocardial infarction undergoing cardiac surgery.

Heparin. The rationale for using heparin in patients with acute evolving myocardial infarction is to establish and maintain patency of the infarct-related artery. However, despite many years of clinical application, its use in this setting remains controversial.[4] Angiographic studies examining the risk:benefit ratio of heparin during acute evolving myocardial infarction are difficult to interpret and compare because of differences in study design (primarily whether or not aspirin and/or thrombolytics also were used). However, the available data suggest that heparin decreases morbidity and mortality rates from reinfarction in patients who do not receive thrombolysis but is of no benefit to patients who receive thrombolysis. Thus, heparin is recommended only in patients who are not candidates for thrombolytic therapy. One exception is tissue plasminogen activator, which it is a more fibrin-specific agent. Because some investigations show that patency rates of infarct-related arteries are higher in patients receiving both tissue plasminogen activator and heparin, heparin is recommended in patients who receive tissue plasminogen activator.

Aspirin. During and after coronary artery plaque rupture, platelets play a vital role in the thrombotic response. The importance of platelets and thrombosis in the pathophysiology of acute coronary syndromes is well established. In addition, thrombi composed predominantly of platelets are more resistant to thrombolysis than are thrombi with lesser numbers of platelets. Therefore, sound scientific basis exists for inhibiting platelet aggregation in patients with acute evolving myocardial infarction, and overwhelming evidence documents the benefits of antiplatelet therapy in this patient population. Although many antiplatelet regimens have been evaluated, the most extensively tested is aspirin, for which the evidence of benefit is most compelling. Aspirin clearly decreases mortality and reinfarction rates when given as short-term therapy for AMI, when given to patients with unstable angina, and when given as long-term secondary preventive therapy in a wide range of patients with established cardiovascular disease. Despite this evidence, studies suggest that aspirin remains underused for treatment of acute coronary syndromes.[5] Dramatic reductions in mortality (as high as 50%) have been observed, and the benefits appear to be greatest in the patients at highest risk. Several studies have demonstrated clearly the beneficial role of aspirin in the treatment of unstable angina. Thus, all patients with acute evolving myocardial infarction should receive aspirin, regardless of whether thrombolysis and/or angioplasty is used. The lowest dose that is known to be effective (160–325 mg for acute cardiovascular events) should be given because higher doses result in higher rates of complications.

The beneficial effects of aspirin appear to be additive to those of thrombolytics. A meta-analysis of 32 trials using aspirin as adjunctive therapy to thrombolysis demonstrated significantly decreased reocclusion rates (11% vs. 25%) and recurrent ischemic events (25% vs. 41%) with aspirin therapy.[6] Despite its demonstrated effectiveness in treating and preventing atherosclerotic disease, aspirin produces only partial inhibition of platelet aggregation; therefore, it is a relatively weak antiplatelet agent. In addition, a minority of patients appear to be relatively resistant to the antiplatelet effects of aspirin, even when it is administered in large doses. Alternative options for inhibiting platelet function continue to be investigated. The most promising appear to be the platelet glycoprotein (GP) IIb/IIIa receptor antagonists, which interfere with the final common pathway for platelet aggregation.[7] GP IIb/IIIa inhibitors are capable of more complete platelet inhibition and are likely to play an increasingly greater role in the treatment of cardiovascular diseases.

Magnesium.   Magnesium is a critical cofactor in over 300 intracellular enzymatic processes, including several that are integrally involved in mitochondrial function, energy production, maintenance of ionic gradients, cell volume control, and resting membrane potential.[8] Patients with acute evolving myocardial infarction may have a total body deficit of magnesium for a wide variety of reasons, including advanced age, low dietary intake, or prior diuretic use. A functional magnesium deficit also may be due to catecholamine-induced increases in free fatty acids, which stimulate adipocyte trapping. Many experimental models have shown that supplemental administration of magnesium before coronary occlusion, during coronary occlusion, coincident with reperfusion, or during a short interval (15–45 minutes) after reperfusion reduces infarct size and prevents myocardial stunning secondary to reperfusion injury. However, delayed administration beyond a short interval (15–60 minutes) after reperfusion is no longer effective in reducing myocardial damage.[9] Because of its trivial cost, ease of administration, widespread availability, and the fact that it has the potential to decrease morbidity and mortality, magnesium supplementation in all patients with acute evolving myocardial infarction should be considered to maintain serum levels of 2.0 mEq/L or more. Magnesium administration may cause vasodilation and hypotension.

Hemodynamic Control

Hemodynamic control prior to myocardial revascularization is of utmost importance to prevent myocardial ischemia and infarct extension. Traditional pharmacologic approaches to prevention and treatment of myocardial ischemia have focused on optimization of the myocardial oxygen supply:demand ratio (Table 2).[10,11] Useful pharmacologic agents for hemodynamic control include beta-adrenergic blockers, angiotensin-converting enzyme (ACE) inhibitors, nitrates, alpha2-adrenoceptor agonists, and calcium channel antagonists.

Beta-adrenergic Blockers.   The use of beta-adrenergic blockers in patients with acute evolving myocardial infarction has proven immediate and long-term benefits. To date, beta-adrenergic blockers are the only well-established means of prophylaxis against myocardial ischemia that reduces morbidity and mortality rates in patients with coronary artery disease undergoing surgery.[12] Immediate beneficial effects include a decrease in myocardial oxygen demand due to reduced heart rate and contractility. The decrease in heart rate increases duration of diastole, enhances coronary perfusion time, increases subendocardial blood flow, and reduces myocardial oxygen consumption. Beta-adrenergic blockers also can cause "reverse" coronary steal by reducing oxygen demand and thus increasing coronary vascular tone in normal regions. They also attenuate the adverse effects of sympathetic nervous system activation, including increases in heart rate and myocardial contractility, decreases in coronary blood flow secondary to constriction of large epicardial coronary vessels, coronary cyclical flow phenomena at the stenosis site generated by platelet aggregation and dispersion, and overall plaque instability. Beta-adrenergic blockers also increase oxygen supply by increasing diastolic time and reducing wall stress, especially in patients with left ventricular hypertrophy. Ventricular arrhythmias may be reduced. In addition, beta-adrenergic blockers may decrease myocardial oxygen consumption by antagonizing the lipolytic effects of catecholamines and decreasing circulating blood levels of free fatty acids. Administration of beta-adrenergic blockers to patients with acute evolving myocardial infarction decreases mortality, probably reduces infarct size, and may decrease the incidence of ventricular rupture and arrhythmias. Beta-adrenergic blockers are antiischemic, protect against myocardial reinfarction, and reduce overall mortality caused by cardiac death and congestive heart failure in both

Table 2.   Optimization of Myocardial Oxygen Supply:Demand Ratio

Decrease myocardial oxygen demand
  Decrease heart rate
  Decrease contractility
  Decrease left ventricular end-diastolic volume
  Reduce afterload

Increase myocardial oxygen supply
  Increase coronary blood flow
    Decrease vasoconstriction
    Decrease thrombosis
    Increase diastolic time
    Increase aortic diastolic pressure
    Reduce ventricular end-diastolic pressure
  Increase blood oxygen content
    Increase hematocrit
    Increase oxygen saturation

the immediate and remote perioperative periods. Thus, use of beta-adrenergic blockers is recommended in all patients with acute evolving myocardial infarction unless contraindications are present (congestive heart failure, bronchospasm, or heart block).

Angiotensin-converting Enzyme Inhibitors.   ACE inhibitors decrease mortality in patients with acute evolving myocardial infarction, have favorable effects on ventricular remodeling, and reduce the subsequent development of congestive heart failure. The mortality benefits are additive to those achieved with aspirin and beta-adrenergic blockers. Thus, use of ACE inhibitors should be considered in all patients with acute evolving myocardial infarction after initiation of reperfusion strategies, aspirin, and beta-adrenergic blockers unless contraindications are present (hypotension or known hypersensitivity).

Alpha$_2$-adrenoceptor Agonists.   Alpha$_2$-adrenoceptor agonists exert beneficial cardiovascular effects by reducing central sympathetic nervous system activity. They prevent tachycardia, hypertension, and increased sympathetic tone perioperatively. They may have a potential advantage over beta-adrenergic blockers because of their ability to attenuate the adverse effects of sympathetic nervous stimulation mediated by peripheral alpha- as well as beta-adrenoceptors. However, large-scale clinical trials have yet to demonstrate convincingly their efficacy in the reduction of morbidity and mortality in patients with coronary artery disease.

Nitrates.   Nitrates are a mainstay in the medical management of myocardial ischemia. Nitroglycerin reduces myocardial oxygen demand by decreasing left ventricular diastolic volume and preload. It increases supply by producing coronary artery vasodilation (large epicardial arteries and collateral conduit vessels) and reducing ventricular end-diastolic volume. Nitroglycerin is also a donor of nitric oxide, which may have direct cardioprotective properties. The physiologic benefits of sodium nitroprusside are similar to those of nitroglycerin, with the added advantage of afterload reduction. However, the precise role of sodium nitroprusside in management of myocardial ischemia is controversial because of the possibility of coronary artery steal (from vasodilation of coronary artery resistance vessels). Although nitrates possess beneficial hemodynamic effects and also may have beneficial antiplatelet effects, their effect on outcome is uncertain. Despite well-established beneficial effects, intraoperative prophylaxis with nitroglycerin has yielded equivocal results in patients with coronary artery disease. Some investigators in the prethrombolytic era revealed reductions in mortality rates, yet no such reductions have been demonstrated since the introduction of thrombolytics. Thus, nitrates are not routinely used in patients with acute evolving myocardial infarction. If they are used, care should be taken to avoid hypotension and reflex tachycardia (especially prominent with sodium nitroprusside), which detrimentally affect the myocardial oxygen supply:demand ratio.

Calcium Channel Antagonists.   Calcium channel antagonists display a wide variety of cardiovascular effects. They decrease myocardial oxygen demand by reducing heart rate and contractility, and they may increase supply via coronary artery vasodilation, increased diastolic time, and reduced wall stress. They are not helpful in the acute phase of myocardial infarction, and concern has arisen over a possible association with increases in mortality. Although somewhat controversial, calcium channel antagonists such as nifedipine or nicardipine may be specifically indicated when coronary artery vasospasm is suspected.

Thoracic Epidural Anesthesia

Thoracic epidural application of local anesthetics has many potential benefits, including intense postoperative analgesia, stress response attenuation, and thoracic cardiac sympathectomy.[13] The myocardium and coronary vasculature are densely innervated by sympathetic nerve fibers that arise from T1 to T5 and profoundly influence total coronary blood flow and distribution. Cardiac sympathetic nerve activation initiates coronary artery vasoconstriction and paradoxical vasoconstriction in response to intrinsic vasodilators. In patients with coronary artery disease, cardiac sympathetic nerve activation disrupts the normal matching of coronary blood flow and myocardial oxygen demand. Animal models show an intense poststenotic vasoconstrictive mechanism mediated by cardiac sympathetic nerve activation that attenuates local metabolic vasodilation in response to myocardial ischemia. Furthermore, myocardial ischemia initiates a cardiocardiac reflex, meditated by sympathetic nerve fibers, that augments the ischemic process. Cardiac sympathetic nerve activation probably plays a central role in initiating postoperative myocardial ischemia by decreasing the myocardial oxygen supply via mechanisms listed above.

Thoracic epidural anesthesia with local anesthetics effectively blocks cardiac sympathetic nerve afferent and efferent fibers. Patients with symptomatic coronary artery disease benefit from cardiac sympathectomy, and application of thoracic sympathetic blockade in the management of angina pectoris was described as early as 1965. Thoracic epidural anesthesia with local anesthetics increases the diameter of stenotic epicardial coronary artery segments without causing dilation of coronary arterioles, decreases determinants of myocardial oxygen demand, improves left ventricular function, and decreases anginal symptoms. Furthermore, cardiac sympathectomy increases the endocardial: epicardial blood flow ratio, improves collateral blood flow during myocardial ischemia, decreases poststenotic vasoconstriction, and attenuates the myocardial ischemia-induced cardiocardiac reflex. In an animal model, thoracic epidural anesthesia with local anesthetics decreases myocardial infarct size after coronary artery occlusion.

In short, thoracic epidural anesthesia with local anesthetics may benefit patients undergoing myocardial revascularization by effectively blocking cardiac sympathetic nerve activity and improving the myocardial oxygen supply: demand balance. However, during emergent myocardial revascularization, time may not allow for catheter placement, and concern persists about epidural hematoma formation when epidural catheters are used in this setting.[14]

Additional Protective Agents

Although controlling systemic and coronary hemodynamics is certainly important, over the past decade an explosion of investigation has provided novel therapeutic strategies that may confer myocardial protection independent of systemic and coronary hemodynamics.[10] These agents (Table 3) are discussed in detail later in this chapter, because most have been applied as adjuncts to cardioplegia solutions. Some, however, also may be used systemically (e.g., magnesium). This listing is by no means complete; focus is directed toward protective agents that at present show the greatest promise of clinical benefit. These agents work via many diverse mechanisms that alter the metabolic, mechanical, and/or electrophysiologic consequences of myocardial ischemia. However, the vast majority are investigational, and there is no "magic bullet" to treat myocardial ischemia. Myocardial ischemia remains multifactorial in

Table 3. Additional Protective Agents

Hypocalcemia	Intravenous and inhalational anesthetics
Magnesium	Glucose
Adenosine	Calcium channel antagonists
Potassium channel openers	Beta-adrenergic blockers
Sodium channel blockers	Growth factors
Aprotinin	Antiplatelet drugs
Bradykinin	Adhesion molecule inhibitors
Opioid delta-receptor agonists	

origin, and one must not lose sight of the importance of traditional hemodynamic management. Primary goals should remain control of heart rate, decrease in myocardial contractility, and preservation of coronary perfusion pressure. These goals may be achieved pharmacologically or mechanically (e.g., intraaortic balloon pump). Once hemodynamics is controlled, one may choose from a long (and growing) list of agents that may or may not provide additional myocardial protection.

Cardioplegia Techniques

During CABG, the heart is subjected to varying periods of myocardial ischemia, depending on technique of revascularization. The decision to induce global myocardial ischemia (i.e., aortic cross-clamp application, cardioplegia administration, cardiac arrest) arose from the surgeon's need for a still, blood-free field to correct the underlying coronary artery lesions. The induction of elective ischemia during CABG on myocardium that is either diseased or has been subjected to previous periods of ischemia causes detrimental effects. Indeed, up to 90% of patients undergoing myocardial revascularization have decreased ejection fraction and/or cardiac index in the immediate postoperative period compared with preoperative values.[15] Such prolonged, reversible postischemic contractile dysfunction (stunned myocardium) is thought to result from decreased responsiveness of cardiac myofilaments to calcium secondary to generation of oxygen-derived free radicals and/or disturbances in calcium homeostasis that lead to intracellular calcium overload.[16] Ischemia-induced intracellular acidosis results in sodium entry into the myocyte. Excessive sodium cannot be removed because of impaired sodium–potassium exchange mechanisims induced by ischemia. Increased intracellular sodium levels cause increased intracellular calcium levels because of facilitated calcium entry and/or decreased calcium removal from the cell via sodium–calcium exchange mechanisms. Intracellular calcium overload then contributes to myocyte injury and causes contractile dysfunction.

Many recent investigations have focused on techniques that initiate myocardial preconditioning (ischemic and/or pharmacologic) to attenuate such postisichemic contractile dysfunction.[17,18] Beneficial effects of myocardial preconditioning appear to be modulated via protein kinase C activation. Protein kinase C activation results in a number of various myocyte intracellular events that beneficially affect ion exchange mechanisms, contractile proteins, gene expression, and intracellular acid-base balance, among others. Many experimental studies have revealed that protein kinase C activation prior to cardioplegic arrest may result in improved myocardial performance after reperfusion. However, although the potential for these applications is great, actual clinical application is in its infancy.

The myocardium is at risk for damage not only during ischemic arrest but also during reperfusion after the period of ischemic arrest.[19] Repurfusion injury can expedite death of vulnerable, yet still viable, myocardium by initiating a series of metabolic events involving cytotoxic reactive oxygen species, complement activation, and/or neutrophil adhesion. Reperfusion initiates an inflammatory response beginning with complement activation, which is followed by recruitment and accumulation of neutrophils into the vulnerable myocardium. Therefore, recent investigations have focused on manipulation of inflammatory response in an attempt to limit reperfusion injury.[20]

Standard Cardioplegia

Opinions vary enormously about what constitutes the "best" cardioplegia solution and the "best" method of delivery.[21,22] Choices during induction, maintenance, and reperfusion of cardioplegia include cardioplegia composition; intermittent vs. continuous, antegrade vs. retrograde, and hypothermic vs. normothermic methods; use of crystalloid vs. blood; method of controlled reperfusion; and whether additional protective agents are used (Table 4). Obviously, the combination of choices is overwhelming, and the fact that so many methods of myocardial protection exist indicates that no clear evidence supports one method over another. Unfortunately, although many important advances have occurred in this field, postoperative myocardial depression remains an important cause of morbidity and mortality, indicating that myocardial protection remains suboptimal.

Most surgeons use intermittent, antegrade, hypothermic, blood cardioplegia. Cardioplegia composition usually is formulated to be hyperkalemic, hypocalcemic, alkaline, and slightly hyperosmotic. Magnesium supplementation also is recommended by many. Hyperkalemic cardioplegia leads to rapid membrane depolarization of cardiac tissue. At this depolarized potential, fast sodium channels are inactivated, resulting in diastolic arrest and rapid cessation of contractile activity (thus reducing metabolic demands within the myocyte). Subsequent alterations in sodium and calcium exchange lead to sodium and calcium influx through membrane sodium–calcium exchange mechanisms and leakage of calcium from the sarcoplasmic reticulum, which causes intracellular calcium overload and myocyte damage and increases the risk of reperfusion damage. Furthermore, high potassium concentrations can directly damage endothelial cells. The depolarizing nature of hyperkalemic cardioplegia, which results in detrimental ionic imbalance caused by continued transmembrane flux, initiates abnormal regulation and activation of intracellular second messenger and enzyme systems and alterations in contractile performance. Probably depolarization is a major factor in postoperative myocardial depression. Recent

Table 4. Methods of Induction, Maintenance, and Reperfusion of Cardioplegia

Cardioplegia composition	Crystalloid vs. blood
Intermittent vs. continuous	Controlled reperfusion
Antegrade vs. retrograde	Additional protective agents
Hypothermic vs. normothermic	

investigation reveals that a potentially beneficial alternative to standard hyper-kalemic depolarized arrest may be induction of a "hyperpolarized" or "polar-ized" arrest, which maintains myocyte membrane potential at or near resting membrane potential.[23] Thus, transmembrane ionic flux should be minimized, resulting in improved myocardial protection. Indeed, use of adenosine and/or potassium channel openers appears to initiate hyperpolarized arrest and has demonstrated improved myocardial protection after myocardial ischemia com-pared with hyperkalamic depolarized arrest.

Modification of Standard Cardioplegia

Cardioplegia Composition. Whether cardioplegia should be crystalloid-based or blood-based and whether it should be supplemented with additional protective agents remain controversial issues.

Intermittent vs. Continuous. Although most surgeons use intermittent de-livery of cardioplegia, the choice remains somewhat controversial. Continuous delivery may present a substantial impediment to visibility during construc-tion of the distal anastomoses.

Antegrade vs. Retrograde. A large amount of research, spanning many years, has focused on the advantages and disadvantages of antegrade and ret-rograde delivery of cardioplegia.[24-26] The major advantages of antegrade car-dioplegia are simplicity and reliability. However, the anatomy of the coronary artery lesions variably influences distribution (and efficacy) of antegrade car-dioplegia. In addition, aortic insufficiency may inhibit adequate delivery of an-tegrade cardioplegia, the possibility of coronary ostial injury and/or coronary artery emboli is always present, and surgery must be interrupted during ad-ministration. Thus, many surgeons also use retrograde cardioplegia delivered into the coronary sinus.

Advantages of retrograde cardioplegia include obviation of operative inter-ruptions, decreased risk of aortic root air, and ability to flush coronary artery debris. Retrograde cardioplegia should not be the sole source of cardioplegia because individual coronary venous drainage patterns vary greatly. As a result, specific cardiac areas (right ventricle and posterior aspect of the interventricu-lar septum) may not receive adequate protection. The right ventricle may be difficult to protect with any type of delivery (antegrade and/or retrograde), es-pecially in the presence of occlusion of the right coronary artery. Thus, some surgeons recommend construction of a saphenous vein graft early during revascularization for delivery of antegrade cardioplegia to protect the right ventricle. Numerous factors affect efficacy of retrograde cardioplegia, includ-ing flow rate (high flows are needed to ensure uniform distribution) and catheter positioning within the coronary sinus (distal positioning may obstruct tributaries, mainly the posterior interventricular vein). Furthermore, the venous drainage system of the heart may possess valves that obstruct flow. The clinical benefits of retrograde cardioplegia may be related to better homoge-nous cooling rather than substrate replenishment. High flows through the coronary sinus are often limited by high coronary sinus pressure, which may induce myocardial edema, perivascular hemorrhage, or direct injury to the sinus. In addition, presence of venovenous shunts and thebesian channels may contribute to nonuniform distribution of retrograde cardioplegia. Some studies have suggested that more than one-half of all retrograde cardioplegia may drain directly into the ventricles via thebesian channels.

Traditionally, homogenous distribution of cardioplegia (antegrade and/or retrograde) was assessed via observation of quiescence of electrocardiogram electrical activity, decrease in myocardial temperature, and direct visualization. More recently, myocardial contrast echocardiography has been used to assess adequacy of cardioplegia distribution. The benefit of myocardial contrast echocardiography is that all myocardial segments may be assessed directly and in real time. Investigations involving myocardial contrast echocardiography have demonstrated the importance of collateral coronary vessels in determining distribution of cardioplegia. If collateral coronary vessels are not present, antegrade cardioplegia without retrograde cardioplegia may not produce sufficient homogenous distribution of cardioplegia. If collateral coronary vessels are present, however, antegrade without retrograde cardioplegia probably produces sufficient homogenous distribution. Myocardial contrast echocardiography appears to be the only reliable method to determine adequacy of collateral coronary vessels during revascularization at the time of cardioplegia delivery. The preoperative angiogram and electrocardiogram are poor predictors of regions at risk for incomplete cardioplegia distribution.

Hypothermic vs. Normothermic.   Theories about the optimal temperature of cardioplegia solutions have evolved over the years.[27] Hypothermic cardioplegia beneficially decreases myocyte metabolic rate but detrimentally affects postoperative myocardial recovery. On the other hand, normothermic cardioplegia detrimentally increases (relative to hypothermia) myocyte metabolic rate but enhances postoperative myocardial recovery. Compared with hypothermic cardioplegia, normothermic cardioplegia is associated with a greater rate of spontaneous return to sinus rhythm and decreased postoperative release of cardiac enzymes, suggesting enhanced myocardial protection. Warm reperfusion enhances immediate myocardial recovery and improves myocardial protection induced by hypothermic cardioplegia. Although normothermic cardiopulmonary bypass (and cardioplegia) may be associated with better myocardial recovery (lower incidence of postoperative low cardiac output syndrome), concern persists about detrimental neurologic effects.

Crystalloid vs. Blood.   Various crystalloid cardioplegia solutions differ in ionic composition, attempting to resemble the intracellular, extracellular, or intermediate environment. Despite promising experimental evidence of superior myocardial protection with use of cardioplegia that resembles the intracellular environment, clinical trials have yielded conflicting results. At the same time, growing experimental evidence suggests a beneficial role for blood cardioplegia (which, in theory, is more "physiologic" than crystalloid cardioplegia). Blood cardioplegia improves oxygen-carrying capacity, enhances myocardial oxygen consumption, preserves myocardial high-energy phosphate stores, facilitates aerobic myocardial metabolism during aortic crossclamping, and reduces anaerobic lactate production.

Controlled Reperfusion.   Controlled reperfusion with warm substrate-enriched cardioplegia (also known as a "hot-shot") attempts to attenuate reperfusion injury.[28,29] After aortic unclamping, the postischemic myocardium is vulnerable to sudden calcium influx. Unprotected calcium entry at this time may cause a hypercontractile state with subsequent sarcolemmal damage. Initial cardioplegia reperfusion maintains arrest and prevents hypercontracture, allowing a brief interval in which ionic balances can recover more normally during immediate reoxygenation. Most clinicians use the cardioplegia composition and method of administration initially described by Buckberg in 1989, which avoids high potassium concentration, limits calcium concentration, controls osmolarity (to limit edema), and tightly regulates flow and pressure parameters.[25] This technique enhances preservation of high-energy phosphates, limits transsarcolemmal pH gradients on reperfusion, limits sodium and calcium overload during reperfusion, and reduces morbidity and mortality rates. Additional recent work indicates that further manipulations during controlled reperfusion (optmization of potassium concentration, limiting of acidosis, replenishing of citric acid cycle, increase in osmolarity) in patients undergoing emergency myocardial revascularization may improve morbidity and mortality rates in this high-risk subset of patients.[20] Other methods of potentially limiting reperfusion calcium damage include use of calcium channel antagonists and sodium ion–hydrogen ion exchange inhibitors. In the future, more comprehensive approaches (e.g., manipulation of neutrophils, use of oxygen free radical scavengers) may be added as new information unfolds.

Additional Protective Agents. As previously stated, the past decade has seen an explosion of investigation that has produced novel therapeutic strategies that may confer myocardial protection (see Table 3). Various manipulations may be performed during induction, maintenance, and/or reperfusion of cardioplegia. Investigations have explored many varied options, including manipulations that modify energy substrates, modify ionic balance, modify cellular acidosis, modify enzyme regulation, and modify the inflammatory response. A wide variety of experimental animal models reveal that myocardial ischemia and reperfusion injury can be attenuated, but clinical application has been minimal. Many studies have shown that optimal concentration of an agent added to cardioplegia can provide myocardial protection, whereas an excess of the same agent may have detrimental effects that limit any benefit. Most recently, molecular aspects of the interaction between vascular endothelium and inflammatory cells have emerged as an important potential mediator of ischemia-reperfusion injury, and the first attempts at gene therapy to modify myocardial responses to stress and ischemia are under way.[30] Such therapy would allow organ-selective, local delivery of higher levels of agents than can be safely achieved via systemic administration.

Intracellular calcium overload plays a major role in myocardial reperfusion injury. Thus, cardioplegia solutions are rendered hypocalcemic to limit calcium entry into the cell. However, calcium-free cardioplegia may damage the myocardium, a phenomenon initially described by Zimmerman in 1967 and termed calcium paradox.[31] The proposed mechanism of calcium paradox is as follows: calcium-free cardioplegia renders membranes more susceptible to calcium influx via sodium–calcium exchangers on re-exposure to calcium-containing solutions. The results are severe tissue damage, mitochondrial swelling, and increases in myocardial water content. The potential for calcium paradox in the clinical setting, however, is a matter of controversy.

Magnesium, the second most abundant intracellular ion, is lost during myocardial ischemia; as a result, magnesium-dependent cellular reactions are impaired.[8,9] Magnesium supplementation of cardioplegia improves myocardial protection (assessed with systolic and diastolic parameters) via a variety of pathways and decreases the incidence of postoperative arrhythmias. Probably the main mechanism of magnesium's beneficial effects is its ability to modulate intracellular calcium levels by inhibiting calcium entry into the cell as well as displacing calcium from sarcolemmal membrane binding sites. This process prevents mitochondrial calcium uptake, which can lead to uncoupling of oxidative phosphorylation and decreased energy production. There is a definite specific interrelationship between magnesium and calcium: magnesium enhances the myocardial protective effects of hypocalcemic cardioplegia but cannot prevent the detrimental effects of normocalcemic cardioplegia. Thus, the optimal magnesium concentration in cardioplegia depends on the calcium concentration since the beneficial effects of magnesium supplementation and hypocalcemia are additive as well as interdependent. Additional beneficial effects of magnesium are prevention of sodium influx (which limits calcium influx) and facilitation of asystole at lower potassium concentration.

Adenosine was introduced as an additive to cardioplegia in 1980, and numerous studies have detailed improved myocardial protection with its use.[32,33] Adenosine has potent vasodilator effects and is a key component of autoregulation of coronary artery blood flow. Adenosine is released tonically by myocytes, endothelium, and neutrophils, and myocyte release into the interstitium increases substantially during ischemia. Fundamental beneficial effects of adenosine include provision of ultrastructural substrates for high-energy phosphate repletion, altered biochemical interactions in myocyte contractile properties, and potentiation of myocyte glycolysis. These beneficial effects are mediated via specific adenosine receptors (at least four subtypes exist). Each adenosine receptor subtype contributes physiologic responses that beneficially influence ischemia and/or reperfusion injury. For example, A_1 receptor stimulation mobilizes protein kinase C, which in turn activates potassium channels, improves anaerobic metabolism and energy status, and attenuates neutrophil-myocyte interactions. A_2 receptor stimulation has direct beneficial effects on neutrophils by inhibiting superoxide anion generation and adhesion molecule expression. It also has a beneficial effect on endothelium by inhibiting activation. Thus, adenosine is useful for preconditioning, treatment during ischemia, and treatment during reperfusion. These cardioprotective effects of adenosine have been suggested to play major roles in reduction of myocardial infarction and apoptosis after myocardial ischemia, cardioplegia-induced arrest, and subsequent reperfusion. Clinically, adenosine-supplemented cardioplegia improves postoperative myocardial functional recovery as assessed by systolic and diastolic parameters. Adenosine supplementation of cardioplegia reduces the time to myocardial arrest compared with hyperkalemic solution alone via initiation of transient hyperpolarization prior to depolarization. Adenosine also reduces potassium-induced intracellular calcium loading, supporting the concept that adenosine exerts a cardioprotective effect. Furthermore, the duration of these beneficial physiologic effects seems to extend well beyond the plasma half-life of the drug.

Numerous experimental drugs act on *adenosine triphosphate-sensitive potassium channels* in cardiac muscle. A large body of literature suggests that openers of this potassium channel exert beneficial effects on ischemic myocardium.[34] The cardioprotective effects of potassium channel openers are thought to result from their properties of reducing action potential duration and inducing cell membrane hyperpolarization by reequilibrating the resting membrane potential closer to the equilibrium constant of potassium. This effect is associated with a reduction in myocardial contractility, attributed to a reduction in intracellular calcium and preservation of high-energy phosphate stores.

Inhaled anesthetics are thought to exert their myocardial protective effects via activation of potassium channels. Potassium channel openers have been used in combination with hyperkalemic cardioplegia solutions, but the results have been conflicting. Some studies have even shown a detrimental proarrhythmic effect. Beneficial physiologic effects include coronary vasodilation and reduction in infarct size. Much like adenosine, potassium channel openers are thought to induce a hyperpolarized arrest.

Sodium channel blockers have been used as cardioplegia adjuvants for many years and are thought to induce a form of "polarized" arrest.[23] Apparently they limit intracellular sodium flux—and thus intracellular calcium flux—after myocardial ischemia. Sodium channel blockers are effective cardioprotective agents against myocardial ischemia and reperfusion injury in various experimental models. Evidence suggests that they may improve myocardial recovery, improve balance of high-energy phosphate levels, and reduce metabolic demands on the ischemic heart compared with the depolarized arrest induced by hyperkalemia.

Aprotinin, administered initially to decrease postoperative bleeding, also may have myocardial protective effects.[35] Investigators have shown myocardial protective benefits of aprotinin in the isolated rat heart subjected to global ischemia and in a model of regional ischemia in dogs. In humans, aprotinin reduces the release of cardiac troponin after myocardial revascularization. The protective mechanism of aprotinin remains unclear but may involve decreases in various inflammatory mediators in the blood and/or decreased degrees of cytotoxicity (resulting in better preservation of selective sarcolemmal permeability and reduced calcium overload). However, routine use of aprotinin during myocardial revascularization is not advocated because of the possibility that the incidence of early vein graft occlusion may be increased, especially in women, in smaller vessels, and in poor-quality distal vessels. However, careful selection of patients based on known risk factors for early graft failure may allow a subgroup to benefit from the myocardial protective action of aprotinin.

Bradykinin exhibits a multitude of beneficial cardiovascular effects. Recent investigation indicates that it plays an essential role in preservation of myocardial structure and function and may improve myocardial tolerance to ischemia through molecular mechanisms probably associated with ischemic preconditioning (protein tyrosine kinase and protein kinase C activation).[36] Bradykinin exerts physiologic effects via interaction with specific receptors: B_1 receptors mediate inflammatory reactions, and B_2 receptors mediate cardiovascular effects. Pretreatment of the heart with bradykinin can preserve myocyte stores of energy-rich phosphates and glycogen, increase coronary blood flow, increase left ventricular contractility, improve left ventricular compliance, decrease reperfusion arrhythmias, and decrease infarct size. In the vasculature, bradykinin stimulates endogenous nitric oxide synthase, leading to increased levels of nitric oxide. In fact, the beneficial clinical effects of angiotensin-converting enzyme inhibitors (improved survival in patients with advanced heart failure or myocardial infarction) may be secondary to decreased degradation of bradykinin (beneficial effects are maintained despite normal plasma and tissue angiotensin II levels). Pretreatment of the myocardium with bradykinin prior to warm cardioplegic ischemia substantially improves postischemic ventricular dysfunction.

Intriguing recent investigation indicates that *opioid delta-receptor agonists* may have myocardial protective effects.[37] This discovery was stimulated by the knowledge that hibernation in animals (during which metabolic processes dramatically slow to approximately 10% of normal levels) appears to be mediated via cyclical variations in endogenous opioid compounds. Furthermore, hibernation can be "reversed" by administration of opioid antagonists. These effects appear to be mediated via the opioid delta receptor. Recent animal studies indicate that cardioplegia supplemented with standard opioid agonists (fentanyl, morphine) confers additional myocardial protection.

Much recent investigation has focused on the potential myocardial protective effects of a wide variety of *intravenous and inhalational anesthetics*.[38] Results indicate that these widely diverse agents may protect the myocardium via many different pathways, including potassium channel activation, inhibition of sodium ion–hydrogen ion exchange, and/or antioxidant effects. Thus, routine administration of intravenous and/or inhalational anesthesia may provide myocardial protection.

Normal myocardium utilizes fatty acids, lactate, and glucose as main substrates for energy. During ischemia, fatty acid metabolism is severely impaired. Oxygen deprivation leads to diminished beta oxidation of fatty acids, but glucose competes favorably with fatty acids for the residual oxygen supplied in lesser amounts. In addition, glycolytic activity is enhanced, leading to lactate accumulation in hypoperfused areas. Restoration of flow after ischemia is associated with decreased fatty acid oxidation and enhanced utilization of carbohydrates (suggesting that postischemic myocardial handling of fatty acids is altered). Thus, in contrast to the normal preoperative state, in which the myocardium preferentially utilizes fatty acids and lactate, the immediate postoperative period after myocardial revascularization is associated with myocardium that preferentially utilizes glucose.[39] Therefore, *glucose supplementation* may provide important metabolic support and improve postoperative myocardial function.

"Beating Heart" Myocardial Revascularization

Minimally invasive myocardial revascularization without cardiopulmonary bypass ("beating heart" surgery) may be beneficial in that the detrimental myocardial effects of cardiopulmonary bypass, aortic cross-clamping, cardioplegia, and ischemia-reperfusion injury are avoided.[40,41] The role of this technique in the usually emergent setting of acute evolving myocardial infarction has not yet been defined and may not be practical. However, in a subset of patients (perhaps those with single-vessel disease), minimally invasive myocardial revascularization without cardiopulmonary bypass may prove to be practical and beneficial.

Conclusion

Myocardial infarction is a dynamic process and almost always is associated with coronary atherosclerosis with superimposed coronary thrombosis. Although recent dramatic technologic advances are responsible for the continuing decrease in mortality due to acute myocardial infarction, it remains fatal in approximately one of three patients. Myocardial protection for patients with acute myocardial infarction is extremely important because infarct size is an important determinent of prognosis. The many efforts to limit myocardial infarct size generally include three often overlapping approaches: early reperfusion, optimization of myocardial oxygen supply:demand ratio, and manipulation of myocardial energy dynamics. Coronary artery bypass grafting is generally reserved for patients in whom other procedures (thrombolysis and/or catheter intervention) have failed. Patients undergoing cardiac surgery with acute evolving myocardial infarction are often hemodynamically unstable (for a wide variety of reasons) and have increased morbidity and mortality rates; therefore, all efforts that improve myocardial protection (i.e., limit infarct size) should be explored.

Prior to the operating room, important myocardial protective agents include heparin, aspirin, and magnesium. Hemodynamic control (focusing on optimization of the myocardial oxygen supply:demand ratio) before myocardial revascularization is of utmost importance to prevent myocardial ischemia and infarct extension. Beta-adrenergic blockers and angiotensin-converting enzyme inhibitors are particularly beneficial and may improve morbidity and mortality rates. Thoracic epidural application of local anesthetics may be beneficial by providing intense postoperative analgesia, stress response attenuation, and thoracic cardiac sympathectomy. Although controlling systemic and coronary hemodynamics is certainly important, over the past decade an explosion of investigation has provided novel therapeutic strategies that may confer myocardial protection independently of systemic and coronary hemodynamics. These agents work via many diverse mechanisms that alter the metabolic, mechanical, and/or electrophysiologic consequences of myocardial ischemia. However, the vast majority of these agents are investigational. There is no "magic bullet" to treat myocardial ischemia.

During coronary revascularization, the heart is subjected to varying periods of myocardial ischemia, depending on the technique of revascularization. The myocardium is at risk for damage not only during ischemic arrest but also during reperfusion after the period of ischemic arrest. Opinion varies enormously as to what constitutes the "best" cardioplegia solution and "best" method of delivery. The various choices for induction, maintenance, and reperfusion of cardioplegia include cardioplegia composition, intermittent vs. continuous, antegrade vs. retrograde, hypothermic vs. normothermic, crystalloid vs. blood, method of controlled reperfusion, and whether additional experimental agents are used. Obviously, the combination of choices is overwhelming and the fact that so many methods of myocardial protection exist indicates that no clear evidence supports one method over another. Most surgeons use intermittent, antegrade, hypothermic, blood cardioplegia. Cardioplegia composition usually is formulated to become hyperkalemic, hypocalcemic, alkaline, and slightly hyperosmotic. Magnesium supplementation also is recommended by many, as is routine use of controlled reperfusion with warm substrate-enriched cardioplegia (also known as a "hot-shot"). Various manipulations may be performed during induction, maintenance, and/or reperfusion of cardioplegia. Investigations have explored many options, including manipulations that modify energy substrates, ionic balance, cellular acidosis, enzyme regulation, and inflammatory response. Unfortunately, although many important advances have occurred, along with many changes in formulation of cardioplegia composition and method of administration, postoperative myocardial depression remains an important cause of morbidity and mortality, indicating that myocardial protection is suboptimal. Perhaps with the recent resurgence of minimally invasive myocardial revascularization without cardiopulmonary bypass ("beating heart" surgery), the detrimental myocardial effects of cardiopulmonary bypass, aortic crossclamping, cardioplegia, and is-chemia–reperfusion injury may be avoided.

References

1. Antman EM, Braunwald E: Acute myocardial infarction. In Braunwald E (ed): Heart Disease; A Textbook of Cardiovascular Medicine, 5th ed. Philadelphia, W.B. Saunders, pp 1184–1288, 1997.
2. Rentrop KP: Thrombi in acute coronary syndromes: Revisited and revised. Circulation 101:1619–1626, 2000.
3. Hirose H, Amano A, Yoshida S, et al: Surgical management of unstable patients in the evolving phase of acute myocardial infarction. Ann Thorac Surg 69: 425–428, 2000.
4. Hirsh J: Drug therapy: Heparin. N Engl J Med 324:1565–1574, 1991.
5. Awtry EH, Loscalzo J: Cardiovascular drugs: Aspirin. Circulation 101:1206–1218, 2000.
6. Roux S, Christellar S, Ludin E: Effects of aspirin on coronary reocclusion and recurrent ischemia after thrombolysis: A meta-analysis. J Am Coll Cardiol 19: 671–677, 1992.
7. Scarborough RM, Kleiman NS, Phillips DR: Platelet glycoprotein IIb/IIIa antagonists: What are the relevant issues concerning their pharmacology and clinical use? Circulation 100:437–444, 1999.
8. Gomez MN: Magnesium and cardiovascular disease. Anesthesiology 89:222–240, 1998.
9. Antman EM: Magnesium in acute MI: timing is critical [editorial]. Circulation 92:2367–2372, 1995.
10. Warltier DC, Pagel PS, Kersten JR: Approaches to the prevention of perioperative myocardial ischemia. Anesthesiology 92:253–259, 2000.
11. Chaney MA, Slogoff S: Perioperative myocardial ischemia and infarction. In Atlee JL (ed): Complications in Anesthesia. Philadelphia, W.B. Saunders, pp 348–350, 1999.
12. Wallace A, Layug B, Tateo I, et al: Prophylactic atenolol reduces postoperative myocardial ischemia. Anesthesiology 88:7–17, 1998.
13. Chaney MA: Intrathecal and epidural anesthesia and analgesia for cardiac surgery. Anesth Analg 84:1211–1221, 1997.
14. Castellano JM, Durbin CG: Epidural analgesia and cardiac surgery: Worth the risk? [editorial]. Chest 117:305–307, 2000.
15. Leung J: Clinical evidence of myocardial stunning in patients undergoing CABG surgery. J Card Surg 8: 220–223, 1993.
16. Gross GJ, Kersten JR, Warltier DC: Mechanisms of postischemic contractile dysfunction. Ann Thorac Surg 68:1898–1904, 1999.
17. Spinale FG: Cellular and molecular therapeutic targets for treatment of contractile dysfuntion after cardioplegic arrest. Ann Thorac Surg 68:1934–1941, 1999.
18. Perrault LP, Menasche P: Preconditioning: Can nature's shield be raised against surgical ischemic–reperfusion injury? Ann Thorac Surg 68:1988–1994, 1999.
19. Park JL, Lucchesi BR: Mechanisms of myocardial reperfusion injury. Ann Thorac Surg 68: 1905–1912, 1999.
20. Schlensak C, Doenst T, Kobba J, Beyersdorf F: Protection of acutely ischemic myocardium by controlled reperfusion. Ann Thorac Surg 68:1967–1970, 1999.
21. Cohen G, Borger MA, Weisel RD, Rao V: Intraoperative myocardial protection: current trends and future perspectives. Ann Thorac Surg 68:1995–2001, 1999.
22. Robinson LA, Schwarz GD, Goddard DB, et al: Myocardial protection for acquired heart disease surgery: Results of a national survey. Ann Thorac Surg 59:361–372, 1995.
23. Chambers DJ, Hearse DJ: Developments in cardioprotection: "Polarized" arrest as an alternative to "depolarized" arrest. Ann Thorac Surg 68:1960–1966, 1999.
24. Aronson S: Cardioplegia delivery: More (or less) than what you see [editorial]. Ann Thorac Surg 68:797–798, 1999.
25. Buckberg GD: Antegrade/retrograde blood cardioplegia to ensure cardioplegic distribution: Operative techniques and objectives. J Card Surg 4:216–238, 1989.
26. Gott VL, Gonzalez JL, Zuhdi MN, et al: Retrograde perfusion of the coronary sinus for direct vision aortic surgery. Surg Gynecol Obstet 104:319–328, 1957.
27. Chocron S, Kaili D, Yan Y, et al: Intermediate lukewarm (20° C) antegrade intermittent blood cardioplegia compared with cold and warm blood cardioplegia. J Thorac Cardiovasc Surg 119:610–616, 2000.
28. Buckberg GD: Substrate-enriched warm blood cardioplegia reperfusion: An alternate view. [editorial]. Ann Thorac Surg 69:334–345, 2000.
29. Chocron S, Alwan K, Yan Y, et al: Warm reperfusion and myocardial protection. Ann Thorac Surg 66:2003–2007, 1998.

30. Allen MD: Myocardial protection: Is there a role for gene therapy? Ann Thorac Surg 68:1924–1928, 1999.
31. Zimmerman ANE, Daems W, Hulsmann W, et al: Morphological changes of heart muscle caused by successive perfusion with calcium-free and calcium-containing solutions (calcium paradox). Cardiovasc Res 1:201–209, 1967.
32. Fogelson BG, Nawas SI, Law WR: Mechanisms of myocardial protection by adenosine-supplemented cardioplegic solution: Myofilament and metabolic responses. J Thorac Cardiovasc Surg 119:601–609, 2000.
33. Vinten-Johansen J, Thourani VH, Ronson RS, et al: Broad-spectrum cardioprotection with adenosine. Ann Thorac Surg 68:1942–1948, 1999.
34. Auchampach JA, Maruyama M, Gross GJ: Cardioprotective actions of potassium channel openers. Eur Heart J 15(Suppl C):89–94, 1994.
35. Hendrikx M, Jiang H, Gutermann H, et al: Release of cardiac troponin I in antegrade crystalloid versus cold blood cardioplegia. J Thorac Cardiovasc Surg 118:452–459, 1999.
36. Feng J, Rosenkranz ER: Bradykinin pretreatment improves ischemia tolerance of the rabbit heart by tyrosine kinase mediated pathways. Ann Thorac Surg 68:1567–1572, 1999.
37. Benedict PE, Benedict MB, Su TP, Bolling SF: Opiate drugs and δ-receptor-mediated myocardial protection. Circulation 100: II-357–II-360, 1999.
38. Mathur S, Farhangkhgoee P, Karmazyn M: Cardioprotective effects of propofol and sevoflurane in ischemic and reperfused rat hearts: Role of K-ATP channels and interaction with the sodium-hydrogen exchange inhibitor HOE 642 (cariporide). Anesthesiology 91:1349–1360, 1999.
39. Pietersen HG, Langenberg CJM, Geskes G, et al: Myocardial substrate uptake and oxidation during and after routine cardiac surgery. J Thorac Cardiovasc Surg 118:71–80, 1999.
40. Chitwood WR, Wixon CL, Elbeery JR, et al: Minimally invasive cardiac operation: Adapting cardioprotective strategies. Ann Thorac Surg 68:1974–1977, 1999.
41. Maslow A, Aronson S, Jacobsohn E, et al: Off-pump coronary artery bypass graft surgery. J Cardiothorac Vasc Anesth 13:764–781, 1999.

21

Mechanical Support for Patients with Acute Coronary Syndromes

RICHARD J. KAPLON, MD
PATRICK M. McCARTHY, MD

Despite advances in the diagnosis and treatment of coronary artery disease during the past several decades, approximately 1.5 million people suffer from acute myocardial infarction (MI) each year in the U.S.[1] Of these, 250,000 patients die within the first hour of onset of ischemia.[1] An appropriate algorithm for the treatment of patients with acute myocardial ischemia includes the possible use of thrombolytics, percutaneous revascularization, or coronary artery bypass grafting (CABG). Unfortunately, despite the improvements seen with urgent revascularization in recent years, the mechanical complications of acute infarction, such as cardiogenic shock, ventricular septal or free wall rupture, and papillary muscle infarction with concomitant mitral regurgitation, continue to challenge physicians. While the overall mortality rate from an acute MI has decreased during the past 30 years (from 17% to 7%), the incidence of cardiogenic shock and its mortality rate have not changed.[2–4]

Patients who remain hemodynamically unstable after an MI despite medical, interventional, or operative attempts at revascularization require mechanical circulatory assistance. Delay in restoring normal systemic hemodynamics and perfusion results in irreversible end-organ dysfunction with poor outcomes. Cardiogenic shock is a clinical definition and includes parameters such as systolic blood pressure < 80 mmHg, urine output < 0.5 ml/kg/min, cardiac index < 1.8 l/min/m², and elevated pulmonary capillary wedge pressure. These changes are usually seen in patients with loss of more than 40% of left ventricular mass and are determined by size of the zone of infarction, collateral circulation, and degree of preinfarction ventricular function.

Specific assist-device selection for patients in cardiogenic shock is based on (1) degree of myocardial dysfunction and amount of support required, (2) likelihood of reversibility of cardiac injury, (3) relative left and right heart dysfunction, (4) likely duration of support, and (5) comorbidities and expectation of meaningful patient recovery. At the Cleveland Clinic Foundation (CCF) and University of Miami/Jackson Memorial Hospital, currently available support devices include intraaortic balloon pump (IABP), extracorporeal life support (ECLS), the Abiomed BVS 5000, the Thoratec ventricular assist device (VAD), and the TCI Heartmate left ventricular assist device (LVAD). Future devices probably will include epicardial compression devices, fully implantable VADs, axial flow pumps, and total artificial hearts.

Intraaortic Balloon Pump

Use of the IABP to treat cardiogenic shock after acute MI was first described by Kantrowitz et al. in 1968.[5] Later reports confirmed its effectiveness.[6,7] Currently, the IABP is the most commonly used cardiac assist device, supporting over 100,000 patients annually.[6,7] Although least invasive and likewise least supportive compared with other cardiac assist devices, the IABP nonetheless has several advantages. It is small, portable, and easily placed and removed percutaneously without the need for operation. Femoral access provides ready placement in the descending thoracic aorta, just distal to the left subclavian artery, in most instances. Relative contraindications to IABP placement include abdominal aortic aneurysm, pregnancy, and aortic valvular insufficiency.

Support from the IABP is based on the principle of intraaortic counterpulsation. Balloon inflation during diastole enhances coronary perfusion; deflation during systole decreases afterload and helps to reduce myocardial oxygen consumption and workload.

Early reports of IABP use for infarction-associated cardiogenic shock demonstrated safety but not efficacy; however, more recent reports have shown that aortic counterpulsation in combination with revascularization increases both survival and coronary patency.[8–10] Further reports suggest that this success translates to "cost-effectiveness" in regard to shorter hospital stay and complication reduction.[11]

Extracorporeal Life Support

Success with ECLS has been demonstrated predominantly in patients with postcardiotomy heart failure; however, favorable outcomes also have been shown in patients with acute MI.[12–15] Muehrcke et al. demonstrated that use of a heparin-coated ECLS circuit permitted 30% of patients requiring postcardiotomy support to be successfully discharged home. Magovern et al. demonstrated that 80% of patients requiring ECLS after coronary bypass surgery were successfully discharged, whereas all patients requiring support after mitral valve surgery died.[12–13] The limitation to survival in the mitral valve group was believed to be persistent left ventricular distention secondary to inadequate ventricular decompression, an issue that clearly has implications with regard to myocardial stunning and ventricular recovery in patients with acute MI.

Although few in number, studies examining the use ECLS for cardiogenic shock after acute MI have shown that approximately 50% of patients may be weaned from ECLS, and 40% enjoy long-term survival.[14–15] Like IABP, ECLS has the advantage of being small, portable, and easily placed and removed percutaneously via the femoral vessels without the need for operation.

Potential limitations include the increase in afterload of the left ventricle in response to retrograde perfusion via the femoral artery and lack of decompression of the left ventricle with venous return solely from the femoral vein. Bavaria et al. demonstrated that ECLS increases left ventricular mural tension and myocardial oxygen consumption by increasing afterload. Muehrke et al.

showed that as many as 56% of patients have persistent ventricular distention, as demonstrated by echocardiography, while they are on ECLS.[13,16]

Allen et al. showed that ventricular decompression after revascularization of ischemic myocardium decreases myocardial oxygen consumption by reducing mural tension and results in decreased muscle damage and improvement in overall functional outcome.[17] Even with concomitant use of an IABP to compensate for the increase in afterload effected by ECLS, as advocated by Lazar et al., postcardiotomy patients on ECLS who had persistent ventricular dilatation did poorly.[13,18] Further studies addressing the long-term impact of this aspect of ECLS on acutely injured myocardium need to be undertaken before the role of ECLS for acute MI can be clearly defined.

Abiomed BVS 5000

The Abiomed BVS 5000 (Abiomed Cardiovascular, Inc., Danvers, MA) is a pneumatically actuated, extracorporeal, pulsatile cardiac assist device that is capable of providing short-term left, right, or biventricular mechanical circulatory support. Approved by the Food and Drug Administration (FDA) in 1992 for postcardiotomy support, this pump has become the second most widely-used assist device, after the IABP.[19] Since its initial FDA approval, indications for use of the Abiomed BVS 5000 have expanded to encompass all forms of recoverable heart failure, including acute MI, myocarditis, and right ventricular support after LVAD placement.

Intracardiac inflow cannulas made of wire-reinforced polyvinyl chloride are readily placed atrially through double-pledgetted polypropylene pursestrings and secured with tourniquets and ties. Drainage also may be achieved from the left ventricular apex or right ventricular diaphragmatic free wall. Pump outflow is typically either to the pulmonary artery or aorta and is facilitated by the presence of a Dacron graft attached to the end of the outflow cannulas. In unusual cases, outflow can be accomplished via a transventricular cannula passed either through the pulmonic or aortic valve for right- or left-sided support, respectively. A Dacron velour coating on the outside of all cannulas helps to promote tissue in-growth at the skin interface and minimizes mediastinal infection.

The console to the device is automated and self-regulating and operates asynchronously with regard to native cardiac function. The pump is preload-dependent and has a constant stroke volume of 80 ml. Changes in pump rate can provide a maximum of 6 L/min flow if preload is adequate.

Advantages of the Abiomed BVS 5000 include ease of placement, pulsatility, and user-friendly console management. As a result, excellent outcomes have been obtained in the form of the "Hub" concept, whereby patients requiring mechanical circulatory support can be placed on this device in the community setting and subsequently transferred to a tertiary care or transplant center better equipped to care for patients with heart failure.[20] Using this scheme, Helman et al. report a 66% survival rate to hospital discharge. Among patients suffering an acute MI, specifically, survival rates up to 70% have been reported.[21]

Although the Abiomed BVS 5000 has been shown to provide excellent, short-term, pulsatile support for all forms of acute, reversible heart failure, its use, particularly for patients with acute MI, is limited.[22] Unlike ECLS, which can be readily placed percutaneously, Abiomed BVS 5000 placement requires sternotomy or thoracotomy. Because VAD insertion necessitates operation, this device is most commonly used as an adjunct to CABG for patients who suffer an acute MI and require postcardiotomy support. Unlike ECLS, however, LVAD support with the Abiomed BVS 5000 completely unloads the left ventricle, minimizing oxygen consumption and work.

Use of the Abiomed BVS 5000 requires full anticoagulation and typically platelet inhibition as well. Although this protocol is advantageous for native coronary and autologous graft patency, bleeding in the perioperative period can be problematic. Moreover, because of device configuration, patient mobility is extremely limited. Typically, patients remain bed-bound, although some may occasionally sit in a chair or ambulate at the bedside in the intensive care unit. As a result, the Abiomed BVS 5000 is best-suited for short-term support, either as bridge-to-recovery or bridge-to-bridge therapy. For patients who remain hemodynamically unstable after CABG for acute MI, this device is an excellent choice to provide support until myocardial recovery or need for long-term mechanical assistance can be determined.

Thoratec Ventricular Assist Device

Like the BVS 5000, the Thoratec VAD (Thoratec Laboratories Corporation, Berkeley, CA) is a pneumatically actuated, paracorporeal cardiac assist device capable of right, left, or biventricular support. Based on the design of William Pierce and James Donachy, this device was first used for postcardiotomy support in 1982 and for bridge to transplant in 1986.[23–25] The Thoratec VAD was approved by the FDA for bridge-to-transplant therapy in 1996, and, like the Abiomed BVS 5000, its role has expanded to encompass all forms of recoverable heart failure. In contrast to the BVS 5000, however, the Thoratec VAD is capable of long-term support.

Pump insertion is accomplished with wire-reinforced polyurethane cannulas. Outflow conduits have a Dacron graft on the end for anastomosis to the aorta or pulmonary artery. Cannulation site selection varies with pathology; higher pump flows have been demonstrated with ventricular cannulation, but factors such as potential ventricular recovery, left ventricular geometry, and presence of ventricular thrombus may influence site selection.[26–28] Velour coating at the skin exit sites helps to promote tissue in-growth and minimize infection.

The VAD blood pump consists of a smooth, seamless pumping chamber made of a proprietary polyurethane polymer (Thoralon), enclosed in a rigid plastic case. Mechanical tilting-disc valves ensure unidirectional flow. Positive and negative pressure from the console via a pneumatic driveline allows the pump to be actuated in "volume" ("fill-to-empty"), "asynchronous" ("fixed-rate"), or "external synchronization" (electrocardiography-driven) modes. Although asynchronous to the heart rhythm, the "volume" mode maintains physiologic blood flow by changing pump rate in response to preload and afterload.

There have been several large reviews of clinical experience with the Thoratec VAD; however, most studies have focused on the outcomes of its use for bridge-to-transplantation therapy or postcardiotomy support.[29–33] Results with the Thoratec VAD for these indications have been similar to the experience reported for other assist devices. Unfortunately, there have been no specific reports addressing use of the Thoratec VAD in the setting of post-MI cardiogenic shock. McBride et al. reported that of 44 patients supported for anticipated recovery, 19 (43%) were weaned from the VAD and 12 (27%) survived;

of 67 patients placed on VAD support as bridge to transplantation, 3 were weaned and 39 (58%) were successfully transplanted.[33] Only 4 patients were placed on VAD support after acute MI.

Hendry et al. reported their experience with mechanical circulatory support for patients with cardiogenic shock due to acute MI.[34] Of 25 patients requiring VADs, 12 received a Thoratec VAD (6 biventricular, 6 left ventricular). The remaining patients were supported with the CardioWest total artificial heart. Twenty-two patients (88%) were transplanted with 1-, 2-, and 5-year survival rates of 71.4%, 71.4% and 51%, respectively. Although the results are not specific to the Thoratec VAD alone, one clearly can extrapolate the success of this device for patients with acute MI.

Limitations to more widespread use of the Thoratec VAD in patients with acute MI are similar to those described for the Abiomed BVS 5000. Device insertion requires sternotomy; therefore, the Thoratec VAD is used more commonly for postcardiotomy support after revascularization. Like the Abiomed device, this pump requires full anticoagulation and typically platelet inhibition as well. Bleeding after device placement is not uncommon. Advantages of this VAD compared with the BVS 5000 include the possibility of long-term support and better patient mobilization and ambulation. Although patients are not routinely sent home on the Thoratec VAD, discharge from the intensive care unit is typical. Recent use of a portable driver may further facilitate patient mobilization and discharge from the hospital setting.[35]

The Thoratec VAD is significantly more expensive than the Abiomed BVS 5000. It is capable of long-term support and therefore requires the patient to undergo only a single procedure if weaning from mechanical assist fails (versus the potential "bridge-to-bridge" phenomenon occasionally seen with the Abiomed pump). It is not clear, however, that more widespread use is justified in patients with acute MI. This device may be best suited to the unusual post-MI patient who clearly requires long-term, biventricular mechanical circulatory assistance as a bridge to recovery or transplant.

TCI Heartmate

The TCI Heartmate LVAD (Thermocardiosystems, Woburn, MA) is an implantable titanium pusher-plate device. It is inserted via median sternotomy. Inflow to the device is from the left ventricular apex; outflow is via a Dacron graft to the ascending aorta. Porcine-valved inflow and outflow conduits ensure unidirectional flow. Maximal stroke volume is approximately 85 ml, and peak flow is 10 L/min. In automatic mode, the Heartmate ejects when the pump chamber is 95% full. The device may be actuated either pneumatically or electrically; the vented-electric model can be pneumatically actuated as well. Because of the textured blood-contacting surfaces, no systemic anticoagulation is necessary. Thromboembolic rates < 3.5% have been reported in patients taking only aspirin, 81 mg/day. The FDA approved the TCI Heartmate for bridge-to-transplant therapy in 1994. Current prospective, randomized trials include use of the device as "destination" therapy (REMATCH: Randomized Evaluation of Mechanical Assistance for Treatment of Congestive Heart Failure) and "salvage" therapy for patients in cardiogenic shock who are not transplant candidates (PRIDE: Patients at Risk of Imminent Death Evaluation).

Lewis et al. described the first experience with an implantable LVAD for hemodynamic support after acute MI.[36] A 47-year-old man who suffered a massive MI complicated by cardiogenic shock and refractory ventricular fibrillation underwent successful placement of a pneumatic Heartmate. Unfortunately, while awaiting an available donor heart, the infarct extended and the patient suffered a ventricular free-wall rupture at the site of the apical cannula, which led to his demise.

Several centers have described successful use of implantable LVADs for mechanical support of cardiogenic shock after acute MI.[34,37–39] Chen et al. reviewed their experience with 25 LVADs placed early (< 2 weeks) or late (> 2 weeks) after MI.[39] The investigators found that patients in the early group had a lower incidence of RVAD placement but a higher incidence of perioperative use of inhalational nitric oxide compared with the late group. Survival to transplant was statistically similar between the two groups (67% and 60%, respectively), as was survival to explant (7% and 0%, respectively). The authors concluded that, in addition to the obvious survival benefit seen with LVAD placement in this setting, "timely application" of LVAD support for post-MI cardiogenic shock may "reveal a subgroup of patients for whom … LVAD insertion may allow for full ventricular recovery."

Theoretical and real advantages to LVAD insertion for post-MI cardiogenic shock include left ventricular decompression, decreased mural tension, diminished left ventricular workload, and enhanced myocardial perfusion. These hemodynamic changes may limit infarct size, facilitate successful bridge-to-transplantation, and improve the likelihood of bridge to recovery.[40–41] Moreover, malignant ventricular arrhythmias, common after acute MI, are well tolerated by patients on LVAD support, which may improve survival rates in such patients.[42–43]

Unpublished data from our experience with implantable LVADs for post-MI cardiogenic shock likewise demonstrated excellent outcomes compared with patients who historically received no mechanical circulatory support. Between 1992 and 1997, 21 patients in cardiogenic shock after acute MI underwent LVAD placement as bridge-to-transplant therapy. Fifteen patients received the TCI Heartmate (8 pneumatic, 7 vented-electric) and 6 received the Novacor N100 electric LVAS (Baxter Health Care, Inc., Oakland, CA). ECLS was required either before LVAD or as an RVAD postoperatively in 5 patients; ECLS placed preoperatively was removed in 3 patients. Complications included bleeding that required reexploration (3 patients), renal failure requiring dialysis (1 patient), respiratory failure requiring prolonged (> 48 hours) ventilator support (6 patients), infection (12 patients), and neurologic events (7 patients). Of the infected patients, 4 had pneumonia and 8 had at least one positive blood culture. Four patients had clinical driveline infections, and one required surgical drainage of the pump pocket. Of the patients suffering a neurologic event, 5 had transient ischemic attacks, 1 had a stroke with complete resolution, and 2 had fatal events. There were no neurologic events among the Heartmate recipients. One patient died from ischemic bowel secondary to a thromboembolic event, one from multisystem organ failure, and one from disruption of the apical inflow cannula. Overall, 16 (76%) patients survived to transplantation, and all were subsequently discharged home.

Controversies about use of an implantable VAD after acute MI have centered on two issues: (1) the risk of placing an apical conduit in freshly infarcted myocardium and (2) the cost-effectiveness of such definitive therapy in patients who may need only temporary support. Despite anecdotal reports of disruption of the left ventricular apical inflow conduit, this complication seems to be rare and probably is not of much concern in the mechanically unloaded left ventricle.[36] Regarding the role of implantable LVADs in patients with acute MI, Oz et al. described a prospective screening scale addressing end-organ dysfunction and operative constraints as a guide for device selection.[44] Points are assigned for urine output < 30 ml/hr (3 points), mechanical ventilation (2 points), prothrombin time > 16 seconds (2 points), central venous pressure > 16 mmHg (2 points), and reoperation (1 point). In their experience, patients with scores < 5 points have a 90% survival rate, whereas patients with scores > 5 points have a 30% survival rate. Patients with lower scores are offered implantable VADs; patients with higher scores receive temporary support. Although a highly aggressive therapy, implantable LVAD placement allows early patient mobilization with possible discharge home. For patients requiring long-term support as bridge to transplant, implantable LVAD placement precludes the need for a second early operation and "bridge-to-bridge" therapy.

Conclusion

Cardiogenic shock complicating acute MI remains a serious problem. Mortality rates are exceedingly high with medical therapy alone; reperfusion and restoration of normal hemodynamics are the only hope for long-term survival.

In our centers, patients who fail thrombolytic therapy undergo urgent percutaneous transluminal coronary angioplasty (PTCA). For patients who are hemodynamically unstable either before or during cardiac catheterization, IABP remains the first-line mechanical therapy. Patients who fail PTCA and have persistent ischemia typically undergo emergent CABG; those who remain hemodynamically unstable despite IABP placement often require ECLS until the operating room can be made available.

After CABG, patients who cannot be weaned from cardiopulmonary bypass or have persistent hemodynamic compromise require further mechanical support. If revascularization was successful and we believe that the patient will require only temporary support, the Abiomed BVS 5000 is our first choice for mechanical circulatory assistance. For patients with left ventricular failure who seem unlikely to have significant short-term myocardial recovery, the TCI Heartmate is implanted. For the unusual post-MI patient with either right ventricular or biventricular failure that appears unlikely to resolve in the near future, the Thoratec VAD is inserted. Patients receiving a Heartmate who later require right ventricular support are placed on either an Abiomed BVS 5000 RVAD (for short-term assist) or Thoratec RVAD (for long-term assist).

The mainstay of therapy for post-MI cardiogenic shock remains myocardial revascularization. However, for patients who cannot maintain normal hemodynamics, mechanical circulatory assistance is necessary to provide adequate end-organ perfusion. None of the currently available cardiac assist devices are without potential risk or complication. Nonetheless, compared with the high mortality rates associated with post-MI cardiogenic shock, these devices offer the best hope for patients who, historically, would not survive.

References

1. American Heart Association: Heart and Stroke Facts: 1995. Statistical Supplement. Chicago, American Heart Association, 1996.
2. Goldberg RJ, Gore JM, Alpert JS, et al: Cardiogenic shock after acute myocardial infarction. N Engl J Med 325:1117, 1991.
3. Sobel B: Coronary thrombolysis and the new biology. J Am Coll Cardiol 14:850, 1989.
4. Hands ME, Rutherford JT, Muller JE, et al: The in-hospital development of cardiogenic shock after myocardial infarction: Incidence, predictors of occurrence, outcome, and prognostic factors. J Am Coll Cardiol 14:40, 1989.
5. Kantrowitz A, Tjonneland S, Freed PS, et al: Initial clinical experience with intraaortic balloon pumping in cardiogenic shock. JAMA 203:113, 1968.
6. Johnson SA, Scanlon PJ, Loeb HS, et al: Treatment of cardiogenic shock in myocardial infarction by intraaortic balloon counterpulsation and surgery. Am J Med 62:687, 1977.
7. Forssell G, Nordlander R, Nyquist O, Schenck-Gustavsson K: Intraaortic balloon pumping in the treatment of cardiogenic shock complicating acute myocardial infarction. Acta Med Scand 206:189, 1979.
8. Scheidt S, Wilner G, Mueller H, et al: Intraaortic balloon counterpulsation in cardiogenic shock. N Engl J Med 288:979, 1973.
9. Waksman R, Weiss AT, Gotsman MS, Hasin Y: Intraaortic balloon counterpulsation improves survival in cardiogenic shock complicating acute myocardial infarction. Eur Heart J 14:71, 1993.
10. Ohman EM, Georges BS, White CJ, et al: Use of intraaortic counterpulsation to improve sustained coronary patency during acute myocardial infarction. Circulation 90:792, 1994.
11. Mehlhorn U, Kroner A, de Vivie ER: 30 years clinical intraaortic balloon pumping: Facts and figures. J Thorac Cardiovasc Surg 47(Suppl 2):298, 1999.
12. Magovern GJ, Magovern JA, Benckart DH, et al: Extracorporeal membrane oxygenation: Preliminary results in patients with postcardiotomy cardiogenic shock. Ann Thorac Surg 57:1462, 1994.
13. Muehrcke DD, McCarthy PM, Stewart RW, et al: Extracorporeal membrane oxygenation for postcardiotomy cardiogenic shock. Ann Thorac Surg 61:684, 1996.
14. Kurose M, Okamoto K, Sato T, et al: Emergency and long-term extracorporeal life support following acute myocardial infarction: rescue from severe cardiogenic shock related to stunned myocardium. Clin Cardiol 17:552, 1994.
15. Jaski BE, Lingle RJ, Overlie P, et al: Long-term survival with use of percutaneous extracorporeal life support in patients presenting with acute myocardial infarction and cardiovascular collapse. ASAIO J 45:615, 1999.
16. Bavaria JE, Furukawa S, Kreiner G, et al: Effect of circulatory assist devices on stunned myocardium. Ann Thorac Surg 49:123, 1990.
17. Allen BS, Rosenkranz ER, Buckberg GD, et al: Studies of controlled reperfusion after ischemia: VII. High oxygen requirements of dyskinetic cardiac muscle. J Thorac Cardiovasc Surg 92:543, 1986.
18. Lazar HL, Treanor P, Yang XM, et al: Enhanced recovery of ischemic myocardium by combining percutaneous bypass with intraaortic balloon pump support. Ann Thorac Surg 57:663, 1994.
19. Guyton R, Schonberger J, Everts P, et al: Postcardiotomy shock: Clinical evaluation of the BVS 5000 biventricular support system. Ann Thorac Surg 56:346, 1993.
20. Helman DN, Morales DL, Edwards NM, et al: Left ventricular assist device bridge-to-transplant network improves survival after failed cardiotomy. Ann Thorac Surg 68:1187, 1999.
21. Grossman D, Levy M, Sears N: Temporary ventricular assist using the Abiomed system as a new option for cardiogenic shock due to myocardial infarction. Heart Failure Summit IV, 1998.
22. Jett GK, Lazzara RR: The Abiomed BVS 5000. In Goldstein DJ, Oz MC (eds): Cardiac Assist Devices. Armonk, NY, Futura, 2000.
23. Pierce WS, Brighton JA, O'Bannon W, et al: Complete left ventricular bypass with paracorporeal pump: Design and evaluation. Ann Surg 180:418, 1974.
24. Pennington DG, Bernhard WF, Golding LR, et al: Long-term follow-up of post-cardiotomy patients with profound cardiogenic shock treated with left ventricular assist devices. Circulation 72:II-216, 1985.
25. Hill JD, Farrar DJ, Hershon JJ, et al: Use of prosthetic ventricle as a bridge to cardiac transplantation for post-infarction cardiogenic shock. N Engl J Med 314:626, 1986.
26. Lohmann DP, Swartz MT, Pennington DG, et al: Left ventricular versus left atrial cannulation for the Thoratec ventricular assist device. ASAIO Trans 36:M545, 1990.

27. Arabia FA, Paramesh V, Toporoff B, et al: Biventricular cannulation for the Thoratec ventricular assist device. Ann Thorac Surg 66:2119, 1998.
28. Holman WL, Bourge RC, Murrah CP, et al: Left atrial or ventricular cannulation beyond 30 days for a Thoratec ventricular assist device. ASAIO Trans 41:M517, 1995.
29. Pennington DG, McBride LR, Swartz MT, et al: Use of the Pierce-Donachy ventricular assist device in patients with cardiogenic shock after cardiac operations. Ann Thorac Surg 47:130, 1989.
30. Korfer R, el-Banayosy A, Posival H, et al: Mechanical circulatory support with the Thoratec assist device in patients with postcardiotomy cardiogenic shock. Ann Thorac Surg 61:314, 1996.
31. el-Banayosy A, Korfer R, Arusoglu L, et al: Bridging to cardiac transplantation with the Thoratec ventricular assist device. J Thorac Cardiovasc Surg 47:307, 1999.
32. Mavroidis D, Sun BC, Pae We Jr: Bridge to transplantation: The Penn State experience. Ann Thorac Surg 68:684, 1999.
33. McBride LR, Naunheim KS, Fiore AC, et al: Clinical experience with 111 Thoratec ventricular devices. Ann Thorac Surg 67:1233, 1999.
34. Hendry PJ, Masters RG, Mussivand TV, et al: Circulatory support for cardiogenic shock due to acute myocardial infarction: A Canadian experience. Can J Cardiol 15:1090, 1999.
35. Farrar DJ, Korfer R, el-Banayosy A, et al: First clinical use of the Thoratec TLC-II Portable VAD Driver in ambulatory and patient discharge settings. ASAIO J 44(7);35A, 1998.
36. Lewis CT, Graham TR, Marrinan MT, et al: The use of an implantable left ventricular assist device following irreversible ventricular fibrillation secondary to massive myocardial infarction. Eur J Cardiothorac Surg 4:54, 1990.
37. Korfer R, el-Banayosy A, Posival H, et al: Mechanical circulatory support: the Bad Oeynhausen experience. Ann Thorac Surg 59(2):S56, 1995.
38. Chua TP, Pepper JR, Fox KM: The use of an implantable left ventricular assist device in a patient with cardiogenic shock following acute myocardial infarction. Int J Cardiol 66:55, 1998.
39. Chen JM, DeRose JJ, Slater JP, et al: Improved survival rates support left ventricular device implantation early after myocardial infarction. J Am Coll Cardiol 33:1903, 1999.
40. Nakatani T, Takano H, Noda H, et al: Therapeutic effect of a left ventricular assist device on acute myocardial infarction evaluated by magnetic resonance imaging. ASAIO Trans 32:201, 1986.
41. Loisance D, Deleuze M, Hillion ML, et al: The real impact of mechanical bridge strategy in patients with severe acute infarction. ASAIO Trans 36:M135, 1990.
42. Oz MC, Rose EA, Slater JP, et al: Malignant ventricular arrhythmias are well tolerated in patients receiving long-term left ventricular assist devices. J Am Coll Cardiol 24:1688, 1994.
43. Holman WL, Roye GD, Bourge RC, et al: Circulatory support for myocardial infarction with ventricular arrhythmias. Ann Thorac Surg 59:1230, 1995.
44. Oz MC, Pepino P, Goldstein DJ, et al: Selection scale predicts patients successfully receiving long-term implantable left ventricular assist devices. Circulation 90:I-308, 1994.

Left Ventricular Free Wall Rupture Complicating Acute Myocardial Infarction

ROQUE PIFARRE, MD

Cardiac rupture complicating acute myocardial infarction (AMI) remains a serious diagnostic and therapeutic challenge. When ventricular free wall rupture after AMI is not followed by sudden death, it is referred to as subacute ventricular rupture. Rupture of the free wall of the left ventricle results in hemopericardium and abrupt hemodynamic deterioration due to cardiac tamponade. The size of the rent is most important. If it is large, tamponade and death ensue rapidly, allowing no time for surgical intervention. If the rent is small, more time than anticipated may be available for management. The diagnosis of subacute ventricular rupture requires a prompt surgical decision, considering that it is a frequent complication after AMI that can be diagnosed and treated successfully.

Myocardial rupture of the left ventricular free wall is a major complication of AMI. However, the incidence has not been clearly established. According to Dellborg et al.,[1] ruptures were found in 17% of 1746 patients who were diagnosed with AMI and died in the hospital. As many as one-third (32%) of the ruptures were subacute; therefore, time would have been available for diagnosis and emergency repair. In a review of 18 published reports before the use of coronary care units, Reddy and Roberts[2] found that the incidence of rupture of the left ventricular free wall or ventricular septum among necropsy cases of AMI ranged from 4% to 24%. Of 648 such patients from their laboratory, 204 (31%) had rupture of the left ventricular free wall or ventricular septum. Of the 204 rupture cases, the site of rupture was the left ventricular free wall in 137 (67%), the ventricular septum in 55 (27%), both left ventricular free and ventricular septum in 7 (4%), and both left ventricular free wall and papillary muscle in 5 (2%).[2]

The first successful operation to repair a free wall rupture was reported by Hatcher and associates in 1970.[3] In 1983, we reviewed the literature and found 12 patients with successful repair of a free wall myocardial rupture who had survived to leave the hospital. To that list we added 4 new cases treated successfully.[4] If the rupture is gradual, the rent may be confined by thrombus formation and pericardial adhesions. A two-way flow of blood may be established through the rupture, and a false aneurysm may develop. The pseudoaneurysm communicates with the ventricular cavity through a relatively small opening.

The outcome of free wall rupture of the left ventricle parallels early recognition and treatment. It is important, therefore, to become familiar with the clinical presentation, diagnosis, and surgical treatment of this frequently lethal complication of AMI.

Etiology

Free wall rupture generally occurs in patients with no history of symptomatic coronary artery disease.[4,5] This finding indicates the absence of long-standing stenotic coronary artery atherosclerosis and collateral circulation. Several autopsy findings have demonstrated a complete thrombotic occlusion of the infarct-related artery. A lack of collateral circulation supplying the infarcted area also was reported.[6,7] Mann and Roberts[8] reported that rupture of the left ventricle is primarily a complication of the first MI and is associated with less coronary narrowing than fatal MI without rupture.

Rupture of the left ventricle free wall generally occurs between 1 and 7 days after myocardial infarction.[9,10] History of pain, time to onset of infarction, and autopsy findings indicate that the peak incidence takes place during the first 1–2 days.[1,5] The Multicenter Investigation of Limitation of Infarct Size (MILIS)[11] study demonstrated that patients with free wall rupture have more extensive infarctions than those with septal rupture. They found that female sex was not associated with a higher risk of rupture.

Several clinical trials have suggested that the survival benefit conferred by thrombolytic therapy may be offset by a paradoxic increase in early deaths due to cardiac rupture.[12] Death from rupture occurred earlier in patients given thrombolytic therapy, with a clustering of events within 24 hours of drug administration. The Late Assessment of Thrombolytic Efficacy (LATE) study evaluated a total of 5711 patients with AMI who were randomized to receive intravenous recombinant tissue-type plasminogen activator (rtPA) or matching placebo within 6–24 hours from symptom onset. In patients treated within 12 hours, the proportion of rupture deaths in the rtPA-treated group was higher than that observed in patients who received placebo, but the difference was not statistically significant. In patients treated after 12 hours, there was no evidence of an increased incidence of rupture with rtPA, and the proportion of deaths due to rupture in this group was lower than that in patients given placebo. The investigators concluded that coronary thrombolysis appears to accelerate rupture events, typically within 24 hours of treatment.[13]

Pathophysiology

Cardiac rupture usually occurs after an AMI involving the left ventricular free wall. The most common locations are anterolateral, anteroapical, posterior, and posterolateral. According to Batts et al., the most common site of rupture is the anterior or lateral wall.[14] The perforation usually occurs in the center of a fresh infarction. The epicardial opening is usually single and varies in size from 1–5 cm in diameter.[5] In all cases, a transmural infarction is present.

Four patterns of rupture have been described.[15] Type I is a direct tear with little dissection or bloody infiltration of the myocardium. Type II has a dissection through the muscle with bloody infiltration. Type III is a rupture with its orifice protected either by thrombus on the ventricular side or by a pericardial symphysis. Type IV is an incomplete rupture; the tear is not transparietal. The tract frequently is located along the interface between viable and necrotic myocardium.[15]

Many patients have no history of coronary artery disease. Often they have single-vessel disease and no collateral circulation. The interval between AMI and cardiac rupture varies from less than 24 hours to 15 days. Most cases occur within the first 5 days.[12] The interval between rupture and death depends on the size of the perforation. The larger the perforation, the shorter the interval. Pericardial adhesions from a previous operation or pericarditis prevent free pericardial bleeding and facilitate the development of a psudoaneurysm. Rupture of the free wall of the heart results in hemopericardium and abrupt hemodynamic deterioration because of cardiac tamponade. The typical patient has a good hemodynamic state after AMI. The pain may recur, and the patient's condition, which was generally stable, suddenly deteriorates. There is an increase in central venous pressure and low cardiac output. Recurrent chest pain accompanied by electromechanical dissociation and clinical signs of pericardial tamponade are highly suggestive of cardiac rupture. Pericardiocentesis is diagnostic and may be life-saving while preparations for operation are being made.

Diagnosis

The diagnosis of ventricular free wall rupture usually is based on a high index of suspicion. In most cases, we are dealing with a healthy patient who suffered an AMI from 1–8 days before the rupture. Continuous pain or reappearance of pain is common.[5] Sudden hypotension, accompanied by paradoxical pulse and increased venous pressure, signals the presence of tamponade. The MILIS study found three clinical characteristics that signaled an increased risk of rupture: lack of history of symptomatic coronary artery disease, large size infarction, and signs of Q-wave infarction in the initial electrocardiogram (EKG).[12]

The fastest and most sensitive diagnostic test to confirm cardiac rupture is transthoracic echocardiography. The most consistent finding is pericardial effusion.[16,17] Purcaro et al. reported a study of 28 cases with subacute free wall rupture.[18] For most cases the diagnosis was based on the demonstration of hemopericardium and cardiac tamponade by echocardiography, cardiac catherization, and pericardiocentesis. In a prospective study of 1247 consecutive patients with AMI, in 33 of whom subacute ventricular rupture was diagnosed at operation, the presence of cardiac tamponade, pericardial effusion, high-density intrapericardial echoes, or right atrial and right ventricular wall compression had a high diagnostic sensitivity and specificity.[19] The EKG appearance of sinus bradycardia followed by nodal rhythm or the presence of electromechanical dissociation is an ominous sign, indicating a large rupture that, most probably, is not amenable to surgical treatment.

Cardiac catherization and coronary angiography are considered by some to be time-consuming and unnecessary.[17] Coronary angiography and coronary artery bypass grafting can be performed later.[20–22] Others believe that cardiac catherization and coronary arteriography, whenever possible, are helpful in assessing left ventricular function and the anatomy of the coronary obstructions.[4,23,24] This knowledge facilitates the planning of the operation and establishes the need for myocardial revascularization, which may be crucial for the patient's survival.

Operative Techniques

The first objective of treatment is to achieve hemodynamic stability. Resuscitation of the patient with rapid infusion of fluids is required, and administration of ionotropic support is often necessary. Repeat pericardiocentesis may improve the patient's condition and, by allowing the time necessary to prepare for surgery, may be life-saving. The use of intraaortic balloon counterpulsation has been helpful in stabilizing the patient. Once the diagnosis of ventricular rupture has been established, surgical treatment should be initiated immediately.

Figueras et al.[25] reported a study of 81 patients with a first transmural AMI who presented with acute hypotension due to cardiac tamponade; 72 also exhibited electromechanical dissociation. Patients with early recovery were managed with prolonged bed rest and blood pressure control with beta blockade, as tolerated. Forty-seven patients died within 2 hours of acute tamponade, and autopsy in 21 showed left ventricular free wall rupture. In 15 others, emergency surgical repair was undertaken; there were 2 survivors. The remaining 19 patients had early recovery with dobutamine and colloid solution; 15 required pericardiocentesis. Four patients died, and autopsy in 3 patients revealed a rupture that was sealed in two. The investigators concluded that long-term survival of selected patients with prompt hemodynamic recovery after left ventricle free wall rupture is possible without surgical repair. The poor results obtained by this method seem to indicate that surgical repair offers a much better prognosis.[4,18,19,26–28]

In 1983, Nuñez and associates reported a 57% survival rate with a technique that consisted of covering the ventricular perforation with a patch fixed to normal myocardium by continuous polypropylene suture.[26] In 1988, Padró et al. reported a case of postinfarction cardiac rupture successfully treated with a sutureless technique.[27] The myocardial perforation was covered with a Teflon patch fixed to the heart surface by a biocompatible glue. In 1993, the two centers reported their combined experience with 13 patients using this technique.[28] The glue—butyl-2-cyanoacrylate manomer—does not require an activating substance because it polymerizes when it comes in contact with tissue moisture. Cardiopulmonary bypass was used only in one patient with a posterior tear. The investigators reported a mean follow-up of 26 months with a 100% survival rate.

Most patients reported in the literature have been treated using cardiopulmonary bypass and closure of the defect by direct suture or patch. Schwarz et al. reported 5 cases with successful surgical repair.[29] They concluded that although the clinical presentation of left ventricular free wall rupture after myocardial infarction is highly variable, close cooperation between experienced echocardiographers and surgeons may allow successful corrections with good long-term results. Reardon et al. concluded that the first objective of treatment is resuscitation of the patient to achieve hemodynamic stability.[30] The next step is pericardiocentesis to relieve tamponade. An intraaortic balloon pump should be inserted early. Surgical repair of the rupture site is the definitive treatment. Feebregts et al. reported success in 5 patients with subacute free wall rupture of the left ventricle after AMI.[31] Infarctectomy with subsequent closure of ruptured area was carried out in 2 patients. Three other patients were treated with direct closure and application of a patch; furthermore, in 2 patients concomitant myocardial revascularization was performed. All patients survived the procedure and were well at a long-term follow-up (mean = 36.4 months). Varbella et al. reported two cases and reviewed the literature.[32] They concluded that if pericardiocentesis yields hemorrhagic fluid, surgical intervention is mandatory, providing both diagnostic confirmation and definitive treatment.

At present, most reports about the management of left ventricular free wall rupture use cardiopulmonary bypass, generalized hypothermia, blood K+ cardioplegia, and decompression of the left ventricle. Whenever possible, the perforation is closed with strips of Teflon felt on each side, using polypropylene sutures (Fig. 1 and 2). In most cases, infarctectomy and patch repair have been used to avoid volume reduction and distortion of the ventricular cavity. The infarcted area around the perforation is resected and replaced with a Dacron patch.[33] The edges of the myocardium are reinforced with pledgets and strips of Teflon felt (Fig 3). Once the repair is completed, it has to be tested for any weak points in the suture line. The ventricle is allowed to contract with some volume in the ventricular cavity to see if any bleeding points require reinforcement stitches. Once the checking is completed, the heart should be supported for another 20–30 minutes to allow the myocardium to recover.

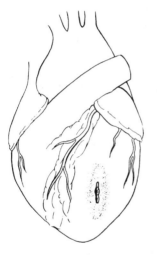

Figure 1. Small perforation in the anterolateral wall of the left ventricle.

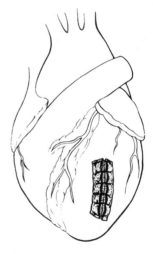

Figure 2. Suture repair of a small perforation with strips of Teflon felt.

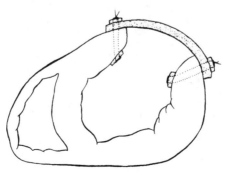

Figure 3. Infarctectomy and patch repair of a free wall rupture.

Results

Long-term survival of patients after repair of free wall ventricular rupture is increasingly common. High suspicion of ventricular rupture, prompt recognition with transthoracic echocardiography and pericardiocentesis, and improved resuscitation and hemodynamic stabilization have contributed to early operation and better survival rates. Because as many as one-third of ruptures may be subacute, time is available for diagnosis and repair.

Padró and associates reported 13 patients treated successfully using a Telfon patch glued on the infarcted area (without the aid of cardiopulmonary bypass in 12 patients).[28] They had no operative deaths. In most other reports, cardiopulmonary bypass was used to repair the free wall ventricular rupture.[3,4,18,19,26,29,34-38]

Although the number of cases in published reports is too small to draw conclusions about the risk of surgery, most of these patients with left ventricular free wall rupture would have died without surgical repair.[39]

Conclusion

After considering our experience and a review of the literature, we conclude that successful management of left ventricular free wall rupture is feasible provided that there is a high degree of suspicion of rupture and the diagnosis is confirmed by echocardiography and, when needed, pericardiocentesis. Once the diagnosis is made, the patient should be supported and stabilized. Early intervention and repair of the free wall rupture is successful in most cases.

All efforts must be directed to the early recognition of the myocardial free wall rupture. Treatment should not be delayed until signs of cardiovascular collapse and electromechanical dissociation appear; by then it may be too late to carry out the repair.

References

1. Dellborg M, Held P, Swedberg K, Vedin A: Rupture of the myocardium: Occurrence and risk factors. Br Heart J 54:11–16, 1985.
2. Reddy SG, Roberts WG: Frequency of rupture of the left ventricular free wall or ventricular septum among necropsy cases of fatal acute myocardial infarction since introduction of coronary care units. Am J Cardiol 63:906–911, 1989.
3. Hatcher CR, Mansour K, Logan WD, et al: Surgical complications of myocardial infarction. Ann Surg 36:163–170, 1970.
4. Pifarré R, Sullivan HJ, Grieco J, et al: Management of left ventricular rupture complicating myocardial infarction. J Thorac Cardiovasc Surg 86:441–443, 1983.
5. Schuster E, Buckley B: Expansion of transmural myocardial infarction: A pathophysiology factor in cardiac rupture. Circulation 60:1532, 1979.
6. Dellborg M, Held P, Swedberg K, Vedin A: Rupture of the myocardium: Occurrence and risk factors. Br Heart J 54:11–16, 1985.
7. London RE, London SB: Rupture of the heart: A critical analysis of 47 consecutive autopsy cases. Circulation 31:202, 1965.
8. Mann JM, Roberts WC: Rupture of the left ventricular free wall during acute myocardial infarction: Analysis of 138 necropsy patients and comparison with 50 necropsy patients with acute myocardial infarction without rupture. Am J Cardiol 62:847–859, 1988.
9. Zahger D, Hammil SC, Edwards WD: A broken heart. N Eng J Med 334:319–321, 1996.
10. Proli J, Laufer N: Left ventricular rupture following myocardial infarction treated with streptrinase. Cathet Cardiovasc Diagn 29:257–260, 1993.
11. Polijola-Sintonen S, Mullen JE, Stone PH, et al: Ventricular septal rupture and free wall rupture complicating acute myocardial infarction: Experience in the multicenter investigation of limitation of infarct size. Am Heart J 117:809–816, 1989.

12. Becker RC, Gore JM, Larubrew C, et al: A comparative view of cardiac rupture in the United States National Registry of Myocardial Infarction. J Am Coll Cardiol 27:1321–1326, 1996.
13. Becker RC, Charlesworth A, Wilcox RG, et al: Cardiac rupture associated with thrombolytic therapy: Impact of time to treatment in the Late Assessment Efficacy (LATE) study. J Am Coll Cardiol 25:1063–1068, 1995.
14. Batts KP, Ackermann DM, Edwards WD: Post-infarction rupture of the left ventricular free wall: Clinicopathiologic correlates in/00 consecutive autopsy cases. Hum Pathol 21:350–355, 1990.
15. Sutherland FWH, Geull FJ, Pateri FL, Naik SK: Postinfarction ventricular free wall rupture: Strategies for diagnosis and treatment. Ann Thorac Surg 61:1281–1285, 1996.
16. Pollak H, Diez W, Spiel R et al: Rare diagnosis of subacute free wall rupture complicating acute myocardial infarction. Eur Heart J 14:640–648, 1993.
17. Raitt MH, Kraft CD, Cardner CJ et al: Subacute ventricular free wall rupture complicating acute myocardial infarction. Am Heart J 126:946–55, 1993.
18. Purcaro A, Costantini C, Ciarupani N, et al: Diagnostic criteria and management of subacute ventricular free wall rupture complicating acute myocardial infarction. Am J Cardiol 80:397–405, 1997.
19. Lopez-Sendon J, Gonzalez A, Lopez de Sa E, et al: Diagnosis of subacute ventricular wall rupture after acute myocardial infarction: Sensitivity and specificity of clinical, hemodynamic and echocardiographic criteria. J Am Coll Cardiol 19:1145–1153, 1992.
20. Eisenman B, Bareiss P, Pacifico AD, et al: Anatomical, clinical and therapeutic features of acute cardiac rupture. J Thorac Cardiovasc Surg 86:78–82, 1978.
21. Mundt ED: Rupture of the heart complicating acute myocardial infarction. Circulation 46:427–429, 1972.
22. Sutherland FWH, Guell FJ, Patter UL, et al:. Post infarction ventricular free wall rupture: Strategies for diagnosis and treatment. Ann Thorac Surg 61:1281–1285, 1996.
23. Hockreister C, Goldstein J, Berer JS, et al: Myocardial free wall rupture after acute myocardial infarction: Survival aided by percutaneous intra-aortic balloon counterpulsation. Circulation 65:1279–1282, 1982.
24. Pappas PJ, Cernaianu AC, Baldino WA, et al: Ventricular free wall rupture after myocardial infarction: Treatment and outcome. Chest 99:892–895, 1991.
25. Figureas J, Cortadella J, Roangelista P, Soler-Soler J: Medical management of selected patients with left ventricular free wall rupture during acute myocardial infarction. J Am Coll Cardiol 29:512–518, 1997.
26. Nunez L, de la Llana R, Lopez-Sendon J, et al: Diagnosis and treatment of subacute free wall ventricular rupture after infarction. Ann Thorac Surg 35:529, 1983.
27. Padro JM, Caralps JM, Montoya JD, et al: Sutureless repair of postinfarction cardiac rupture. J Cardiac Surg 3:491–493, 1988.
28. Padro JM, Mesa JM, Silvestre J, et al: Subacute cardiac rupture: Repair with a sutureless technique. Ann Thorac Surg 55:20–24, 1993.
29. Schwarz CD, Punzengruber C, Ng CR, et al: Clincial presentation of rupture of the left ventricular free wall after myocardial infarction: Report of five cases with successful surgical repair. Thorac Cardiovasc Surg 44:71–75, 1996.
30. Reardon MJ, Carr CL, Diamond A, et al: Ischemic left ventricular free wall rupture: Prediction, diagnosis and treatment. Ann Thorac Surg 64:1509–1513, 1997.
31. Feebregts CJ, Noyez L, Hemsen AG, et al: Surgical repair of subacute left ventricular free wall rupture. J Cardiac Surg 12:416–419, 1997.
32. Varbella F, Bongioanm S, Sibona MA, et al: Subacute left ventricular free wall rupture in early course of acute myocardial infartion: Clinical report of two cases and review of the literature. Giornale Italiano di Cardiologia 29(2):63–70, 1999.
33. Pappas, PJ, Cernaianu AC, Baldino WA, et al: Ventricular free wall rupture after myocardial infarction: Treatment and outcome. Chest 99:892–895, 1991.
34. Windsor HM, Change VP, Shanahan MX: Postinfarction cardiac rupture. J Thorac Cardiovasc Surg 84:755–761, 1982.
35. Fitzgibbon GM, Hooper GD, Heggtveit MA: Successful surgical treatment of postinfarction external cardiac rupture. J Thorac Cardiovasc Surg 63: 622–630, 1972.
36. Anagnostopoulos E, Bentler S, Levett M, et al: Myocardial rupture: Major left ventricular infarct rupture treated by infarctectomy. JAMA 238: 2715–2716, 1977.
37. Pierli C, Lisi G, Mezzacapo B: Suacute left ventricular free wall rupture: Surgical repair prompted by echocardiographic diagnosis. Chest 100:1174–1176, 1991.
38. Bojar RM, Overton JWJ, Medoff VM: Successful management of left ventricular rupture following myocardial revascularization. Ann Thorac Surg 44:312–314, 1987.
39. Siegel M, Zimmerh SH, Robicsek F: Left ventricular rupture following coronary occlusion treated by streptokinase infusion: Successful repair. Ann Thorac Surg 44:413–415, 1987.

Ventricular Septal Rupture Secondary to Acute Myocardial Infarction

ALVARO MONTOYA, MD

Cardiac rupture, acute mitral insufficiency secondary to papillary muscle rupture, ventricular septal rupture, and left ventricular aneurysms are mechanical complications accounting for 20% of deaths following acute myocardial infarction (AMI). Ventricular septal rupture (VSR) is one of the most serious. Medical treatment carries a mortality rate of 50% at 1 week and 90% at 2 months.[1] Aggressive medical management, prompt diagnosis, temporary stabilization using intraaortic balloon counter pulsation and early surgical repair have improved patient survival.

VSR originally was diagnosed at postmorten examination.[2-6] The first antemortem diagnosis was made by Brunn in 1923, and in 1934 Sager established the current diagnostic criteria, stressing the association between coronary artery disease and VSR.[7,8] Surgical correction of VSR was first performed by Cooley in 1956.[9] Delay of surgery was recommended to allow recovery of the injured myocardium and formation of scar tissue to facilitate the repair. By the late 1960s early surgical repair was advocated for clinically deteriorating patients.[10,11] Technical advances, including the use of intraaortic balloon pump (IABP)[12] and myocardial protection with improved perioperative anesthesia, contributed to the decrease in early mortality.

New techniques in repair, approaching the defect through the infarcted myocardium,[10-13] use of prosthetic material to patch the septum,[14] a free wall patch to decrease the amount of tension in the suture line,[15-17] and exclusion of the defect by endocardial patch have increased the survival rate.[43,52] The mortality rate continues to be 11%, despite significant increases in early intervention (within 1 week) after infarction. Since 1982, emergency intervention to repair a VSR within 24 hours of diagnosis has been recommended.[18]

Pathogenesis

One to two percent of patients who die from an AMI exhibit septal rupture at autopsy.[19,20] Such patients present with a characteristic triad of hypertension (41%), first-time myocardial infarction (86%), and one-vessel coronary artery occlusion (54%), with minimal collateral formation to the infarcted area.[21-25] Septal rupture occurs through a zone of necrotic tissue within 10 days of the

MI, before myocardial healing begins.[26] Ruptures can occur early with thrombolytic therapy, decreasing the time between infarction and rupture. The amount of necrotic tissue is greater in hearts with postinfarction VSR than in hearts without this complication.[20,27] Massive transmural necrosis and septal perforation follow the complete occlusion of a major coronary artery supplying the septum. Left ventricular infarction is more extensive in patients with anterior septal rupture. Right ventricular infarction occurs more often with posterior rupture. Sixty percent of ruptures occur anteriorly and are almost always in the distal two-thirds of the ventricular septum. Forty percent occur posteriorly, often with compromised right ventricle caused by occlusion of a large right coronary artery or dominant left circumflex coronary artery.

Two types of rupture may occur: a simple through-and-through perforation located anteriorly or a complex serpiginous dissection of a posterior septum. Defects may be multiple in 5–11% of cases. Complex ruptures are more likely to be associated with rupture of other structures, such as the free wall of the heart or papillary muscle, and consequently have a worse prognosis. Eighty percent of inferior ruptures are complex, whereas 73% of anterior ruptures are simple.[28] Ventricular aneurysms often are associated with VSR because of the nature of transmural MI, ranging in incidence from 35% to 70%.[13,22] The average age of patients with this complication is increasing (62 years). VSR affects men (60%) more often than women.

Clinical Presentation

Abrupt deterioration in the clinical condition of a post-infarction patient, leading to congestive heart failure and cardiogenic shock, is suggestive of VSR. Recurrence of chest pain, fall in arterial blood pressure and biventricular heart failure (right more prominent than left) initiate the rapid downhill course. The sudden appearance of a holosystolic murmur, loudest in the third, fourth, and fifth intercostal spaces near the left border of the sternum and radiating to the axilla, clearly indicates the possibility of VSR. This sign is present in 90% of cases.[29–31] A thrill is palpated in 60% of patients.[31] A diastolic murmur also may be detected and usually is associated with a large defect or a left ventricular aneurysm.[1] These findings occur from 24 hours to 2 weeks after AMI but are observed most often around the third or fourth day.[30–32]

Sudden decline in the patient's condition, congestive heart failure, and cardiogenic shock are explained not only by the amount of myocardial damage but also by the magnitude of the left-to-right shunt created by the septal rupture. A low cardiac output syndrome develops, induced by overload of the already compromised right ventricle and leading to multiorgan failure.

Electrocardiographic (EKG) findings and rhythm abnormalities are not specific to the diagnosis of VSR. EKG abnormalities may indicate the location of the infarct and perforation.[33] Persistent ST-segment elevation may suggest left ventricular aneurysm. Pleural effusions, increased vascularity, and cardiac enlargement are found on the plain chest radiograph,[24] but no findings are specific to VSR. Echocardiography aids the immediate diagnosis of mechanical complications in hemodynamically compromised patients with AMI. Two-dimensional transthoracic echocardiography enables direct visualization of ventricular septal rupture in up to 80% of cases, and combined two-dimensional Doppler echocardiography is diagnostic in 95%.[34] Echocardiography demonstrates an echo-free area of the septum, dyskinesia, or ventricular aneurysm. It is helpful in differentiating VSR, papillary muscle rupture, and mitral regurgitation.

The quickest technique to diagnose a shunt at the ventricular level is bedside insertion of a Swan-Ganz balloon-tip catheter into the right side of the heart to measure oxygen saturation at the levels of the superior vena cava and pulmonary artery. Step-up greater that 9% between the two samples is diagnostic of VSR in patients with a new murmur after AMI.[35] Shunt size, as calculated from oxygen saturations and pulmonary-to-systemic flow ratio, is correlated with the size of the defect. Pressure measurements give the degree of ventricular failure. Elevation of right ventricular pressure, although not as high as systemic pressure, indicates right-side failure and is common in post-infarction VSR. Pulmonary edema and left ventricular failure are associated with rupture of the papillary muscle.

Left-heart catheterization is essential to obtain the information necessary for an adequate surgical approach. Left ventricular function, location of the defect, and mitral valve function may be assessed. However, definition of the coronary anatomy and quality of the arteries is most important to survival. Early and late survival rates are improved when revascularization of the myocardium is performed at the time of VSR repair.[36]

Differential Diagnosis

The sudden appearance of a loud systolic murmur after an acute MI is strongly suggestive of VSR or acute mitral insufficiency secondary to rupture of a papillary muscle.[7] Patients with VSR present with severe heart failure and a pansystolic murmur. The murmur is located to the left of the sternal border and often is accompanied by a parasternal thrill.[1] The murmur of a ruptured papillary muscle is more toward the apex and has no thrill. EKG evidence of an inferior wall MI without a conduction defect may lead to the diagnosis of a ruptured papillary muscle.[1] The diagnosis of VSR is established by demonstrating a left-to-right shunt (with oxygen step-up at the right ventricle level). Limited cardiac catheterizaton is performed at the bedside using a flow-directed balloon catheter. The presence of a left-to-right shunt confirms the existence of septal rupture. Right ventricular infarction with tricuspid insufficiency, mitral regurgitation due to left ventricular dilatation or true aneurysm, massive pulmonary embolism with right-heart failure, and an evolving pericardial rub also should be considered in the differential diagnosis of VSR.

Management

The diagnosis of post-infarction VSR is an indication for prompt surgical repair, regardless of the patient's condition.[18,29,30,32,37,38] A short interval between infarction and operation is a significant factor in survival. Cardiogenic shock can develop rapidly, and death can occur without warning. The natural history of VSR is progressive deterioration and death if intervention is delayed. Once diagnosis is confirmed by clinical presentation, echo color Doppler flow imaging, and bedside right-heart catheterization, immediate pharmacologic therapy is instituted to decrease afterload and reduce systemic vascular resistance, while maintaining adequate systemic blood pressure. Vasodilators may decrease the left-to-right shunt and increase cardiac output. All of these measures should be done simultaneously with insertion of an IABP to provide counter-pulsation, reduce left ventricular afterload, increase cardiac output, and decrease the QP/QS ratio.[12]

Although balloon pumping produces a temporary overall improvement in the patient's condition, complete hemodynamic correction cannot be obtained. Peak improvement lasts for a short period without further benefit, and unexpected deterioration may occur.[32] Cardiogenic shock and organ failure are responsible for the poor outcome of patients with VSR. Shortening the duration of shock by immediate surgery is the best plan. It is therefore necessary to proceed with cardiac catheterization. Thorough knowledge of the heart's condition, including coronary anatomy, allows the surgical team to perform complete repair.

Surgical Approach

Early mortality associated with surgical repair of VSR has decreased gradually, despite the fact that patients undergo earlier surgery after AMI and often are in cardiogenic shock. Skillington reported a 11% mortality rate in 36 patients undergoing surgical repair of VSR.[18] Better understanding of the anatomy and pathophysiology of VSR, coupled with aggressive medical therapy and prompt surgical intervention, have contributed to this improvement. Technical advances also have been important. Perioperative use of an IABP, excellent cardiac anesthesia, improved techniques to protect the myocardium during aortic cross-clamping, complete repair of the defect, and correction of any associated cardiac pathology are mandatory.

After arrest of the heart with cardioplegia, the coronary arteries are inspected. Aortocoronary bypasses, as indicated by angiography, are performed at this time to provide full revascularization, lessen the degree of myocardial ischemia, and facilitate off-pump recovery. Bypass of significantly diseased vessels, especially those supplying viable parts of the left ventricular myocardium, lower the early and late risks of surgery. Coronary artery disease is etiologically related to post-infarction septal perforation. Therefore, survival is improved when the underlying cause is corrected.[27]

The method of repair is determined by the location of the rupture, size of the septal perforation, and quality of the myocardial tissue. The defect is commonly approached through the infarcted myocardium, thus avoiding damage to uninvolved muscle. In the past, VSR was repaired through a right atriotomy or right ventriculotomy. This approach proved to be inadequate because limited exposure of the septum led to technical difficulties and residual shunts.[39] Minimal debridement of the edges of the defect is now recommended. Careful, meticulous placement of repair sutures should take into account the friable and necrotic muscle. Good bites through healthy tissue and reinforcement with Teflon avoid tearing of the muscle and recurrence of the defect. Closure of the defect without tension, which requires the use of a prosthetic material or a bovine pericardial patch, makes a significant contribution to technical success.[40] Use of the free wall patch to close the left ventriculotomy incision, thus decreasing the tension in the suture line, is also a major advance in technique. Good results are obtained with all methods of closure when these principles are followed. Surgical repair is performed according to the type of pathology.

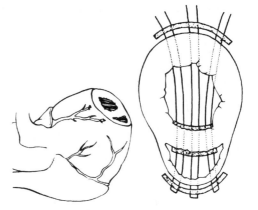

Figure 1.   Repair of apical septal rupture.

Apical defects, once visualized, are repaired by incorporating the apex of the septum into the apical portion of the right and left ventricular free walls of the ventriculotomy incision, using mattress sutures reinforced by Teflon strips (sandwich technique)[37] (Fig. 1).

Large defects may require the use of a septal prosthetic patch in the closure. The approach to an anterior infarction with a large septal perforation differs somewhat from the approach to an apical defect. The septum is visualized through an incision in the infarcted muscle, and the perforation is assessed. A prosthetic patch is used to close the defect between the septum and the free margin of the right ventricle. Mattress sutures reinforced with Teflon are passed through healthy tissues of the septum away from the defect. Subsequently these sutures are placed through a Dacron or bovine pericardium and tied down, making sure that all corners are covered.[14] The anterior border of the patch is then incorporated into the ventriculotomy closure (Fig. 2A). When a large anterior perforation is encountered, a second prosthetic patch is necessary to close the left ventricular free wall, thus decreasing the amount of tension on the suture line. It also helps to preserve the geometry of the left ventricle[15,16,41] (Fig. 2B).

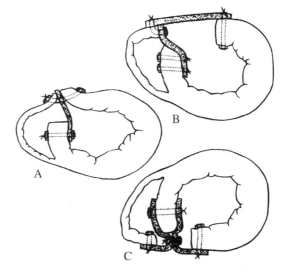

Figure 2.   *A,* Repair of a small anterior septal perforation. *B,* Repair of a large anterior septal perforation. *C,* Repair of a large posterior septal rupture.

Successful repair of inferior/posterior defects associated with myocardial infarctions in these areas is the greatest technical challenge. The same general principles are followed to repair a large anterior defect. The septal perforation is identified through an opening made through the infarcted myocardium. The mitral valve is inspected carefully to rule out damage to the valve mechanism. The mitral valve is replaced only in patients with frank papillary muscle rupture. The reported incidence of this additional procedure is as high as 8%.[18,42,43] Valve replacement increases the mortality rate when it is added to septal repair. Septal and free wall patches are used to repair defects with the technique described for large anterior perforations (Fig. 2C).

Infarct exclusion is also used to repair VSR after AMI. A bovine glutaraldehyde-preserved patch is secured to the endocardium of the left ventricle, completely surrounding the necrotic myocardium, to exclude the VSR and infarcted muscle from the left ventricular cavity. The left ventricular cavity is entered through the infarcted myocardium, and the defect is assessed. A bovine pericardial patch 2 cm larger that the infarcted area is secured to the noninfarcted muscle of the septum using continuous 3-0 polypropylene sutures with a large stitch. Care must be exercised not to tear the muscle. This patch is secured to the bottom of the septum and sutured to the upper septum. Once the anterior wall is reached, another 3-0 polypropylene suture is used to secure the patch to the endocardium of the anterior wall. The ventriculotomy is closed with two layers of sutures reinforced with Teflon strips. David used this technique in 52 patients, with a surgical mortality rate of 19%. The defect recurred in only 3 patients[43,52] (Figs. 3 and 4). Associated cardiac corrections are made at this time, such as resection of a ventricular aneurysm.[13] Complete repair of the defect is assessed once cardiopulmonary bypass is terminated. Blood samples for oxygen saturations are obtained from the superior vena cava and pulmonary artery. If a

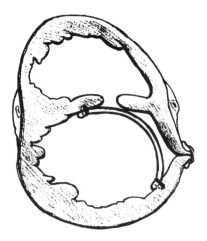

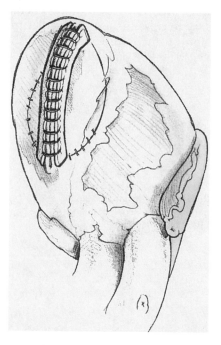

Figures 3 and 4. Repair of anterior VSR by endocardial patch with infarct exclusion.

residual shunt is detected and hemodynamic parameters are poor, further repair is recommended.

When recurrence is suspected postoperatively, diagnosis is confirmed with color Doppler flow mapping. Recurrent defects are repaired when symptoms and signs of congestive heart failure are present. When these defects are small and the patient is asymptomatic, a conservative approach with close observation is indicated.[18]

Survival Rates

Cardiogenic shock as a result of a septal rupture and myocardial infarction represents the most important and serious risk factor determining survival. The early mortality rate is high (70%),[44] and only urgent measures will improve results. Immediate insertion of an IABP and prompt surgical repair provide the only chance for survival.[30,32,45] Patients with VSR without cardiogenic shock have a better prognosis with an excellent outcome after surgery.[21,44]

Timing of surgical repair is also a primary factor in determining survival. An aggressive approach with early surgery gives better results. If surgical intervention occurs within 48 hours of septal rupture, 80% of patients survive. Delaying surgery from 48 hours to 4 weeks increases mortality rates. Many patients deteriorate suddenly while waiting for surgery, and their chance of survival is low. Delayed surgery often results in multiorgan failure secondary to hemodynamic deterioration, which usually is caused by enlargement of the defect. In this setting, surgical risk is increased.[32] Waiting for hemodynamic stabilization with medical treatment, including intraaortic balloon counter pulsation, leads to an increased number of deaths before surgical treatment and a high surgical mortality rate.[32]

Location of the infarction and septal perforation also affects survival, regardless of the timing of surgery. Anterior and apical perforations have a better prognosis after surgical repair.[30,33,46,47] Inferior infarctions and perforations are often associated with right ventricular infarction and failure.[48] Cardiogenic shock is common and increases the mortality rate. Surgical repair of inferior perforations is technically challenging. Perforations associated with inferior infarctions are usually complex[28] because of their proximity to the mitral valve mechanism, and surgical repair becomes more complicated.[18,38]

Improved survival rates also are related to surgical techniques. The myocardium must be protected at all times. Meticulous surgical technique minimizes the incidence of disruption of the suture line. Minimal debridement of the edges of the defect is mandatory. Extreme care in placing the sutures around the muscle and defect decreases the incidence of recurrence. Reinforcement with Teflon pledgets is essential, with good bites through healthy tissue. Use of patches in the septum as well as free wall to decrease tension in the suture line has increased survival rates from 60% to 85%.[16,18,30,32,33,49,50] Exclusion rather than excision of the infarcted septum by endocardial patch has recently been described with excellent results. This technique avoids additional damage to the myocardium, remodels the acutely infarcted ventricle, and enhances survival rates.[43,52]

Coronary artery stenosis in addition to the occluded artery that caused the infarction is often present. A coronary angiogram is performed before surgical intervention, thus offering the benefit of complete revascularization at the time of repair. In patients with post-infarction VSR, coronary stenosis is etiologically related to the septal defect. Myocardial revascularization improves long-term survival rates.[40]

Ages does not appear to be a significant factor in survival. A mortality rate of 12.5% has been reported for patients over the age of 70.[18] Excellent hospital survival rates are explained by improvements in perioperative anesthesia, myocardial protection, and surgical techniques. Residual ventricular septal defect has been reported in up to 28% of survivors undergoing surgical repair[51] and is associated with a high mortality rate. Surgical repair of the recurrent defect when the patient is unstable improves survival. Small residual defects are well tolerated.

Conclusion

Ventricular septal rupture after an AMI is now a rare event. It is caused by occlusion of a major coronary artery that supplies the septum, with inadequate collateral circulation. The sudden hemodynamic deterioration of a patient recovering from an AMI, with the appearance of a new systolic murmur over the precordium, is indicative of a ruptured septum. Echocardiography aids in immediate diagnosis. Two-dimensional echocardiography and Doppler enable direct visualization of the septal defect. The diagnosis is confirmed by bedside right-heart catheterization, using a Swan-Ganz catheter, that demonstrates a blood oxygen saturation step-up at the ventricular level.

Immediate hemodynamic stabilization is achieved with inotropic agents in conjunction with intraaortic balloon counterpulsation. Cardiac catheterization and coronary angiogram provide information about other coronary lesions that need to be addressed.

Prompt surgical intervention is mandatory to prevent hemodynamic deterioration, which occurs suddenly and unexpectedly. Basic technical principles must be followed to provide adequate repair and decrease the chance of recurrence. Myocardial revascularization and correction of other associated anomalies give better results. Ventricular septal rupture is no longer a condition with a prohibitive mortality rate, even in elderly patients. Surgical survival is high, and functional status is excellent once the patient is discharged.

References

1. Sanders RJ, Kern WH, Blount SG: Perforation of the interventricular septum complicating myocardial infarction. Am Heart J 51:736–748, 1956.
2. Beith AJ: A case of septal rupture. Trans Pathol Soc London 3:69, 1850.
3. Grosse GJ: Ein Fall von Ruptur de Herzkammerscheide Wand mit Retrograder Emboli in der Leber. Inang, Dissert, Rostock, C. Bolat, 1906.
4. Peacock DL: A case of rupture of the septum. Trans Pathol Soc London 5:102, 1854.
5. Pergami E: Ulcera perforante del setto del cuore: Morte subitanea. Ann Univ de Med e Chir 42:237, 1876.
6. Younmans JB: Perforation of the interventricular septum of the heart, with report of a case. Arch Intern Med 28:495, 1921.
7. Brunn F: Rupture of the interventricular septum. Wein Arch F Inn Med 66:533–544, 1923.
8. Sager RV: Coronary thrombosis: Perforation of the infarcted interventricular septum. Arch Intern Med 53:140–148, 1934.
9. Cooley DA, Belmonte A, Benjamin A, et al: Surgical repair of ruptured interventricular septum following acute myocardial infarction. Surgery 41:930, 1957.
10. Daggett WM, Buckley MJ, Akins CW, et al: Improved results of surgical management of post-infarction ventricular septal rupture. Ann Surg 196:269, 1982.

11. Stinson EB, Becker J, Shumway N: Successful repair of post-infarction ventricular septal defect and biventricular aneurysm. J Thorac Cardiovasc Surg 58:20–24, 1969.
12. Gold HK, Leinbach RC, Sander ChA, et al: Intra-aortic balloon pumping for ventricular septal defect or mitral regurgitation complicating acute myocardial infarction. Circulation 47:1191–1196, 1973.
13. Javid H, Hunter JA, Najafi H, et al: Left ventricular approach for the repair of ventricular septal perforation and infarctectomy. J Thorac Cardiovasc Surg 63:14–24, 1972.
14. Iben AB, Pupello DF, Stinson EB, Shumway NE: Surgical treatment of post-infarction ventricular septal defects. Ann Thorac Surg 8:252–262, 1969.
15. Collins HA, Collins IS: Replacement of left ventricular myocardium. Circulation 37(Suppl):18–23, 1968.
16. Daggett WM, Mundth ED, Gold HK, et al: Early repair of ventricular septal defect complicating inferior myocardial infarction. Circulation 50(Suppl 3):112–116, 1974.
17. Daggett Wm, Buckly MJ, Austen WG: Improved results of surgical management of post-infarction ventricular septal rupture. Ann Surg 196:269–277, 1982.
18. Skillington PD, Davies RH, Luff AJ, et al: Surgical treatment for infarct-related ventricular septal defects. J Thorac Cardiovasc Surg 99:798–808, 1990.
19. Cummings RG, Reimer KA, Califf R, et al: Quantitative analysis of right and left ventricular infarction in the presence of post-infarction ventricular septal defect. Circulation 77:33–42, 1988.
20. Moore CA, Nygaard TW, Kaiser DL, et al: Post-infarction ventricular septal rupture: The importance of location of infarction and right ventricular function in determining survival. Circulation 74:45–55, 1986.
21. Lemery R, Smith HC, Giuliani ER, Gersh BJ: Prognosis in rupture of the ventricular septum after acute myocardial infaraction and role of early surgical intervention. Am J Cardiol 70:147–151, 1992.
22. Hill JD, Lary D, Kerth WJ, Gerbode F: Acquired ventricular septal defects: Evolution of an operation, surgical technique and results. J Thorac Cardiovasc Surg 70:440–450, 1975.
23. Lee FA: Treatment of the hemodynamically unstable patient. Cardiol Clin 6:63–79, 1988.
24. Miller SW, Drusmore RE, Greene RE, Daggett WM: Coronary ventricular and pulmonary abnormalities associated with rupture of the interventricular septum complicating myocardial infarction. Am J Roentgenol 131:571–577, 1978.
25. Radford MJ, Johnson RA, Daggett WM, et al: Ventricular septal rupture: A review of clinical and physiologic features and analysis of survival. Circulation 3:545–553, 1981.
26. Mallory GK, White PD, Salcedo-Salgar J: The speed of healing of myocardial infarction. Am Heart J 18:647, 1939.
27. Crosby IK, Craver JM, Crampton RS, et al: Resection of acute posterior ventricular aneurysm with repair of ventricular septal defect after acute myocardial infarction. J Thorac Cardiovasc Surg 70:57–62, 1975.
28. Edwards BS, Edwards WD, Edwards JE: Ventricular septal rupture complicating acute myocardial infarction: Identification of simple and complex types in 53 autopsied hearts. Am J Cardiol 54:1201–1205, 1984.
29. Madsen JC, Daggett WM: Repair of post-infarction ventricular septal defects. Semin Thorac Cardiovasc Surg 10:825–832, 1998.
30. Montoya A, McKeever LS, Scanlon P, et al: Early repair of ventricular septal rupture after infarction. Am J Cardiol 45:345–348, 1980.
31. Swithinbank JM: Perforation of the interventricular septum in myocardial infarction. Br Heart J 21:562–566, 1959.
32. Scanlon PJ, Montoya A, Johnson SA, et al: Urgent surgery for ventricular septal rupture complicating acute myocardial infarction. Circulation 72(Suppl 2):185–190, 1985.
33. Daggett WM, Burwell LR, Lawson DW, Austen WG: Resection of acute ventricular aneurysm and ruptured interventricular septum after myocardial infarction. N Engl J Med 283:1507–1508, 1970.
34. Kishon Y, Iqbal A, Oh JK, et al: Evolution of echocardiographic modalities in detection of post myocardial infarction ventricular septal defect and papillary muscle rupture: Study of 62 patients. Am Heart J 125:667–675, 1993.
35. Hillis LD, Firth BG, Winniford MD: Variability of right-sided cardiac oxygen saturations in adults with and without left-to-right intracardiac shunt. Am J Cardiol 58:129–132, 1986.
36. Muehrcke DD, Blank S, Daggett WM: Survival after repair of post-infarction ventricular septal defects in patients over the Age of 70. J Card Surg 7:290–300, 1992.
37. Montoya A: Ventricular septal rupture secondary to acute myocardial infarction. Card Surg State Art Rev 6:425–433, 1993.
38. Held AC, Cole PL, Alpert JS: Rupture of interventricular septum complicating acute myocardial infarction. Am Heart J 116:1336–1366, 1988.

39. Kitamura S, Mendez A, Kay JH: Ventricular septal defect following myocardial infarction. J Thorac Cardiovasc Surg 61:186–189, 1971.
40. Muehrcke DD, Daggett WM: Current surgical approach to acute ventricular septal rupture. Adv Card Surg 6:69–90, 1996.
41. Schumacker HB: Suggestions concerning operative management of post-infarction septal defects. J Thorac Cardiovasc Surg 64:452–459, 1972.
42. Gaudiani VA, Miller DC, Shumway NE: Post-infarction ventricular septal defect: An argument for early operation. Surgery 89:48–55, 1981.
43. David T, Armstrong S: Surgical repair of post-infarction ventricular septal defect by infarct exclusion. Semin Thorac Cardiovasc Surg 10:105-110, 1998.
44. Matsui K, Kay JH, Mendez M, et al: Ventricular septal rupture secondary to myocardial infarctions: Clinical approach and surgical results. JAMA 245:1537, 1981.
45. Giuliani ER, Fuster V, Gersh BJ, et al: Cardiology: Fundamentals and Practice. St. Louis, Mosby-Year Book, 1991, pp 1407–1413.
46. Gaudiani VA, Miller DC, Stinson EB, et al: Post-infarction ventricular septal defect: An argument for early operation. Surgery 89:48–55, 1989.
47. Kahn JC, Rigaud M, Gandjbakhch I, et al: Posterior rupture of the interventricular septum after myocardial infarction: Successful early surgical repair. Ann Thorac Surg 23:483–486, 1977.
48. Zehender M, Kasper W. Kauder E: Right ventricular infarction as an independent predictor of prognosis after acute myocardial infarction N Engl J Med 328:981–988, 1993.
49. Brandt B III, Wright CB, Ehrenhaft JL: Ventricular septal defect following myocardial infarction. Ann Thorac Surg 27:580, 1979.
50. Miyamoto AT, Lee ME, Kass RM, et al: Post-myocardial infarction ventricular septal defect. J Thorac Cardiovasc Surg 86:41, 1983.
51. Baillot R. Pelletier C, Trivino-Marin J: Post-infarction ventricular septal defect: Delayed closure with prolonged mechanical circulatory support. Ann Thorac Surg 35:138–142, 1983.
52. David TE, Dale L, Sun Z: Post-infarction ventricular septal rupture: Repair by endocardial patch with infarct exclusion. Thorac Cardiovasc Surg 110:1315–1322, 1995.

24

Repair of Left Ventricular Aneurysm

ROQUE PIFARRE, MD

Left ventricular aneurysm is the most common mechanical complication after an acute myocardial infarction (AMI). Its frequency has been reported at various times between 3.8% and 15%.[1] Faxon et al. reported an incidence of 7.6% using data from the coronary artery surgery study (CASS).[2] Lately, the incidence has been reduced by new methods of therapy for AMI. Beta-adrenergic blocking agents, intravenous heparin, angiotensin-converting enzyme (ACE) inhibitors, intraaortic balloon counterpulsation, thrombolytic agents, and percutaneous transluminal coronary angioplasty (PTCA) have contributed to its reduction.[3] Approximately 50% of left ventricular aneurysms that occur after an AMI appear within 48 hours of the onset of chest pain; the remainder appear within 2 weeks. Serial noninvasive imaging in patients with AMI clearly demonstrates that formation of left ventricular aneurysm results from the expansion of infarcted myocardium within 2–14 days of the AMI.[4]

Visser et al. studied 158 consecutive patients after their first AMI with echocardiography at 5 days, 3 months and 1 year. They found that an aneurysm developed in 35 patients: in 27 of 84 (31%) patients with anterior infarctions, 6 of 68 (9%) patients with posterior infarction, and 2 of 6 patients with anteroposterior infarction.[5] The aneurysm developed during the first months after the AMI. Left ventricular aneurysm most commonly results from AMI. AMI and left ventricular aneurysm may result from coronary artery disease, trauma to the left anterior descending coronary artery, coronary arterial emboli, or anomalous origin of the left coronary artery from the pulmonary artery.[6]

Historical Background

The surgical repair of ventricular aneurysm has evolved significantly since 1955 when Likoff and Bailey reported the first closed resection of a ventricular aneurysm.[7] A large clamp was applied to the neck of the aneurysm, and a segment was resected after the base of the aneurysm had been sutured. In 1958 Cooley and associates reported the first open resection using cardiopulmonary bypass.[8] This method—resection of the aneurysm and linear closure of the ventriculectomy—remained unchanged for almost three decades. The advent of coronary arteriography made possible the combination of the ventricular aneurysm repair with myocardial revascularization and, therefore, improved long-term results. Using this combination, we reported in 1973 a reduction in the postoperative mortality rate.[9] In 1985 Jatene described the use of purse-string suture and a Dacron patch to close the resected aneuyrsm.[10] In 1989 Dor reported a new surgical technique called endoventricular circular plasty.[11] The same year Cooley described the technique of ventricular endoaneurysmorrhaphy.[12] By using a Dacron patch, these techniques do not reduce the size of the ventricular cavity and preserve the anatomy of the left ventricle. Left ventricular function is improved and, as an end result, so is the late survival rate.

Incidence and Natural History

The incidence of left ventricular aneurysm following a transmural MI has been reported to be 3.5– 20%.[1,13] Cosgrove and associates noted that the incidence of chronic aneurysms is decreasing.[3] The morbidity and mortality rates of patients with ventricular aneurysm are difficult to estimate. There are variations between autopsy and clinical series. Schlichter reviewed 102 autopsy cases and determined that 73% of the aneurysms had been present for less than 3 years and 88% for less than 5 years.[1] Proudfit reported a group of 74 patients with ventricular aneurysms as demonstrated with ventriculogram.[14] The survival rate and quality of life have been significantly improved with myocardial revascularization and repair of the ventricular aneurysms. The latest techniques of ventricular reconstruction with a patch represent a breakthrough that has significantly reduced the mortality rate seen with the old technique of linear reconstruction of the ventricle.[10–12] Shapira and associates reported that, although linear repair had a similar effect on left ventricular geometry, endoaneurysmorrhaphy resulted in a greater increase in postoperative left ventricular ejection fraction and a substantially improved long-term clinical outcome.[15] Komeda et al. reported excellent long-term results after repair of left ventricular aneurysms.[16] They added that the newer techniques of repair are valuable in patients with poor left ventricular function.

Pathophysiology

The pathophysiology of ventricular aneurysm is explained on the basis of a noncontractible (akinetic) area that may progress into a paradoxically pulsating (dyskinetic) area.[17] Large dyskinetic areas dissipate most of the contractile force of the heart and require it to generate a greater tension to achieve the same intraluminal pressure as dilatation occurs. During systole, the aneurysm wall (scar) fails to contract, leading to reduced ejection fraction and cardiac output. In diastole the aneurysm wall does not distend normally, resulting in elevated left ventricular end-diastolic pressure. Klein observed that when an aneurysm is greater than 20% of the left ventricular surface, left ventricular end-diastolic pressure and volume increase, with decreases in isometric rate of pressure rise and mean fiber-shortening velocity and distance, according to the law of Laplace. Dilatation leads to increased intracavitary pressure, which results in yet more dilatation.[18] With 20% of the myocardium inactive, fiber-shortening distance must exceed physiologic limits to maintain the same stroke volume. To compensate for the loss of shortening distance, the heart must enlarge and, indeed, cardiomegaly is usually seen in the presence of a large aneurysm. Energy is not expended effectively. The forces of contraction of the unaffected myocardium dissipate in the aneurysmal sac, resulting in a reduction of the stroke volume and cardiac output and eventually congestive heart failure.

Postinfarction aneurysms of the left ventricle have been classified as two general types. The first type is characterized by extensive endocardial fibroelastosis. In the second type, a layered thrombus has formed. The normally smooth endocardial surface is transformed into a damaged surface that promotes platelet adherence and aggregation.[19] Hochman correlated these types with clinical symptoms.[20] He found that fibroelastosis was associated with arrythmias, whereas thrombotic aneurysms were associated with systemic embolization.

Jatene emphasized the importance of collateral circulation.[10] The effect of a coronary occlusion depends on the size of the occluded artery and the presence of collateral circulation. Lack of collateral circulation results in a much larger infarction and development of a ventricular aneurysm. Inoue et al. reported that the culprit lesion of the myocardial infarction was severe and that the collateral circulation was nonexistent or poor.[21] Banerjee et al. reported that the size of the aneurysm was significantly larger in the absence of collateral circulation.[22]

Diagnosis

The history of a previous MI is practically always present. A ventricular aneurysm should be suspected when the patient has a stormy recovery after an AMI, especially with the advent of congestive heart failure. The appearance of cardiac enlargement or diastolic gallop, hypotension, thromboembolic episodes, and rupture of the septum are suggestive of a ventricular aneurysm. Angina pectoris, congestive heart failure, or both are usually present. Life-threatening ventricular arrythmias are common.

Our experience showed that 50% of patients complained of angina alone, 14% had congestive heart failure, 26% had angina and congestive heart failure, and 10% had ventricular arrythmias.[23] In some cases, the chest radiograph shows an enlarged and distorted left cardiac shadow (Fig. 1); in other cases, it

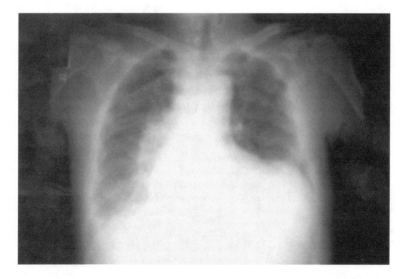

Figure 1. Chest radiograph of a patient with ventricular aneurysm.

may not be helpful. The electrocardiogram usually shows Q waves in the precordial leads. Persistent ST-segment elevation is a common finding. Two-dimensional echocardiography is comparable to cineangiography for the detection, localization, and determination of resectability of true ventricular aneurysms. However, contrast ventriculography remains the single most useful test for diagnosis of a ventricular aneurysm and planning of the operation. According to Viser et al., septal involvement was best detected by echocardiography.[5] Left ventricular angiography is better than echocardiography to define the type and extent of the aneurysm. True aneurysms are differentiated from pseudoaneurysms by the fact that the mouth of a true aneurysm is almost as wide as the body.

Coronary angiography is mandatory in all cases to determine the need for myocardial revascularization. When the diagnosis of ventricular aneurysm is made, concomitant aneurysmectomy and myocardial revascularization are recommended.

Surgical Technique

The classic technique of left ventricular aneurysm repair calls for the removal of the fibrotic area, leaving a margin of 1–2 cm of fibrous tissue to place the stitches. The standard linear closure of the left ventricle is accomplished using interrupted mattress sutures placed through strips of Teflon felt. A reinforcing over-and-over suture has been used by most surgeons (Fig. 2). This approach may be acceptable for small aneurysms, but in most cases it results in ventricular dysfunction due to alteration of ventricular geometry. The linear closure technique reduces the size of the ventricular cavity and alters the anatomy of the remaining left ventricular muscle. The end result is manifested by tachycardia, low cardiac output, and left ventricular failure.

In 1985 Jatene described a technique to reshape the left ventricular cavity using a patch. The healthy muscle is brought to its normal position, leaving an

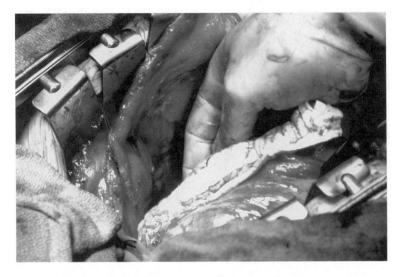

Figure 2.   Completed repair showing suture reinforcement with Teflon felt strips (classic repair).

akinetic area the size of the original infarcted area, and then replaced by the patch.[10] Emphasis is placed on the need to determine the size of the aneurysm, careful removal of the thrombi from the ventricular cavity, elimination of septal paradoxical motion, and careful ventricular reconstruction with a prosthetic patch. The aneurysmal surface is reduced using a pursestring suture placed to reduce the aneurysmal orifice.

The technique of ventricular endoaneurysmorrhaphy was described by Cooley in 1989.[12] This technique restores normal shape, contour, and ventricular volume. It is done with a patch that restores the geometry of the left ventricle. The operation is performed using cardiopulmonary bypass, moderate total body hypothermia, and cold blood cardioplegia. The aneurysm is opened longitudinally, and all thrombi are removed. An elliptical patch graft is fashioned to replace the fibrotic area of the aneurysm. The patch is sutured to the transition zone between viable myocardium and the fibrotic area that constitutes the aneurysmal sac. The fibrous edges of the aneurysmal sac are used to cover the patch by direct suture. Myocardial revascularization is performed when indicated. We find this technique useful and practical. At present it is considered the technique of choice by most surgeons (Fig. 3).

Regardless of the technique used, it should be emphasized that the presence of thrombus in the ventricular cavity is common. Manipulation of the left ventricle before arresting the heart should be avoided to prevent dislodgment of fragments of the thrombus that may embolize into the systemic, mesenteric, or cerebral circulation (Fig.4).

When malignant tachyarrythmia is present, intraoperative mapping should be carried out, and the arrythmiogenic focus should be localized. Endocardial resection or cryoablation is performed as indicated.

Results

The reported operative mortality rate varies significantly from series to series. At Loyola University Medical Center, we operated on 113 patients with ventricular aneurysms between 1984 and 1988, with a 30-day mortality rate of 8.8%. During 1989 and 1990, we repaired 36 ventricular aneurysms using the new reconstructive techniques, with a mortality rate of 2.8%. At the time of surgery, 30 patients received one bypass, 18 received two bypasses, 3 received three bypasses, and 1 received four bypasses. Three patients underwent mapping and endocardial stripping or cryoablation. Using the new technique Jatene reported a reduction in mortality from 11.6% to 4.3%.[10] Cooley and associates used the new technique in 136 patients.[24] They reported a 6-month survival rate of 90.5% and a 1-year survival rate of 85.3%. In 1993, Mills et al. reported their experience with repair of 61 left ventricular aneurysms.The mortality rate was 3.3%.[25] They changed from the standard linear repair to routine use of a modified endoventricular repair. Prate et al. reported the use of bovine pericardium instead of Dacron for grafting with the endoaneurysmorrhaphy technique.[26] They concluded that this technique provides excellent initial results and believe that the use of bovine pericardium for grafting produces better functional results than the use of Dacron. Sinatra and associates compared conventional aneurysmectomy and direct closure of the ventricular wall with the endoventricular patch plasty.[27] They reviewed 118 patients, 87 using the conventional technique and 31 patients with the endoventricular patch plasty technique. The hopsital mortality

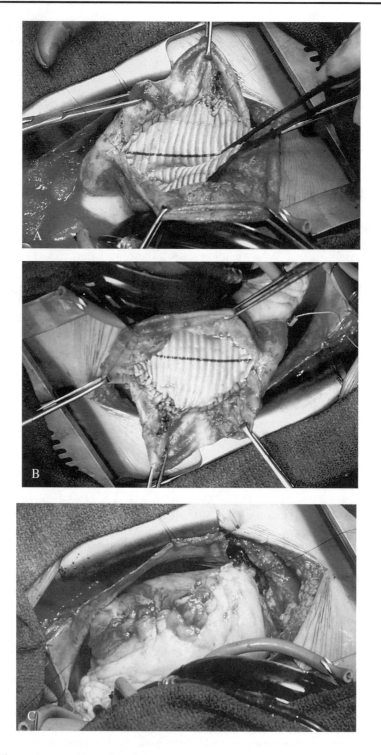

Figure 3. *A,* Suturing the patch and preserving the aneurysmal sac. *B,* Completing patch suture. *C,* Aneurysmal sac sutured on top of the patch (Cooley's endoaneurysmorrhaphy technique).

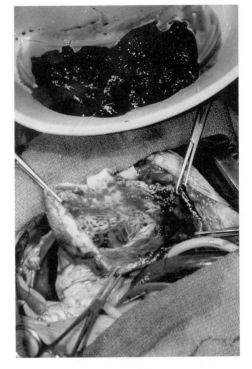

Figure 4.   *Top,* Large amount of thrombus removed from the aneurysm. *Bottom,* Left ventricular aneurysmal sac open.

rate in the conventional group was 10.3%, whereas in the endoventricular patch plasty group no hospital deaths occurred (p < 0.05). They concluded that patch plasty associated with complete myocardial revascularization results in a better outcome for patients undergoing left ventricular aneurysmectomy.

Shapira et al. compared the clinical outcomes and echocardiographic measurements of left ventricular volume and spherity in 27 patients who underwent endoaneurysmorrhaphy and 20 patients who had linear repair.[15] They concluded that endoaneurysmorrhaphy resulted in a greater increase in postoperative left ventricular ejection fraction and a substantially improved long-term clinical outcome. Rastergar et al. described the reconstruction of the left ventricle with a pericardial patch combined with mapping-guided subendocardial resection for recurrent ventricular tachycardia in 25 patients over a 5-year period.[28] There was no operative or postoperative (30-day) mortality. They concluded that endoaneurysmorrhaphy with a pericardial patch combined with mapping-guided subendocardial resection frequently cures recurrent ventricular tachycardia with low operative mortality and improvement of ventricular function. Long-term follow-up demonstrates low rates of sudden cardiac death. Dor and associates reported the hemodynamic, electrophysiologic, and clinical results in 171 patients 1 year after endoventricular circular patch repair and coronary grafting for postinfarction left ventricular dyskinetic or akinetic aneurysm.[29] Results at 1 year demonstrated a significant increase in ejection fraction and a significant reduction in ventricular volumes. They believe that patients who benefit most from the operation are those with more severe preoperative left ventricular dysfunction, more frequent ventricular arrythmias, and larger ventricular volumes.

Risk Factors

Several clinical and hemodynamic variables have been examined for relevance as risk factors. In our experience, only mean pulmonary artery pressure and cardiac index were found to be of significant value as risk factors for both mortality and eventual clinical improvement.[23] If the mean pulmonary artery pressure was higher than 45 mmHg and the cardiac index less than 2 L/min/m², the mortality rate was higher and the chances of clinical improvement were reduced.

Cosgrove et al. reported their experience with ventricular aneurysm resection with a mortality rate of 8%.[30] They found that the significant risk factors were emergent procedures, advanced age, left main disease, and history of congestive heart failure. Burton et al. reported that poor left ventricular function had a poor prognosis.[31] Barratt-Boyes and associates identified New York Heart Association (NYHA) function class, presence of congestive heart failure, and extensive coronary artery disease as risk factors for early mortality.[32] Najafi et al. identified recent MI and incomplete revascularization as risk factors for increased operative mortality.[33] Komeda et al. identified poor left ventricular function, age greater than 60 years, previous myocardial infarction, lack of angina pectoris, and NYHA functional class IV as independent predictors of operative mortality.[16]

From all the reported series and our own experience, it is clear that poor ventricular function continues to be the main cause of death. The importance of complete revascularization should not be overlooked.

Pseudoaneurysms

A postinfarction left ventricular pseudoaneurysm occurs when rupture of the ventricular free wall is contained by overlying, adherent pericardium. A postinfarction aneurysm, in contrast, is caused by scar formation that results in thinning of the myocardium.[34] Histologic examination of the resected pseudoaneurysm reveals no evidence of myocardial wall components. Containment of the disrupted myocardium is secured by the pericardium and formation of organized thrombus as the wall of the false aneurysm. This wall has little strength and may rupture. It has been reported that 20–45% of false aneurysms eventually rupture.[35] Therefore, urgent operative management has to be considered, even in asymtomatic patients.[36] The false aneurysm does not form part of the perimeter of the left ventricular cavity and communicates with it through a relatively small orifice.

Komeda and David reported 12 patients who underwent repair of false aneurysms of the left ventricle.[37] Congestive heart failure was the most common clinical presentation. Most patients had three-vessel coronary artery disease. The false aneurysm was located posteriorly in 10 patients and anteriorly in two. Four patients were treated by resection and primary closure of the false aneurysm. In 8 patients the closure was accomplished with a patch. Mitral valve replacement was performed in 3 patients, and 9 patients underwent coronary artery bypass. There were 3 operative deaths, and 1 additional patient died after 2 months. Eight patients survived the operation and remained well after a mean follow-up period of 62 months.

Frances et al. evaluated the clinical presentation, diagnostic accuracy of imaging modalities, results of therapy, and prognosis of 290 patients with left ventricular psuedoaneurysms.[38] Congestive heart failure, chest pain, and dyspnea were the most frequently reported symptoms, but more than 10% were asymptomatic. A murmur was present in 70% of patients. Left ventricular angiography was the definitive test. Regardless of treatment, patients with left ventricular pseudoaneurysms had a high mortality rate, especially those who did not undergo surgery.

The coincidence of true and false aneurysm is quite rare. Only 7 cases have been reported.[39,40] Das et al. reported a case of false aneurysms emanating from a posterior true aneurysm of the left ventricle. The diagnosis was made preoperatively by transesophageal echocardiography and confirmed at surgery. The aneurysms were successfully resected and the ventricle repaired.[40]

Both true and false aneurysms of the left ventricle are complications of myocardial infarction. Because pseudoaneurysms have a tendency to rupture, it is important to make an accurate diagnosis, followed by surgical repair.

References

1. Schlichter J, Hellerstein HK, Katz LN: Aneurysm of the heart: A correlation study of one hundred and two cases. Medicine 33:43–46, 1954.
2. Faxon DP, Ryan TJ, Davis KB, et al: Prognostic significance of angiographically documented left ventricular aneurysm from the Coronary Artery Study (CASS). Am J Cardiol 5:157–164, 1982.
3. Cosgrove DM, Lytte, BW, Taylor PC, et al: Ventricular aneurysm resection: Trends in surgical risk. Circulation 79 (Suppl I): 97–101, 1989.
4. Raton LW, Weiss JL, Buckley BH, et al: Regional cardiac dilatation after acute myocardial infarction: Recognition by two-dimensional echocardiography. N Engl J Med 300:57–62, 1979.
5. Visser CA, Kan G, Meltzer RS, et al: Incidence, timing and prognostic value of left ventricular aneurysm formation after acute myocardial infarction: A prospective, serial echocardiographic study of 158 cases. Am Heart J 57:729–732, 1986.
6. Pifarré R, Grieco J, Garibaldi A, et al: Acute coronary occlusion following blunt chest trauma. J Thorac Cardiovasc Surg 83:122–126, 1982.
7. Likoff W, Bailey CP: Ventriculoplasty, excision of myocardial aneurysm. JAMA 158:915–920, 1955.
8. Cooley DA, Collins HA, Morris GC, et al: Ventricular aneurysm after myocardial infarction: Surgical excision with use of temporary bypass. JAMA 167:557–560, 1958.
9. Pifarré R, Caralps JM, Tormes FR, et al: Ventricular aneurysm after myocardial infarction. Surgical excision with use of temporary bypass. JAMA 167:557–560, 1958.
10. Jatene AD: Left ventricular aneurysmectomy: Resection or reconstruction? J Thorac Cardiovasc Surg 89:321–331, 1985.
11. Dor V, Saalo M, Coste P, et al: Left ventricular aneurysm: A new surgical approach. Thorac Cardiovasc Surg 37:11–19, 1989.
12. Cooley DA: Ventricular endoaneurysmorrhaphy results of an improved method of repairs. Texas Heart Inst J 16:72–75, 1989.
13. Dubnow MH, Burchell HB, Titus JL: Postinfarction ventricular aneurysm: A clinico-morphologic and electro-cardiographic study of 80 cases. Am Heart J 70:753–760, 1965.
14. Proufit WL, Bruschue AG, Sones FM, Jr: Natural history of obstructive coronary artery disease: Ten years of 601 nonsurgical cases. Prog Cardiovasc Dis 21:53–78, 1978.
15. Shapira OM, Davioloff R, Hilkert RJ: Repair of left ventricular aneurysm: Long-term results of linear repair versus endoaneurysmorrhaphy. Ann Thorac Surg 63:701–705, 1997.
16. Komeda M, David TE, Malik A, et al: Operative risks and long-term results of operation for left ventricular aneurysm. Ann Thorac Surg 53:22–29, 1992.
17. Cooley DH, Frazier OH, Duncan JM et al: Intracavitary repair of ventricular aneurysm and regional dyskinesia. Ann Surg 215:417–423, 1992.
18. Klein MD, Herman MN, Gorlin R: Hemodynamic study of left ventricular aneurysm. Circulation 35:614–630, 1967.
19. Ba'albaki HA, Clements SD Jr: Left ventricular aneurysm: A review. Clin Cardiol 12:5–13, 1989.
20. Hochman JD, Platia EV, Bulkley BH: Endocardial abnormalities in the left ventricular aneurysms: A clinicopathologic study. Ann Intern Med 100:29–35, 1983.
21. Inoue T, Morookas S, Hayashi T, et al: Features of coronary artery lesions related to left ventricular aneurysm formation in anterior myocardial infarction. Angiology 44:593–598, 1993.

22. Benerjee AK, Madan Mohan SK, Ching GW, et al: Functional significance of coronary collateral vessels in patients with previous Q1 wave infarction: Relation to aneurysm, left ventricular end diastolic pressure and ejection fraction. Int J Cardiol 38(3):263–271, 1993.

23. Moran JM, Scanlon PJ, Neurickas R, Pifarré R: Surgical treatment of postinfarction ventricular aneurysms. Ann Thorac Surg 21:107–113, 1976.

24. Cooley DA, Frazier OH, Duncan JM, et al: Intracavitary repair of ventricular aneurysm and regional dyskinesia. Ann Surg 215:417–423, 1992.

25. Mills NL, Everson CT, Hockmuth DR: Technical advances in the treatment of left ventricular aneurysm. Ann Thorac Surg 55:792–800, 1993.

26. Prates PR, Vitola D, Sant'anna JR, et al: Surgical repair of ventricular aneurysms. Early results with Cooley's technique. Texas Heart Institute J 20:19–22, 1993.

27. Sinatra R, Maerinaf, Braccio M, et al: Left ventricular aneurysmectomy; comparison between two techniques, early and late results. Eur J Cardio-Thorac Surg 12:291–297, 1997.

28. Rastegar H, Link MS, Foote CB, et al: Perioperative and long-term results with mapping-guided subendocardial resection and left ventricular endoaneurysmorrhaphy. Circulation 94:1041–1048, 1996.

29. Dor V, Sabatier M, DiDonato M, et al: Late hemodynamic results after left ventricular patch repair associated with coronary grafting in patients with postinfarction akinetic or dyskinetic aneurysm of the left ventricle. J Thorac Cardiovasc Surg 110:1291–1299, 1995.

30. Cosgrove DM, Lytle BW, Taylor PC, et al: Ventricular aneurysm resection: Trends and surgical risk. Circulation 79:97–101, 1989.

31. Burton NA, Stinson EB, Oyes PE, Shumway NE: Left ventricular aneurysm: Preoperative risk factors and long-term postoperative results. J. Thor Cardiovasc Surg 77:65–75, 1979.

32. Barratt-Boyes BG, White HD, Agnew TM, et al: The results of surgical treatment of left ventricular aneurysms: An assessment of risk factors affecting early and late mortality. J Thorac Cardiovasc Surg 87:87–98, 1984.

33. Najafi H, Neng R, Javid H, et al: Postmyocardial infarction left ventricular aneurysm. Cardiovasc Clin 12:81–91, 1982.

34. Brown SL, Gropler RJ, Harris KM: Distinguishing left ventricular aneurysm from pseudoaneurysm. A review of the literature. Chest 111:1403–1409, 1997.

35. Gobel FL, Visudh-Arom K, Edwards JE: Pseudoaneurysms of the left ventricle leading to recurrent pericardial hemorrhage. Chest 59:23–27, 1971.

36. Stewart S, Huddee R, Stuard I, et al: False aneurysm and pseudo-false aneurysm of the left ventricle: Etiology, pathology, diagnosis, and operative management. Ann Thorac Surg 31:259–265, 1981.

37. Komeda M, David TE: Surgical treatment of postinfarction false aneurysm of the left ventricle. J Thorac Cardiovasc Surg 106:1189–1191, 1993.

38. Frances C, Romero A, Grady D: Left ventricular pseudoaneurysm. J Am Coll Cardiol 32:557–561, 1998.

39. Martin RH, Almond CH, Saab S, et al: True and false aneurysms of the left ventricle following myocardial infarction. Am J Med 62:418–424, 1977.

40. Das AK, Wilson GM, Furnary AP: Coincidence of true and false left ventricular aneurysm. Ann Thorac Surg 64:831–834, 1997.

25

Surgery for Ischemic Mitral Regurgitation

BRYAN K. FOY, MD

Of the potential mechanical complications or sequelae of coronary artery disease, severe ischemic mitral regurgitation (IMR) is among the most clinically daunting. The spectrum of clinical presentations is vast and includes a host of variables related to acuity, associated myocardial infarction, cardiogenic shock, and multiple organ system dysfunction as well as the ordinary panoply of medical problems associated with this patient cohort. The challenge for the cardiologist and cardiovascular surgeon is to identify the existence of IMR, quantitate its severity and acuity, and define which patients can best be treated medically vs. surgically. Fortunately, both medical and surgical armamentaria are substantial. The outcome for patients with IMR identified and treated appropriately can be dramatically improved compared with patients receiving no specific therapy. Notwithstanding, IMR remains a serious therapeutic and diagnostic challenge in a group of high-risk patients.

Definition

IMR actually describes a group of physiologically related entities. The term implies that the mitral valve and its chordae tendineae are structurally free of significant mechanical abnormalities. The insufficiency across the mitral valve is due primarily to coronary disease and the resultant ischemia or infarction of the myocardium that may be present. IMR, therefore, may be caused by rupture of an infarcted papillary muscle as the most extreme or acute presentation or by annular dilatation and restricted leaflet motion due to general left ventricular dilatation and related clinically to myocardial infarction or ischemic fibrosis. In addition, an intermediate presentation in fact may be related to intermittent ischemia, primarily of the posterolateral or posteroinferior walls of the heart. However, IMR implies a mitral valve and chordae that are morphologically intact; it also implies that regurgitation is related primarily to myocardial disease mediated by coronary atherosclerosis.

Anatomy

The anatomy of the mitral valve has been described extensively elsewhere but merits notation in the context of IMR. The papillary muscles are generally termed posteromedial (posterior) and anterolateral (anterior). The posteromedial papillary muscle usually is supplied by branches of the posterolateral circumflex coronary artery or posterolateral right coronary artery. When papillary muscle rupture occurs, it most commonly affects the posteromedial papillary muscle; in rare cases, the anterolateral papillary muscle also is affected. Papillary muscle rupture is a fairly uncommon cause of IMR. More typically, acute syndromes are caused by acute infarction of the posterior wall of the heart related to infarctions mediated by occlusion of the circumflex or right coronary artery, depending on coronary dominance. Annular dilatation or restricted leaflet motion, on the other hand, may be related to global change in left ventricular volume or shape, which may be mediated by disease of the left anterior descending or left main coronary arteries. The chordae and leaflets have no discrete blood supply and, therefore, are unaffected by ischemia per se.

Pathology

IMR is associated with the pathologic spectrum of myocardial ischemia and infarction. There are no discernible pathologic abnormalities of the mitral valve itself. The myocardium may be entirely normal in patients who have only exercise-induced ischemia and IMR. The myocardium may demonstrate any of the phases of infarction and necrosis when IMR presents in this setting, or the pathology of the myocardium may demonstrate a pattern of mixed fibrosis and cellular disarray when examined at a time remote from the acute infarction. The degree of IMR is not well correlated to the degree or extent of ischemia or infarction, nor to the acuity of presentation.

Physiology

Several classification schemes have been developed to describe mitral insufficiency. By and large, they are independent of the underlying cause (e.g., rheumatic, infectious, traumatic, myxomatous, ischemic). Typically, mitral regurgitation is graded from 0 to 4+, although in this particular context perhaps significant vs. trivial, surgical vs. medical, or fixed vs. reversible may be more helpful categories.

The most helpful categorization of IMR to the clinician is based on patient presentation. Specifically noteworthy are acute vs. chronic presentation, fixed vs. reversible IMR, and mild or severe symptoms:

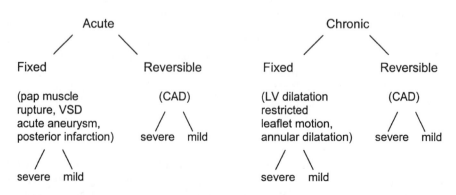

VSD = ventricular septal defect, CAD = coronary artery disease, LV = left ventricular.

In fact, the presenting symptom complex may be viewed as a three-dimensional matrix:

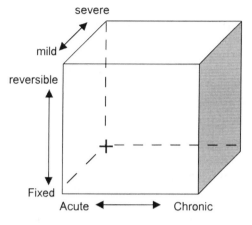

Mortality and prognosis may be viewed quickly in this format. Note especially that patients in the back lower left of the box (acute, fixed, severe) have the worst overall prognosis, whereas patients on the upper right front corner (chronic, mild, reversible) have the best prognosis.

In general, the more acute, the more severe, and the more fixed the problem, the greater likelihood that surgical treatment of the mitral valve itself will be required. This cohort of patients is also at highest risk during surgical intervention.

Diagnosis

Patients with IMR often present for medical care and are misdiagnosed or dismissed with no specific diagnosis. The most common misdiagnosis relates to early pulmonary edema masquerading and treated as pneumonia. The murmur of IMR often is hard to auscultate or intermittent and therefore missed altogether. Hepatomegaly, jugular venous distention, ascites, or ankle edema may be present in extreme cases. The gold standard for diagnosis is echocardiography, preferably transesophageal, wherein precise evaluation of the mitral leaflets, prolapse or restriction, left atrial size, left ventricular size, regional wall motion abnormalities, reversal of pulmonary vein flow, and pulmonary artery pressures may be assessed. The electrocardiogram may be normal or show ischemia, injury, infarction, or arrhythmias such as atrial fibrillation or flutter. Chest radiographs may be normal or show varying degrees of pulmonary congestion or cardiomegaly.

Cardiac catheterization typically reveals multivessel coronary artery disease (CAD), especially of the right coronary and circumflex arteries; varying degrees of mitral regurgitation; and associated left ventricular dysfunction. Right-heart catheterization demonstrates pulmonary hypertension, with a large V-wave on the pulmonary capillary wedge pressure tracing in severe cases.

Medical Therapy

The armamentarium of medical treatment modalities is fairly extensive and may be applied to all forms of IMR. The degree to which these therapies are applied and the rapidity with which they are instituted depends on the severity and acuity of presentation.

Digitalis. All patients not in renal failure should receive digitalis to prevent rapid conduction of supraventricular arrhythmias via the atrioventricular node. The role of digitalis in preventing atrial fibrillation in this setting is controversial.

Diuretics. Loop diuretics should be used as needed to reduce circulatory blood volume and pulmonary capillary wedge pressures. One should attempt to idealize the preload based on an individually constructed Starling curve of preload vs. cardiac output.

Angiotensin-converting enzyme (ACE) inhibitors. ACE inhibitors are highly useful in promoting afterload reduction and also may play a protective role in preventing adverse postinfarction remodeling, which may cause IMR. The severity of IMR may be mitigated significantly with appropriate doses of ACE inhibitors; functional improvement of one or two New York Heart Association (NYHA) classes is not unusual. Higher than normal doses of ACE inhibitors may be required to achieve the maximal benefit, and renal function must be monitored. Other vasodilators, such as sodium nitroprusside and nitroglycerin, may be beneficial on an acute basis; they should be administered intravenously.

Phosphodiesterase inhibitors. Milrinone and amrinone offer significant clinical improvement in fairly acute IMR by improving left ventricular function overall and functioning as both a pulmonary and peripheral vasodilator. This therapy is best tolerated acutely with measurement of right-sided heart pressures and cardiac output. Benefit also has been noted subacutely.

Rhythm control. The most frequent arrhythmia is atrial fibrillation, which can be highly deleterious in terms of both cardiac output and reduction of myocardial perfusion via rapid ventricular response rates. All efforts need to be directed toward restoring and/or maintaining normal sinus rhythm with appropriate antiarrhythmic therapy. Our own approach favors use of intravenous amiodarone, with a fairly low threshold for electrocardioversion of unstable patients.

Beta blockers. Beta blockers are highly effective in reducing ischemic episodes, even in patients with fairly poor left ventricular function. Coreg has shown particular promise in the ventricle with IMR and low ejection fraction but requires close monitoring of titration.

Percutaneous transluminal coronary angioplasty (PTCA)/lytics. Interventional techniques are appropriate in IMR as in any coronary syndrome. Multivessel applications share the same limitations as in the general population of patients with CAD. Varying degrees of success have been noted with PTCA or lytics in reversing IMR. Some reports have documented complete reversal of IMR and acute pulmonary hypertension.[1,2] In patients in whom myocardial infarction is complete and transmural, PTCA or lytics probably will be of little help. Surgery should be considered sooner in severe acute cases.[3]

Swan-Ganz catheterization. Right-heart catheterization with complete hemodynamic monitoring is particularly helpful in severe acute cases of IMR. Pharmacologic, interventional, and respiratory therapies may be guided more precisely. The need for intraaortic balloon pump insertion may be recognized earlier.

Transesophageal echocardiography (TEE). TEE is extremely valuable in assessing numerous variables related to IMR. One can clearly evaluate the presence of leaflet prolapse or restriction, papillary muscle rupture, associated ventricular septal defect or aneurysm, mural thrombus, and degree of left ventricular dysfunction as well as evaluate pulmonary artery pressures.[4,5]

Because the degree of IMR seems to vary during the acute and convalescent phases of acute myocardial infarction, one should not become wedded to a single study demonstrating little or no IMR when the patient's condition later deteriorates.[6]

Surgical Therapy

Indications

Patients should be considered as candidates for surgical correction when severe IMR cannot be controlled by medical therapy. The ultimate expression includes cardiogenic shock and fulminant pulmonary edema in an intubated patient receiving inotropic and balloon pump support. Despite the extreme presentation, surgical correction probably will save the patient's life. When medical therapy has been exhausted or is judged unlikely to control symptoms, patients should be approached surgically. Two subsets of patients with IMR need to be addressed separately:

1. **Intermittent IMR.** Some patients have intermittent symptoms of severe IMR, which may be provoked by stress testing. Particularly helpful in this area is stress echocardiography, with which IMR may be visualized under stress, often in association with regional wall motion abnormalities. If coronary angiography reveals anatomy that correlates with exercise physiology and if no mitral regurgitation is present at rest, coronary bypass alone or PTCA may reasonably be expected to resolve the IMR.[7]

2. **Severe CAD with mild mitral regurgitation.** Patients who require coronary artery bypass grafting (CABG) with mild-to-moderate mitral regurgitation present a difficult group surgically. Clearly, if left ventricular function is significantly depressed (ejection fraction < 25%), CABG alone should be undertaken without surgically addressing the mitral valve, provided that the IMR is no more than moderate.[8]

Note, however, that in the presence of poor left ventricular function with an ejection fraction < 25%, severe IMR (grade 3 or 4), and severe CAD, the mitral valve must be addressed during CABG.[9] The relative merits of repair vs. replacement are discussed below. Suffice it to say that severe mitral regurgitation, regardless of left ventricular function, must be corrected concurrently with CABG.[10]

Preoperative Considerations

Enthusiasm is growing for the use of preoperative intraaortic balloon pumping in patients with severe IMR, especially on the heels of acute myocardial infarction. Heart failure should be controlled and hemodynamic performance optimized to the extent possible, usng all medical means. Elective endotracheal intubation often improves oxygenation dramatically.

Operative Considerations

In addition to preoperative efforts to optimize heart function, Swan-Ganz catheterization, TEE, and the usual host of intravenous pharmacologic agents are mandatory. In addition, we have found that the use of inhaled nitric oxide, beginning at 20 ppm, is a useful adjunct in this difficult patient group.

Operative Approach

We favor bicaval cannulation, moderate hypothermia, and a lateral approach to the previously unoperated mitral valve. The transseptal approach is best in patients with prior mitral valve repair or replacement.

Meticulous myocardial protection is paramount. Antegrade and retrograde cold blood cardioplegias are routinely used. In addition, cardioplegia delivery via completed saphenous bypass grafts may be supplemented.

In the setting of relatively acute-onset IMR, the left atrium may be rather small, and exposure may be limited.

If the subvalvar apparatus is intact and leaflet motion is not restricted or prolapsed, mitral ring annuloplasty alone probably will be adequate. Adequacy of repair, however, must be assessed postoperatively via TEE.

If papillary muscle rupture has occurred or if leaflet motion is restricted, mitral valve replacement with some chordal preservation is more expedient than complex repair.

In patients with posterior leaflet prolapse and an otherwise intact subvalvar apparatus, quadrangular resection of the posterior leaflet with ring annuloplasty is appropriate.

Again, if the IMR is mild to moderate, most surgeons consider CABG alone to be appropriate because long-term survival and functional capacity are not improved with mitral repair or replacement.

Repair vs. Replacement

Several studies—primarily retrospective— have tried to determine the superiority of one approach over another in IMR. Some have demonstrated improved long-term results with repair over replacement, although often at some increase in acute operative mortality rate. Others have not been able to demonstrate any difference in long-term or short-term survival between mitral repair and replacement. Both acute and long-term results seem related more closely to the patient's preoperative condition and comorbid variables than to the technique of mitral surgery. It is reasonable to conclude that the appropriate operative technique is the one with which the operating surgeon is most comfortable and facile, so that operating times may be minimized with predictable results.

Surgical Results

Keeping in mind that most patients undergoing surgical treatment of IMR are essentially medical failures, the surgical results seem reasonable. Factors leading to the highest operative mortality rates are poor left ventricular function with an ejection fraction < 25%, recent AMI, papillary muscle rupture, advanced age, diabetes, respiratory failure, and cardiogenic shock. Mortality rates in this troubling group may be as high as 30–50%. Thus, another consideration to keep in mind for appropriate candidates is cardiac transplantation. In general, operative mortality rates for cardiac transplantation in this group are about 12%.

For patients with slightly better ventricular function and an ejection fraction > 25%, mortality rates plummet to an acceptable 5–15%. Clearly, advances in myocardial protection, anesthetic techniques, pharmacologic support, and preoperative echocardiographic evaluation have affected surgical results positively.

Conclusion

Ischemic mitral regurgitation describes a range of physiologic disturbances from mild insufficiency to catastrophic shock and pulmonary edema. Degree of insufficiency, mode of presentation (from acute to chronic), and degree of reversibility affect mortality rates and influence the appropriate form of therapy. Cases that are most severe, acute, and irreversible usually are related to infarction and rupture of the posteromedial papillary muscle and typically require surgical correction at considerable risk. Lesser degrees of insufficiency, particularly those that are chronic and/or reversible, are more likely to be amenable to medical therapy. The vast array of available medical tools includes digoxin, diuretics, ACE inhibitors, antiarrhythmics, and newer beta blockers.

The underlying pathophysiologic disturbance in IMR is myocardial dysfunction related to CAD. As such, the armamentarium of medical, interventional, and surgical techniques to treat CAD is directly relevant. Chronic IMR in association with severe CAD requiring CABG probably requires direct surgical therapy only when insufficiency is severe. Lesser degrees of insufficiency are best treated with the combination of CABG for severe CAD and medical therapy. This approach is particularly relevant for patients with an ejection fraction below 25%, in whom lengthy, complicated operations increase significantly the risks of morbidity and mortality. Short of frank rupture of a papillary muscle, conventional repair techniques are warranted. Expeditious valve replacement should be considered in papillary muscle rupture, particularly if CABG also is indicated.

Advances in medical and surgical therapies for ischemic mitral regurgitation have improved outcomes significantly. Notwithstanding, prevention, screening, and earlier treatment of underlying coronary artery disease hold the greatest promise to reduce the incidence of this often challenging and frequently fatal condition.

References

1. Karim MA, Hailu A, Deligonul U: Instantaneous resolution of ischemic mitral regurgitation and pulmonary hypertension by angioplasty. Int J Cardiol 47 :183–186, 1994.
2. LeFeuvre C, Metzger JP, Lachurie ML, et al: Treatment of severe mitral regurgitation caused by ischemic papillary muscle dysfunction: Indications for coronary angioplasty. Am Heart J 123(4 Pt 1): 860–865, 1992.
3. Lehmann KG, Francis CK, Sheehan FH, Dodge HT: Effect of thrombolysis on acute mitral regurgitation during evolving myocardial infarction: Experience from the thrombolysis in myocardial infarction (TIMI) trial. J Am Coll Cardiol 22:714–749, 1993.
4. Smith MD, Cassidy JM, Gurley JC, et al: Echo Doppler evaluation of patients with acute mitral regurgitation: Superiority of transesophageal echocardiograph with color flow imaging. Am Heart J 129:967–974, 1995.
5. Horstkotte D, Schulte HD, Reinhard N, et al: Diagnostic and therapeutic considerations in acute, severe mitral regurgitation: Experience in 42 consecutive patients entering the intensive care unit with pulmonary edema. J Heart Valve Dis 2:512–522, 1993.
6. Moursi MH, Bhatnagar SK, Vilacosta I, et al: Transesophageal echocardiographic assessment of papillary muscle rupture. Circulation 94:1003–1009, 1996.
7. Peteiro J, Freire E, Monserrat L, Castro-Beiras A: The effect of exercise on ischemic mitral regurgitation. Chest 114:1075–1082, 1998.
8. Christenson JT, Simonet F, Bloch A, et al: Should a mild to moderate ischemic mitral valve regurgitation in patients with poor left ventricular function be repaired or not? J Heart Valve Dis 4 :484–488, 1995.
9. Oury JH, Cleveland JC, Duran CG, Angell WW: Ischemic mitral valve disease: Classification and systemic approach to management. J Card Surg 9(2 Suppl):262–273, 1994.
10. Hausmann H, Siniawski H, Hetzer R: Mitral valve reconstruction and replacement for ischemic mitral insufficiency: Seven years' follow-up. J Heart Valve Dis 8:536–542, 1999.

Index

Page numbers in **boldface** type indicate complete chapters.